Anatomy in Diagnostic Imaging

'To our inquiring students'

PETER FLECKENSTEIN
&
JØRGEN TRANUM-JENSEN

ANATOMY IN DIAGNOSTIC IMAGING

MUNKSGAARD • COPENHAGEN

North and South America
W. B. SAUNDERS COMPANY
Philadelphia, London, Toronto

Anatomy in Diagnostic Imaging
1st edition, 3rd printing 1995

Layout and typesetting, graphic designer: Tegneren Jens ApS
Cover layout: Munksgaards Tegnestue
Reproduction: Repro Centret, Vejle, Denmark
Printer: AiO Print as, Odense, Denmark

ISBN 0-7216-4000-1

PREFACE

Diagnostic imaging means visualization of internal structures in the human body by a number of different techniques applied in clinical practice for the diagnosis of human disorders. The field of diagnostic imaging has long entailed the use of X-rays, but has been expanded in recent years by a number of new imaging techniques, based on alternative physical principles, e.g. nuclear magnetic resonance, ultrasound reflection and isotope emissions.

Full advantage of the diagnostic possibilities in clinical imaging is only possible with a sound knowledge of gross anatomy. Consequently, training in image interpretation begins early in the preclinical curriculum of many medical schools.

We have collected this atlas of typical normal images, primarily for the medical student as a guide to the interpretation of images in terms of gross anatomical structures, but the atlas will be found useful by all medical personnel working with diagnostic imaging. It is an all-round reference collection covering the essentials of imaging with conventional and digitalized X-ray techniques, computed X-ray tomography (CT), magnetic resonance tomography (MR), ultrasound sonography and isotope scintigraphy.

The introductory chapter gives a synopsis of the principles and concepts that underlie the imaging and examination techniques and which are prerequisites for the interpretation of the images. The following chapters together cover all the body regions and the organ systems of the human body. The collection includes imaging of intrauterine life, examples of bone development in childhood, and bones of old age.

All the images are presented in their original form together with an identical copy on which the image is interpreted and labelled in terms of the visualized gross anatomical structures. Emphasis has been placed on correct anatomical terminology.

Copenhagen May 1993

Peter Fleckenstein
Jørgen Tranum-Jensen

Acknowledgments

Without the generous help of many collegues it would not have been possible to compile this book. We feel especially indebted to Margrethe Herning, Hvidovre Hospital, for spending many hours with us selecting most of the MR scans. Similarly, Hans Pedersen and Fritz Efsen, Rigshospitalet, Copenhagen, provided many of the angiographic images. Flemming Roald Jensen and senior nurse Vibeke Fleckenstein Jacobsen, Rigshospitalet, Copenhagen, provided us with most of the obstetric ultrasound images, and Annegrete Veje, M.Sc., at the Holbæk Community Hospital helped us with the scintigrams.

We are grateful to many other collegues who offered their time producing and selecting images from their files: Poul Erik Andersen, Odense Hospital; Adel Ibrahim Belal, Cairo University; Jens Bang, Rigshospitalet, Copenhagen; Sven Dorph, Herlev Hospital; Henrik Egeblad, Skejby Hospital; Mogens Eiken, Gentofte Hospital; Inger Fledelius, Frederikssund Hospital; Ole Henriksen, Hvidovre Hospital; Lise Ingemann Jensen, Herlev Hospital; Agnete Karle, Bispebjerg Hospital; Anna Marie Nehen, Aalborg Hospital; Jørgen Nepper-Rasmussen, Odense Hospital; Sten Levin Nielsen, Herlev Hospital; Knud Olesen, Bispebjerg Hospital; Karen Damgaard Pedersen, Herlev Hospital; Arne Rosenklint, Gentofte Hospital; Henrik Schmidt, Nykøbing Falster Hospital (knee arthrography); Charlotte Strandberg, Gentofte Hospital; Ib Sewerin, School of Dentistry, University of Copenhagen; Peter Theilade, Institute of Forensic Pathology, University of Copenhagen; Christian Torp-Pedersen, Gentofte Hospital.

Marion Wulff, now at the X-ray Clinic, Hvidovre, followed the project from its beginning at the Skt. Lukas Hospital, and has given us many valuable and positive critical appraisals throughout. We owe a special debt of gratitude to the staff of the X-ray Department of the former Skt. Lukas Hospital, notably the radiographers, Liisa Marthin and Kirsten Strauss, who produced most of the X-rays. Similarly, radiographer Ester Klausen, Gentofte Hospital, helped us produce most of the CT scans.

Special thanks are due to photographer Birgit Risto at the Department of Medical Anatomy of the Panum Institute, who spent many hours with us in the darkroom, during week-ends and holidays, devoting all her skills to the production of the many photographic prints on which all of the illustrations are based. Special thanks are due also to Lis Sharwany, who typed the manuscript with its tormenting wealth of anatomical names, and who, patiently, accepted the many revisions.

M.E. Matthiessen at the Department of Medical Anatomy of the Panum Institute read the manuscript on the atlas part with careful scrutiny, saving us some embarassing errors.

Ib Leunbach, University of Lund, Sweden , likewise read the technical chapters and gave us valuable suggestions.

The chapter on ultrasound was in addition kindly reviewed by Margit Mantoni, Gentofte Hospital, and Jan Fog Pedersen, Glostrup Hospital.

We also wish to thank the Munksgaard Publishing Company for excellent collaboration throughout the project. This applies particularly to the editor Finn V. Andersen, and to Jens Lund Kierkegaard, who was in charge of lay-out.

Finally, we owe our most sincere gratitude to our wives and children, who did not exercise their obvious rights to revolt against husbands and fathers using all week-ends and most of their holidays for about two years in the preparation of this book.

Copenhagen, May 1993
Peter Fleckenstein
Jørgen Tranum-Jensen

Contents

Spine

Cervical spine

Thoracic spine

Lumbar spine

Head

Skull

Ear

Orbita

Paranasal sinuses

Temporomandibular joint

Principles and Techniques

Several physical principles are utilized in diagnostic imaging to visualize the internal structure, composition and functions of the living body. An elementary understanding of the imaging techniques and the basic physical principles is a prerequisite for full recognition of the diagnostic possibilities and for thorough and critical image interpretation.

This chapter may serve as an introduction to the basic physical principles, the techniques and the concepts used in diagnostic imaging, avoiding undue technical details and strenuous mathematical formalisms.

Techniques based on X-rays

The production and nature of X-rays

X-rays occupy a range of the electromagnetic wave spectrum. For purposes of diagnostic imaging, useful wavelengths are between 0.06 and 0.006 nm. Unlike visible light, X-rays cannot be deflected by lenses or analogous devices. Diffraction and wave optics can therefore largely be ignored in diagnostic imaging with X-rays. It is useful to picture X-rays as linearly propagating streams of indivisible quanta of energy, *photons*. Accordingly, X-rays are commonly characterized by their photon energies rather than by their wavelengths or their wave frequencies. Because X-rays are generated by conversion of the energy acquired by electrons accelerated through an electrical field gradient in the kilovolt (kV) range, the convenient unit of X-ray photon energies is the kilo-electron-volt (keV), the diagnostically relevant range being 20-200 keV (fig. 1).

The X-ray tube

The source of X-rays for diagnostic imaging is the *X-ray tube* (fig. 2) in which a narrow beam of electrons, emitted from an electrically heated tungsten filament (the cathode), is accelerated in vacuo and focused electrostatically to impinge the target anode that emits a small fraction (0.2-2%) of the incident electron energy as X-rays. The rest of the energy dissipates as heat in the anode, which usually is made from a tungsten alloy with high thermal stability, shaped as a disc and rotating at high speed to spread the thermal load evenly over a large area.

The energy (wavelength) of the X-rays generated

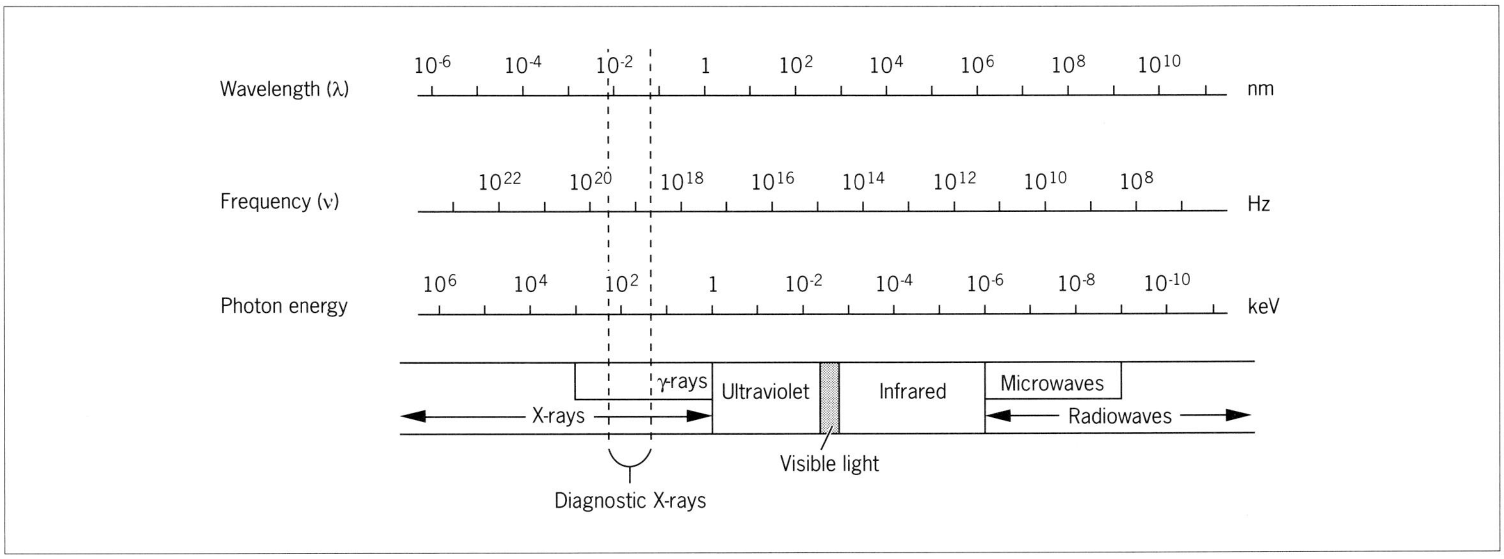

Fig. 1. The electromagnetic wave spectrum, given by wavelength, frequency and photon energy.

The propagation velocity (c) of electromagnetic waves is constant (in vacuo): 3×10^{17} nm $\times$ sec^{-1}, and relates to wavelength (λ) and frequency (ν) by: $c = \lambda \times \nu$.

Electromagnetic waves are emitted as discrete quanta of energy (photons). The energy (E) of a photon relates to its frequency (ν) by: $E = h \times \nu = \frac{h \times c}{\lambda}$, where h is Planck's constant. If energy, E is expressed in keV and wavelength, λ in nanometers, the relation becomes: $E = \frac{1{,}24}{\lambda}$

One electron volt (eV) is the energy acquired by an electron accelerated through a gradient of one volt. 1000 eV = 1 keV.

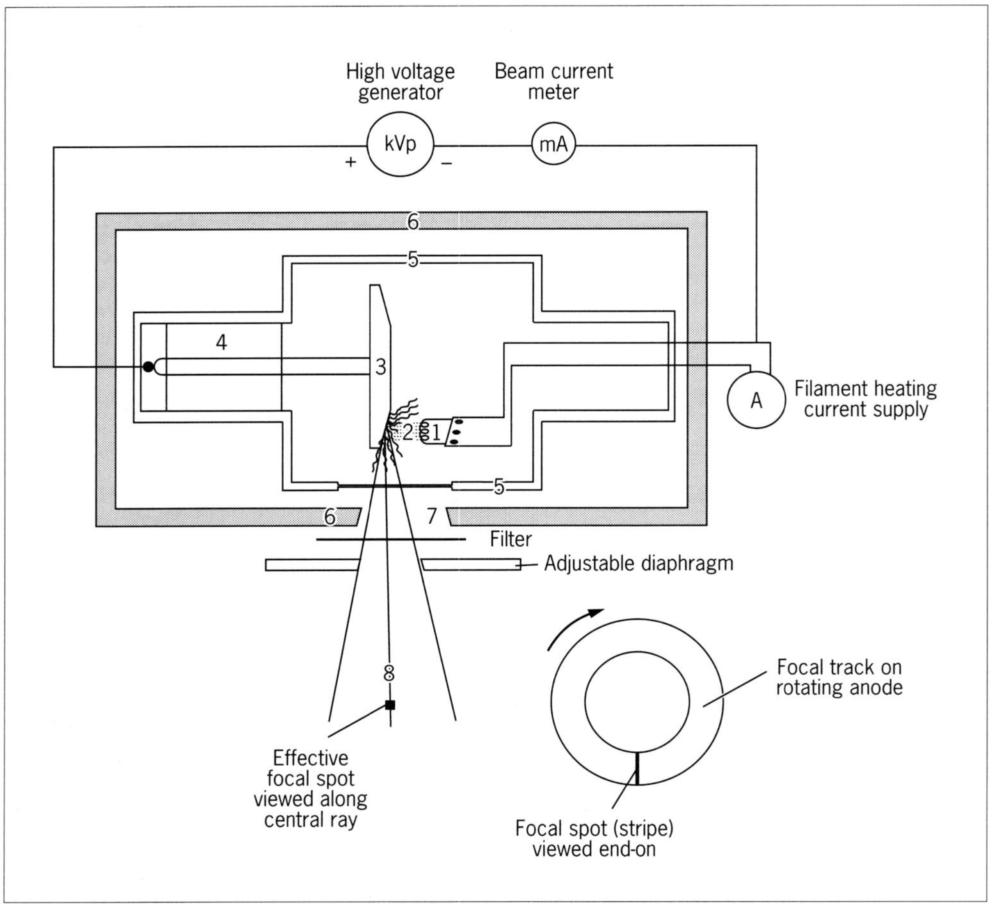

Fig. 2. Diagrammatic presentation of the basic elements of a diagnostic X-ray tube.

Details of circuitry are not given.
1: Cathode filament
2: Electron beam
3: Rotating anode
4: Anode motor drive
5: Vacuum tube
6: Lead shield
7: Window
8: Central ray

by the tube is primarily controlled by adjustment of the electrical potential difference between the cathode and the anode, *the accelerating voltage.* In all commonly used tubes, the high voltage is generated by rectification and high voltage transformation of alternating current. Evening-out is incomplete and the high voltage is rippled. Mean accelerating voltage may be only 30-50% of the peak voltage in the cycle. The high voltage setting of an X-ray unit usually refers to the peak voltage and is denoted *kVp* to indicate this fact.

The intensity of X-rays produced by the tube at a given high voltage setting is determined by the number of electrons hitting the anode, and is expressed as a milli-amperes (mA) current carried through the vacuum by the electron beam from the cathode to the anode, *the beam (tube) current.* For accelerating voltages above some 40 kV (the saturation voltage), the beam current is largely determined by the cathode filament temperature only, and this in turn is regulated by the filament heating current supply.

The quantity (dose) of X-rays delivered by the tube is proportional to the time during which the beam current flows and is conveniently expressed as milli-ampere-seconds (mAs).

The X-ray photons emitted by the anode distribute with varying intensity over a spectrum, with a maximum set by the peak accelerating voltage of the tube. Thus, the X-ray beam is polychromatic. Even if the accelerating voltage is constant the beam is still highly polychromatic due to the nature of the process by which X-rays are generated at the anode ("Bremsstrahlung"), not to be elaborated here.

Photons with energies below some 20 keV are generally useless for radiography because they cannot penetrate the body parts examined. Still, they are harmful because their energy is absorbed superficially in the irradiated tissue (especially the skin). Insertion of thin aluminum or copper plates, *filters*, in the path of the X-ray beam removes these unwanted low energy photons (fig. 3). The mean photon energy thereby increases; the beam is said to be *hardened.*

The X-ray tube is surrounded by a lead shield with a window that permits passage of the X-rays. The size and shape of the window, *the aperture*, can be varied by means of adjustable *diaphragms* (fig. 2).

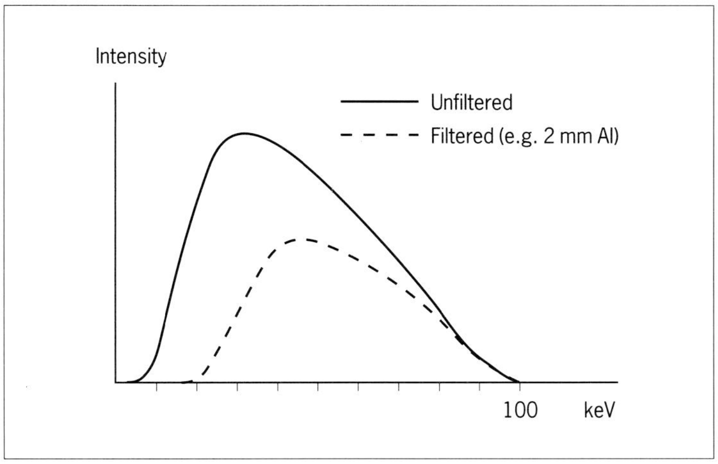

Fig. 3. The effect of filtering on the distribution of photon energies in the X-ray beam from a 100 kVp tube.

Even the unfiltered beam has been "filtered" by passage through the wall of the X-ray tube whereby the lowest energies have been rejected. Additional filtering lowers the overall intensity, but increases the mean photon energy.

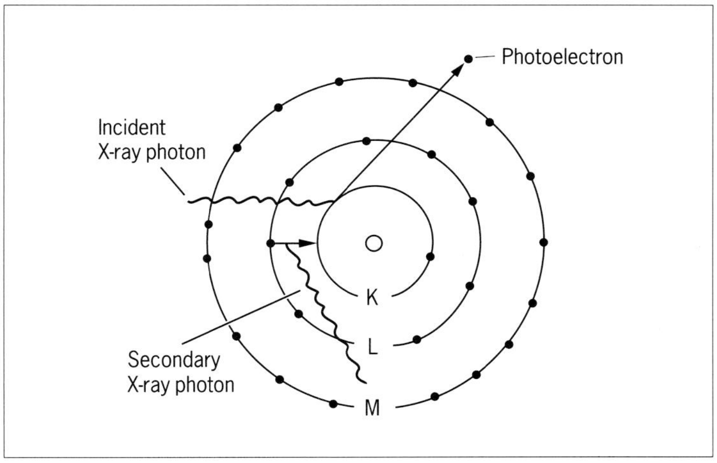

Fig. 4. The photoelectric interaction.

The X-rays radiate from the tube as a diverging bundle originating from the area of the anode hit by the electron beam, the "focus", and limited by the tube exit aperture. The axis of this bundle is called the *central ray*, and the focus viewed along this axis is called the *effective focal spot* (fig. 2). The smaller this spot, the better the obtainable resolution in the radiograph. It is usually in the order of 1 mm^2 or less. The X-ray beam should always be restricted by the diaphragms to "illuminate" the minimally required area of the body. This adjustment is called *collimation*.

Interactions of X-rays with matter

At the X-ray energies applied in diagnostic imaging, three types of interaction are to be considered: elastic scatter, the photoelectric effect, and inelastic (Compton) scatter.

Elastic scatter is an interaction whereby photons undergo a change of direction without loss of energy. This type of scatter takes place at all diagnostically relevant photon energies, but accounts for only a few per cent of the total scatter.

The photoelectric effect (fig. 4) is an interaction in which the incident photon delivers all of its energy to an atom which in turn releases this energy in the form of an electron, a *photoelectron*, which is ejected from one of the inner electron shells of the atom at high speed. An electron from one of the outer shells soon "falls in" to fill the vacancy, and energy is concomitantly released in the form of a new X-ray photon, emitted in a random direction and with an energy that is characteristic of the particular element. This secondary photon is of lower energy than the exiting photon. It may emerge as secondary radiation from the object, but is mostly absorbed by new interactions. The atom is left ionized, and the released photoelectron collides with other atoms and causes a large number of secondary ionizations. The photoelectric effect is strong when the incident photon energy is just moderately higher than the binding energy of an inner shell electron. Only the two electrons in the innermost shell, the K-shell, have binding energies sufficiently high to engage in photoelectric interactions within the diagnostic X-ray energy range. The photon energy that is just sufficient to release a photoelectron from the K-shell is denoted a *K-edge*, because the X-ray attenuation increases steeply as a threshold phenomenon at this energy level (fig. 5). The K-edges have characteristic values for the different elements (table 1). In soft tissues composed of lighter elements (C,N,O), photoelectric attenuation becomes quantitatively

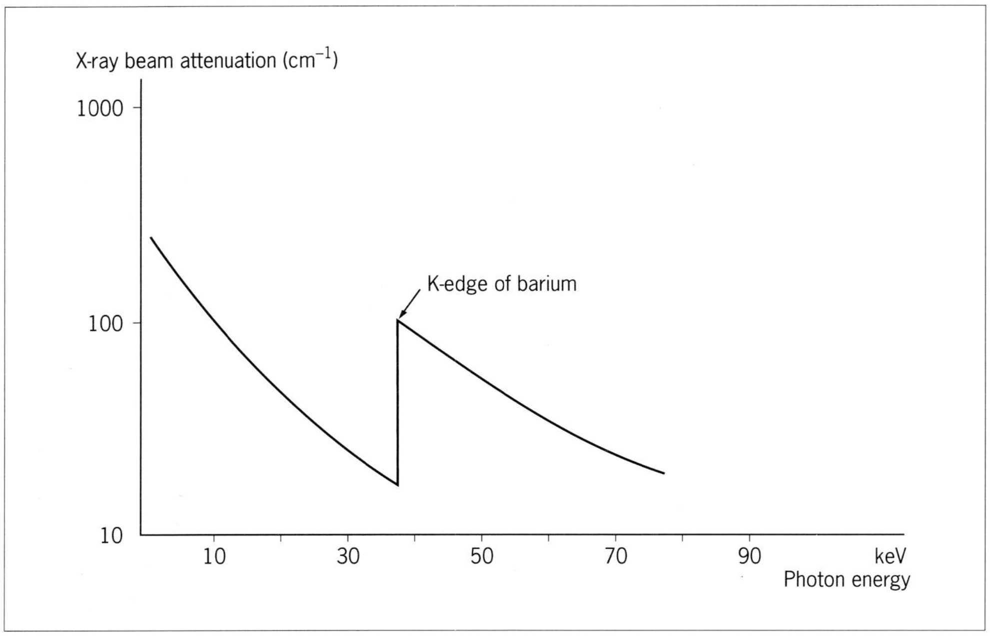

Fig. 5. The K-edge effect.

X-ray absorption increases steeply at photon energies equal to the binding energy of the K-shell electrons of an element, a so-called K-edge.

Table 1

Element	K-edge (keV)
Carbon	0.3
Nitrogen	0.4
Oxygen	0.5
Phosphorus	2.1
Calcium	4.0
Iodine	33.2
Barium	37.4
Lead	88.1
Iron	7.1

unimportant at photon energies above some 35 keV. Because the binding energy of K-shell electrons is higher for higher elements (like calcium), the photoelectric effect remains quantitatively important for bone imaging up to some 50 keV. Barium and iodine have their K-edges at 37 keV and 33 keV, respectively. It is these high K-edges that are utilized when barium and iodine are used in contrast media.

The inelastic (Compton) scatter (fig. 6) results from interaction of X-ray photons with outer shell electrons which are ejected (recoil electrons) to leave the atom ionized, while the incident photon proceeds with reduced energy and with a concomittant change of direction. An X-ray photon may engage in several such events of inelastic scatter on its path through an object, eventually giving up all of its energy, i.e. it becomes absorbed in the tissue. Compton scatter accounts for most of the scatter in diagnostic radiology. It depends primarily on the number of electrons per unit volume of tissue, and this in turn correlates almost linearly with the mass density of the tissues. It is independent of atomic number, and this is why the contrast of bone relative to soft tissues decreases at higher X-ray energies, where the photoelectric effect disappears.

Both the photoelectric effect and inelastic scatter result in a loss of electrons from atoms. This may cause the breakage of chemical bonds, and because the ionized atoms (notably those of C, N and O) are chemically highly reactive, new chemical bonds are established that are alien to the tissue. It is the X-rays' ability to cause ionizations that includes them in the family of *ionizing radiation*, and it is these ionizations and their derived chemical reactions that cause the biological damage from such radiation.

The differential ability of different tissues to scatter and absorb X-ray photons, no matter by which mechanism, is given by their *linear attenuation coefficient (cm^{-1})*, which expresses the fractional reduction in beam intensity along the linear beam path after passage through one centimeter of the tissue. The

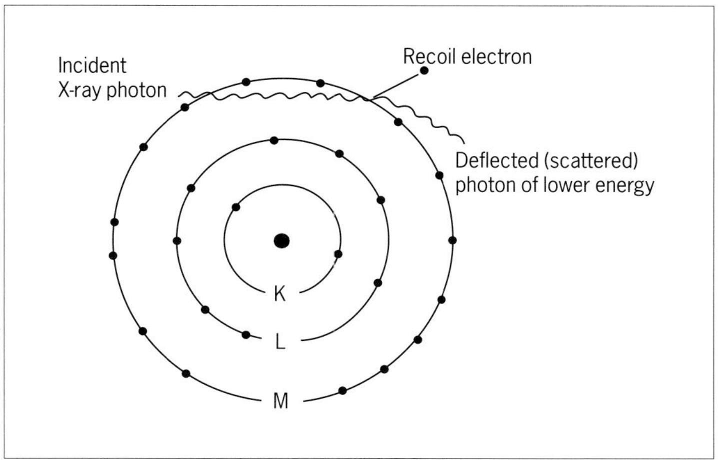

Fig. 6. Inelastic (Compton) scatter.

Units of absorbed dose and biological effect of ionizing radiation

The quantity of energy absorbed by the tissues is expressed in unit *gray* (Gy). One gray is equal to absorption of 1 joule/kg. The former unit of absorbed dose, *rad*, relates to gray by 1 Gy = 100 rads.

A practical measure of the biological effect (damage) of ionizing radiation is given in unit *sievert* (Sv), which is the absorbed dose in gray multiplied by a "quality factor" for the specific type of radiation in question. The quality factor for diagnostic X-rays and γ-emitting isotopes is around 1, while it is about 10 for α-radiation and 2 for slow β-radiation. Though α- and β-radiation penetrate tissues poorly they can inflict serious damage if delivered by isotopes present within the body and perhaps even concentrated in certain tissues, e.g. in bone marrow.

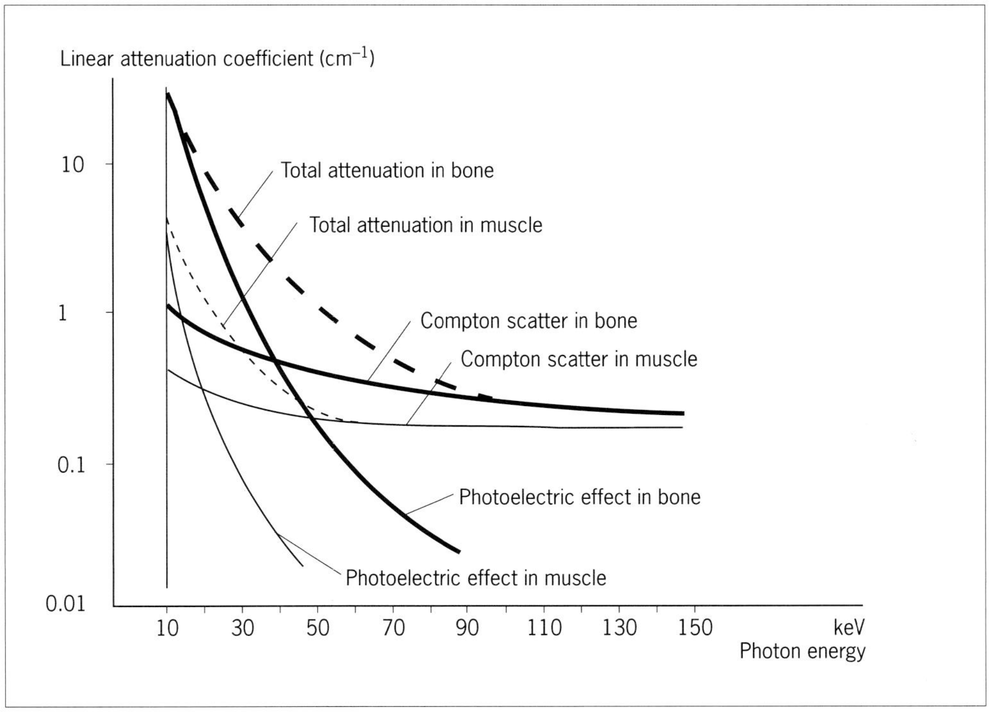

Fig. 7. The relative contribution of the photoelectric effect and of Compton scatter to attenuation of X-rays in bone and muscle.

linear attenuation coefficient of a given tissue varies with the X-ray energy, being high for lower energies where the photoelectric effect prevails and levelling off for higher X-ray energies where Compton scatter dominates, and hence the mass density rather than the atomic composition of the material becomes the prime determinant of attenuation (figs. 7 and 8).

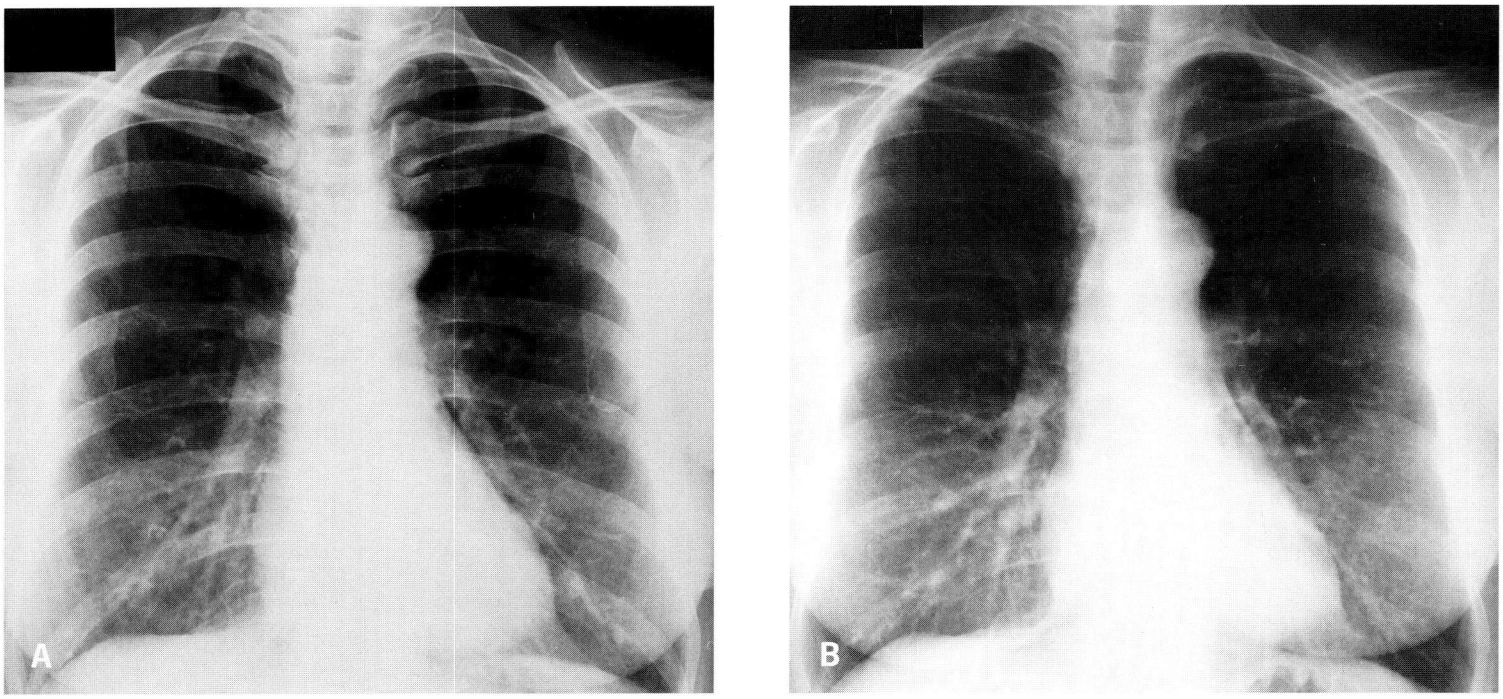

Fig. 8. The effect of X-ray energy on image contrast between bone and soft tissues.

Image A is recorded with a high voltage setting at 50 kVp, B at 150 kVp. The lower beam energy in (A) yields higher contrast between bone and soft tissues, because of the contribution of photoelectric interactions in bone imaging at low kVp.

Conventional imaging with X-rays

The basic set-up for conventional imaging with X-rays is very simple (fig. 9). The X-ray tube focal spot acts as a point source. The body part examined is composed of structural elements with different transparencies (attenuation coefficients) for X-rays, and the image appears as a 2-D projection of the 3-D object, much like a shadow-figure, following the simple geometric rule of central projection. Thus, X-ray imaging is very different from optical imaging which implies a distinct focal plane in the object and a distinct image plane.

The diverging bundle of collimated and filtered X-rays leaving the tube has approximately the same intensity throughout a cross-section of the bundle. Accordingly, the intensity decreases proportionally as the square of the distance from the focal spot. The streams of linearly propagating X-ray photons ("rays") are variously attenuated by scatter and absorption along different linear paths through the object, depending on the thickness, the mass density and the elemental composition of the structural details passed. The emerging bundle of X-rays, modulated during passage through the object, conveys information in the form of variations in beam intensity within a cross section of the bundle. This modulated bundle of X-rays emerging from the object is sometimes referred to as the *aerial image*, and it can be recorded on a film or a fluorescent screen inserted anywhere across the bundle.

Imaging geometry

It follows from the principle of central projection that *the image is always magnified.* The magnification increases when the object-to-film distance is increased, and the magnification decreases when the focus-to-object distance is increased. This implies that relative dimensional distortions are inherent in the image because structural details located closer to the focus will appear more magnified than details from a more remote location within the object (fig. 9b). This effect becomes more pronounced the

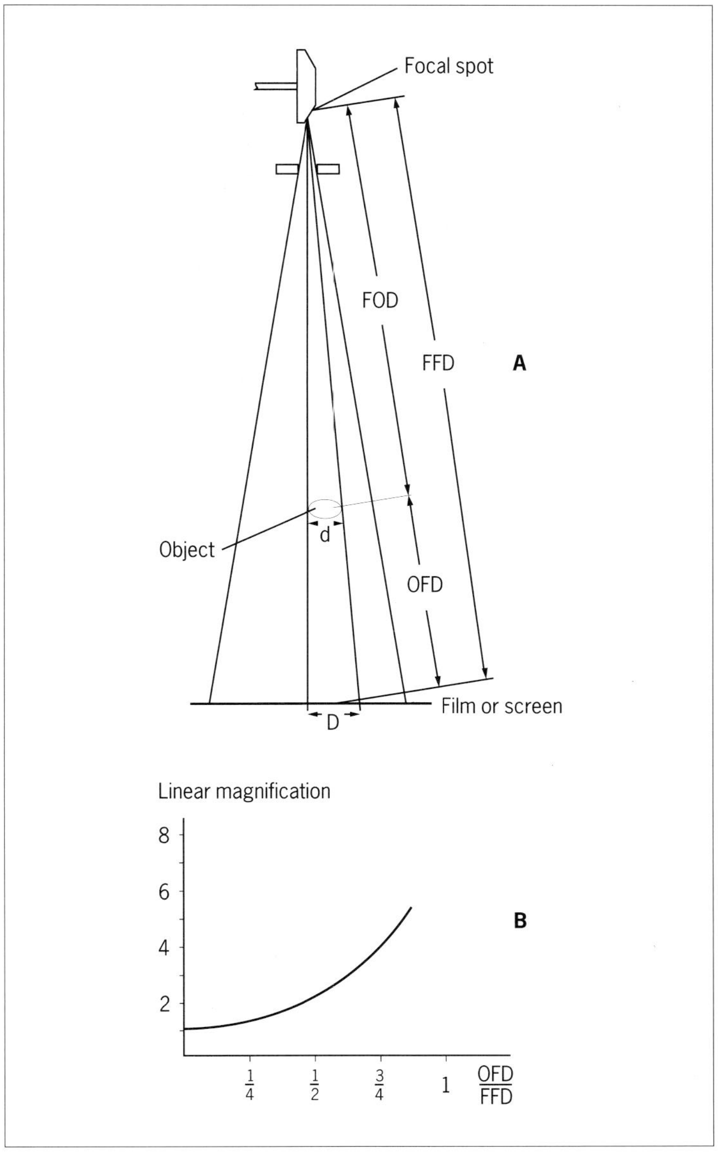

Fig. 9. X-ray imaging geometry.

A) Linear magnification $M = \frac{D}{d} = \frac{FFD}{FOD} = \frac{FFD}{FFD - OFD}$

B) Magnification as a function of the object-to-film distance (OFD) relative to the focus-to-film distance (FFD).

thicker the object is relative to the focus-to-film distance. Inherent in the imaging principle is also that structural elements along the same linear path are all superimposed, and information on their relative depth in the object is not contained in the image.

The contour sharpness of an imaged object (e.g., a trabecula of bone) is highly dependent on the size of the focal spot as well as the object-to-film distance relative to the focus-to-film distance (fig. 10).

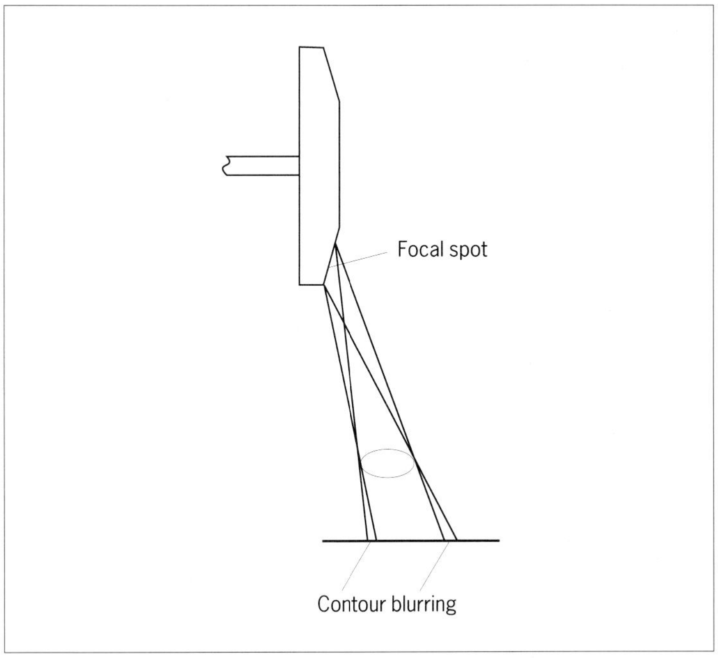

Fig. 10. The influence of focal spot size on image sharpness.

Scattered radiation

The interaction of the incident X-rays with the object causes random scatter of X-ray photons. This scatter is, on the one hand, a major contributor to the ray-attenuation on which X-ray imaging is based, but on the other hand is a nuisance if the scattered photons reach the image recorder (film) because they spread randomly over the field and impair image contrast and resolution. Preventing scattered X-rays from reaching the film is a major concern in radiology, and one or more of the following measures are employed to this end:

1. Collimation of the beam to that minimally necessary for imaging the object in question, thereby eliminating scattered radiation from irrelevant structures. This is an important measure also from a radiation hygienic point of view.

2. The length of the beam path through the body part examined may be reduced by appropriate positioning, sometimes supplemented with compression as used in mammography.

3. Increasing the air gap between the object and the film causes more of the scattered photons to miss

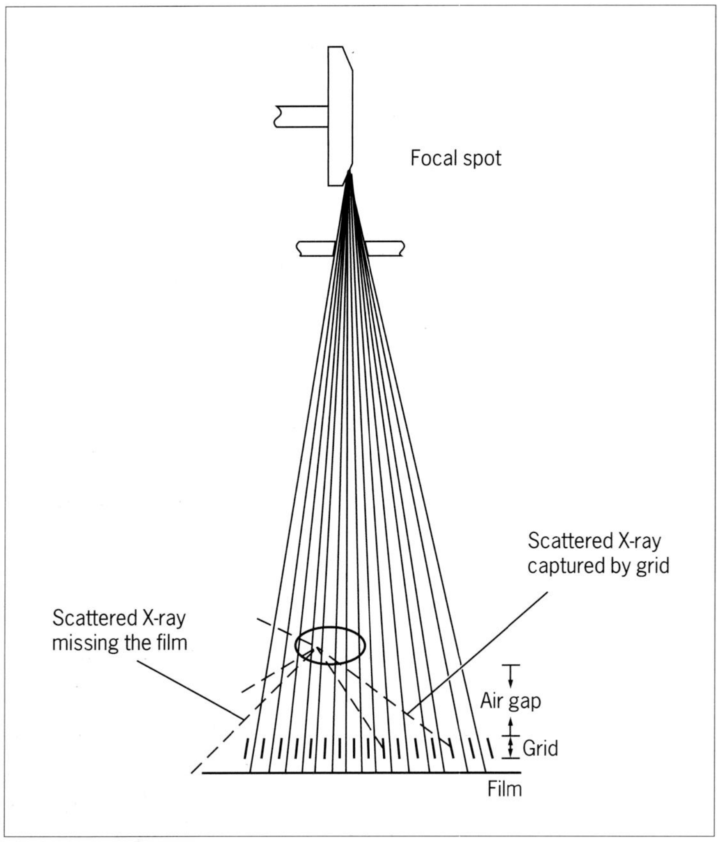

Fig. 11. Exclusion of scattered radiation by air-gap and grid.

The depicted grid is of the "focussed" type with angled lamellae, designed to a certain film-to-focus distance.

the film. Magnification is thereby increased, but this may be compensated by an increase of the focus-to-object distance.

4. Choosing an appropriate kVp setting relative to the elemental composition of the object in order to maximize photoelectric interactions (in, e.g., bones or contrast media) greatly improves contrast.

5. An effective and commonly applied measure to exclude scattered photons is the use of *grids* inserted in the beam path in front of the film. Grids are built from closely spaced thin lead strips interspersed by a material that is freely permeable to X-rays. The lead strips will absorb X-rays which are not arriving parallel, or near parallel, to the strips. The strips are often arranged at angles to match the direction of the (unscattered) X-rays throughout the image plane (fig. 11). The grid superimposes fine parallel lines on the image. For some applications this is tolerable, for others it is not, and the lines can then be eliminated by transversal motion of the grid during the exposure of the film. The mechanical device used to guide this motion is commonly designated a *Bucky mechanism*.

Conventional X-ray tomography

Tomography means "drawing of a slice", and denotes a special X-ray technique to image only structures contained in a predetermined plane of interest within the body part examined, while structures above and below this plane are blurred out. Tomography is often used as a supplement to an ordinary X-ray examination to clearly visualize and to ascertain the location of an observed structure.

The basic principle of conventional tomography is, during the exposure, to move the X-ray tube and the film cassette synchronously but in opposite directions relative to a stationary axis (fig. 12). The movements may be just straight line translational or may follow more complicated paths. The location of the axis determines the tomographic plane. The angular movement relative to the axis, known as the *tomographic angle*, determines the thickness of the tissue "slice" to be imaged sharply. The larger the angle, the thinner the slice.

Special tomographic machines can produce a panoramic image of a curved plane, best known from *Orthopantomograms* of the dental arches (see p. xx).

X-ray films

Films for X-ray imaging are manufactured to optimize their efficiency as detectors of the X-ray image. This is achieved with special photographic emulsions layered on both sides of the film base. This double coating slightly reduces the resolution of the film and, for special purposes where high resolution is important (e.g. in mammography), single coated films are used. The efficiency of X-ray photons in exposing the photographic emulsion is only moderate, but is increased (up to a factor of 100) by sandwiching the film between two layers of "*intensifying screens*" within the *cassette*, which is a lightproof but X-ray-transparent box containing the film. The intensifying screens are thin foils, which are freely permeable to the X-rays, and which contain a substance that emits multiple lower energy photons (within the visible range of the electromagnetic spectrum) when hit by a single high-energy X-ray photon.

The performance of an X-ray film (with associated intensifying screens) as a recorder of the X-ray image is expressed in the *characteristic curve* for the film (fig. 13). The characteristic curve varies with the kVp setting and the development conditions applied. The two key parameters of the film are the *speed* and the *contrast*. The speed denotes the exposure needed to obtain a specified optical density (O.D.), usually 1. The contrast is given by the slope of the linear part of the characteristic curve, denoted "*gamma* (γ)", and it expresses the exposure range which will be displayed on the grey tone scale between white and black. The lower the gamma, the larger the exposure range to be covered but the smaller will be the difference on the grey-tone scale between closely spaced doses of exposure, i.e. less image contrast between two structures that transmitted the X-rays with only a small difference in attenuation.

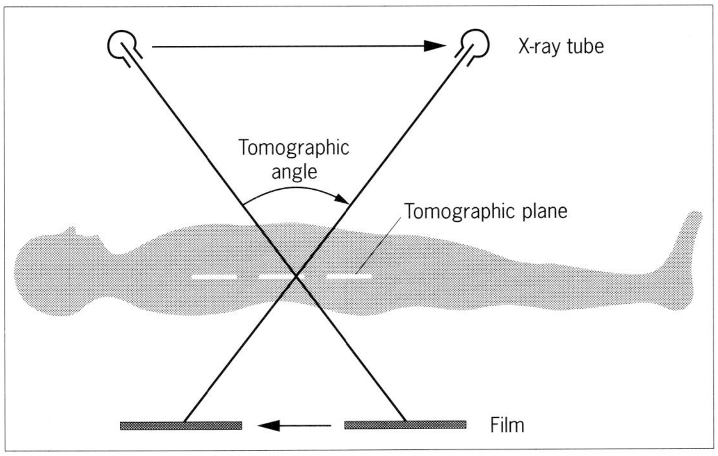

Fig. 12. Principle of conventional X-ray tomography.

Fluorescent screens and image-intensifying tubes

The image conveyed by the X-ray bundle emerging from the patient may be viewed directly on a screen coated with a substance, a "*phosphor*", which emits visible light (fluoresces) when hit by X-rays. Observation of the X-ray image on such a screen is called

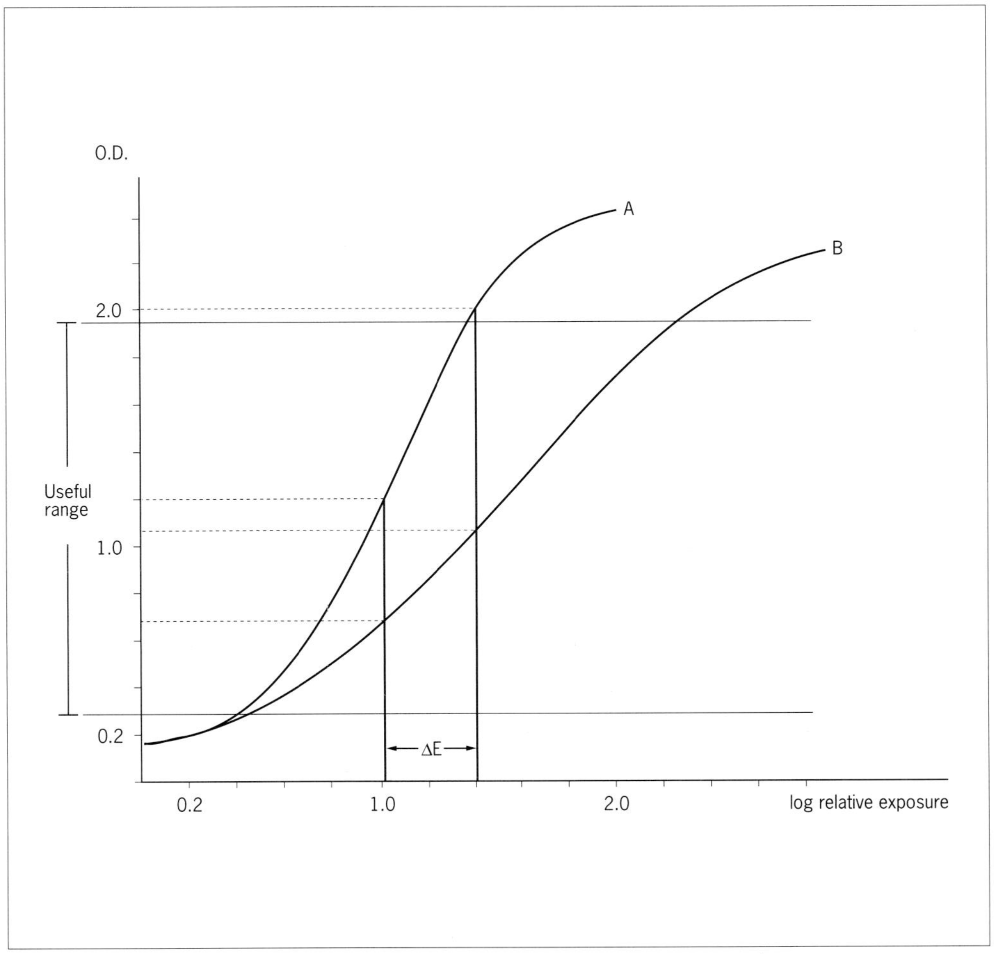

Fig. 13. Characteristic curve of two different films.

Film A has a higher speed (is more sensitive) than film B. Film A also gives more contrast than B because a given narrow exposure range (ΔE) is differentiated over more grey-tones by film A. Film B, on the other hand, will display a broader exposure range within the useful range of film densities (O.D. ~ 0.25 - 2.0).

The optical density (O.D.) of a transparent object, e.g. an X-ray film viewed on a light box, is defined by

$$\text{O.D.} = \log \frac{I_i}{I_e}$$

where I_i and I_e denote the intensity of incident and transmitted light, respectively. Thus, an O.D. of 2 means that only 1/100 of the incident light from the box is transmitted, which means nearly black.

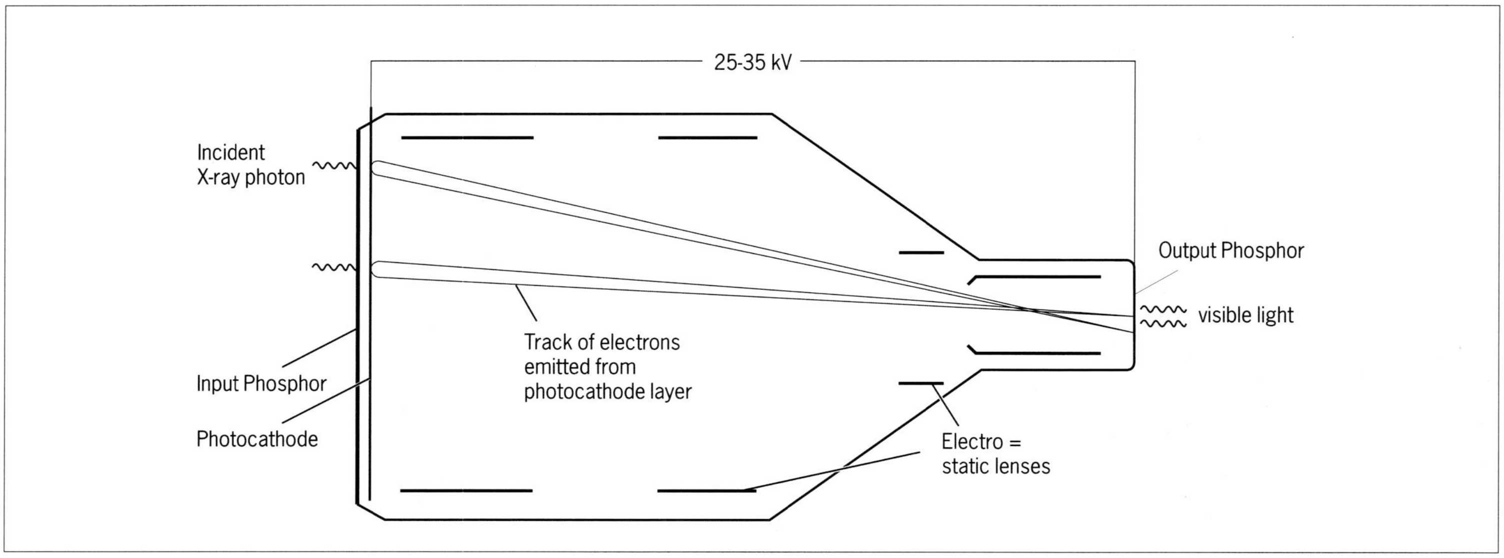

Fig. 14. The basic design of an image intensifier tube. For explanation, see text.

fluoroscopy, or just *"screening"*. The advantage of fluoroscopy is that motion may be observed directly, e.g. the swallowing of contrast medium through the pharynx and down the oesophagus. The light yield of such screens is rather low, and quite high patient doses of X-rays are needed to obtain an image of sufficient brightness to be viewed directly with the eye. Formerly, radiologists spent long hours in dim light viewing such screens. Though protected behind leaded glass, this led to undue radiation exposures of the radiologists. Fluoroscopy was greatly aided by the advent for the *image intensifying tube* (fig. 14). The input screen of this tube receives the X-rays from the patient and emits multiple lower energy photons from a phosphor. These photons in turn elicit release of electrons from an adjacent photocathode layer. These electrons are accelerated through a high voltage gradient along the tube and are at the same time focussed by an electrostatic lens arrangement to hit a smaller screen at the other end of the tube. This screen is coated with a phosphor that emits visible (yellow-green) light with high efficiency when hit by electrons. The gain in screen brightness, the intensification, from the input to the output screen is in the order of several thousand-fold. The image on the output screen is usually viewed with a videocamera and displayed on a TV-monitor, and may be recorded on film as well.

Digital subtraction X-ray imaging

The principle of image subtraction is especially applied in angiography. It involves the recording of one plain image before and a sequence of images during or after intravascular injection of a contrast medium. The first image is used to make a "mask" with reversed contrast. When this mask is superimposed on one of the following images all the image details that were stationary between the exposures cancel out, leaving only those structures (e.g. arteries) that have been delineated by the contrast medium in the second image. The contrast of this subtraction image may subsequently be increased to display the vascular ramifications with great clarity (see e.g. p.180). The procedure of image subtraction may be performed purely photographically, but is now mostly executed in a computerized image processor after digitalization of the images.

The success of this sort of image subtraction is heavily dependent on effective immobilization of the body part examined so that the two images are truly identical except for the injected contrast.

The principle of image subtraction may also be applied to two images recorded in rapid succession

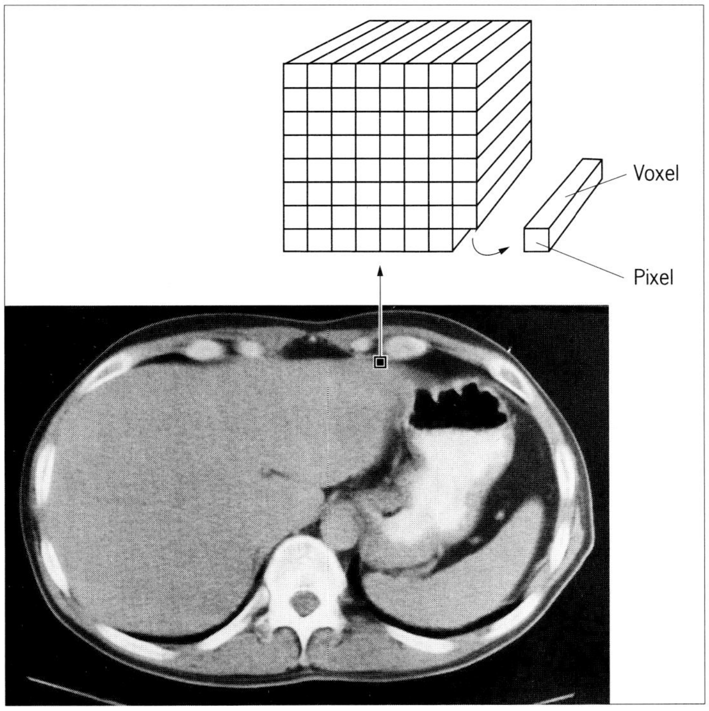

Fig. 15. An image composed of pixels, each representing a volume element, a voxel.

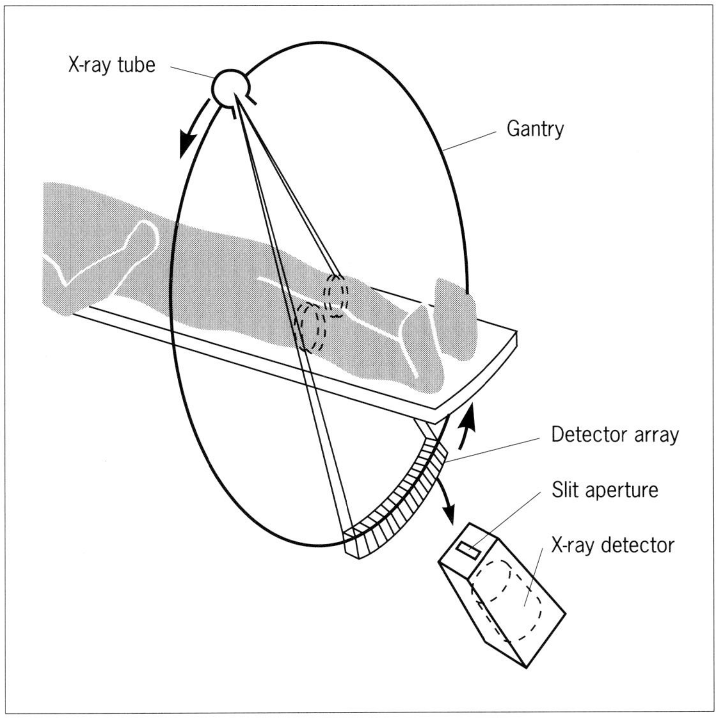

Fig. 16. The basic design of a CT-scanner with synchronous rotating X-ray tube and detector array.

but at different kVp settings (e.g. 60 and 150 kV) in order to enhance the contrast of structures whose attenuation coefficient changes markedly between the two kV settings, e.g. of bones or contrast medium.

Computed X-ray tomography

A computed X-ray tomography (CT) image is a squared matrix of picture elements, *pixels*. Each pixel represents a small volume element, a *voxel*, within an imaginary "section" or "slice" of the body part examined (fig. 15). The average linear X-ray attenuation coefficient of each voxel has been derived by computation from a series of measurements collected by the CT-scanner, and has been assigned a grey-tone value linearly related to its magnitude. Highly attenuating structures are shown in white, and slightly attenuating structures in black, i.e., as they would appear in conventional X-ray imaging. Thus, the CT-image is a map of the spatial distribution of calculated X-ray attenuation coefficients.

The CT scanner

The basic design of a commonly used type of CT scanner is shown in fig. 16. The X-ray tube is set in motion on a circular rail, the "*gantry*", surrounding the patient, who is positioned on a couch centrally in the gantry. The X-ray beam is collimated to a thin fan that intersects the patient. The angular width of the fan determines the field to be imaged. The intensity of the X-rays emerging after passage of the patient is recorded by an array of closely spaced detectors mounted on the rail to follow in synchrony the circular motion of the tube. Each of the detectors is equipped with diaphragms defining a slit aperture, and is precisely aligned to accept only such photons as have travelled a linear path from the X-ray tube focal spot. The length of the slit defines the thickness of the section from which measurements are derived. During one revolution of the tube the detectors record the intensity of transmitted X-rays along a very large number of linear paths, in the order of one million or more. All these measurements are collected over a short period (1-3 seconds in most scanners). The kVp of the X-ray tube is usually set so high (120-140 kV) that inelastic (Compton) scatter is the only quantitatively import-

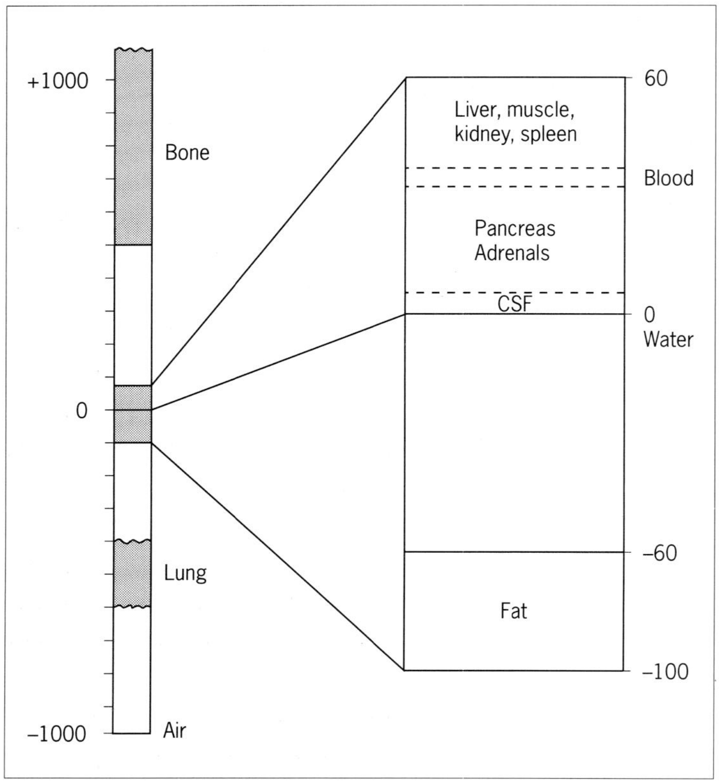

Fig. 17. The Hounsfield scale.

Approximate CT numbers of some tissues and organs are indicated.

ant process that attenuates the beam. This implies that the CT-image can, with good approximation, be read as a map of tissue mass densities.

After completion of one "section" the couch moves a predetermined length and the next set of measurements is collected. Section thickness may be varied from 2 to 20 mm on most scanners, and sections may be sampled consecutively or sequentially.

The CT scanner may also be used to collect an image analogous to a conventional X-ray image if the X-ray tube and the detector array are kept stationary while the patient, lying on the couch is moved longitudinally through the gantry. Such a "*scout view*" is usually taken at the beginning of an examination and used for planning of the subsequent tomography sequence and as a reference on which the positions of the tomograms are indicated. Mostly, CT tomograms are sampled perpendicular to the long axis of the body, but the gantry may be tilted as well as turned some 25° on most scanners to obtain oblique sections.

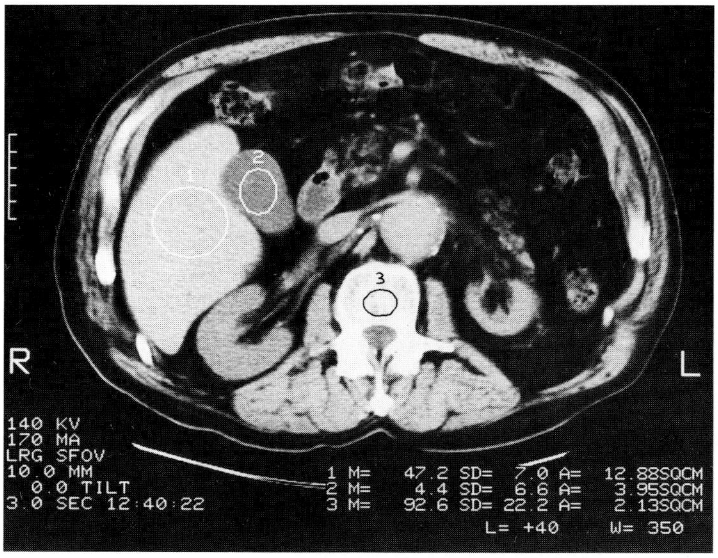

Fig. 18. CT image of abdomen.

R and L denote patient's right and left. A centimeter scale to the left in the image gives the linear calibration. The image is displayed with settings of level and window of 40 and 350, respectively. The X-ray tube has been operated at 140 kVp with a tube current of 170 mA. The tomographic slice thickness is 10 mm, and the data to construct the image have been collected over a period of 3 seconds. Three locations have been selected for display of numerical figures of X-ray attenuation. Location 1 is in the liver and has an area of 12.88 square centimeter, and an average CT number of 47.2 with a standard deviation (SD) of 7.0. Location 2 is in the gall bladder, location 3 is in the cancellous bone of a vertebral body. Note the high SD of the latter. Atherosclerotic calcifications are present in the aorta and right renal artery.

To overcome movement artefacts in cardiac CT imaging, the data sampling may be gated on the ECG to within a particular phase of the cardiac cycle. Respiratory movement artefacts are usually overcome simply by asking the patient to suspend breathing during the short period of data collection.

Image construction

The attenuation of X-rays recorded along one of the numerous paths through each section is the sum of contributions from all the voxels passed, and all the voxels in the section have been intersected by a multitude of beam paths. By a computational procedure, known as *filtered back projection*, the average linear attenuation coefficient of each voxel can now be calculated. The attenuation coefficients are calculated relative to that of water and for convenience are multiplied by a constant to make them large whole numbers. The coefficient of water is by definition zero, and the constant is chosen so that the coefficient for air becomes -1000. This brings dense bone to values around +1000. This scale of attenuation coefficients spanning 2000 units is the *Hounsfield scale*, and one unit is called a *CT-number* or a *Hounsfield unit*. The scale is shown in fig. 17, where the positions of some tissues and materials are given.

Most CT scanners have facilities to display in numerical figures the average CT-numbers and their standard deviation within a small area of the image that may be selected with a cursor, and to display the CT-numbers of the individual pixels (fig. 18).

The human eye will not discriminate more than about 20 steps on a grey-tone scale. Because many tissues differ only by a few Hounsfield units they will only be differentiated in the image if a small range of the Hounsfield scale is displayed on the grey-tone scale. The number of Hounsfield units differentiated on the grey-tone scale in the image is denoted the *window width(W)*, and the midpoint value of the window is denoted the *level(L)*. If the window is chosen to cover e.g. 100 units, to be discriminated on a 20 step grey-tone scale, each step will cover 5 units. All voxels with a CT number that is higher than the upper limit of the window will be displayed in white, and all below will be in black. The effects on the image of varying the window width around a fixed level, and of varying the level with a fixed window is shown in fig. 19. It is obvious that the window and level must be chosen appropriately for discrimination of the structures of interest, and certain combinations may be referred to as standard *bone settings*, *soft tissue settings* and *lung settings* (fig. 20).

It is important to bear in mind that the CT-number of a voxel and the derived grey-tone of the corresponding pixel is set by the average attenuation within that voxel. This imaging principle implies that the dimensions of a structure may be appreciably distorted, especially where tissues of widely differing CT-numbers meet, e.g. bone and brain. If a voxel contains say 10% dense bone and 90% brain by volume, the average CT-number may be around 120. If now the image is displayed with a window of 100 and a level of 40, the upper limit of the window will be at 90 and the pixel is consequently shown in white, which means that the bone will appear thicker than it is. If the level were raised to, say, 150, the CT numbers differentiated on the 20-step grey-tone scale would span from 100 to 200, i.e., it would include the voxel of 120 which would be displayed as a dark grey pixel as if it were all brain. Such dimensional distortions in CT-images are referred to as the *partial volume effect*, and they become more pronounced the thicker the sections are. The effect is very pronounced also at the borders between airways and air. Thus, the diameter of a bronchus will appear too small with a setting that resolves the smaller lung vessels.

As the X-rays penetrate tissues they become increasingly "hardened", because the lower energy photons are preferentially absorbed and scattered. The linear attenuation coefficient therefore decreases. The computing program of the CT-scanner takes this effect into account, albeit on the basis of expected averages. If a piece of metal (e.g. a dental filling) is included in the section, gross artefacts arise, so-called *beam hardening artefacts*. Such artefacts are seen also in images of soft tissues encased in thick bone, e.g. in the posterior cranial fossa.

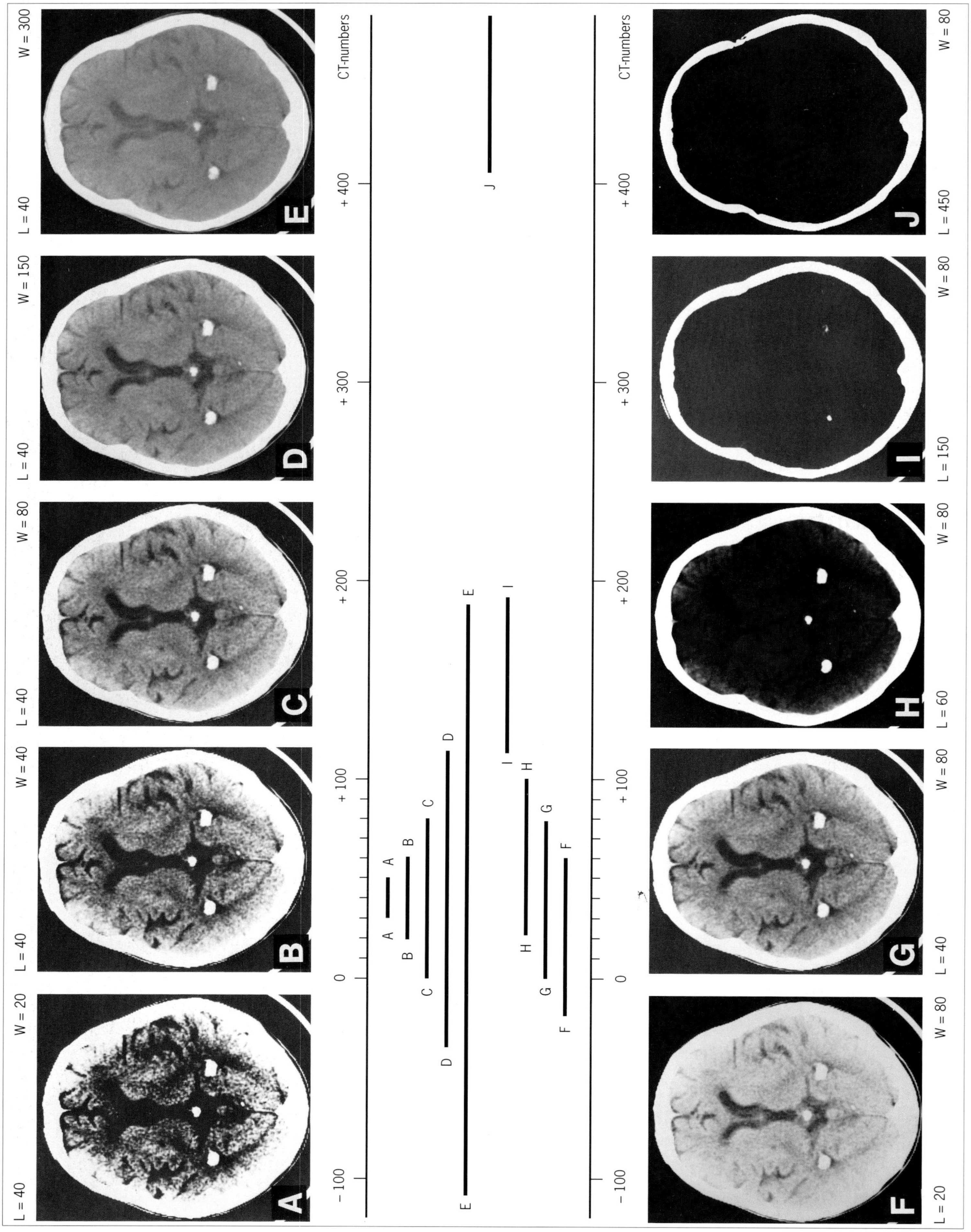

A
L = 40
W = 20
B
L = 40
W = 40
C
L = 40
W = 80
D
L = 40
W = 150
E
L = 40
W = 300
−100
0
+100
+200
+300
+400
CT-numbers
F
L = 20
W = 80
G
L = 40
W = 80
H
L = 60
W = 80
I
L = 150
W = 80
J
L = 450
W = 80

⇐ **Fig. 19. Effects of level and window setting in imaging of the brain by CT.**

The upper panel shows the tomogram displayed with a constant level (40) and increasing window from left to right. The lower panel shows the tomogram displayed with a constant window (80) and increasing level from left to right.

Note calcifications in pineal body and choroid plexus.

⇒ **Fig. 20. Standard "tissue settings" in a CT slice of the thorax.**

Upper frame (A): "Lung settings" (L = -700/W = 1000).
Middle frame (B): "Soft tissue settings" (L = 40/W = 500).
Lower frame (C): "Bone settings" (L = 250/W = 500).

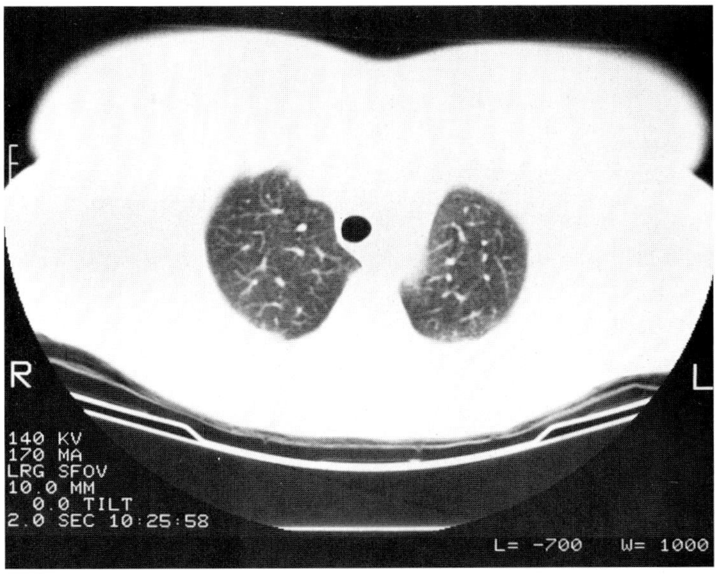

A

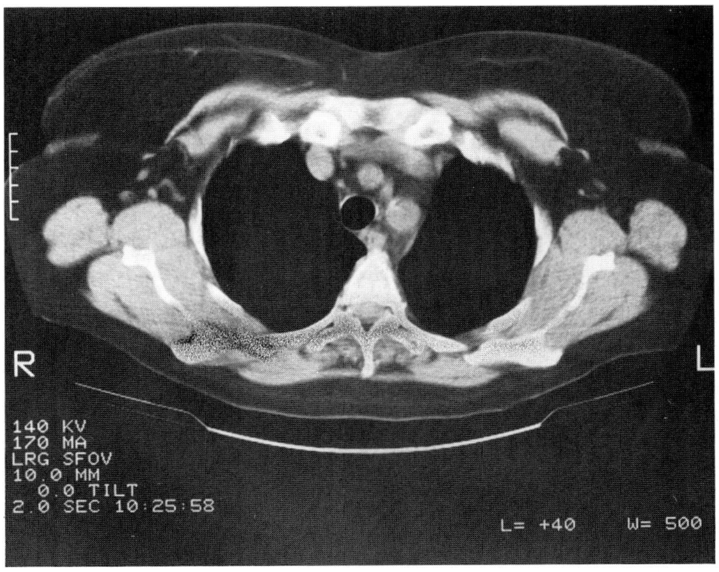

B

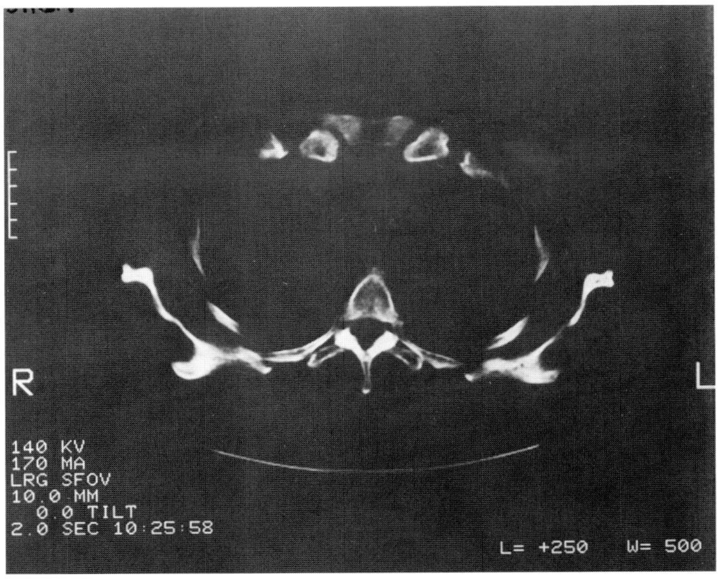

C

X-ray contrast enhancing media

Contrast media are used to either increase or to decrease the X-ray attenuation coefficient of a tissue or an organ in order to make it stand out in positive or negative contrast relative to its surroundings.

All positive contrast media now in use contain iodine or barium. These elements have K-absorption edges at 33 and 37 keV, respectively (fig. 5 and table 1). This means that they effectively absorb X-ray photons by photoelectric interaction in the 33 (37) to about 55 keV energy range, which is well represented in the beam from an X-ray tube operated at 80-100 kVp. At high kVp settings, e.g. 150 kVp, the positive contrast effect of these elements is considerably lowered because Compton scatter then dominates. So, when the concentration of contrast medium is low, lower voltage settings are generally used.

Barium

Barium is used as suspensions of fine particles of barium sulphate for imaging of the alimentary tract. Formulations differ with respect to barium content, viscosity and "stickiness", according to purpose.

The pharynx and oesophagus may be examined during the act of swallowing a gulp of barium suspension. The stomach, duodenum and small intestine may similarly be examined after ingestion of a barium meal. For examination of the stomach, sodium bicarbonate is often given in order to produce an image where the sticky barium suspension lines the wall of the stomach which has been distended by carbon dioxide gas liberated from the bicarbonate. This is a so-called *double contrast examination*, where gas serves as the negative contrast agent. This examination may yield fine resolution of details in the gastric mucosal surface. Barium suspensions given as enemas are widely used for examination of the rectum, the colon and the terminal ileum, and are often combined with insufflation of air to produce a double contrast image for improved visualization of mucosal details (see e.g. p. 267).

Iodine

Iodine is used in stable covalent binding to various organic molecules. *Iodinated oils* have for most of their original applications been replaced by water-soluble media, and are now only used for lymphography (see e.g. p. 111) and sometimes for hysterosalpingography (HSG).

The development of atoxic and *water-soluble, iodinated contrast media* that are tolerated by intravascular or subarachnoid injection and which are rapidly cleared from the circulation by renal excretion was a major breakthrough in radiology. There exists a wealth of preparations developed over more than 50 years of improvements in the chemistry and formulation of these media.

From a practical point of view, and disregarding details of their chemistry, the water soluble contrast media are commonly grouped into *ionic* versus *non-ionic* and *high-osmolality* versus *low-osmolality media*.

The contrast enhancement produced by any of the media is determined by the number of iodine atoms encountered by an X-ray photon along a linear path through the object. If the path is short, e.g. across a small vessel or duct, the concentration of the medium must be correspondingly high. This can often be achieved only at concentrations of the medium well above normal plasma osmolality (300 mOsm/kg), for some applications going as high as 1500-2000 mOsm/kg, which frequently causes adverse reactions. This problem is especially pronounced with ionic media because they dissociate to produce two or more osmotic effectors in solution. By various non-ionic substitutions and by increasing the number of iodine atoms per molecule it has become possible to develop *non-ionic, low-osmolality contrast media* which have become especially useful for angiography and myelography. It is possible with these media to keep the peak intravascular osmolality below some 500 mOsm/kg or less in high-resolution arteriography.

A major concern in *urography* is that the contrast medium should have a high renal clearance rate resulting in a high urinary concentration (see e.g. p. 282). The media may be given by fairly slow intravenous injection and in lower concentrations, and the intravascular osmolality may therefore be kept low even with ionic media.

Water-soluble, iodinated contrast media are used for a variety of other purposes, e.g. sialography (p. 156), dacryocystography (p. 149), direct pyelography and cystography, hystero-salpingography (p. 291), direct cholangiography (p. 269), arthrography (p. 97) and bronchography. They are used also to visualize the gastrointestinal tract, especially in CT-imaging.

A special class of iodinated contrast media are the *cholecystographic media*, some of which are given orally and others intravenously, and which are excreted with the bile in sufficient concentration to visualize the gall bladder and biliary ducts, the latter only properly with the intravenous cholecystographic media.

Gas

Air or carbon dioxide are used as *"negative" contrast media*. Their use in combination with barium for gastrointestinal double contrast examinations has already been mentioned. Air is used also for double contrast examination of joint cavities. Retroperitoneal or mediastinal gas insufflation may serve to separate and improve the visualization of organs and vessels at these sites, but is now seldom used. Introduction of air in the subarachnoid cavity and the brain ventricles for their visualization, *pneumoencephalography*, is now also largely out of use.

Techniques based on nuclear magnetic resonance

Principles of MR scanning

The nuclear magnetic dipole moment

An electrical charge which has an angular momentum, *a spin*, creates a *magnetic dipole moment* aligned with the axis of spin. This applies to electrons and protons, which have both a spin and a charge, but also to neutrons because the component electrical charges of this particle are non-uniformly distributed within its volume. Two identical and closely packed particles, e.g. two protons or two neutrons within an atomic nucleus, will align their spins so as to cancel out their magnetic dipole moments. Therefore, only nuclei with an odd number of protons and/or neutrons possess a magnetic dipole moment for the nucleus as a whole. Among the biologically relevant atomic nuclei with magnetic dipole moments, that of hydrogen,the single proton, is by far the quantitatively dominating species, and it is also ubiquitously present in living matter. Some rare isotopes of other biologically relevant elements, e.g. ^{13}C, ^{23}Na and ^{31}P, also have nuclear magnetic dipole moments and may be utilized experimentally, especially if an organism has been artificially enriched with the isotopes.

Nuclear magnetic resonance imaging (MRI, "NMR" or just "MR") is based on manipulation of nuclear magnetic dipole moments by means of externally applied magnetic fields and subsequent recording and analysis of radiosignals emitted from the nuclei in response to these manipulations. The phenomenon of nuclear magnetic resonance (NMR) has long been exploited as a fruitful analytical tool in chemistry. The development of diagnostic imaging techniques based on NMR required the construc-

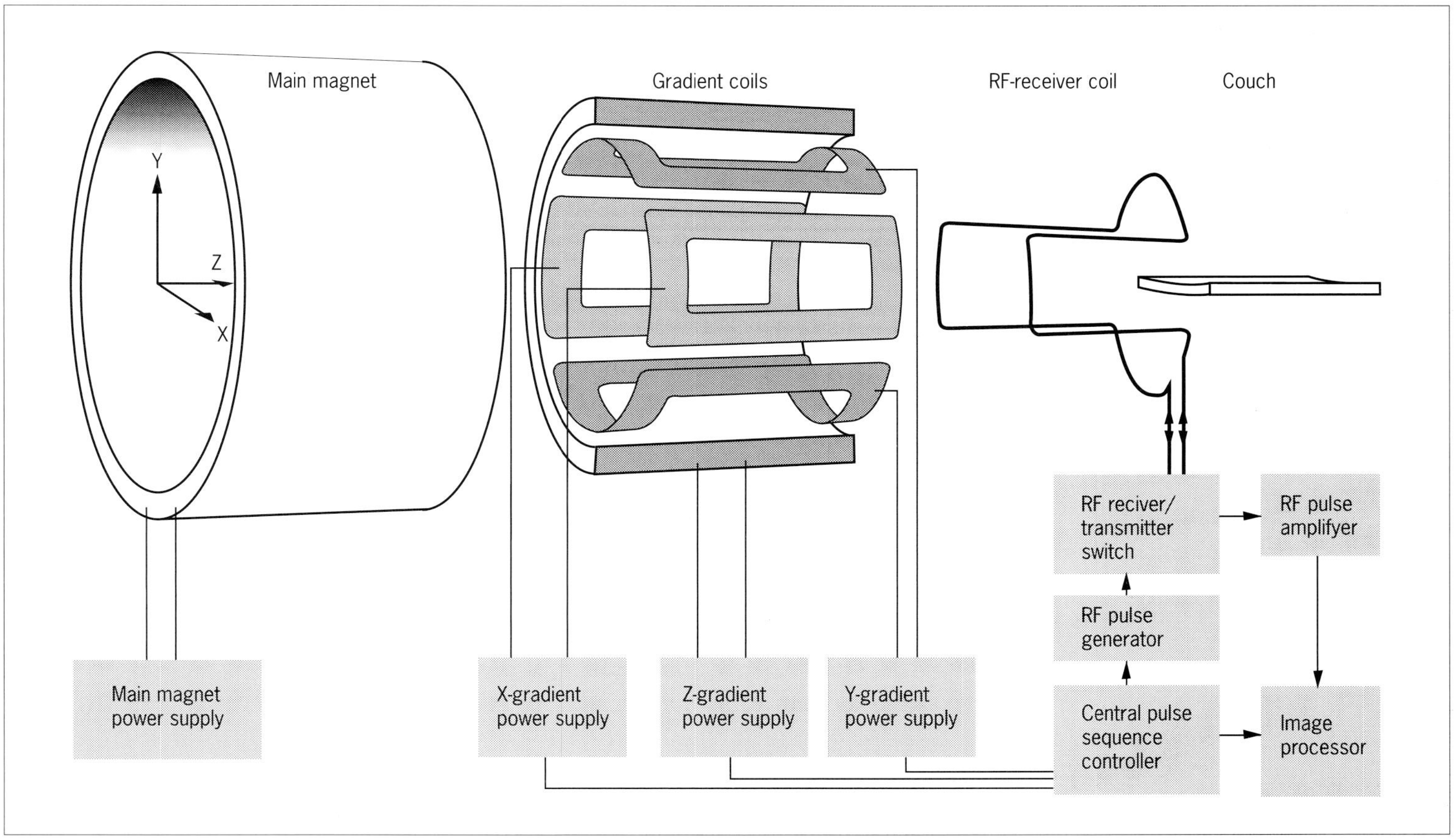

Fig. 21. The basic design of an MR scanner.

tion of apparatuses for the generation of strong and uniform magnetic fields, large enough to accomodate a whole person, and the development of methods to resolve the topological origin of the complex MR radiosignals emitted from within the body. Electron spin resonance (ESR) cannot be similarly utilized in diagnostic imaging because of technical problems, not yet solved.

Because virtually all diagnostic MR imaging thus far has been concerned with NMR of protons (hydrogen), the following account will refer to the proton, but the principles and concepts apply to any nucleus with a magnetic dipole moment.

The MR-scanner

The basic components of an MR-scanner are shown in simplified diagrammatic form in fig. 21. The *main magnet* produces a very strong and homogeneous field of 0.2 - 2T inside the bore of the magnet. This field must be extremely stable in time, and is commonly produced with superconducting coils cooled with liquid helium. Some MR-scanners employ resistive coils, others are constructed over permanent, ferromagnetic magnets, but none of these can produce fields as strong as those made with superconducting coils.

Inside the bore of the main magnet are installed three sets of coils used to produce *magnetic field gradients*, one in the direction of the main field (the Z-axis), and two perpendicular to this (the X- and Y-axes). The gradient field strengths over the entire patient are only a few percent of the main field strength and can be rapidly varied in time. Inside the gradient coil assembly is mounted a *radiofrequency (RF) transmitter/receiver coil.* For some applications the receiver coil is separate and is placed directly on the surface of the body part to be examined and denoted a *surface coil.* The patient is finally installed on a couch centrally in the bore. A central *pulse sequence controller* operates the gradient coil power supplies and the transmitter-receiver switch of the RF coil through the complex sequences used for the various MR imaging modes. The received RF signals are analyzed by Fourier transformation and spatially decoded in the image processor to be displayed as an image, which is a map of the amplitude of RF signals emitted from small volume elements in an imaginary slice of the patient.

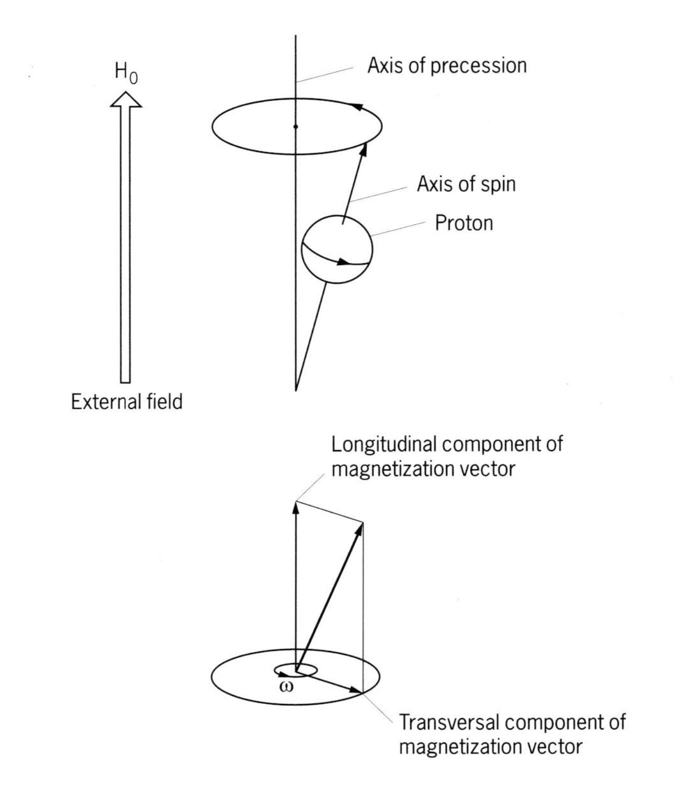

Fig. 22. Proton spin and precession.

The Larmor equation: $\omega = \gamma T$

where ω is the frequency of precession, T is the external magnetic field strength, and γ is a constant (the gyromagnetic ratio).

Tesla (T), is the unit of magnetic field strength. One Tesla is defined as the field which exerts a force of 1 Newton (N) on a one meter length of conductor carrying one ampère of current perpendicular to the magnetic field.

Proton magnetization

When a proton is exposed to a steady external magnetic field, a force will act on its magnetic dipole moment so as to orient it in parallel with the external field, but, due to the spin, it does not swing in as a compass needle would do. Instead it performs a maintained circular movement, called *precession*, in which its own axis of spin rotates at an angle around another axis that is parallel with the external field, much like a toy spinning top, in the gravitational field (fig. 22). The magnetic dipole moment of the precessing proton has a magnitude and a direction

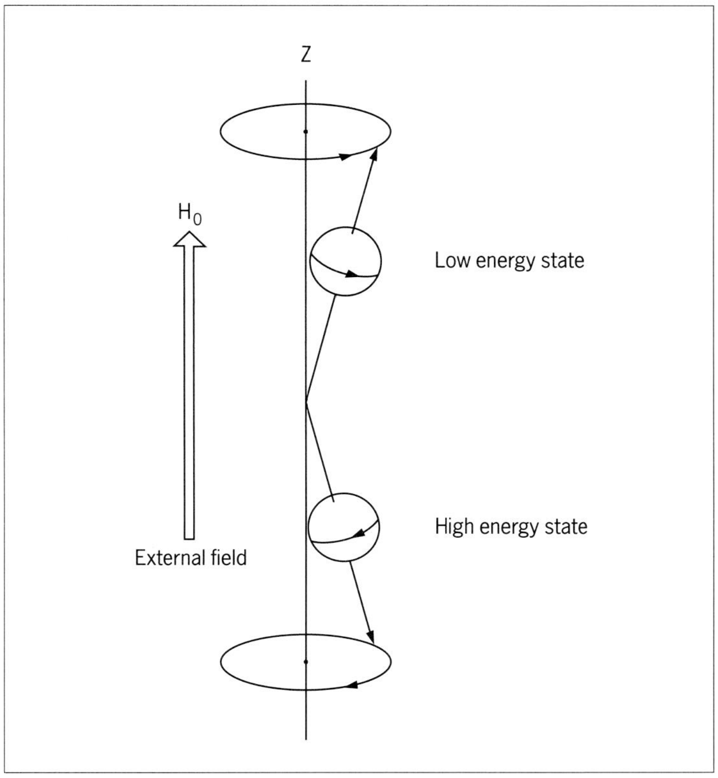

Fig. 23. Illustration of proton spin levels.

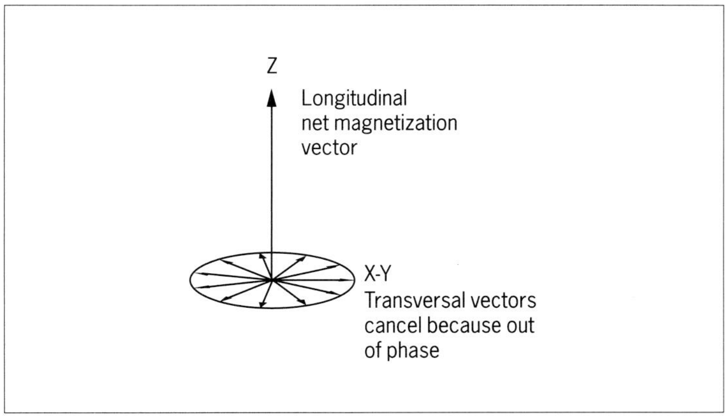

Fig. 24. Pictorial representation of the net magnetization vector.

and may therefore conveniently be expressed by a vector. This vector may be resolved in one component aligned with the axis of precession, "the longitudinal component", and a second component, oriented perpendicular to the external field and rotating with the frequency of precession, "the transverse component" (fig. 22).

The frequency of precession, the *Larmor frequency*, is linearly related to the strength of the external field as expressed by the Larmor equation (fig.22). The unit of magnetic field strength is *tesla* (T), and the precessional frequency of protons is 42.6 MHz/T, a constant denoted the *gyromagnetic ratio* (γ) of the proton (hydrogen). The Larmor frequency is actually not exactly the same for all protons, but may differ by a few ppm depending on the chemical bonds they have established. Thus, the Larmor frequency of protons in water and in aliphatic fatty acid chains differs by about 3 ppm (~ 130 Hz) in a 1T field. Such differences are designated *chemical shifts*.

Exposed to the external field, the spin of the proton may be at one of two discrete energy levels, according to principles of quantum mechanics not to be elaborated here. At the one spin-energy level the longitudinal component of the magnetic vector points in the same direction as the external field, at the other energy level it points in the opposite direction (fig. 23). The fractional distribution of protons between these two states depends on the temperature and the strength of the external magnetic field. A difference manifests itself as a *net magnetization* of the population of protons in the material/tissue within the field. Even at the high field strengths applied in diagnostic imaging (0.1 - 2T), the net magnetization of protons at 37°C is weak, with only a small surplus of protons (a few ppm) being at the low spin-energy level.

The net magnetization may, just as the magnetic dipole moment of the individual protons, conveniently be described by a vector (fig. 24). It is important to note that this *net magnetization vector* represents the statistical equilibrium of a huge population of protons which are constantly influenced by thermal (Brownian) motion, and shifting between the two spin-energy levels. The equilibrium net magnetization vector is aligned parallel (longitudinal) to the external field. The transverse, rotating vectors of the individual protons cancel out by averaging because they are out of phase in the equilibrium state.

Resonance

When a body part/tissue has been installed in the strong, steady and uniform magnetic field of the MR-scanner, the equilibrium state, represented by the net magnetization vector, becomes established within seconds. This equilibrium may be disturbed

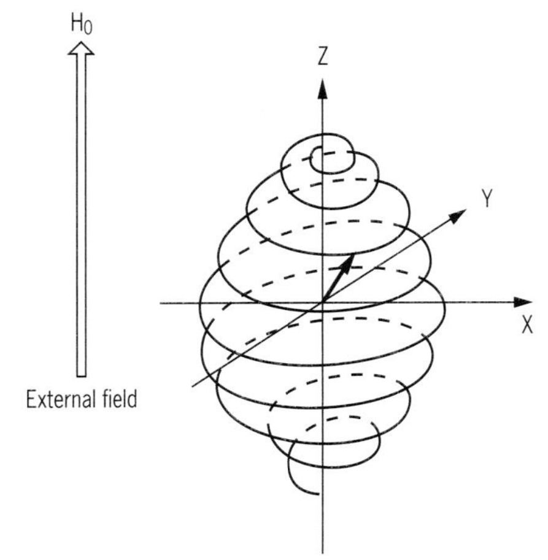

Fig. 25.

Diagrammatic illustration of the gradual change of the net magnetization vector under the influence of an increasing input of energy, delivered by RF-waves at the Larmor frequency.

and shifted by a pulse of electromagnetic waves at the Larmor frequency of the protons (42.6 MHz in a 1T field) entering perpendicular to the main field. This frequency is within the radiofrequency (RF) region of the electromagnetic spectrum (fig. 1). RF waves (photons) of precisely this frequency (energy) will transfer energy by *resonance* to the precessing protons. In principle, a bar magnet oriented perpendicular to the main field and rotating at 42.6×10^6 revolutions per second would do the same job. This resonance transfer of energy has *two* effects on the precessing protons.

Firstly, protons at the low spin-energy level, having absorbed the energy of an RF photon, shift to the high energy level accompanied by a shift in the orientation of their magnetic dipole moments. The magnitude of the *longitudinal net magnetization vector* decreases as more and more protons shift to the high energy level. At a certain RF energy input the longitudinal vector has disappeared. By further input of RF energy a surplus of protons is lifted to the high spin-energy level whereby the longitudinal vector reappears, but now in the opposite direction.

The second effect of the RF pulse is to force the protons into coherent ("in phase" or "synchronous") precession. This is manifested by the appearance of a *transverse net magnetization vector* that rotates with the Larmor frequency.

The net magnetization vector is, at any given moment, the resultant of the longitudinal and the transverse magnetization vectors. Thus, with an increasing RF-energy input, the longitudinal vector decreases and the transverse vector grows. The net magnetization vector is therefore tilted more and more towards the transverse orientation while rotating at the Larmor frequency (fig. 25). An RF pulse, delivering energy just sufficient to tilt the net magnetization vector into the transverse orientation, is called *a 90° pulse*. An RF pulse of twice this magnitude will cause the reappearance of a longitudinal vector, but in the opposite direction, and will also cause the transverse vector to rotate in the opposite direction relative to the main field. Such a pulse is called a *180° pulse*. The duration of such excitatory RF pulses used in MR imaging is in the order of a few milliseconds, to give an idea of the time scale.

Relaxation

When the RF pulse is turned off, the excited protons return over a period of time to the initial equilibrium state. This process is called *relaxation*. Now, importantly, the recovery of longitudinal magnetization and the decay of transversal magnetization follow different and independent time courses, both according to simple exponential functions, but with different time constants, denoted $\mathbf{T_1}$ for recovery of longitudinal magnetization, and $\mathbf{T_2}$ for decay of transversal magnetization. T_1 is the time at which the longitudinal magnetization has recovered 63% of its equilibrium magnitude. T_2 is the time at which the induced transversal magnetization has decayed by 63% (to 37%) of its maximum strength (fig. 26). The two relaxation processes reflect two types of interactions between the precessing protons and their surroundings.

Recovery of longitudinal magnetization implies loss of energy whereby those protons that were lifted to the high spin-energy level during magnetization give up this energy and fall back. This loss of energy is largely of thermal nature with a molecular basis in random collisions with surrounding molecules, collectively called "the lattice". The longitudinal relaxation process is therefore, according to its nature, sometimes referred to as *"the thermal relaxation time"* or *"the spin-lattice relaxation time"*. It is a fast process in pure liquids (T_1 in the order of a few seconds) and even faster in impure liquids, and is much slower in solids where random molecular motion is more restricted and collision events are therefore less frequent.

Decay of transverse magnetization implies loss of phase coherence between the precessing protons. This process has its origin in mutual magnetic interactions between the protons, and between the protons and local field inhomogeneities, e.g. due to the presence of other atoms with magnetic dipole moments precessing at other frequencies, or due to microinhomogeneities/instabilities in the external field. Because interactions between nuclei with different spins is a major contributor to the transversal relaxation process, this is often referred to as *"the spin-spin relaxation time"*. In pure liquids, characterized by mobile molecules, intrinsic and local field variations are rapidly fluctuating and tend to average out. In solids, molecules are more fixed and local intrinsic field inhomogeneities therefore more permanent, causing protons to systematically dephase. Therefore T_2 tends to be short in solids (milliseconds) and longer in liquids (seconds).

T_1 will generally be longer than T_2, but, especially in liquids, they may approach the same value. Tissues may, simplified, be regarded as complex mixtures of solids, solutes in solvent (water), and fat which at body temperature is something in between solid and liquid. Water and the fatty acid chains of fat are by far the dominating contributors to the proton MR-signals utilized in diagnostic imaging. The other elements may be simply regarded as parts of a complex "lattice" which shapes the thermal relaxation, expressed by T_1, and which creates local (intrinsic) field inhomogeneities which shape the spin-spin relaxation, expressed by T_2. T_1 and T_2 of a given tissue therefore become sort of averages. Actual figures for T_1 vary between soft tissues from about 200 msec in fatty tissue to about 800 msec in grey matter of the brain. T_1 of pure water is for comparison about 2500 msec. T_2 similarly varies between some 40 msec in liver and muscle to about 90 msec in pure fat and white matter of the brain. The chemical shift (~ 3 ppm) between protons of water and protons of fatty acids causes especially rapid decay of transverse magnetization in tissues where fat and "watery" tissue are intimately mixed, e.g. in bone marrow. The mineralized bone tissue contains too few mobile protons to yield detectable MR-sig-

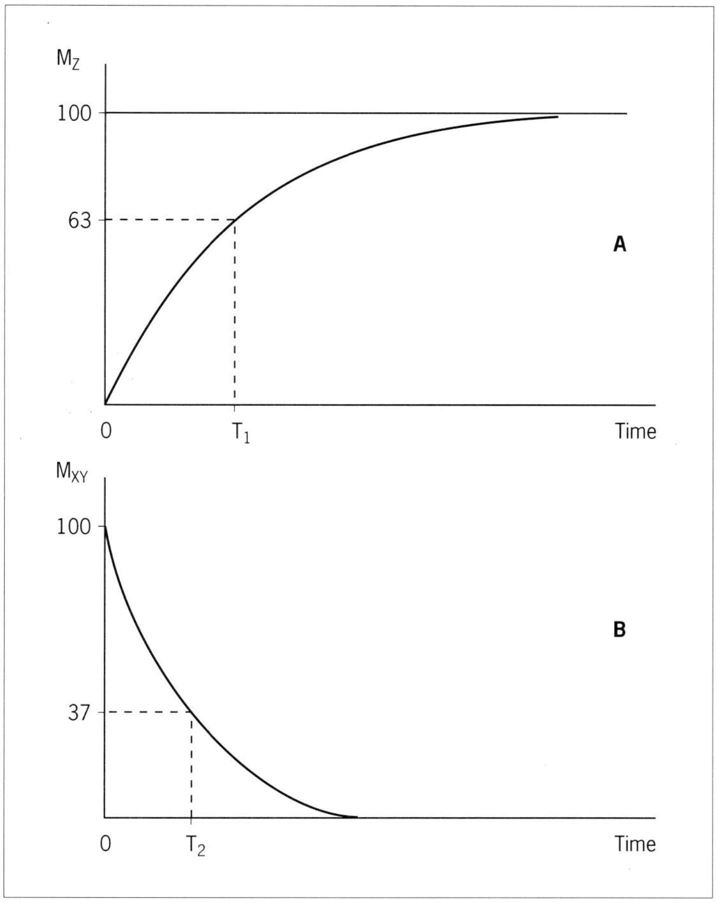

Fig. 26.

A) The exponential recovery of the longitudinal net magnetization vector (M_Z) after termination of a 90° RF-pulse at time 0.

The magnitude of $M_Z = M_0\ (1 - e^{-t/T1})$,

where M_0 is the magnitude of the net magnetization vector at equilibrium. T_1 is the time constant of the recovery process.

B) The exponential decay of the transversal, rotating net magnetization vector (M_{XY}) after termination of a 90° RF-pulse at time 0.

The magnitude of M_{XY} as a function of time (t) is given by: $M_{XY} = M_0\ e^{-t/T2}$,

where T_2 is the time constant of the decay process.

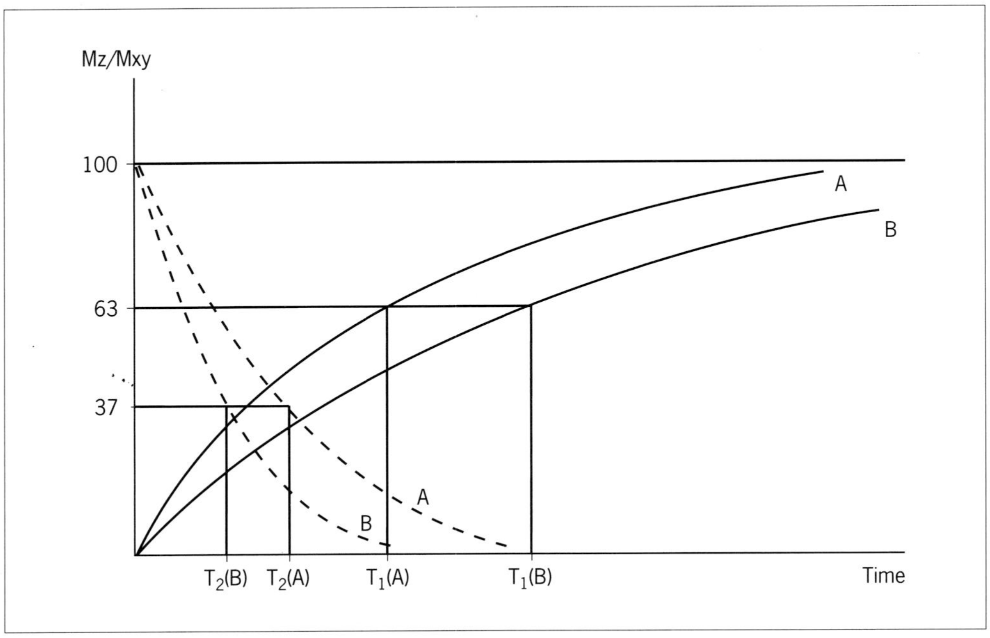

Fig. 27.

Recovery of longitudinal magnetization (M_Z, full line) and decay of transversal magnetization (M_{XY}, broken line) in two tissues, A and B. Tissue A has the shortest T_1 and the longest T_2.

nals in diagnostic imaging. MR imaging is directed at detection and visualization of differences in parameters such as T_1 or T_2 between different tissues and fluids within the body (fig. 27).

During the period of relaxation of the magnetized tissues an electromotive force can be induced in an appropriately situated receiver coil as an RF signal in synchrony with the precessing protons. This RF signal is analyzed and encoded to be displayed as an image. Importantly, only protons that precess in phase give rise to detectable radiosignals. This means that the induced radioemission from a volume element ceases when the transverse component of the net magnetization vector in that volume element has decayed, even though the longitudinal component has typically not yet recovered. Thus, to detect differences in T_1 between tissues, and also to fully exploit differences in T_2, complex excitatory pulse sequences are applied, to be detailed in due course.

MR contrast media

The relaxation times (expressed by T_1 and T_2) of a given tissue will be shortened if a paramagnetic substance is targeted to that tissue, because the paramagnetic substance creates local field inhomogeneities due to their unpaired electrons. This principle is applied in MR imaging utilizing the rare earth *gadolinium*, chelated to DTPA. Gd-DTPA will not cross the normal blood-brain barrier and is used to detect defects in this barrier. Gd-DTPA is excreted in the urine and may be utilized in urological MR imaging. Gd-DTPA is so far the only MR contrast medium in routine clinical use, but several others will undoubtedly soon follow. Thus, magnetized iron oxide particles (MIOP) will, after intravenous administration, be taken up by the macrophages in liver, spleen and bone marrow and shorten the relaxation time in these organs, but not in tumors lodged in these tissues.

Methods for obtaining spatial (tomographic) resolution of the MR signals

The final MR image is, as was the CT image, a squared matrix of *pixels*, each representing a small volume element, a *voxel*, within an imaginary "slice" of the patient. Each pixel has been assigned a greytone value proportional to the amplitude of the radiosignal emitted from the corresponding voxel in a defined period of time following a sequence of RF excitations, chosen to maximize differences between tissues with respect to a particular parameter, e.g. T_1 or T_2.

To achieve the required spatial resolution, three coordinates need to be known for each voxel. To select the position of the tomographic section (the first coordinate, Z) a magnetic field gradient is established along the patient (fig. 28A). In consequence of this gradient, a given radiofrequency will resonate only with protons located within a narrow cross-section of the gradient. Changing the frequency of the excitatory RF pulse will move the cross section to

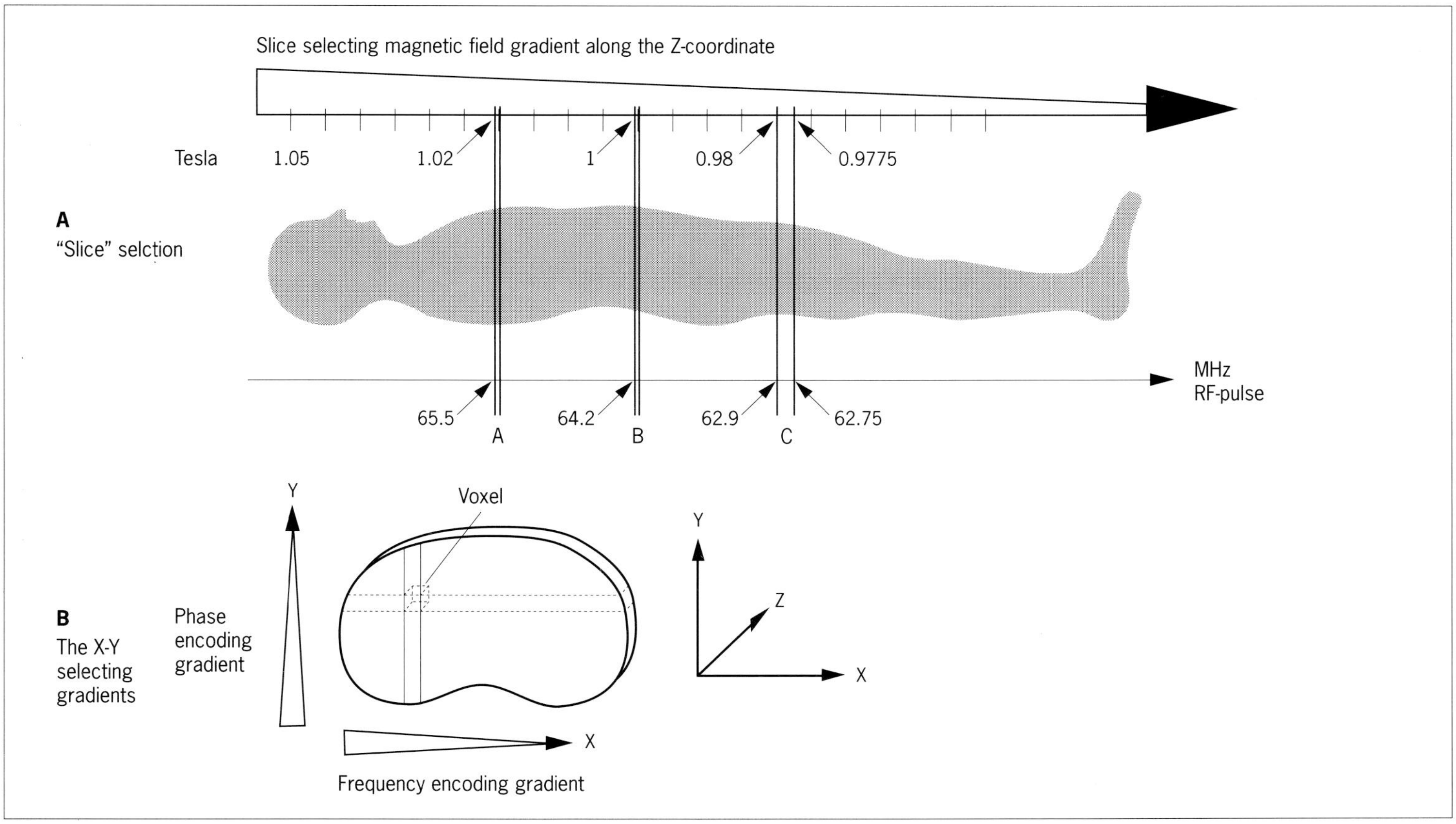

Fig. 28. Principle of spatial resolution.

A thin slice (A) will be excited by an RF-pulse of e.g. 65.5 MHz. Changing the RF-pulse to 64.2 MHz moves the excited section to position B. If the RF-pulse has a bandwidth from 62.75 to 62.9 MHz, a thicker slice at position C becomes excited.

another position along the gradient where it matches the Larmor frequency of the protons. The steeper the gradient and the narrower the bandwidth of the RF pulse, the thinner the slice to be excited by resonance at the Larmor frequency. Usually the gradient and the bandwidth are adjusted to obtain excitation of a slice about 10 mm thick. *This slice-selecting gradient* is present during the RF pulse and defines the position of the tomographic section.

The two additional coordinates (X and Y) needed to define the voxel may be obtained by various methods. A common method applies two additional weak gradients, the frequency-encoding gradient and the phase-encoding gradient.

The frequency-encoding gradient is established perpendicular to the slice-selecting gradient and is switched on immediately after the excitatory RF pulse has been sent in. This gradient will have the effect of establishing a continuous increase in precessional (Larmor) frequencies from one edge of the section to the opposite edge, so that a particular frequency derives from a particular row of voxels across the slice (fig. 28B).

The phase-encoding gradient is applied at right angles to both the slice-selecting and the frequency-encoding gradient, and it is switched on for only a very short period of time after the excitatory RF pulse has been switched off. It has the effect of producing a continuous change in precessional phase across the slice, so that a particular phase derives from a particular row of voxels oriented perpendicular to the rows defined by the frequency-encoding gradient (fig. 28B).

Now, when the complex radiosignal emitted by the excited cross-section of the patient is picked up by the receiver coil and subjected to a Fourier analysis, which means resolution into a number of component elementary sine waves, the frequency and the phase of each of these elementary waves define together the coordinates of the voxel from which the wave originated. The amplitude of the elementary wave can now be assigned a grey-tone that is proportional to its magnitude and is displayed as the corresponding pixel in the image. By convention, high signal amplitudes are displayed towards white and low amplitudes towards black on the grey-tone scale. As in CT imaging, the scale has about 20 steps, and the "window width" and the "level" can be varied. Sometimes additional color-encoding is used.

The three gradients used to obtain spatial resolution of the MR signals can be interchanged, so that axial, sagittal and coronal sections may freely be produced without moving the patient. It is possible also to excite and sample radiosignals simultaneously from several appropriately spaced sections to speed up the collection of a long series of sections, e.g. by simultaneous collection of every fourth section in a series of 32.

Flow effects and movement artefacts in MR imaging

Flow in blood vessels and CSF may influence MR imaging in very complex ways. Depending on the RF-pulse sequences applied, the presence of flow may give rise to weaker or stronger signals than expected had the blood been immobile. Without going into detail, it appears clear that a fast flow perpendicular to the section may have the effect of carrying away those protons that should have given a signal during the RF-signal sampling period, whereby the blood vessel becomes "signal void" and displayed in black on the image. In other situations, protons with "spuriously" strong signals may be carried into the section by flow. Flow in the plane of the section may disturb the spatial X-Y encoding/decoding and give rise to artefacts. Therefore, wherever flowing blood is imaged one must anticipate that the signal intensity from the blood may be spurious, and that peculiar positional artefacts may be present. These are often seen as blurred streaks through a vessel, extending across the image in the direction of the phase-encoding gradient.

Movement artefacts are much more of a problem than in CT, because MR sampling times are considerably longer. Thus, to obtain useful cardiac imaging the data collection has to be gated on the ECG. Also, gating on the respiratory cycle may be necessary, because many patients may have difficulty in suspending their breathing for sufficiently long periods of time. Finally, and regrettably, intestinal peristalsis is often a major obstacle to abdominal MR imaging.

MR imaging modes and pulse sequences

There are three basic MR imaging modes routinely used in diagnostic practice:

1. *Proton density-weighted imaging* is directed at visualizing differences between tissues in their density of protons, irrespective of their chemical bonds and differences in T_1 and T_2. Thus, the contrast between pixels can be translated into differences in proton density between voxels. Proton density-weighted images are obtained with a simple pulse sequence, but many tissues are not well discriminated.

2. *T_1-weighted imaging* is directed at visualizing differences between tissues in the time course of recovery of the longitudinal equilibrium magnetization after it has been disturbed by an RF pulse. Thus, the contrast between pixels can be translated into differences in T_1 between voxels. T_1-weighted images generally give the best all-round anatomical resolution, and are therefore used almost throughout the atlas part of this book.

3. *T_2-weighted imaging* is directed at visualizing differences between tissues in the time course of decay of transverse magnetization after it has been induced by an RF pulse. Thus, the contrast between pixels can be translated into differences of T_2 between voxels. T_2-weighted images are particularly useful for distinction of CSF (fig. 29).

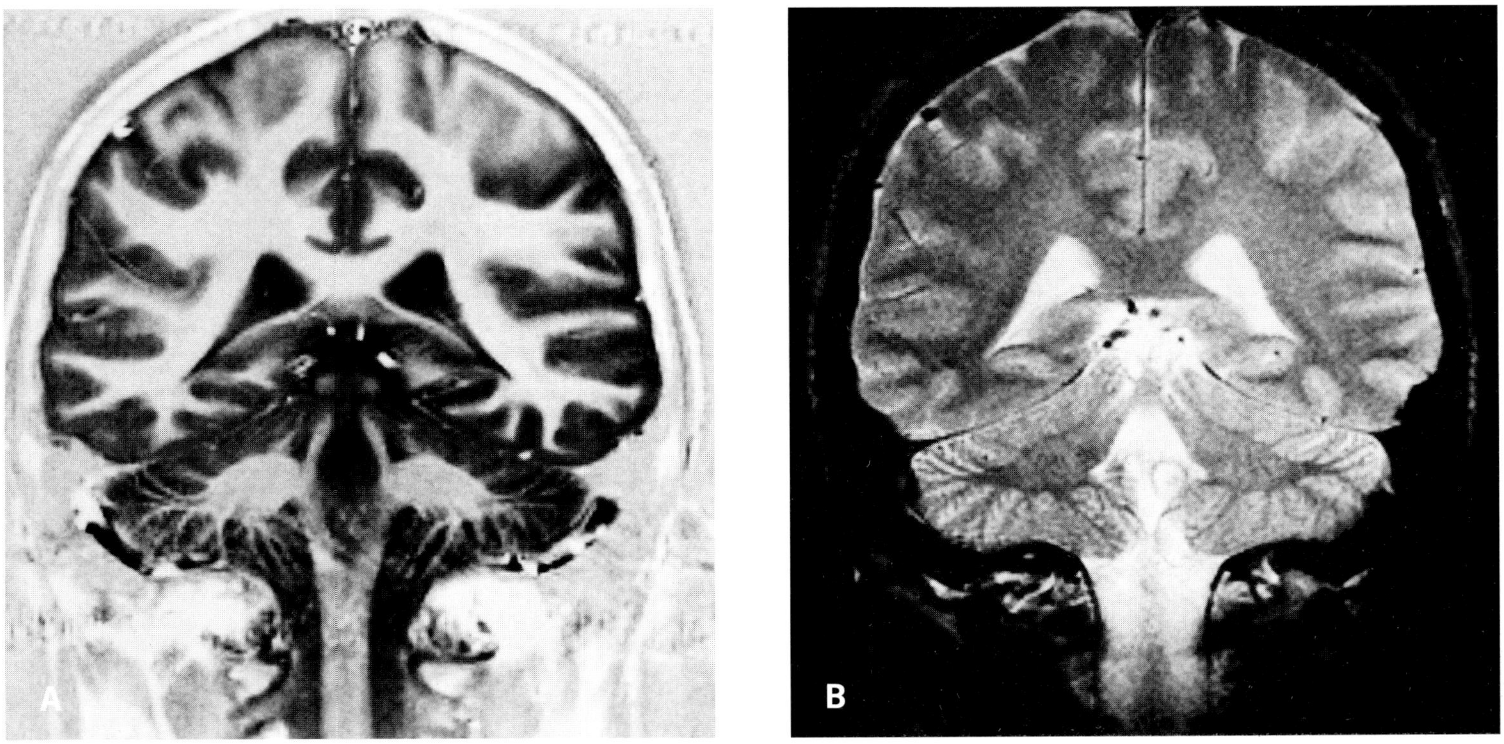

Fig. 29. Difference between T_1- and T_2-weighting in MR brain imaging.

The same coronal section of the brain shown in a strongly T_1-weighted recording (A), and a strongly T_2-weighted recording (B). Note that the contrast between white and grey matter is reversed betweeen these imaging modes, and that the cerebrospinal fluid gives a strong signal (white) by T_2-weighting and no signal (dark) by T_1-weighting.

Besides the above three basic imaging modes there are others, e.g. directed at visualization and quantitation of flow, or directed at visualization of specific chemical (metabolic) parameters, so-called spectroscopic imaging, but these specialized techniques will not be elaborated here.

MR pulse sequences

In the equilibrium state, no radiosignals are emitted from the tissues, which have become magnetized by the main field. This is because the longitudinal magnetization vector is directed along the main field (and is therefore silent) and because the rotating transversal vectors of the individual protons are out of phase. Radiosignals are detected only when the net magnetization vector has a rotating transversal component, i.e. that a sufficient number of protons precess in phase.

To obtain radiosignals specifically related to the proton density, the T_1 or the T_2 parameters of the tissues, it is necessary to employ various excitatory RF pulse sequences, called *MR pulse sequences*. These pulse sequences are repeated until enough signals have been collected from all voxels. Usually, several signals are sampled from each voxel and averaged.

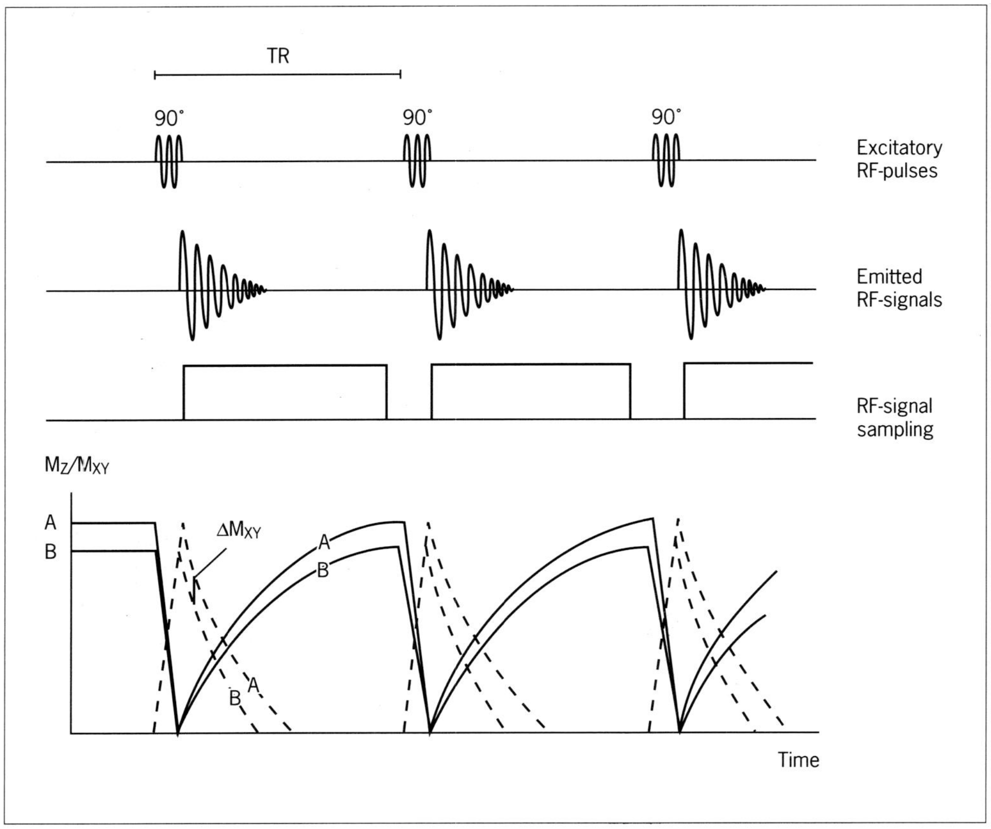

Fig. 30. Saturation recovery pulse sequence.

The lower graph illustrates the time-dependent variation in magnitude of longitudinal (M_Z, full line) and transversal (M_{XY}, broken line) magnetization in two tissues, A and B, of which A has the highest proton density. The magnitude of the RF-signals sampled after termination of the excitatory 90° RF-pulses is higher from voxels of tissue A than from voxels of tissue B, the difference being proportional to the maximum difference (ΔM_{XY}) in magnitude of the M_{XY} vectors in the two tissues.

There are four standard pulse sequences:

1. *The "saturation" recovery pulse sequence* (fig. 30). This pulse sequence consists of 90° pulses repeated at intervals, TR, i.e. "repetition time", chosen to be long (seconds) enough so that the equilibrium state is reestablished between pulses. The 90° pulses "flip" the longitudinal net magnetization vector of all the voxels into the transversal plane. The radiosignals emitted from the voxels in response to this manoeuvre are at their maximum amplitude right after the 90° pulse has been switched off, because the protons precess in phase, but decay exponentially as the protons loose coherence. This signal is often called *"free induction decay" (FID).* At its maximum amplitude this signal is directly proportional to the number of precessing protons, and an image based on these maximum signals will be a proton-weighted image.

   Importantly, at the time the FID signal has decayed to silence in all voxels, the longitudinal magnetization vectors may not yet have recovered. Differences between voxels in the time course of longitudinal magnetization recovery may be disclosed if the next 90° pulse is applied before the equilibrium is reached. This maneuver is denoted:

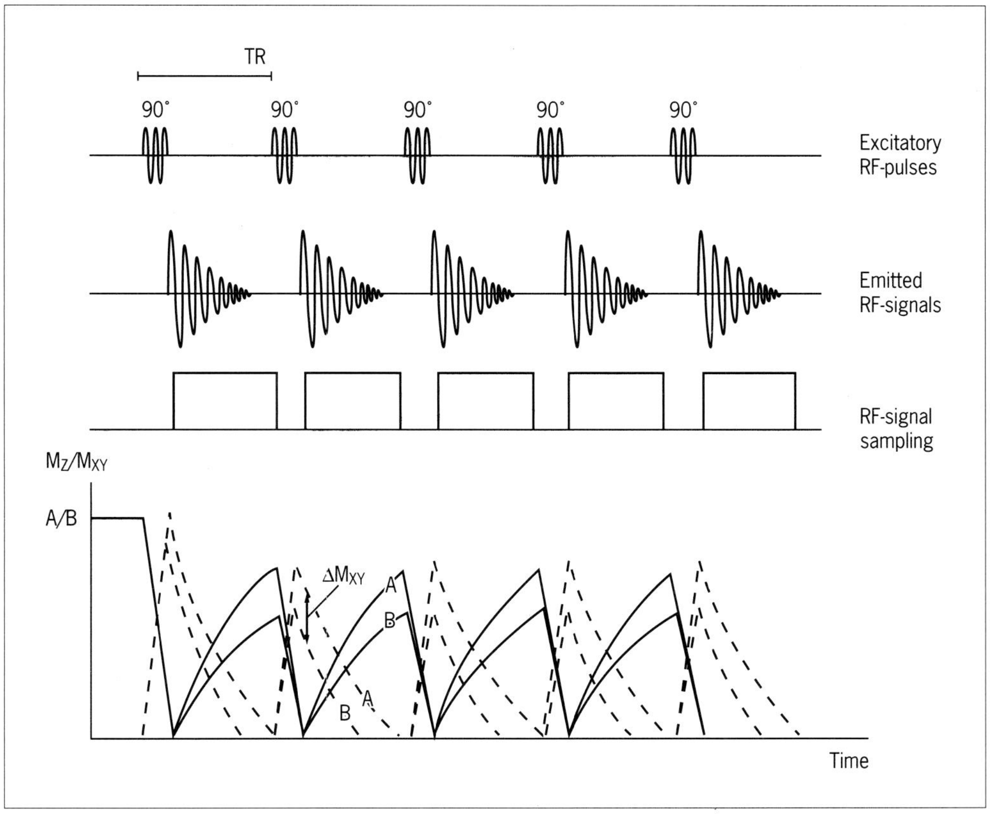

Fig. 31. Partial saturation recovery pulse sequence.

The lower graph illustrates the time-dependent variation in magnitude of longitudinal (M_Z, full line) and transversal (M_{XY}, broken line) magnetization in two tissues, A and B, having an equal proton density but differing in T_1. The difference in magnitude of longitudinal magnetization during recovery becomes expressed in the difference (ΔM_{XY}) in magnitude of the signal-giving transversal vectors.

2. *The partial saturation recovery pulse sequence* (fig. 31).
   This pulse sequence differs from the previous sequence only with respect to TR, which is chosen to be so short that the longitudinal magnetization vectors of the voxels have not fully recovered. The following 90° pulse will flip them back to the transversal plane, and the radioemissions resume with amplitudes proportional to the magnitude of the "flipped" vectors. Thus, voxels differing in the rate at which their longitudinal magnetization recovers, i.e. they differ in T_1, will now emit signals of different amplitude - those with the fastest recovery (shortest T_1) emitting with the highest amplitude. An image based on radiosignals called forth by a 90° pulse will therefore display differences in T_1 between voxels, i.e. be T_1-weighted.

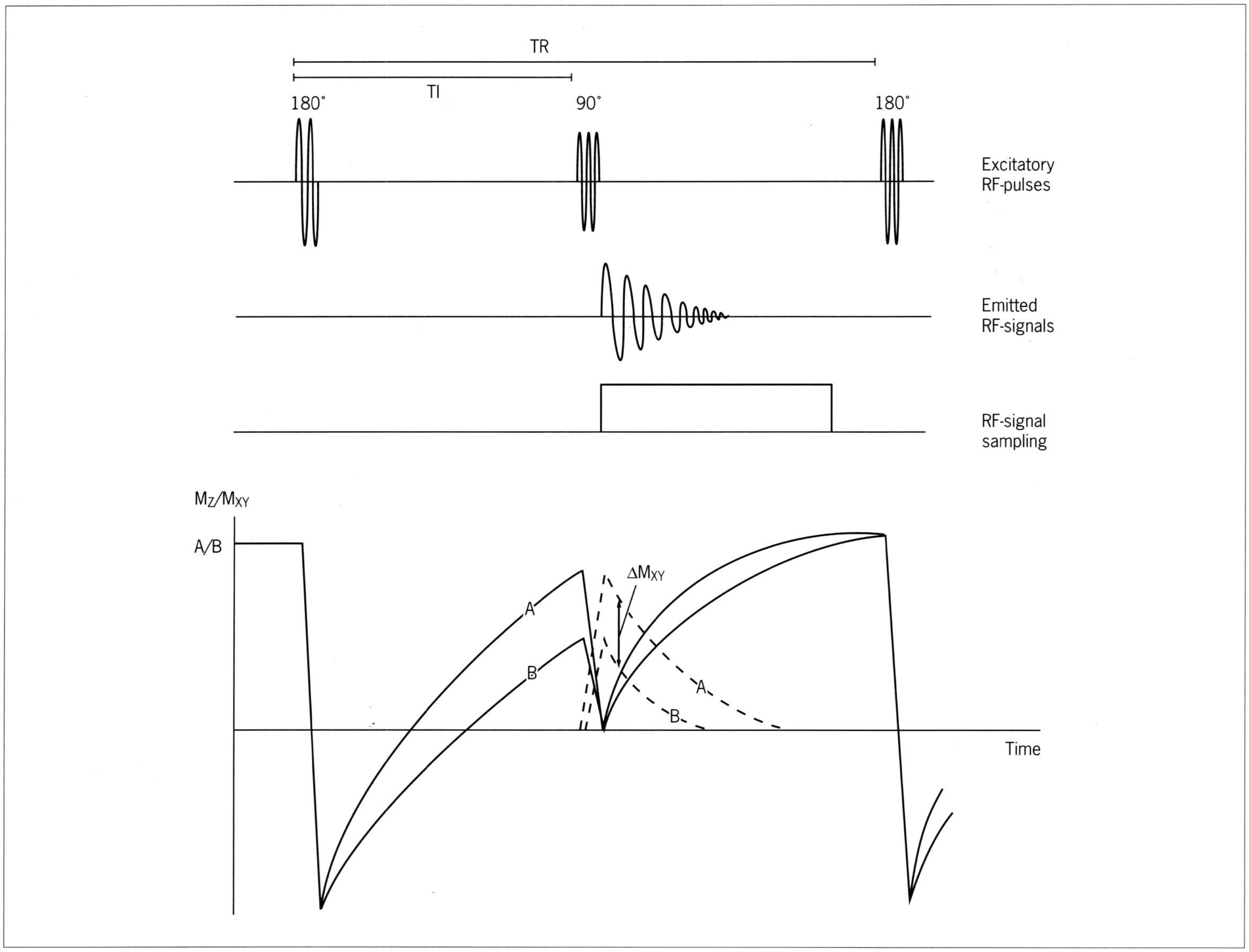

Fig. 32. Inversion recovery pulse sequence.

The lower graph illustrates the time-dependent variation in magnitude of the longitudinal (M_Z, full line) and transversal (M_{XY}, broken line) magnetization of two tissues, A and B, having an equal proton density but differing in T_1. This difference becomes expressed as ΔM_{XY} of the transversal magnetization.

3. *The inversion recovery pulse sequence* (fig. 32).
This pulse sequence consists of a series of 180° pulses each followed after an interval by a 90° pulse. Time to repeat of the 180° pulse is denoted TR and time to initiation of the 90° pulse is denoted TI (*"inversion time"*). The 180° pulse delivers energy to invert the net magnetization vector relative to the main field. From this position it will recover with a time course determined by T_1. Because the road back to equilibrium is long, differences in T_1 between voxels will yield pronounced differences in the magnitude of their longitudinal vectors during recovery. When the 90° pulse is applied at time TI, the longitudinal vectors are flipped and differences in their magnitude become expressed in the amplitude of the radiosignals emitted by the voxels just after cessation of the 90° pulse. An image based on these radiosignals therefore becomes strongly T_1-weighted.

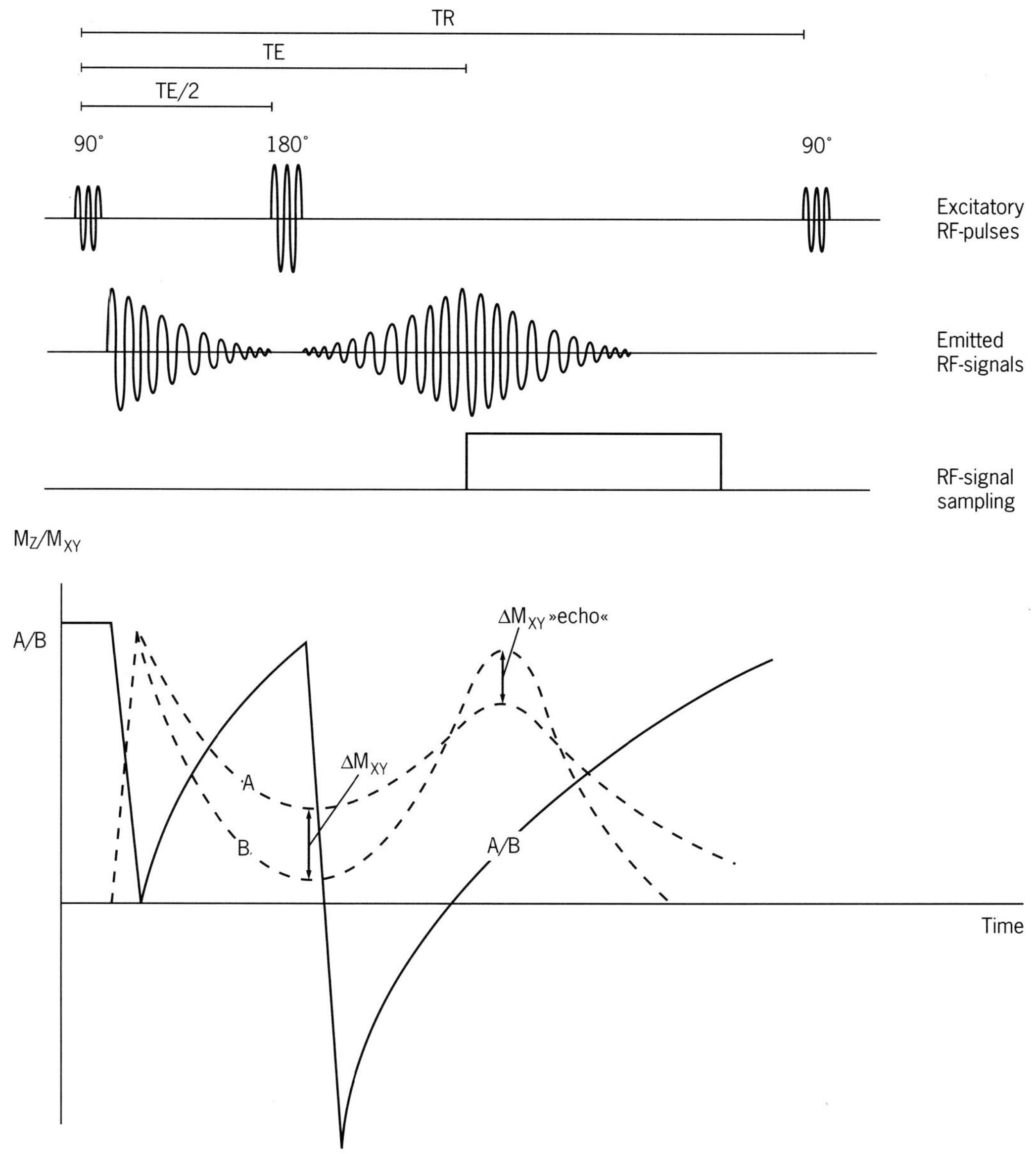

Fig. 33. Spin-echo pulse sequence.

The lower graph illustrates the time-dependent variation in magnitude of longitudinal (M_Z, full line) and transversal (M_{XY}, broken line) magnetization vectors in two tissues, A and B, which for the sake of simplicity have the same proton density and the same T_1 but differ in T_2. Following the initial 90° pulse, the difference in T_2 becomes expressed and reaches its maximum ΔM_{XY} after time TE/2. The signals at this time are very weak, however. The 180° pulse "refocussess" the dephasing protons, and the difference in T_2 now becomes expressed at a much higher signal intensity, labelled ΔM_{XY}"echo". Another virtue of the echo signal is that it is not influenced by local (and static) field inhomogeneities.

4) *The spin-echo pulse sequence* (fig. 33).

This sequence is composed of a series of 90° pulses each followed at time TE/2 by a 180° pulse. The time TE/2 is so denoted because it is half the time TE till sampling of the radiosignal, called the "echo". The strategy in this pulse sequence is to tilt the longitudinal magnetization vector by 90° into the transversal plane. Initially, following this pulse the protons will precess in phase, but soon begin to lose coherence because some protons precess faster than others, observed as the decaying radiosignal (FID). The 180°

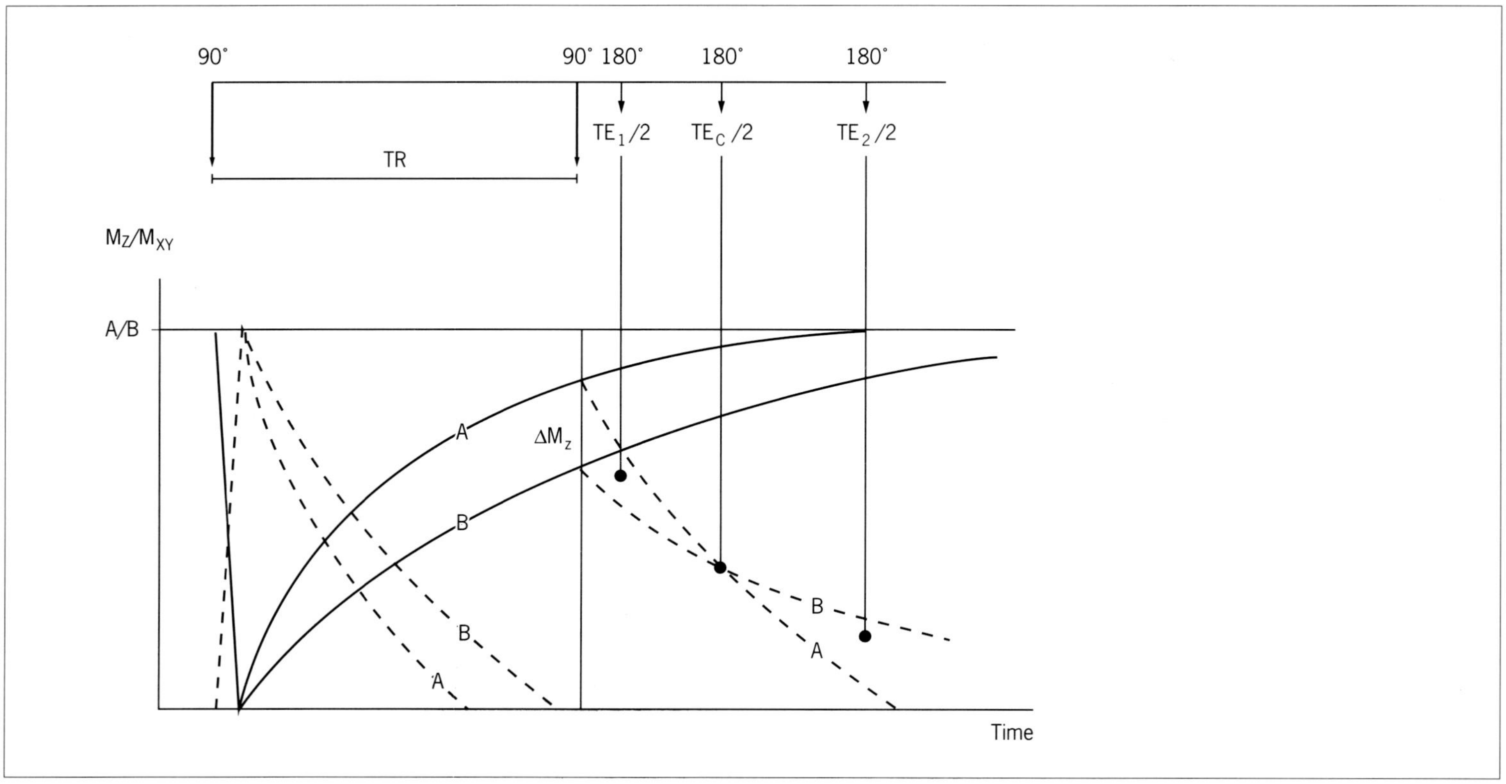

Fig. 34. Graph to illustrate how the proper choice of TR and TE can be used to construct T_1-weighted and T_2-weighted images by a spin-echo sequence.

The two tissues, A and B, have the same proton density but differ in T_1 as well as T_2 as shown by the time course of recovery of longitudinal (M_Z, full lines) and decay of transversal (M_{XY}, broken lines) magnetization, following a 90° pulse. At time TR when the longitudinal magnetization of the tissues has not yet recovered (differ by ΔM_Z), another 90° pulse is applied. During the subsequent decay of transversal magnetization, a 180° pulse is applied at time TE/2, and the echo-signal is sampled at time TE (see fig. 33). If TE/2 is chosen to hit at the time $TE_1/2$ indicated, the echo-signals at time TE_1 from A and B will be proportional to their difference in T_1. If the 180° pulse is applied at time $TE_2/2$, the echo-signals at time TE_2 will be proportional to the difference in T_2 between the tissues. If the 180° pulse was applied at time $TE_c/2$, the echo-signals would be of equal magnitude from the two tissues.

pulse inverts the longitudinal vector and has the additional effect that the protons now precess "the other way round" relative to the direction of the main field. Those protons that precessed a little faster than others now keep pace with the slower ones; the protons are said to "refocus". This elicits a radiosignal, an "echo", that increases in amplitude until the point of maximum refocussing is reached and then levels off again. Depending on the choice of TR and TE, the "echo" radiosignals can be used to construct T_2- as well as T_1- and proton-weighted images, as explained in fig. 34.

Techniques based on ultrasound reflection

The production and nature of ultrasound

Ultrasound waves are *mechanical waves*, bound to propagate in matter. Their propagation through a material has its basis in coherent oscillatory movements of the constituent molecules, considered as particles, *longitudinal* to the direction of propagation of the sound wave front. The material is best viewed as being composed of small units of mass, *"sound particles"*, that need not have a uniform molecular composition, which they seldom do. The individual particles oscillate about an equilibrium position fixed in space, like balls elastically suspended between two springs. The number of oscillations undergone by the particles in one second is the *frequency* of the sound in Hertz (Hz).

The coherent particle oscillations spread through the material by mechanical transfer of energy from one particle to the next giving rise to alternating bands of compressions and rarefactions that propagate through the material with a *propagation velocity* which is constant and specific to the material. The distance between successive compressions (or rarefactions) is denoted the *wavelength* of the sound. Thus, the propagating sound waves are characterized by their frequency (ν), wavelength (λ) and propagation velocity (c) through the relation
$c = \nu \times \lambda$, as are other types of waves.

The frequencies utilized in diagnostic ultrasound imaging are in the 2 - 10 MHz(megahertz) range. The wave propagation velocity (the speed of sound) in soft tissues, blood and water varies by only a few percent around an average value of 1540 m $\times$ sec^{-1}, with corresponding wavelengths of about 0.75 mm at 2 MHz, decreasing to 0.15 mm at 10 MHz. The propagation velocity is much higher in dense bone (about 3500 m $\times$ sec^{-1}) and much lower in air (300 m sec^{-1}).

The property of a material that determines the velocity (c) with which sound waves are propagated is the *acoustic impedance* (Z), which is related to the mass density (ρ) and the modulus of elasticity/stiffness (E) through the relation:

$$Z = \sqrt{\rho \times E} = \rho \times c.$$

It is important to distinguish the propagating acoustic wave phenomenon from the coherent oscillatory motions of the individual particles in the material. The maximum velocity of the particles, as they pass their equilibrium positions, relates to the energy transported by the acoustic wave through the material. At the energy inputs applied in diagnostic ultrasound imaging, the maximum particle velocities in soft tissues are only 3-4 cm $\times$ sec^{-1} or less, and the excursion of the particles to either side of their equilibrium positions, denoted the *elongation*, is in the order of 2 nm (nanometers) or less, not to be confused with the wavelength (λ) of the sound.

The source of ultrasound for diagnostic imaging is the *piezoelectric ultrasound transducer* (fig. 35). The key component of this assembly is a disc of a special ceramic material made up of orderly aligned molecules that have the property of electrical dipoles. A thin layer of electrically conducting metal has been plated onto both sides of the disc, so that an electrical field can be set up across the disc, which is often called the *"crystal"*. In response to such a field the molecular dipoles realign and the disc consequently changes its thickness. When a high frequency alter-

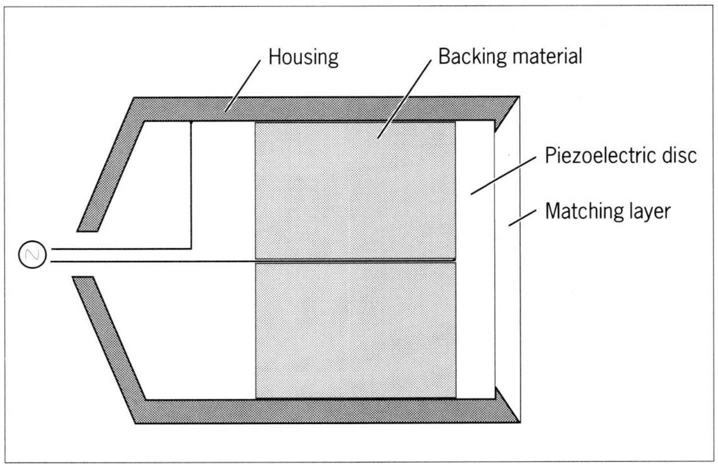

Fig. 35. The basic design of an ultrasound transducer.

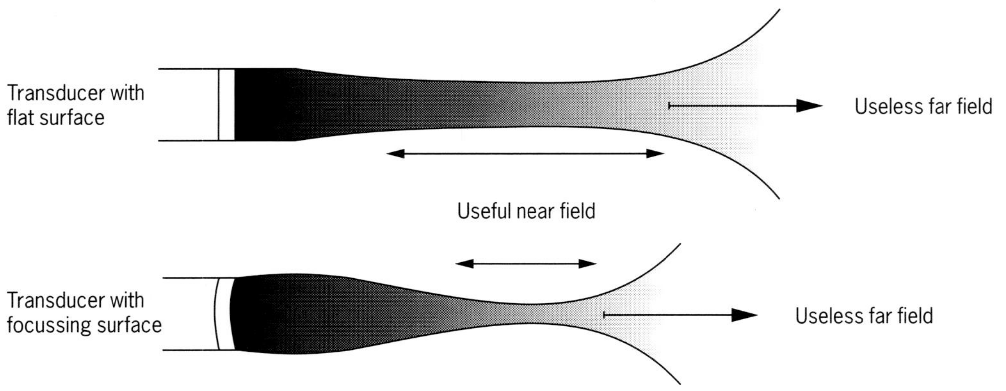

Fig. 36. The shape of ultrasound "beams" produced by an unfocussed and a focussed transducer.

nating voltage is applied, the crystal oscillates, and these oscillations become particularly forceful and uniform at a single frequency, *the resonance frequency*, which is determined by the thickness of the disc. When the voltage is turned off, the crystal continues to oscillate at the resonance frequency. It is the job of the "backing" material in the transducer to quickly damp this "after-ringing". It is essential that the ultrasound pulse lengths are extremely short (less than a μ-second) because the axial ("depth") resolution in the final image decreases with increasing spatial pulse length. Reduction of the wavelength also reduces the spatial pulse length and improves resolution. Typical frequencies of transducers for imaging are 2.5, 3.5, 5 and 7.5 MHz.

The transducer is covered with a thin layer ("the matching layer") of a material with an acoustic impedance in between that of the ceramic disc and that of skin. When the transducer is held against the skin the acoustic contact is further improved with a gel substance spread in advance over the skin.

The piezoelectric transducer also functions in the reverse direction as the receiver of ultrasound echoes. When the "listening" transducer is hit by incoming ultrasound waves, the disc is slightly deformed and electrical potentials are set up across the disc. These electrical signals are the ones used to construct the image.

The crystal disc of the transducer acts as a vibrating piston producing a "beam" of ultrasound waves (fig. 36). If the disc is plane this beam is almost rod-shaped out to a certain distance from the disc (the *"near field"* or Fresnel zone), and the beam intensity falls off steeply along the edge of the beam. This is the useful part of the beam. At a certain distance from the crystal the beam spreads out in a cone (the *"far field"* or Fraunhofer zone), which is useless for imaging. The physics governing the shape of the beam is rather complex, but depends primarily on the diameter of the crystal and the sound frequency. The piezoelectric disc may be concave shaped or an acoustic lens may be inserted to make the near field beam converge towards a "focus", but this reduces the length of the near field (fig. 36). The lateral resolution in the ultrasound image depends on the width of the beam. Focussing improves resolution, but reduces the thickness of tissue that can be imaged. A compromise is usually chosen, depending on the purpose.

It should be noted that when the transducer is used for imaging, the waves are sent off in very short "trains" followed by a pause where the transducer "listens" to echoes. The spatial length of a train is only 2 mm or less, but it follows the path of the "continuous" beam as a propagating cross section of it.

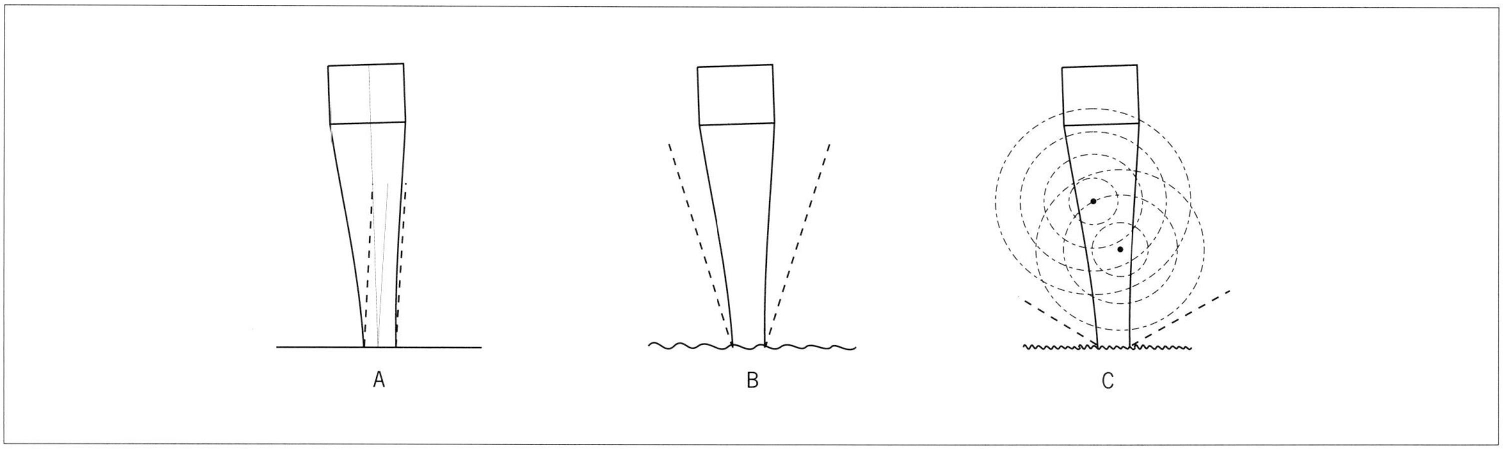

Fig. 37.

A) Specular reflection.
The angle of incidence equals the angle of reflection. If the angle deviates more than little from perpendicular, the reflected sound waves will miss the transducer.

B) Reflection from a ruffled surface.
The reflected waves spread over an angle so that only a smaller fraction reaches the transducer.

C) Diffuse scatter.
Small corpuscles or a finely rippled surface will spread the sound waves in all directions so that only a very small fraction returns to the transducer.

Interactions of ultrasound with tissues

At all frequencies and intensities of ultrasound applied in diagnostic imaging, three types of interactions are relevant: 1) Absorption, 2) Reflection, and 3) Diffuse scatter, all contributing to *attenuation* of the ultrasound beam intensity. Additionally, refraction and diffraction phenomena take place, but they are of minor significance. At beam intensities much higher and of longer duration than those used for imaging, various destructive effects occur in the tissues, not to be elaborated here.

Absorption

Absorption of ultrasound in tissues means transfer of energy from the coherent particle oscillations into disordered particle motions, which translates into *heat*, caused by internal friction between the constituent molecules of the tissue. Absorption is the dominant contributor to ultrasound beam attenuation. The intensity of the beam decays exponentially with distance and is therefore conveniently expressed in decibels (dB). Decibel (dB) is a measure of relative intensities of sound defined as: $dB = 10 \log \frac{I_1}{I_2}$. Additionally, the absorption increases linearly with the frequency in soft tissues. On average, the absorption amounts to 1 dB/cm/MHz. Thus, at a depth of 10 cm the intensity of a 5 MHz beam will have been reduced by 50 dB which translates into a 100,000-fold reduction. Considering that an echo from this depth will have to travel another 10 cm back to the transducer, the signal received will have decayed by about 100 dB relative to an echo-signal received from a structure superficially in the skin. A signal reduced by this amount is virtually useless. Therefore, for imaging of tissues in depth, e.g. in the abdomen, lower frequencies are used, but this is at the expense of axial resolution. Absorption in urine is significantly lower than in tissue. A filled bladder may therefore conveniently be utilized as a "window" to pelvic viscera.

Reflection

When the propagating ultrasound wave encounters

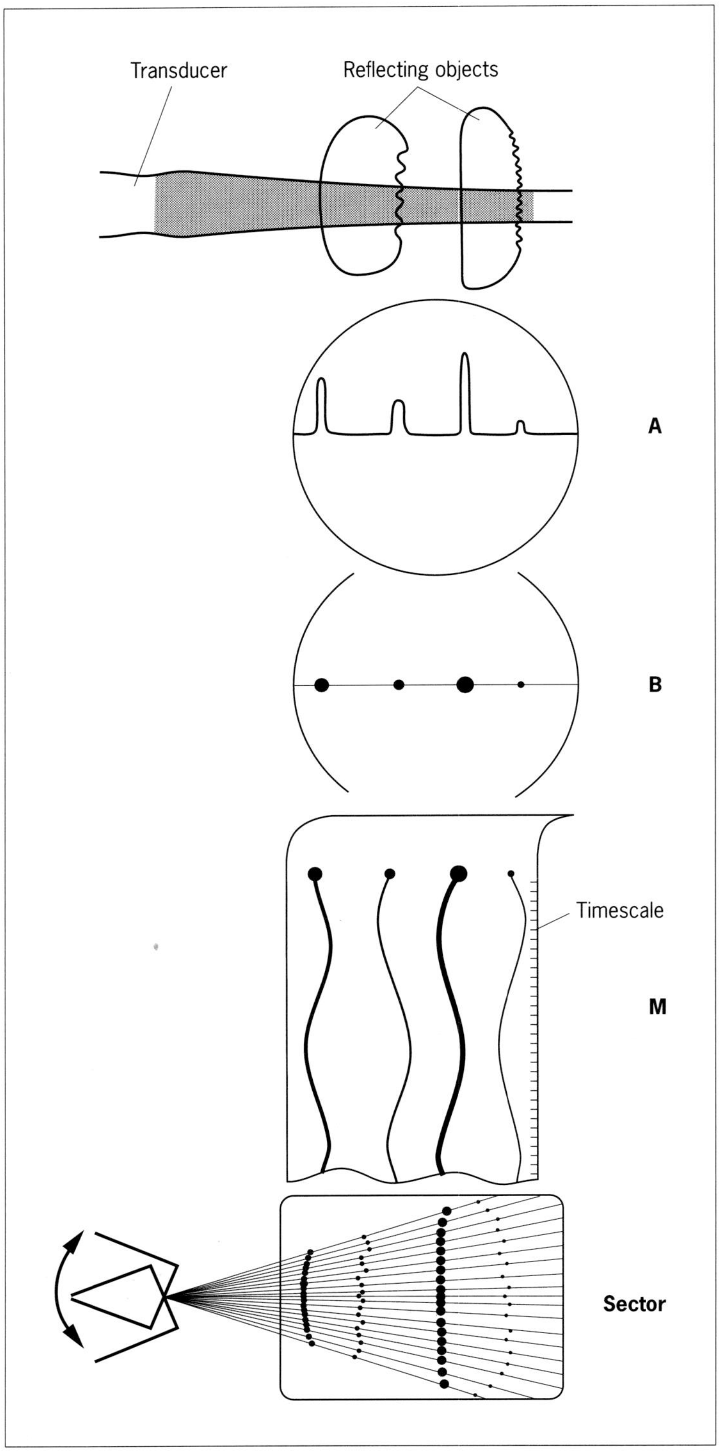

Fig. 38. Ultrasound imaging modes.

Ultrasound beam passing various reflecting surfaces.

A-mode display, "amplitude mode".
The echoes are displayed on an oscilloscope screen as deflections with amplitudes and positions corresponding to the reflecting surfaces.

B-mode display, "brightness mode".
The echoes are displayed as dots with brightness and positions corresponding to the reflecting surfaces.

M-mode display, "motion mode".
The echoes are recorded in the B-mode on a strip chart. If the reflecting surfaces move, their movements are recorded as waving curves. Periodicity and amplitude of movements are clearly visualized.

Tomographic imaging mode, "sector scanning".
The echoes are displayed in the B-mode on a videoscreen as the transducer scans back and forth through an angle (a "sector").

an interface between two tissues of different acoustic impedance, part of the wave energy is reflected as an echo. If the acoustic impedances of the two tissues are identical, no echo is produced. If the difference is very large, as betweeen soft tissues and bone or air, virtually all the wave energy is reflected, producing a strong echo and an *"acoustic shadow"* behind the bone or the airfilled organ. This effect makes it impossible to image the brain through the skull. (But the neonatal brain may be imaged through the fontanelles). It also makes it impossible to image lungs and gasfilled intestines.

It is primarily the reflections – echoes – from interfaces between tissues with small or moderate differences in acoustic impedance which are utilized for ultrasound imaging. If the interface is perfectly smooth and of sufficient size the wave is reflected as by a mirror, denoted *specular reflection* (fig. 37a). This implies that if the interface is at an angle to the beam, the echo may miss the transducer. Thus, very

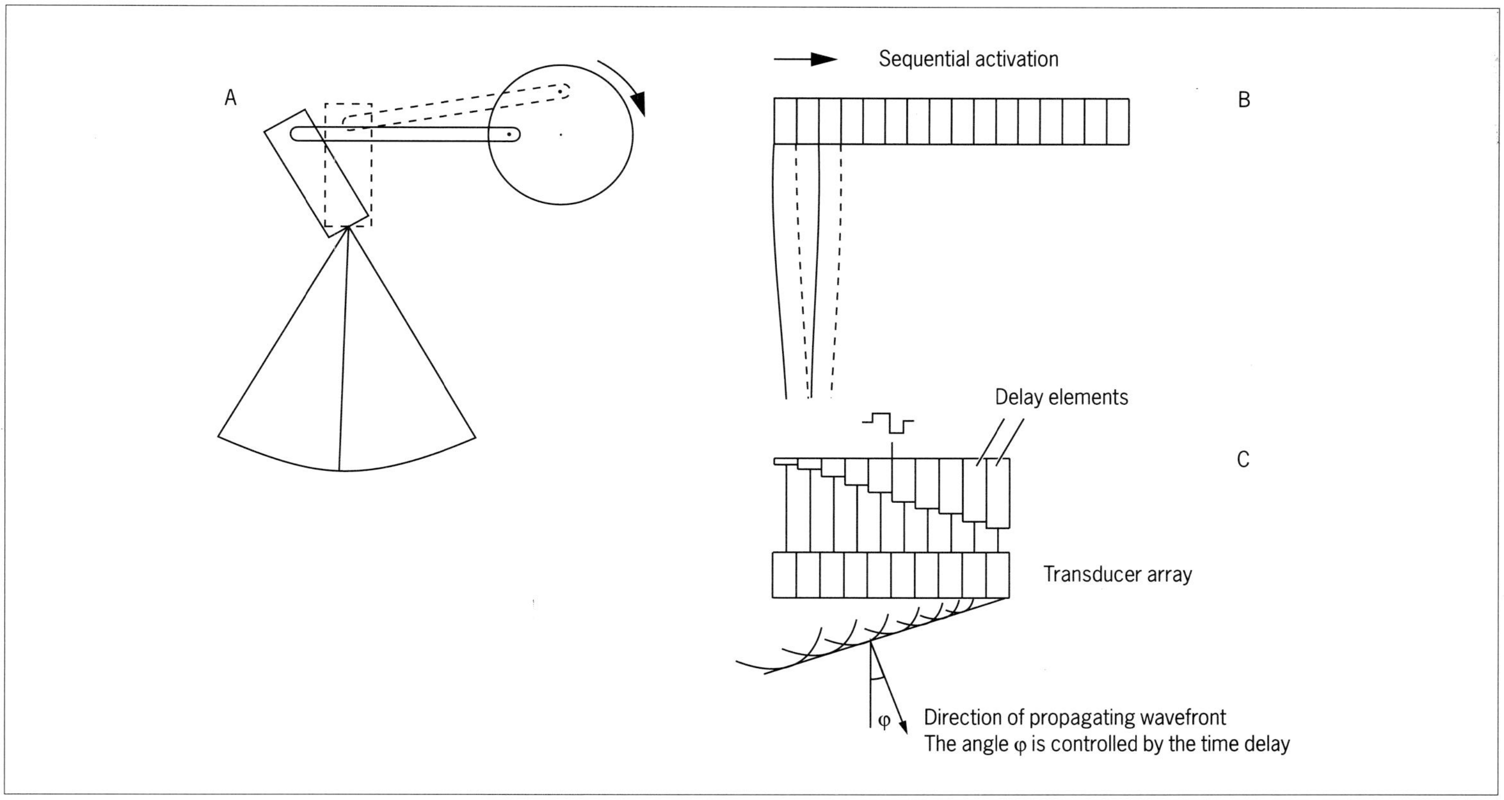

Fig. 39. Ultrasound scanning principles.

A) Simple mechanical device to produce sector scanning.
B) Linear transducer array.
C) Phased array transducer.

smooth surfaces, e.g. an umbilical cord, will be imaged only where parts of its surface are perpendicular to the beam. If, however, the surface is ruffled, the reflected wave takes various directions, but part of it may be captured by the receiving transducer (fig. 37b). This is why curved organ surfaces are usually imaged, albeit with decreasing contrast the more steeply the surface is angled relative to the beam.

Diffuse scatter

When the ultrasound waves encounter a finely rippled surface or corpuscles which are small relative to the wavelength, e.g. small blood vessels, and the acoustic impedance of the material differs from the surroundings, the corpuscles give rise to diffuse scatter in the form of spherical waves originating from the corpuscle (fig. 37c). Only a very small fraction of these waves reaches the receiving transducer, but they contribute to the finely speckled appearance of parenchymatous organs like the liver, spleen, and uterus as well as skeletal muscles.

Ultrasound imaging modes

Assuming a constant velocity of sound (1540 m × sec^{-1}) through soft tissues – and this is almost true – the time taken from emission of a 1 μsec pulse to receipt of an echo can be directly tranlated into twice the distance to (and from) the reflecting structure. This is exactly analogous to what a fisherman does when he estimates the depth of a shoal of herring with his sonar. Time to echo from 10 cm depth will be some 130 μsec, so the time resolution needs to be accurate.

The echoes received from a stationary transducer may be displayed on an oscilloscope trace as deflections proportional to the magnitude of the echoes. This is denoted amplitude – or *"A-mode" imaging* (fig. 38). Instead of deflections, the intensity of the oscilloscope beam may be modulated along the trace to produce dots of different brightness along the trace. This is denoted brightness – or *"B-mode" imaging* (fig. 38). If the distance to the reflecting ob-

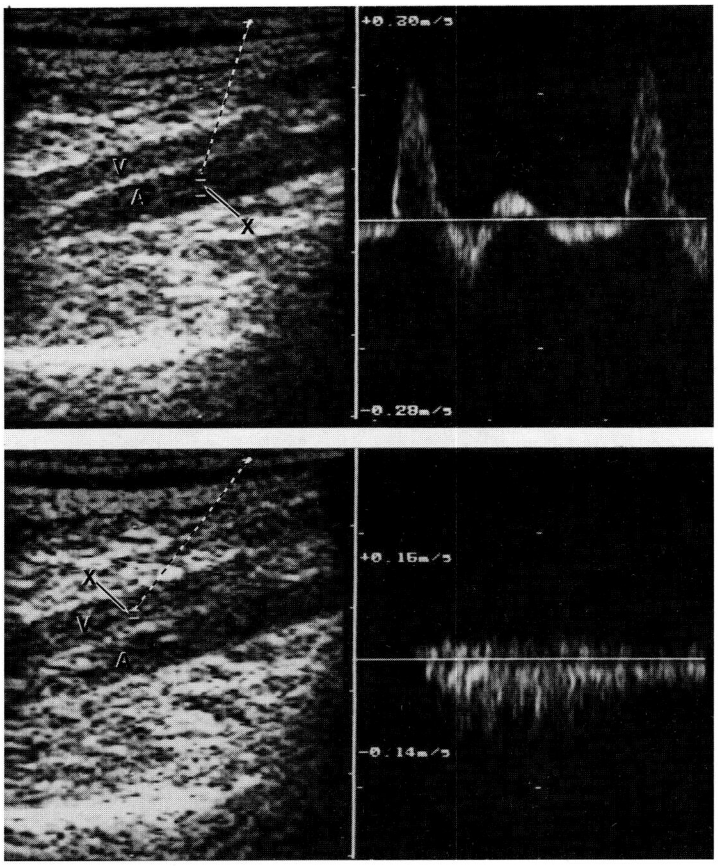

Fig. 40. Ultrasound duplex scanning of the popliteal artery (upper frame) and vein (lower frame).

The curves to the right in the images display the flow pattern recorded from measurement of Doppler shifts at the recording site (X) in the artery (A) and in the vein (V), selected on the tomographic scanning image to the left. The stippled lines indicate the directions along which Doppler shifts have been measured.

jects changes, then the dots will move back and forth along the oscilloscope trace. So, when the trace is recorded on a strip chart recorder, curves will be drawn that show the motion of the reflectors. This is denoted motion – or *"M-mode" imaging*, which is very much in use in cardiology for the study of, e.g., ventricular wall and valve motions (fig. 38).

None of the above techniques produces real images. If, however, the transducer beam is set to scan back and forth through an angle, a "sector", at a constant angular speed, sufficient to scan the sector some 20 times per second, and the echoes are displayed in B-mode along a line that scans synchronously over a sector of a videomonitor screen, then a true, real time, tomographic image is obtained from the ultrasound echoes (fig. 38).

The angular scanning motion is commonly produced with a mechanical construct that involves moving parts (fig. 39A). Scanning may also be performed by sequential activation of a long linear array of stationary transducers to yield a rectangular scan field (fig. 39B). It is possible also from a linear array of stationary transducers to produce a beam that sweeps an angular sector, as with a mechanical scanner. This is obtained by a very accurately timed sequence of activation, utilizing Fresnel interference between the waves from neighboring transducers (fig. 39C). Such a construct is called a *"phased array transducer"*.

Because ultrasound wave energy is absorbed exponentially as the wave travels through the tissues, the echoes from deeply located structures will be much weaker than echoes from identical but more superficially located structures. To obtain an equally weighted image, all ultrasound scanners are equipped with a facility called *"time-gain-control"* (TGC), which is an amplifier that enhances the echo-signals relative to their timing and inverse to the exponential decay which is due to absorption. Besides this, most scanners are equipped with additional controls to enhance or to suppress signals arriving according to a selected timing, i.e. from selected depths.

The Doppler effect and Doppler imaging

Sound reflected from an object moving away from the transducer will return to the transducer with increased wavelength (decreased frequency), and conversly with an increased frequency if the object is moving towards the transducer. Such shifts in frequency are called *Doppler shifts*, and they are extensively utilized for the measurement of flow rates in vessels, where the blood corpuscles constitute the reflectors in the flowing blood. Precise quantitation of flow rate requires that the angle between the ultrasound beam and the direction of flow is known.

If the angle is 90° no Doppler shift will be observed. It is possible, in analogy to real-time ultrasound scan-imaging, to produce an image constructed from echoes with positive and/or with negative Doppler shifts and to superimpose these images according to a color coding, e.g. blue and red, on an ordinary and simultaneously recorded grey-tone image. This composite image is denoted a *"color-flow Doppler" image*, and it is of enormous value in cardiovascular diagnosis. Measurement of Doppler shifts are used in *"duplex" scanning* where the site of measurement of Doppler shift can be selected on a simultaneously recorded real-time scan-image (fig. 40).

Techniques based on radioisotope emissions

Scintigraphy

Diagnostic scintigraphic imaging involves the following basic elements: a suitable *radioisotope* given in an appropriate chemical and pharmaceutical formulation that assigns it a specific target within the body, and a recording system that can map the distribution of the radioisotope and which, for most purposes involves the *gamma camera*.

Suitable radioisotopes

Radioisotopes used for routine diagnostic imaging are all emitters of γ-photons with energies in the 80 - 200 keV range, i.e. equivalent to usual diagnostic X-ray photon energies (fig. 1). The designations γ-rays and X-rays refer only to the origin of the photons: X-rays derive from processes confined to the electron shells of atoms, while γ-rays arise from processes in the nuclei of certain unstable isotopes.

The photons of γ-radiation have discrete energies specific to the nuclear reactions they stem from, i.e. the radiation is monochromatic, while photons from an X-ray tube are polychromatic in a continuous spectrum. The monochromaticity of γ-emissions is important because it can be utilized to distinguish the origin of γ-photons by analysis of their energies.

Photons of energies in the above-mentioned range penetrate tissues very well and may easily escape the body and be recorded by an external detector.

Radioisotopes that emit α– and β^--radiation are generally useless for diagnostic imaging because these types of radiation are effectively absorbed in the tissues, and also because their radiation elicits many secondary ionizations, i.e., biological damage. Some radioisotopes which emit favorable γ-radiation must be rejected for diagnostic purposes because their decay products are harmful β^--emitters. Positron (β^+)-emitters have special applications (PET) to be briefly touched upon at the end of this chapter.

Clearly, the radiation dose received by the patient must be kept to a minimum. For this reason, the *half-life* (T½) of the radioisotope should be so short that the needless radiation received after the examination soon levels off. A T½ of half to twice the time needed for performing the clinical examination may be considered appropriate. In some applications, the elimination becomes further accelerated by excretion via the kidneys or lungs. In general, the radiation received by the patient during scintigraphic diagnostic imaging is about equal to that of X-ray examinations.

Further requirements of an ideal radioisotope are that it should be pharmacologically atoxic in the doses required, and that it should have a chemistry favorable for binding to pharmaceuticals, allowing its targeting to specific tissues and organs in the body. Finally, it should be readily available at a reasonable cost. Radioisotopes that meet these requirements and which are extensively used in diagnostic practice include: iodine ^{123}J (T½ ~ 13 hours), thallium ^{201}Tl (T½ ~ 3 days), Xenon ^{133}Xe (T½ ~ 5 days) and technetium ^{99m}Tc (T½ ~ 6 hours). Several others are available and are used alternatively or for special purposes.

Pharmaceutical formulations of radioisotopes

For most purposes, radioisotopes are used in special chemical formulations or attached as a label to a pharmaceutical in order to target the isotope to a special tissue, a metabolic pathway or a physiological/pathophysiological phenomenon.

^{123}J is used for thyroid scintigraphy, given as iodide. Because iodine is easy to couple covalently to various molecules, e.g. albumin, it is frequently used as a radiolabel. It has, together with ^{131}J, had a long-standing application in *renography*, coupled to hippuran which has a high renal clearance rate and is well suited for evaluation of renal function. Recording and quantitation of the time course of renal excretion is an important part of the renographic examination, besides the basic scintigraphic imaging.

^{201}Tl, given as chloride, has a special application for evaluation of myocardial ischemia.

^{133}Xe is used, inhaled as a gas, for examinations of lung ventilation.

^{99m}Tc takes up a dominant position in diagnostic imaging because the half-life of this isotope (6 hours) is just right, and the emitted γ-photon has an energy (140 keV) that penetrates tissues very well and is favorable for detection with the gamma camera. The decay product, ^{99}Tc, decays further with ß-emission to a stable ruthenium isotope, but the half-life of this transition is so long (2×10^5 years) that it may be considered biologically insignificant. Finally, ^{99m}Tc is readily available from a handy generator (a molybdenum $^{99}/_{42}$Mo-"cow", which can be milked every day) in the form of pertechnetate (TcO_4^-) which has a chemistry that is favorable for a number of coupling reactions. Thus, ^{99m}Tc may be used coupled to phosphate compounds, e.g. as diphosphonate, for bone scintigraphy; coupled to HIDA for biliary scintigraphy; coupled to albumin for scintigraphic perfusion studies, e.g. lung perfusion; coupled to colloids for labelling of macrophages in liver, spleen and bone marrow; and coupled to glucoheptonate for brain scintigraphy, to mention a few applications. ^{99m}Tc-pertechnetate is suitable also for thyroid scintigraphy, because it concentrates in the thyroid analogous to perchlorate.

The gamma camera

The basic design of a typical gamma camera, as used for diagnostic scintigraphic imaging, is shown in fig. 41. The γ-photon detector is a large single crystal of sodium iodide, doped with thallium. Typical dimensions are 40 cm diameter and 5-10 mm thickness. A *"collimator"* consisting of a lead plate with numerous closely spaced parallel holes is mounted in front of the crystal. This collimator absorbs γ-photons which do not travel parallel – or near parallel – with the axis of the holes. Thus, the collimator defines, for each point in the crystal, a direction of incident γ-photons.

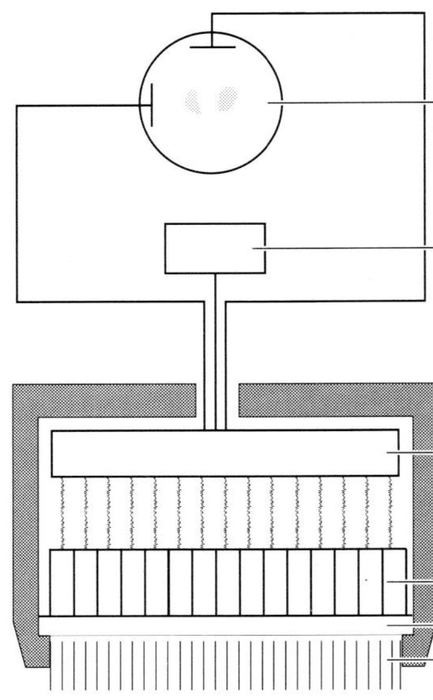

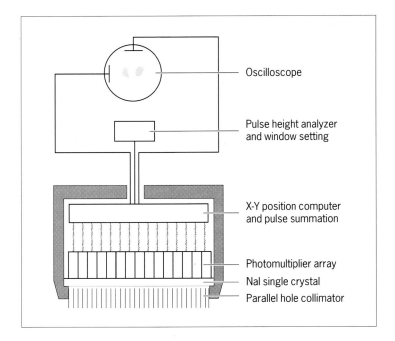

Fig. 41. The basic design of a gamma camera with parallel hole collimator.

When hit by γ-photons in the relevant energy range, the crystal emits (scintillates) quanta of blue light in a number proportional to the energy of the incident γ-photon. The evoked light emission is picked up by a hexagonal array of up to a hundred photomultipliers mounted in good optical contact with the back of the crystal. The photomultiplier signals are fed into a computer facility which performs two basic calculations. Firstly, the position (X-Y coordinates) of the scintillation event is calculated by comparing the signal intensities to find the position of the maximum. Secondly, the "pulse height" is calculated as the sum of all the signals belonging to a single scintillation event. The sum is proportional to the energy of the incident γ-photon, which in turn is specific to the radioisotope. If the pulse height is lower than "expected" it is likely to derive from a γ-photon that was scattered, losing energy and direction *en route* to the camera. An adjustable "*window*" is set to reject scintillations with less than, say, 90% of the expected maximum pulse height. The recorded and accepted scintillations are displayed according to their X-Y coordinates on an oscilloscope screen, from where it may be photographically recorded. A modern camera has the capacity to process some 50,000 scintillations per second. Reasonable image quality requires sampling of some 10^6 scintillations.

The resulting scintigram is a two-dimensional projection of the spatial distribution of the isotope within the body. Two geometric factors are of special importance when the image is evaluated. Firstly, the longer the distance between the patient and the camera the poorer will be the lateral resolution because the collimator discriminates only the angles of incoming photons. Secondly, because the intensity of γ-radiation in a given direction decreases with the square of the distance from the source, the number of photons reaching the detector from a deeply located source will be smaller than if the same source was more superficially located. This difference is further augmented by the fact that a γ-photon from a deep source is more likely to be absorbed on its way, or to be scattered and lose direction and energy to such an extent as to be rejected by the collimator or the pulse height analyzer. Therefore, a scintigram will image structures close to the body surface and close to the detector with markedly better contrast and resolution than deep and remote structures. It is therefore common practice in many examinations to collect images both from the back and the front of the patient.

Single photon emission computed tomography (SPECT) and positron emission tomography (PET)

It is possible to obtain a tomographic image with ordinary γ-emitting isotopes if the gamma camera is rotated around the patient through 180° or 360° in steps of a few degrees, e.g. 6°, and data are collected at each position. By a computational procedure analogous to CT-imaging, a tomographic image of the spatial distribution of the isotope is produced. The data acquisition time is quite long, and the resolution is often rather low.

The radiation produced by *positron emitting isotopes* is remarkable. The positron emitted from the nucleus will, after traversing a very short path, be annihilated by fusion with a random electron, and the joint mass of the positron and the electron will thereby be converted into pure energy in the form of two photons, each of very high energy (0.511 MeV), that leave the site of annihilation in exactly opposite (180°) directions.

This phenomenon is utilized for tomographic imaging (PET). The PET-scanner consists of a ring of detectors, the plane of the ring defining the tomographic section. The signals received by the detectors are analyzed for coincidence, because coincidence derives from the capture of both of the high-energy photons from an annihilation event which has taken place along the straight line joining the two detectors. When a sufficient number of annihilation events have been recorded in this way, it is a relatively simple computational procedure to derive a tomographic image of the isotope distribution. PET has great potential, but the method is seriously hampered by the fact that the relevant positron emitting isotopes are very shortlived ($T\frac{1}{2}$ in the order of a few minutes). Thus far, the technique has almost exclusively been used as a research tool.

Principles of nomenclature and positioning

The vocabulary used in diagnostic imaging to indicate planes, directions, and locations is largely identical to the established anatomical nomenclature which refers to the "anatomical standard position", i.e., standing erect, arms by the sides and palms facing forwards. By tradition, in diagnostic imaging, some anatomical terms are replaced by synonymous "radiology terms", and the anatomical vocabulary has been supplemented.

Anatomical *planes* are commonly designated *sections*, with reference to tomographic imaging.

The *median section* (fig. 42A) divides the body in two halves which are symmetric on the body surface.

A *sagittal section* denotes any section parallel to the median section. The median section is sometimes denoted the mid-sagittal section.

A *paramedian section* is a sagittal section close to the median section.

A *frontal section* (fig. 42B) denotes any vertical section perpendicular to the median section. In diagnostic imaging, frontal sections are commonly denoted *coronal sections*, because they are about parallel to the plane of the coronal suture.

A *transversal section* (fig. 42C) is perpendicular to both the coronal and the sagittal sections. It is sometimes denoted a *horizontal section*, but the established term in radiology is an *axial section*, so denoted because it is the image that would be produced if a transversal slice of the body was conventionally imaged by an X-ray beam oriented along the axis of the body.

In axial tomographic imaging of the head, the standard tomographic planes are parallel to the *orbito-meatal plane*, which is defined by the lateral canthus of the eye and the center of the external auditory meatus; both easy to identify. This plane is virtually identical to the *Frankfurter plane* ("German horizontal"), defined by the lower margin of the orbit and the upper edge of the external auditory meatus.

In conventional X-ray imaging, the inherent magnification of an object depends on its location in the beam path between the X-ray tube focal spot and

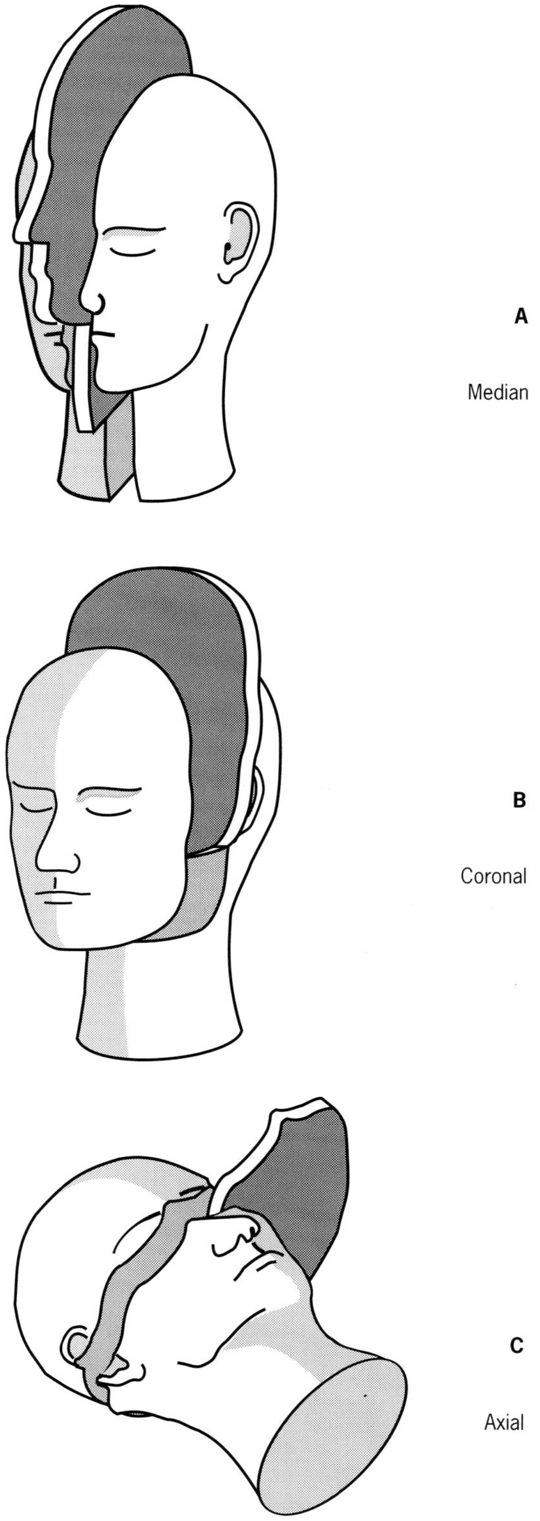

Fig. 42. Tomographic planes.

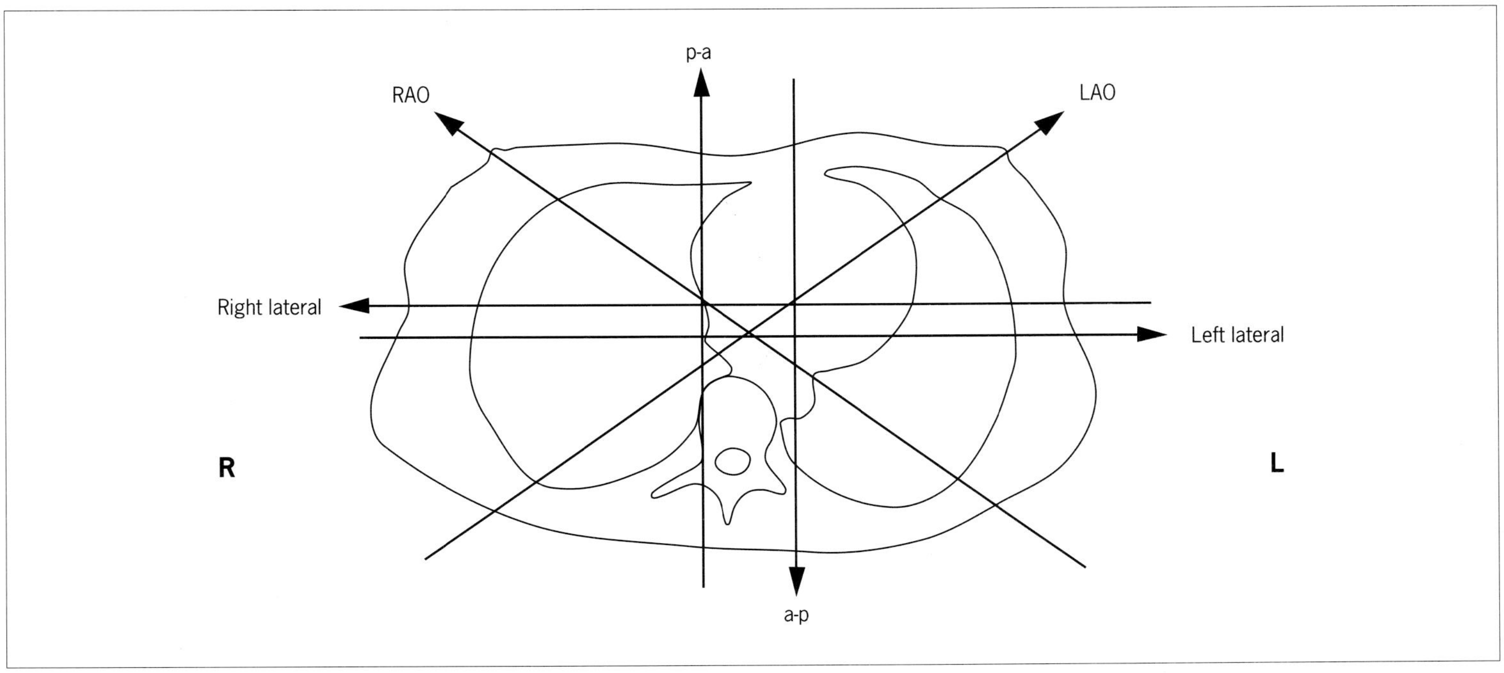

Fig. 43. Denotations of directions in conventional X-ray imaging.

the film. Thus, an X-ray of the cranium taken with the beam entering the stern to expose a film placed behind the occiput will show the frontal sinuses at higher magnification than with the reverse beam direction. It is therefore common practice to indicate the direction of the beam path using the following terms (conf. fig. 43):

An antero-posterior (a-p) X-ray is taken with a beam entering the anterior (ventral) side of the body to expose a film placed on the posterior (dorsal) side. A *postero-anterior (p-a) X-ray* is the opposite of an a-p X-ray.

A left lateral X-ray is taken with a beam entering the right lateral side to expose a film placed to the left of the body. A *right lateral X-ray* is the opposite.

An *axial X-ray* is taken with a beam passing along the axis of the body (cranially or caudally) to expose a film located in a transversal plane.

A *tilted X-ray* is taken with a beam which is angled relative to a transversal plane.

An *oblique X-ray* is taken with a beam which is angled relative to a sagittal plane.

A *right anterior oblique (RAO) X-ray* is taken with the film placed on the right anterior side of the body, to be exposed by a beam entering the left dorsal side of the body.

A *left anterior oblique (LAO) X-ray* is analogous to the above with left and right interchanged.

An X-ray of the hand, wrist and lower arm is often taken with a beam entering the dorsum of the hand to expose a film below the volar face of the hand, and is denoted a *dorso-volar X-ray*. An analogous X-ray of the foot is denoted a *dorso-plantar X-ray*.

Conventions of image presentation used in the atlas part of this book:

Conventional X-rays

A-p and p-a X-rays are shown as if the patient was facing the observer.

Lateral X-rays are shown with the left side of the patient towards the observer.

Supine and prone X-rays are shown with the patient's head towards the left or upwards.

Tomographic sections

Axial sections are seen from below. This is international convention.

Coronal sections are seen from the patient's front.

Sagittal sections are seen from the patient's left.

Upper Limb

Shoulder and upper arm

Elbow

Lower arm

Wrist

Hand

Arteries and veins

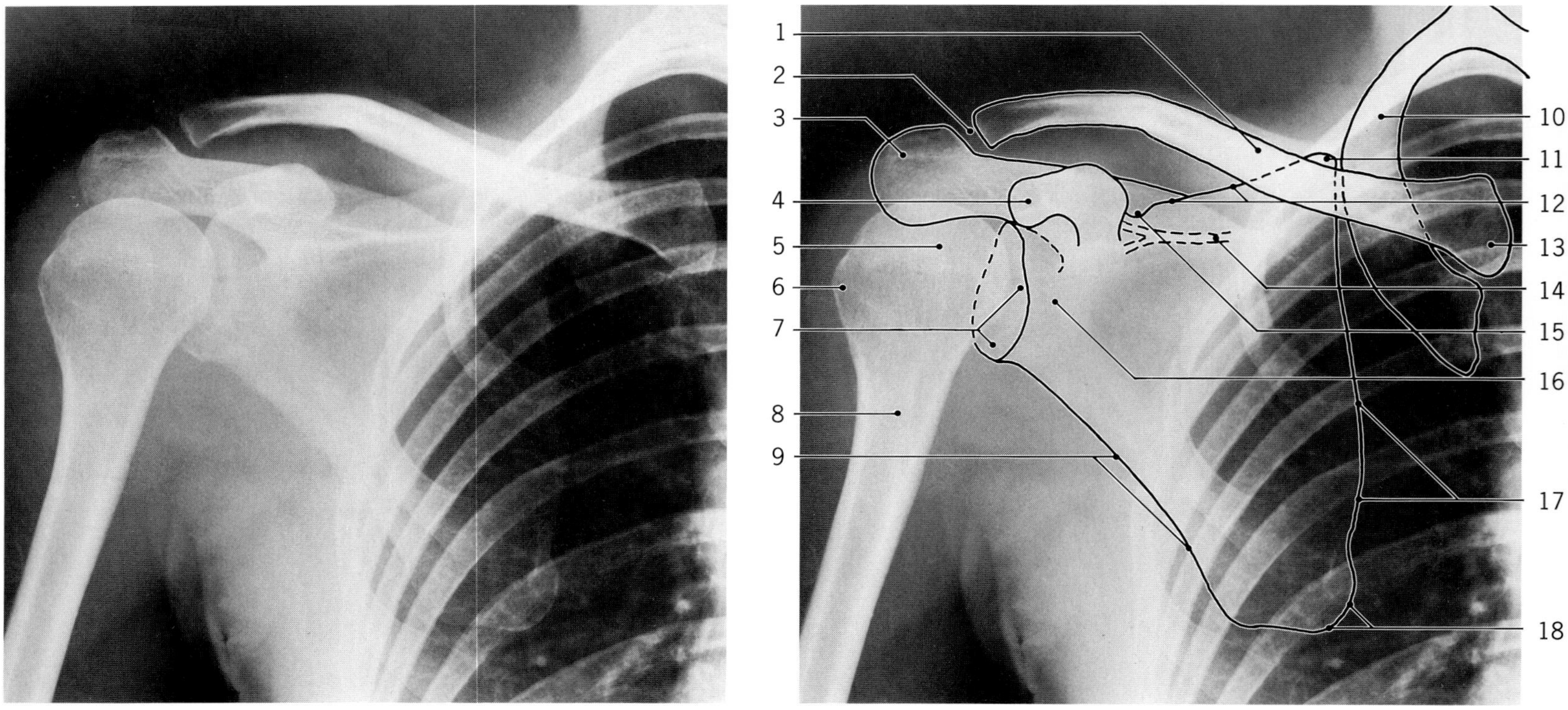

Shoulder, a-p X-ray

1: Clavicle
2: Acromioclavicular joint
3: Acromion
4: Coracoid process
5: Humeral head
6: Greater tubercle
7: Glenoid cavity
8: Surgical neck of humerus
9: Lateral border of scapula
10: First rib
11: Superior angle of scapula
12: Superior border of scapula
13: Sternal end of clavicle
14: Spine of scapula
15: Scapular notch
16: Neck of scapula
17: Medial border of scapula
18: Inferior angle of scapula

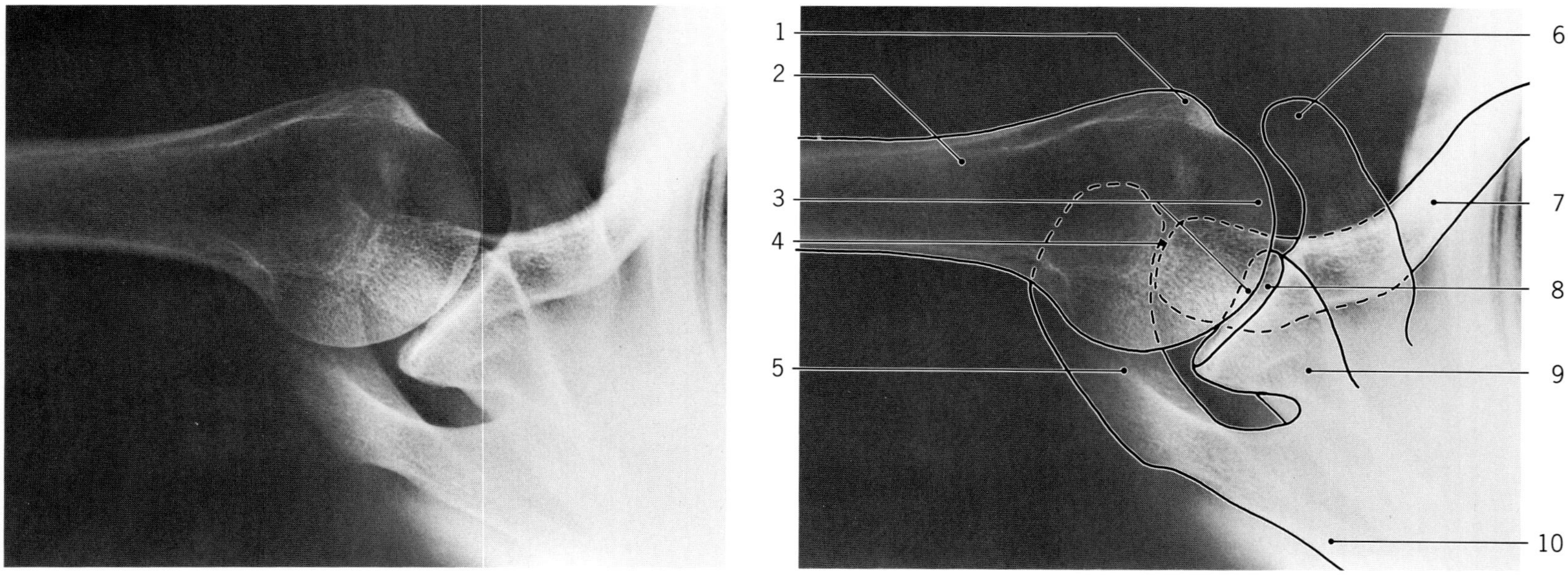

Shoulder, axial X-ray

1: Greater tubercle
2: Surgical neck of humerus
3: Humeral head
4: Acromioclavicular joint
5: Acromion
6: Coracoid process
7: Clavicle
8: Glenoid cavity
9: Neck of scapula
10: Spine of scapula

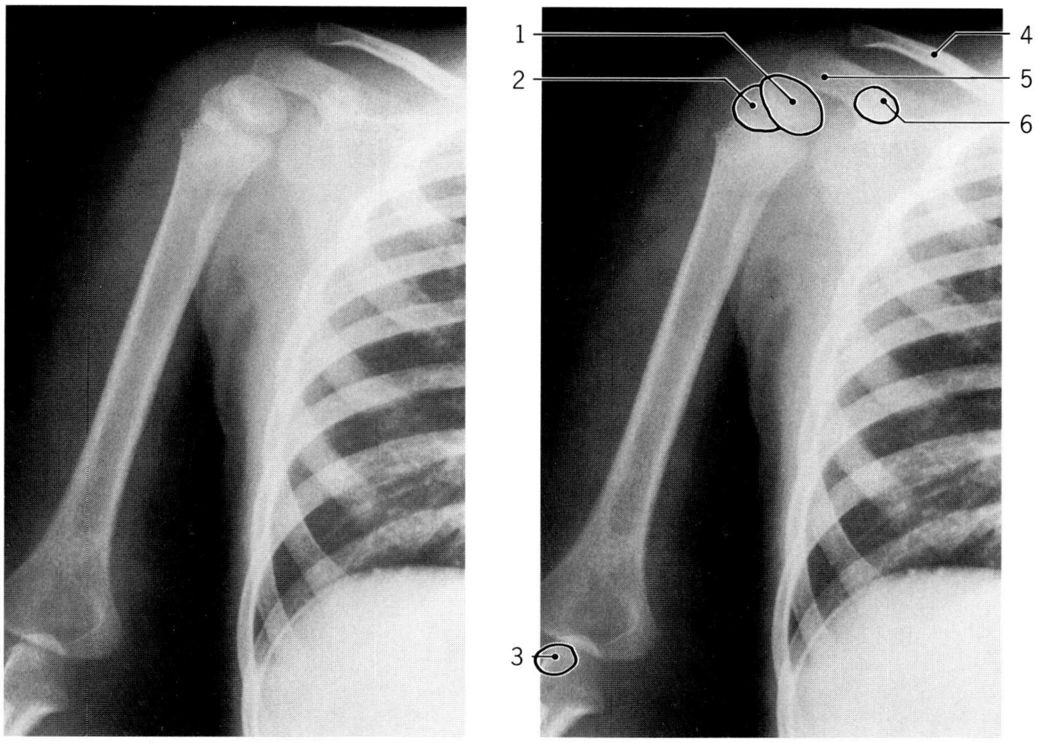

Shoulder, a-p X-ray, child 5 years

1: Humeral head (ossification center)
2: Greater tubercle (ossification center)
3: Capitulum (ossification center)
4: Clavicle
5: Acromion
6: Coracoid process (ossification center)

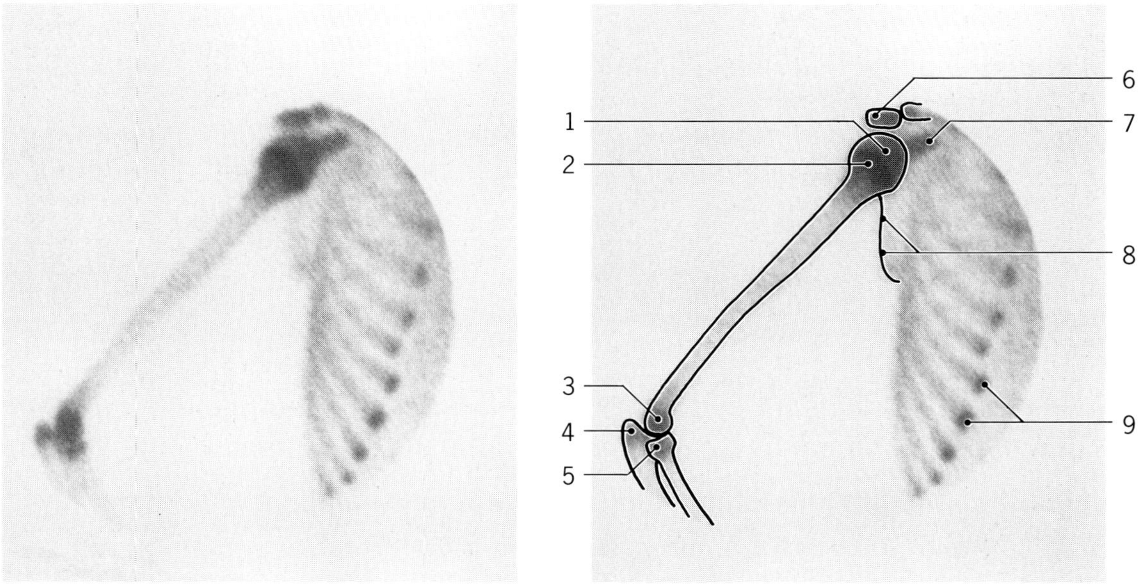

Shoulder and upper arm, ^{99m}Tc-MDP, scintigraphy, child 12 years

1: Humeral head
2: Growth plate of proximal epiphysis of humerus
3: Trochlea and capitulum
4: Olecranon
5: Head of radius
6: Acromion
7: Coracoid process
8: Lateral margin of scapula
9: Osteochondral transition of ribs

Scout view

1: Coracoid process
2: Right humeral head, inward rotated
3: Sternal end of clavicle
4: Left humeral head, outward rotated
5: Plane of section

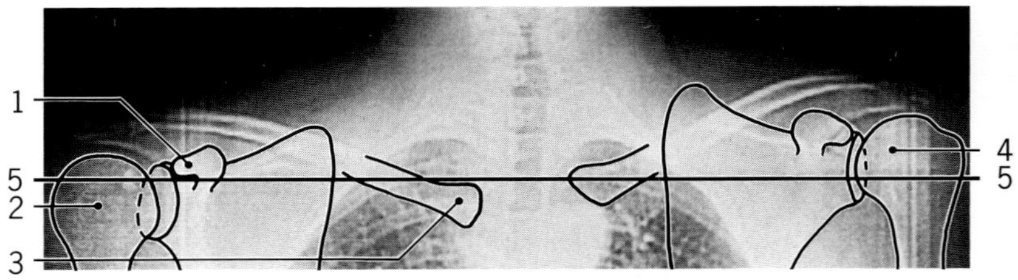

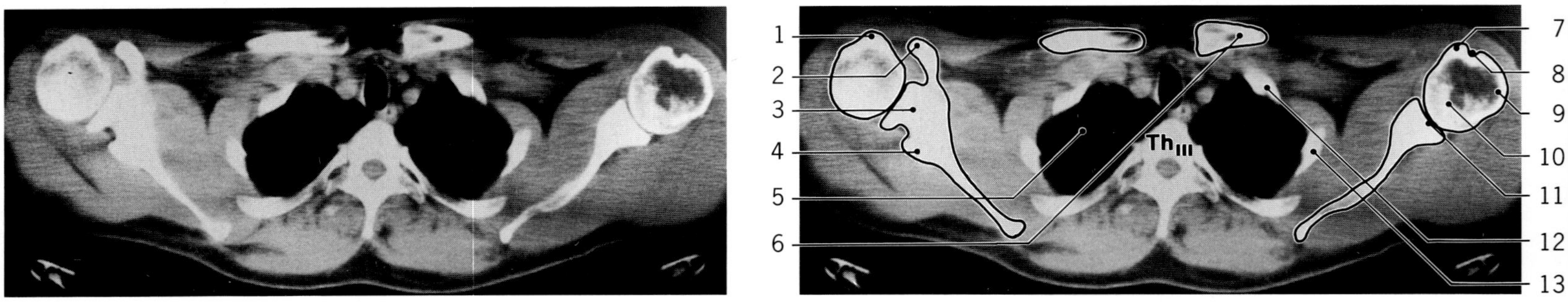

Shoulder, axial CT

1: Greater tubercle
2: Coracoid process
3: Neck of scapula
4: Spine of scapula
5: Apex of lung
6: Sternal end of clavicle
7: Minor tubercle
8: Intertubercular groove
9: Greater tubercle
10: Humeral head
11: Glenoid cavity
12: First rib
13: Second rib

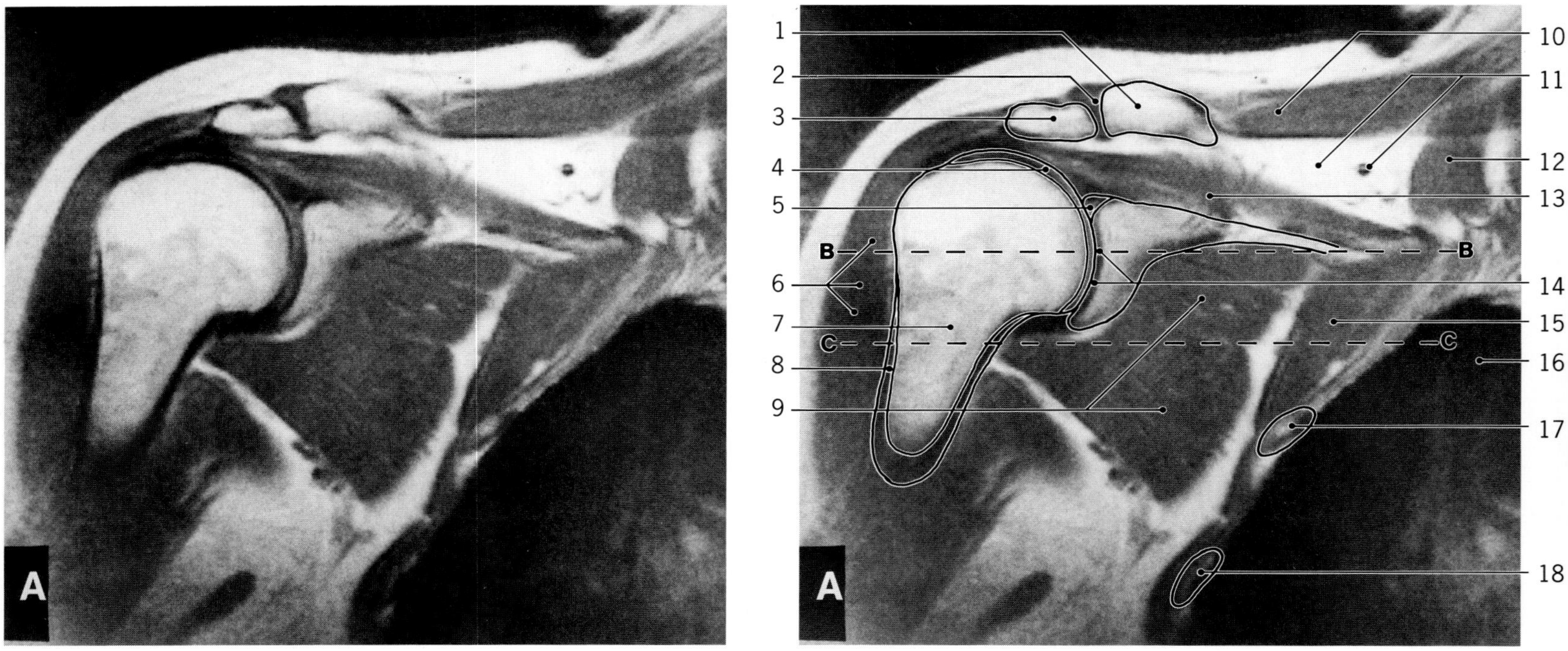

Shoulder, coronal MR

Plane of sectioning indicated on section B

1: Acromial end of clavicle
2: Acromioclavicular joint with discus
3: Acromion
4: Articular cartilage of humeral head
5: Labrum glenoidale
6: Deltoideus
7: Red and yellow bone marrow
8: Compact bone of humeral shaft
9: Subscapularis
10: Trapezius
11: Apex of axilla with fat and vessels
12: Levator scapulae
13: Supraspinatus
14: Glenoid cavity
15: Scalenus medius
16: Apex of lung
17: First rib
18: Second rib
B-B and C-C: Plane of sections on following page

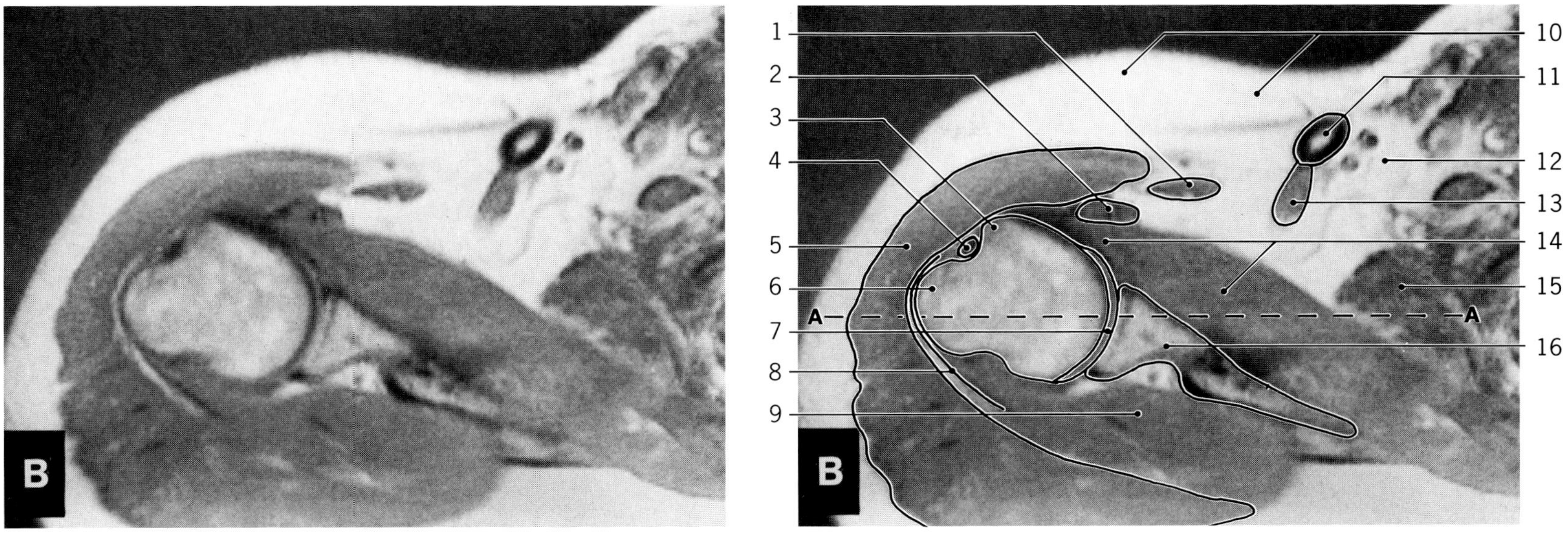

Shoulder, axial MR

Plane of sectioning indicated on section A

1: Pectoralis minor
2: Coracobrachialis, and biceps, short head
3: Minor tubercle
4: Biceps, long head
5: Deltoideus
6: Greater tubercle
7: Articular cartilage
8: Subdeltoid bursa
9: Infraspinatus
10: Subcutaneous fat
11: Clavicle
12: Apex of axilla with fat, vessels and nerves
13: Subclavius
14: Subscapularis
15: Scalenus medius
16: Neck of scapula
A-A: Plane of section (A) on previous page

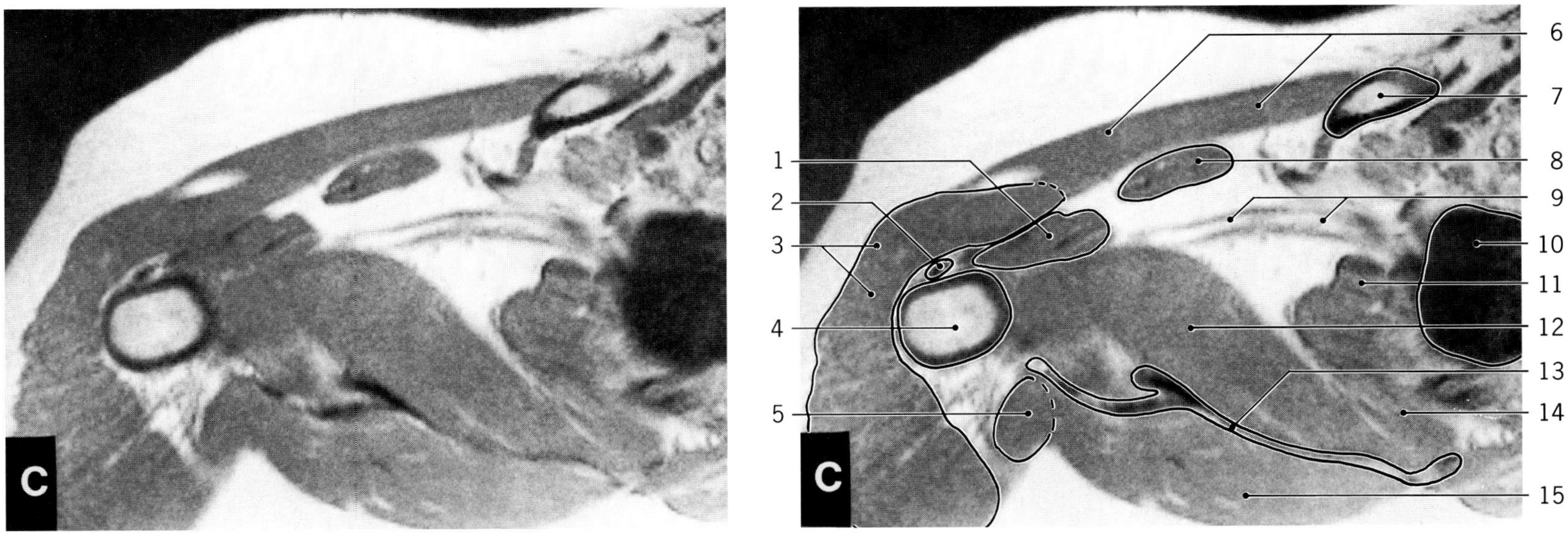

Shoulder, axial MR

Plane of sectioning indicated on section A

1: Coracobrachialis, and short head of biceps
2: Biceps, long head
3: Deltoideus
4: Surgical neck of humerus
5: Triceps, long head
6: Pectoralis major
7: Clavicle
8: Pectoralis minor
9: Axillary artery and brachial plexus
10: Apex of lung
11: Scalenus medius
12: Subscapularis
13: Scapula
14: Serratus anterior
15: Infraspinatus

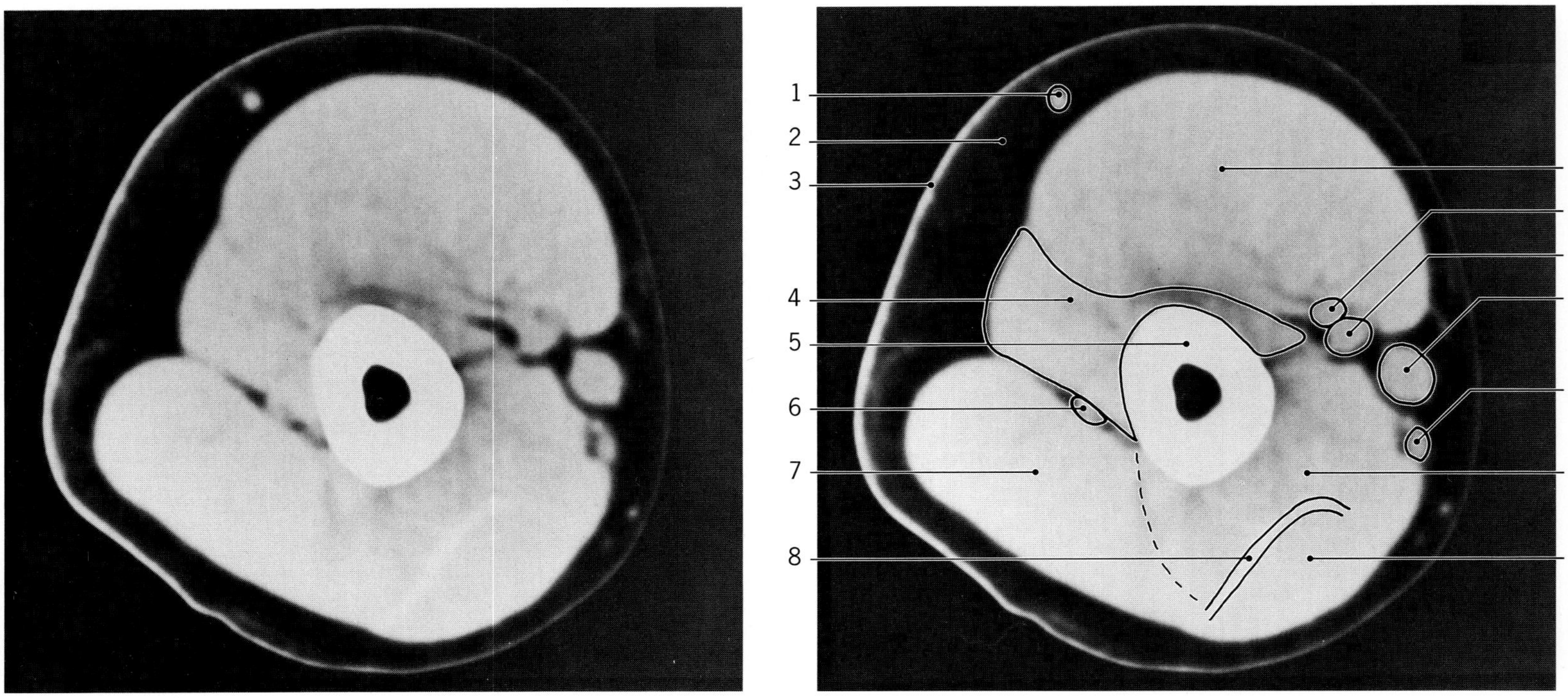

Upper arm, middle, axial CT

1: Cephalic vein
2: Subcutaneous fat
3: Skin (thick laterally)
4: Brachialis
5: Humerus
6: Radial nerve
7: Triceps, lateral head
8: Intramuscular tendon
9: Biceps
10: Median nerve
11: Brachial artery
12: Brachial vein
13: Ulnar nerve
14: Triceps, medial head
15: Triceps, long head

Scout view for elbow, axial CT
on opposite page

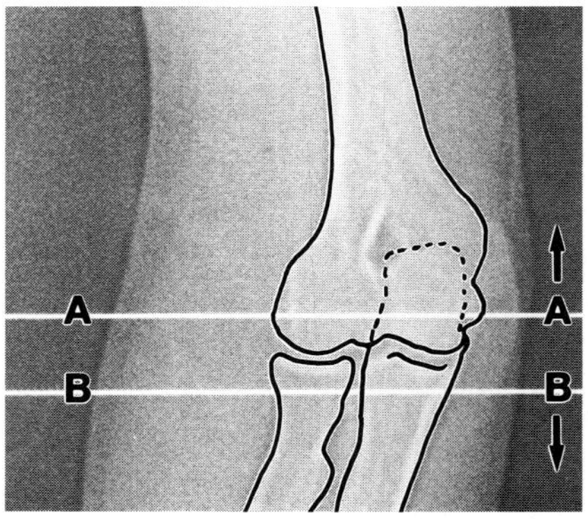

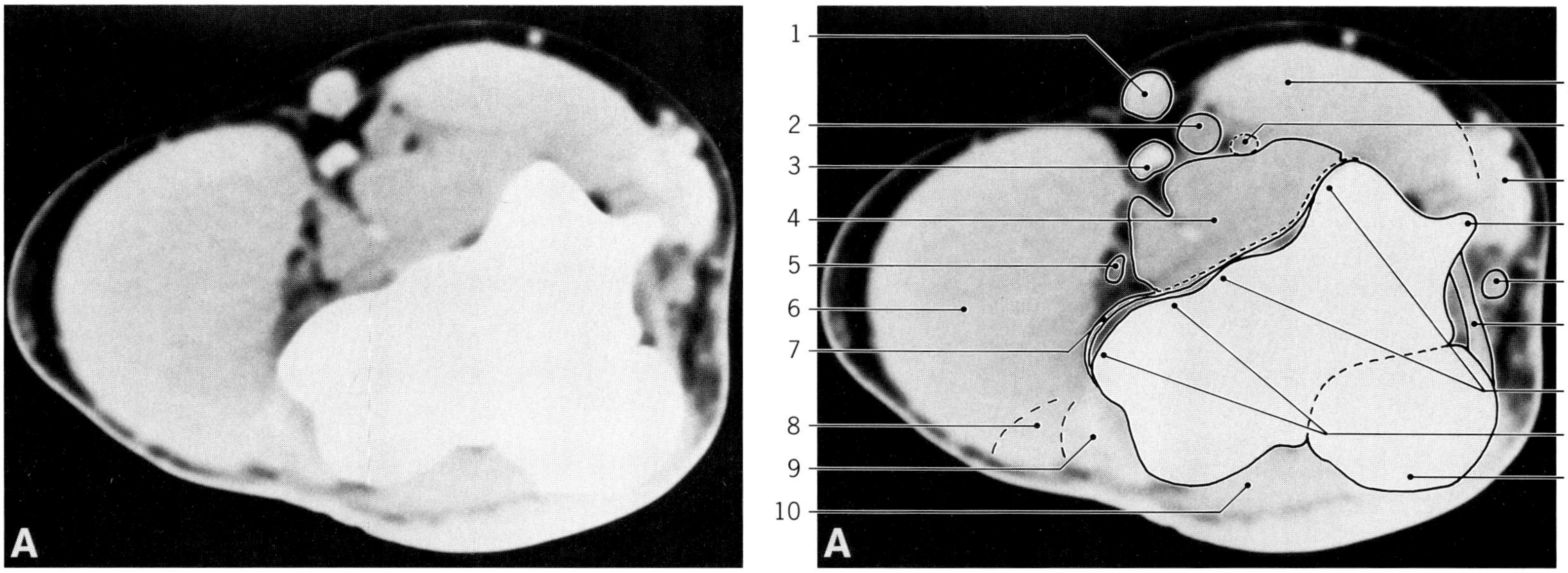

Elbow, axial CT

1: Median cubital vein
2: Brachial artery
3: Biceps (tendon)
4: Brachialis
5: Radial nerve
6: Brachioradialis
7: Articular capsule
8: Extensor carpi radialis longus
9: Common extensor tendon
10: Anconeus
11: Pronator teres
12: Median nerve
13: Common flexor tendon
14: Medial epicondyle
15: Ulnar nerve
16: Medial collateral ligament
17: Trochlea
18: Capitulum
19: Olecranon

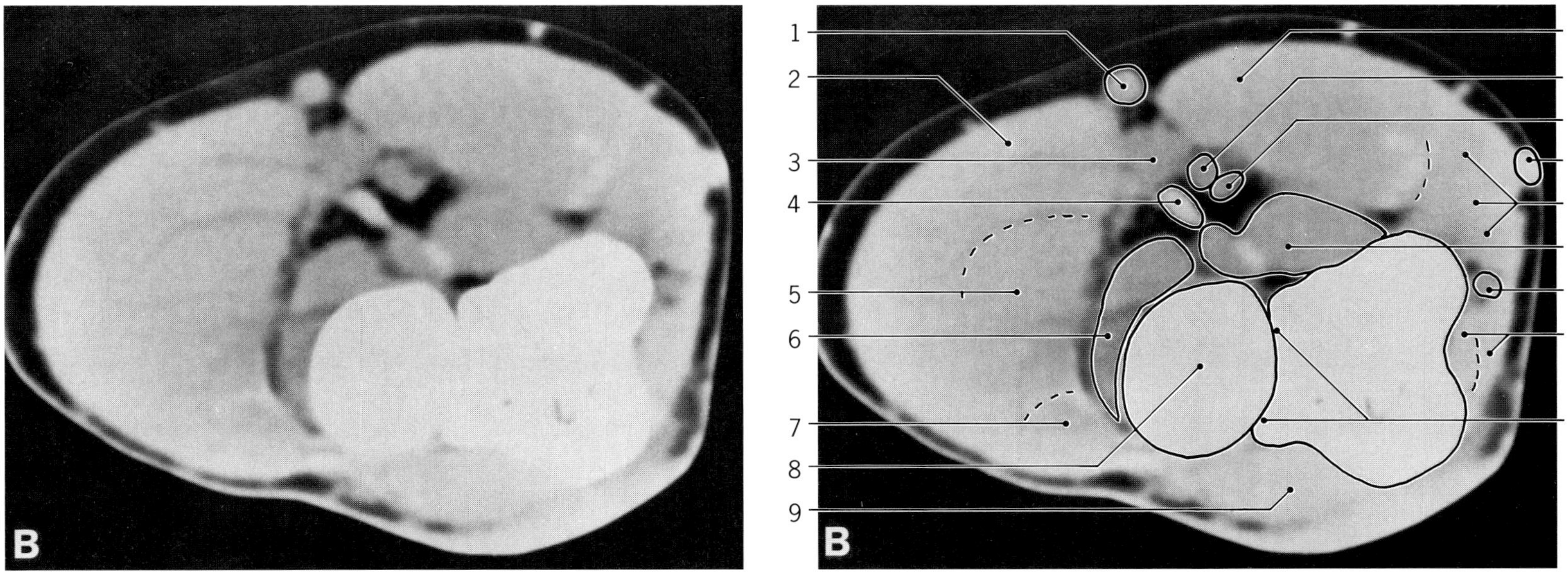

Elbow, axial CT

1: Median cubital vein
2: Brachioradialis
3: Cubital lymph node
4: Biceps (tendon)
5: Extensor carpi radialis longus
6: Supinator
7: Extensor carpi radialis brevis
8: Head of radius
9: Anconeus
10: Pronator teres
11: Brachial artery
12: Median nerve
13: Basilic vein
14: Extensor carpi radialis, palmaris longus, and flexor digitorum superficialis
15: Brachialis
16: Ulnar nerve
17: Flexor digitorum profundus, and flexor carpi ulnaris
18: Proximal radio-ulnar joint

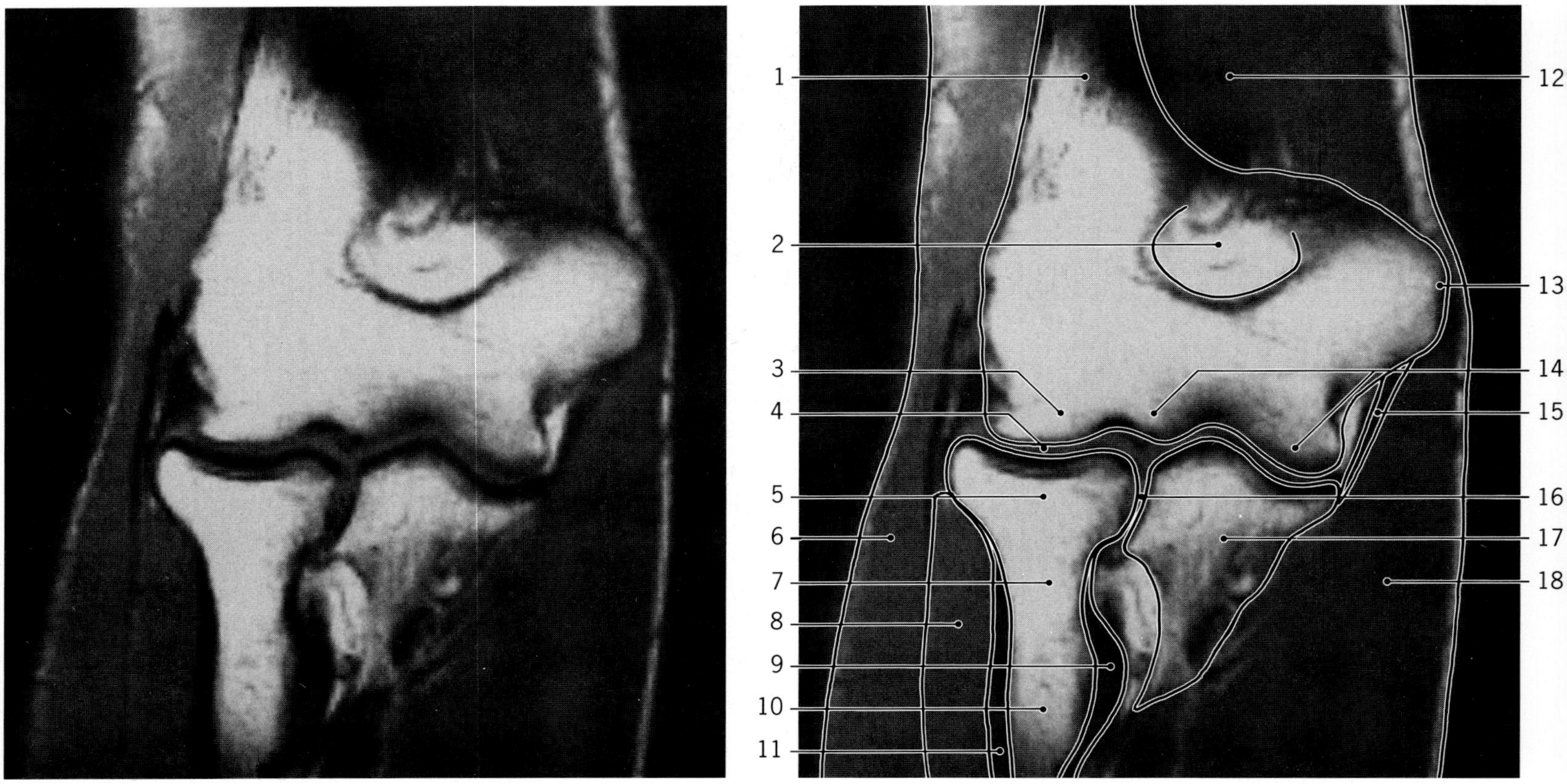

Elbow, coronal MR

1: Humeral shaft
2: Olecranon fossa
3: Capitulum
4: Humeroradial joint
5: Head of radius
6: Brachioradialis
7: Neck of radius
8: Supinator
9: Radial tuberosity
10: Yellow bone marrow
11: Compact bone
12: Triceps brachii
13: Medial epicondyle
14: Trochlea
15: Medial collateral ligament
16: Proximal radio-ulnar joint
17: Ulna
18: Flexor muscles of forearm

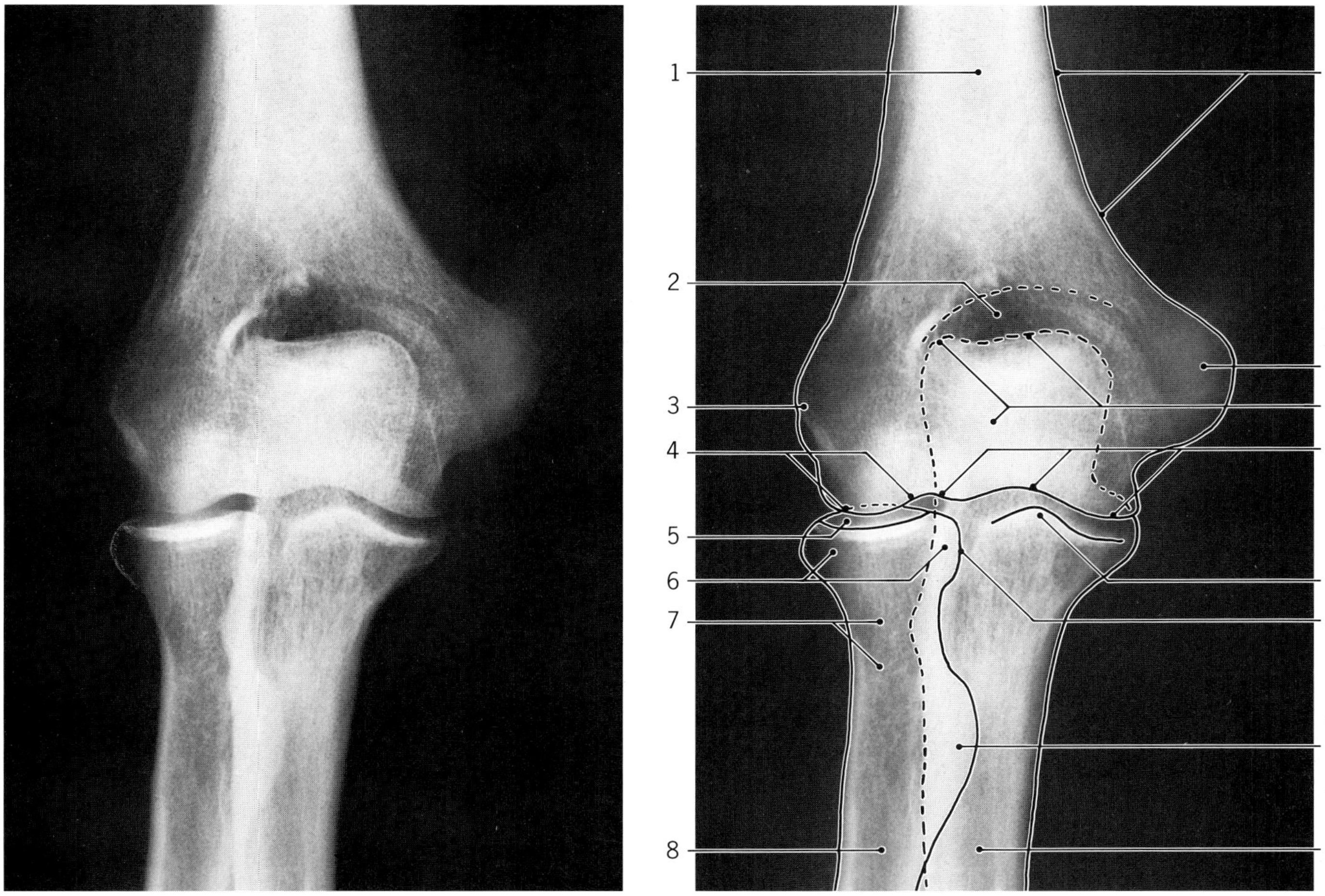

Elbow, a-p X-ray

1: Shaft of humerus
2: Olecranon fossa, and coronoid fossa (superimposed)
3: Lateral epicondyle
4: Capitulum
5: Humero-radial joint
6: Head of radius
7: Neck of radius
8: Shaft of radius
9: Medial supracondylar ridge
10: Medial epicondyle
11: Olecranon
12: Trochlea
13: Coronoid process
14: Articular circumference of radius
15: Radial tuberosity
16: Shaft of ulna

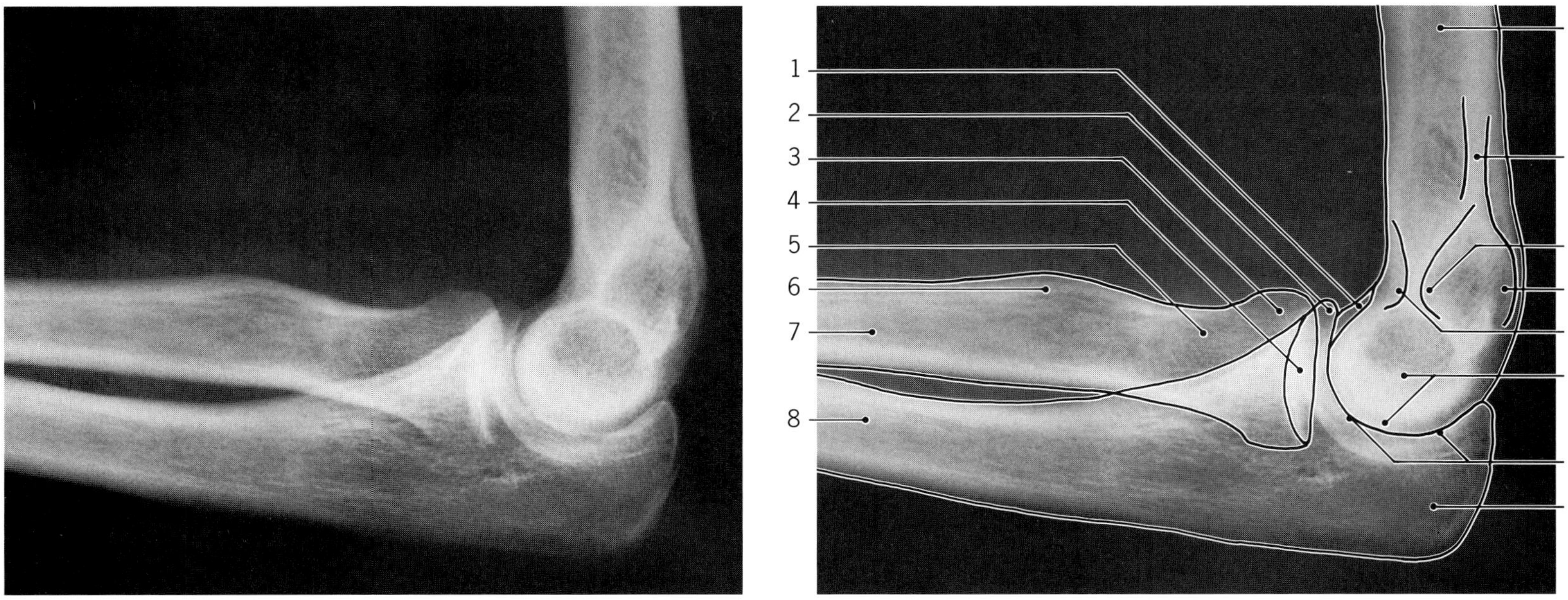

Elbow, lateral X-ray

1: Capitulum
2: Coronoid process
3: Head of radius
4: Articular fovea of radius
5: Neck of radius
6: Radial tuberosity
7: Shaft of radius
8: Shaft of ulna
9: Shaft of humerus
10: Medial supracondylar ridge
11: Olecranon fossa
12: Medial epicondyle
13: Coronoid fossa
14: Trochlea
15: Humero-ulnar joint
16: Olecranon

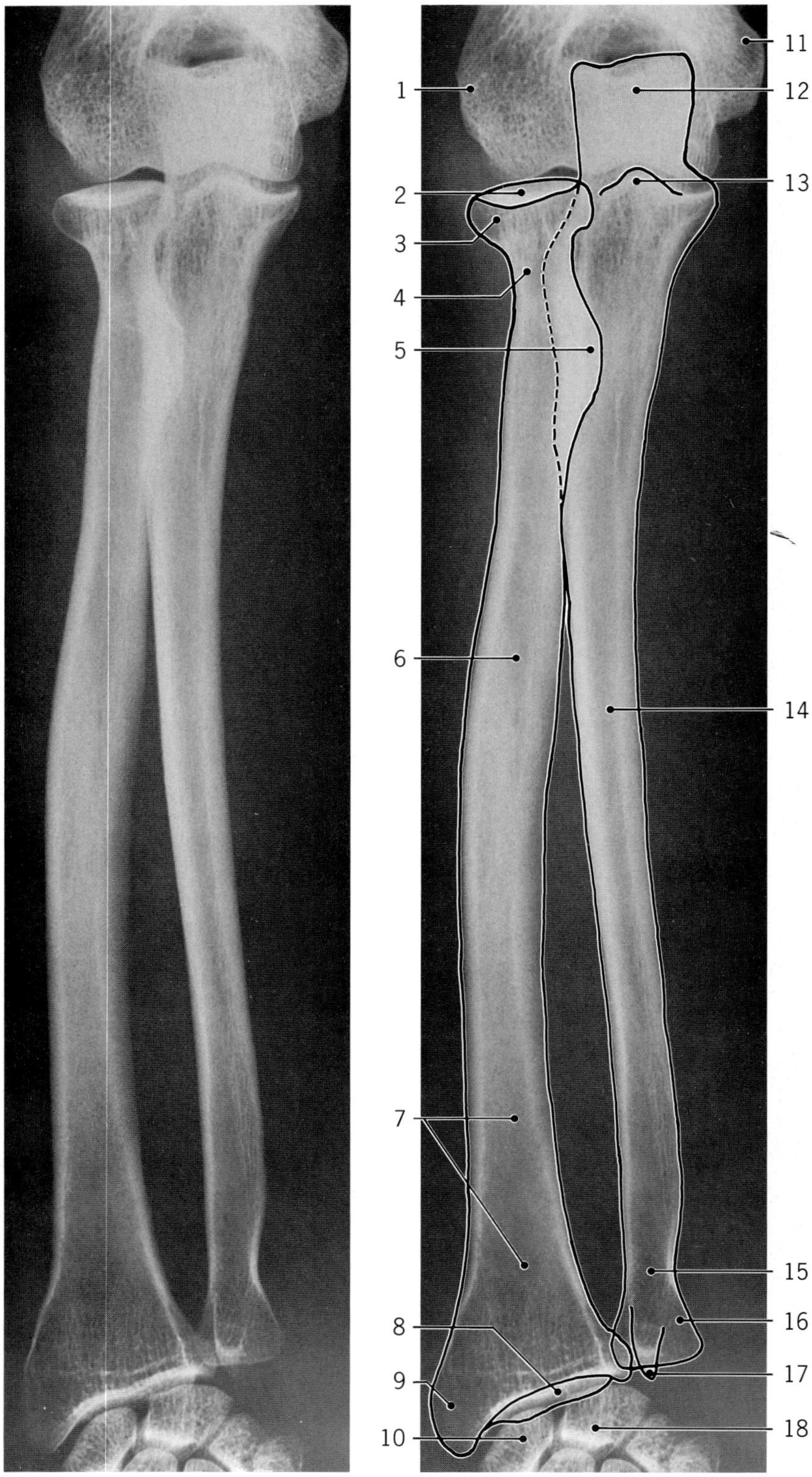

Lower arm, a-p X-ray

1: Lateral epicondyle
2: Articular fovea of radius
3: Head of radius
4: Neck of radius
5: Tuberosity of radius
6: Shaft of radius
7: Distal end of radius
8: Carpal articular surface of radius
9: Styloid process of radius
10: Scaphoid bone
11: Medial epicondyle
12: Olecranon
13: Coronoid process
14: Shaft of ulna
15: Neck of ulna
16: Head of ulna
17: Styloid process of ulna
18: Lunate bone

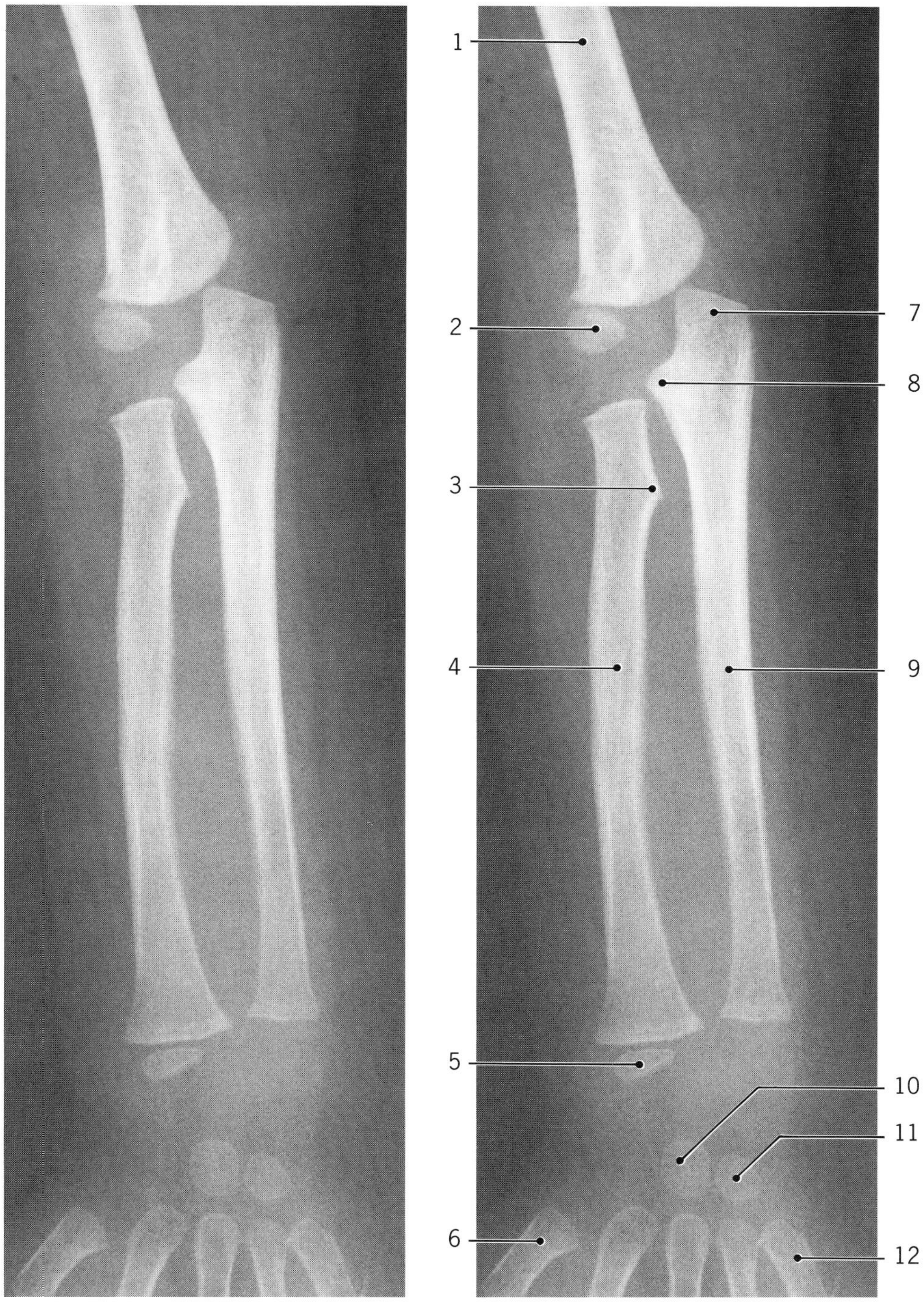

Lower arm, a-p X-ray, child 2 years

1: Diaphysis of humerus
2: Capitulum (ossification center)
3: Tuberosity of radius
4: Diaphysis of radius
5: Distal epiphysis of radius (ossification center)
6: First metacarpal bone
7: Olecranon
8: Coronoid process of ulna
9: Diaphysis of ulna
10: Capitate bone (ossification center)
11: Hamate bone (ossification center)
12: Fifth metacarpal bone

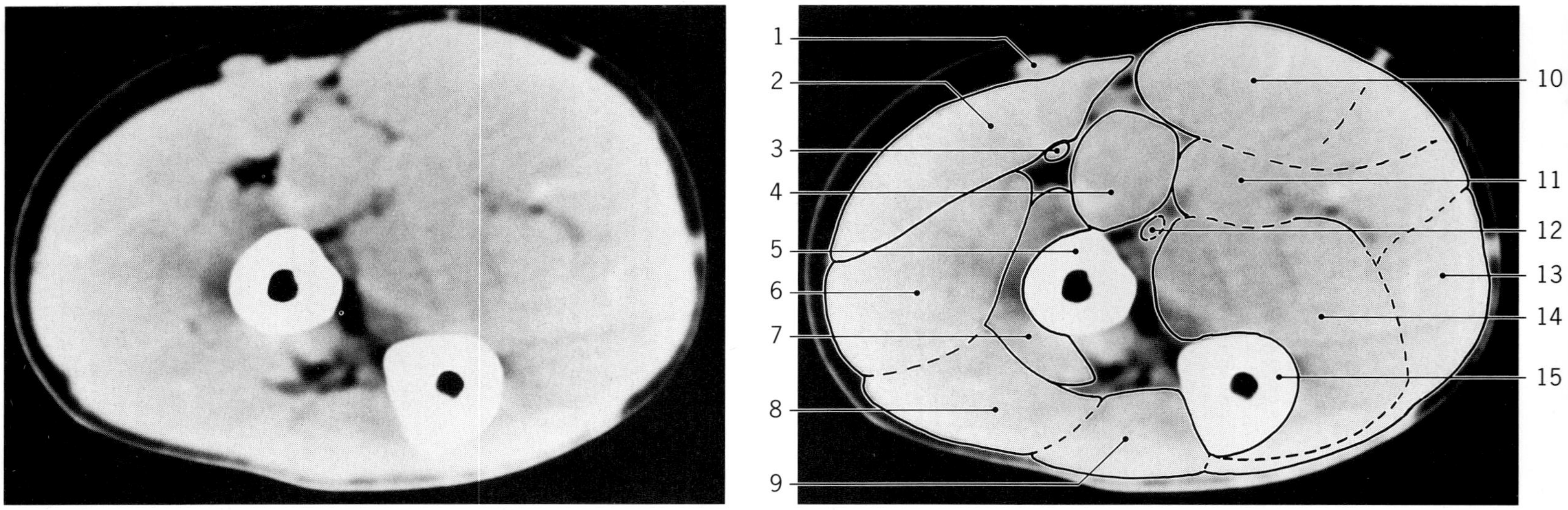

Lower arm, supinated, middle, axial CT

1: Subcutaneous vein
2: Brachioradialis
3: Radial artery
4: Pronator teres
5: Radius
6: Extensor carpi radialis longus, and brevis
7: Supinator
8: Extensor digitorum
9: Extensor carpi ulnaris
10: Flexor carpi radialis, and palmaris longus
11: Flexor digitorum superficialis
12: Median nerve
13: Flexor carpi ulnaris
14: Flexor digitorum profundus
15: Ulna

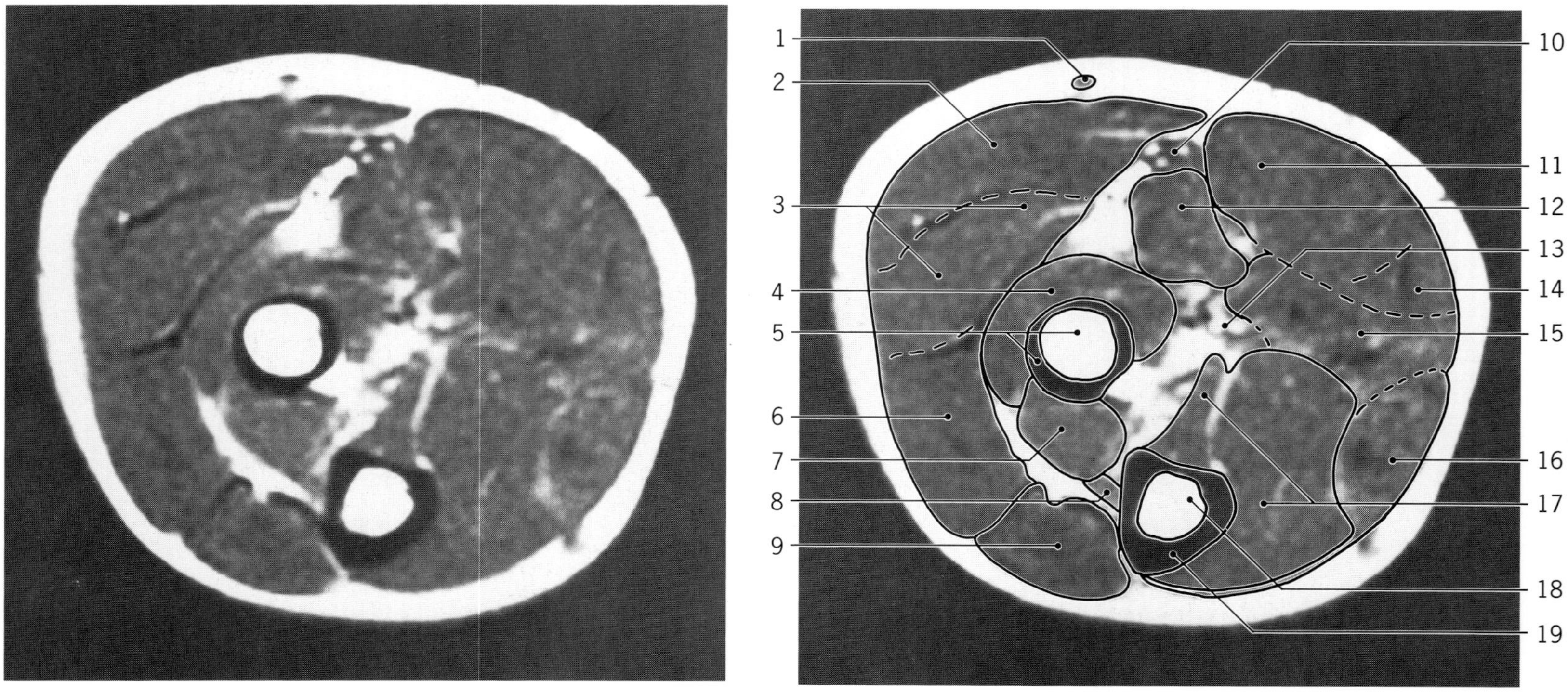

Lower arm, pronated, middle, axial MR

1: Cephalic vein
2: Brachioradialis
3: Extensor carpi radialis longus and brevis
4: Supinator
5: Shaft of radius
6: Extensor digitorum
7: Abductor pollicis longus
8: Extensor pollicis brevis
9: Extensor carpi ulnaris
10: Radial artery and veins
11: Flexor carpi radialis
12: Pronator teres
13: Ulnar artery and veins
14: Palmaris longus
15: Flexor digitorum superficialis
16: Flexor carpi ulnaris
17: Flexor digitorum profundus
18: Shaft of ulna (bone marrow)
19: Compact bone

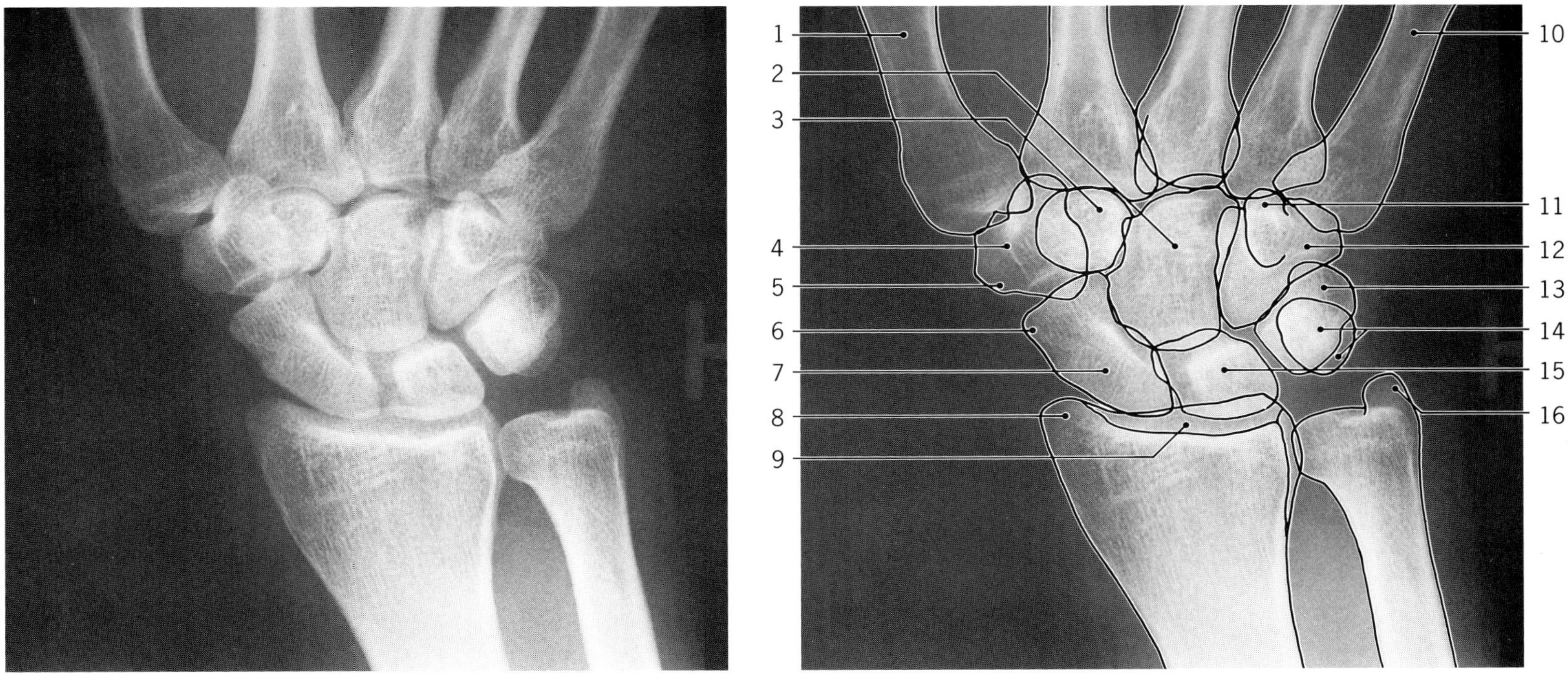

Wrist, dorso-volar X-ray

1: First metacarpal bone
2: Capitate bone
3: Trapezoid bone
4: Trapezium
5: Tubercle of trapezium
6: Tubercle of scaphoid bone
7: Scaphoid (navicular) bone
8: Styloid process of radius
9: Carpal articular surface of radius
10: Fifth metacarpal bone
11: Hamulus of hamate bone
12: Hamate bone
13: Triquetral bone
14: Pisiform bone
15: Lunate bone
16: Styloid process of ulna

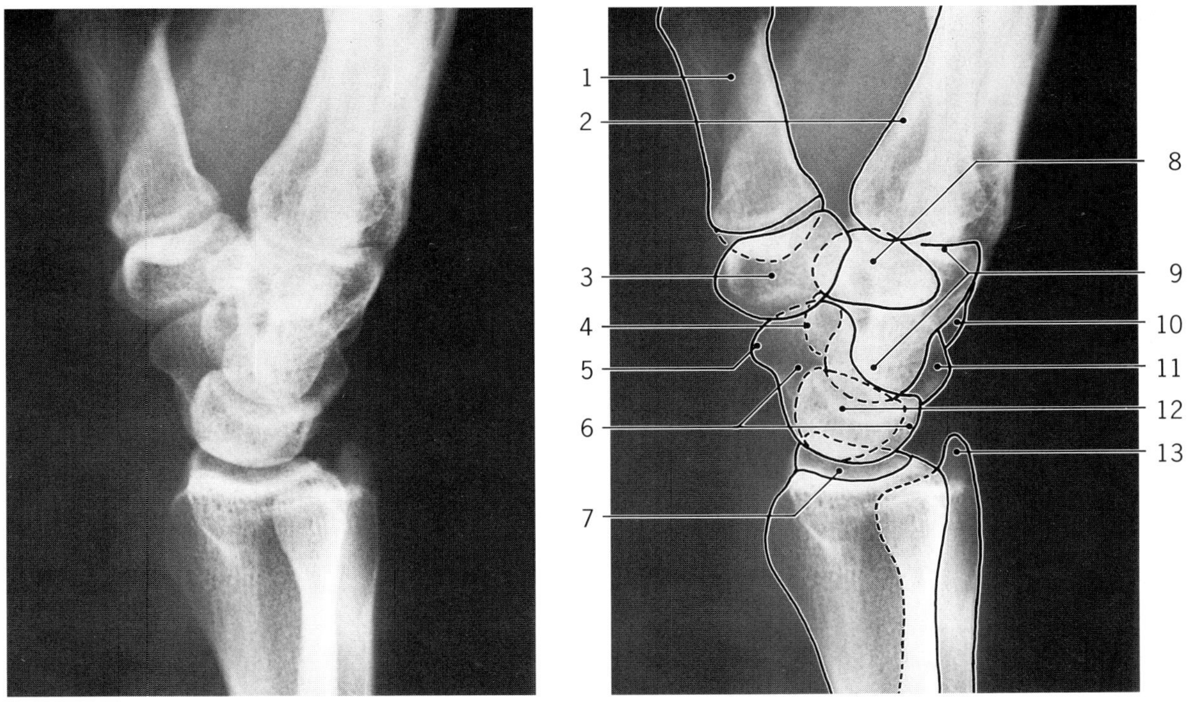

Wrist, lateral X-ray

1: First metacarpal bone
2: Second metacarpal bone
3: Trapezium
4: Pisiform bone
5: Tubercle of scaphoid bone
6: Scaphoid bone
7: Carpal articular surface of radius
8: Trapezoid bone
9: Capitate bone
10: Hamate bone
11: Triquetral bone
12: Lunate bone
13: Styloid process of ulna

Scout for wrist, axial CT

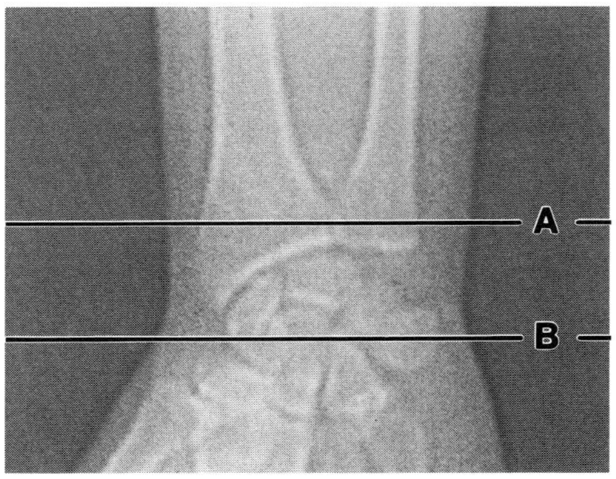

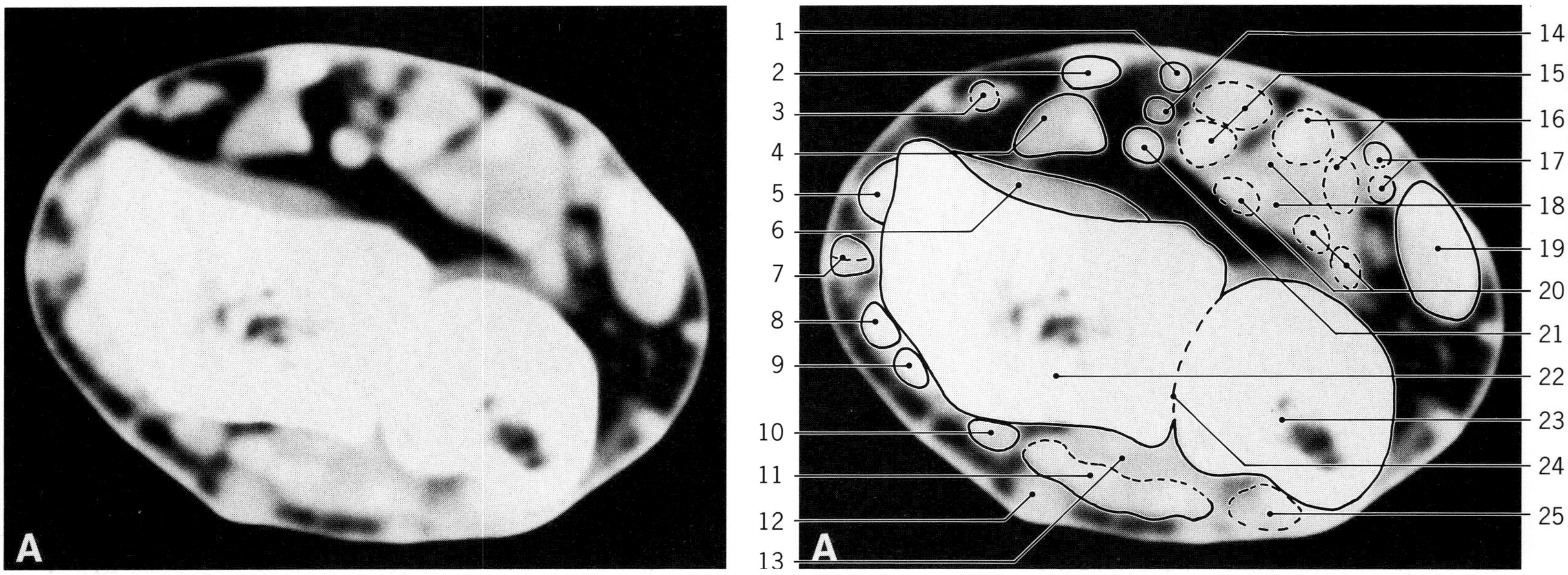

Wrist, axial CT

1: Palmaris longus (tendon)
2: Flexor carpi radialis (tendon)
3: Radial artery with comitant veins
4: Flexor pollicis longus (tendon)
5: Brachioradialis
6: Pronator quadratus
7: Abductor pollicis longus, and extensor pollicis brevis (tendons)
8: Extensor carpi radialis longus (tendon)
9: Extensor carpi radialis brevis (tendon)
10: Extensor pollicis longus (tendon)
11: Extensor digitorum, and extensor digiti minimi (tendons)
12: Cephalic vein
13: Extensor indicis (tendon)
14: Median nerve
15: Flexor digitorum superficialis tendons to 2. and 3. finger
16: Flexor digitorum superficialis tendons to 4. and 5. finger
17: Ulnar artery and nerve
18: Synovial bursa
19: Flexor carpi ulnaris
20: Flexor digitorum profundus tendons to 3., 4. and 5. finger
21: Flexor digitorum profundus tendon to 2. finger
22: Distal end of radius
23: Head of ulna
24: Distal radio-ulnar joint
25: Extensor carpi ulnaris (tendon)

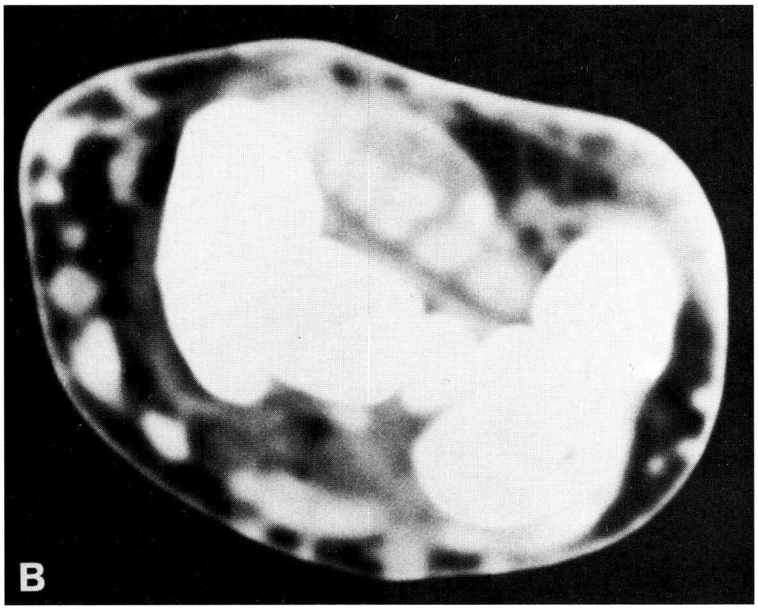

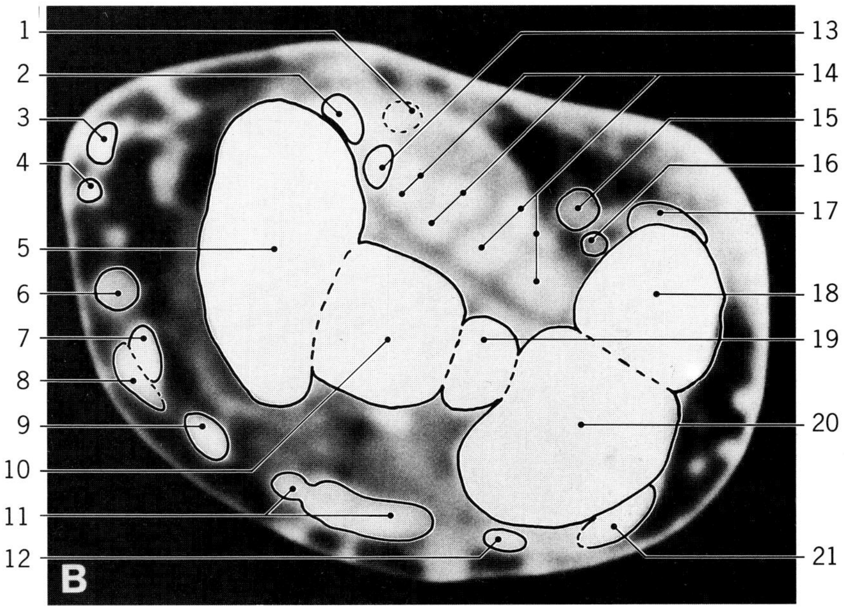

Wrist, axial CT

1: Median nerve
2: Flexor carpi radialis (tendon)
3: Abductor pollicis longus (tendon)
4: Extensor pollicis brevis (tendon)
5: Scaphoid bone
6: Radial artery
7: Extensor carpi radialis longus (tendon)
8: Extensor pollicis longus (tendon)
9: Extensor carpi radialis brevis (tendon)
10: Lunate bone
11: Extensor digitorum, and extensor indicis (tendons)
12: Extensor digiti minimi (tendon)
13: Flexor pollicis longus (tendon)
14: Tendons of flexor digitorum superficialis, and profundus in synovial bursa
15: Ulnar artery
16: Ulnar nerve
17: Flexor carpi ulnaris (insertion)
18: Pisiform bone
19: Hamate bone
20: Triquetral bone
21: Extensor carpi ulnaris (tendon)

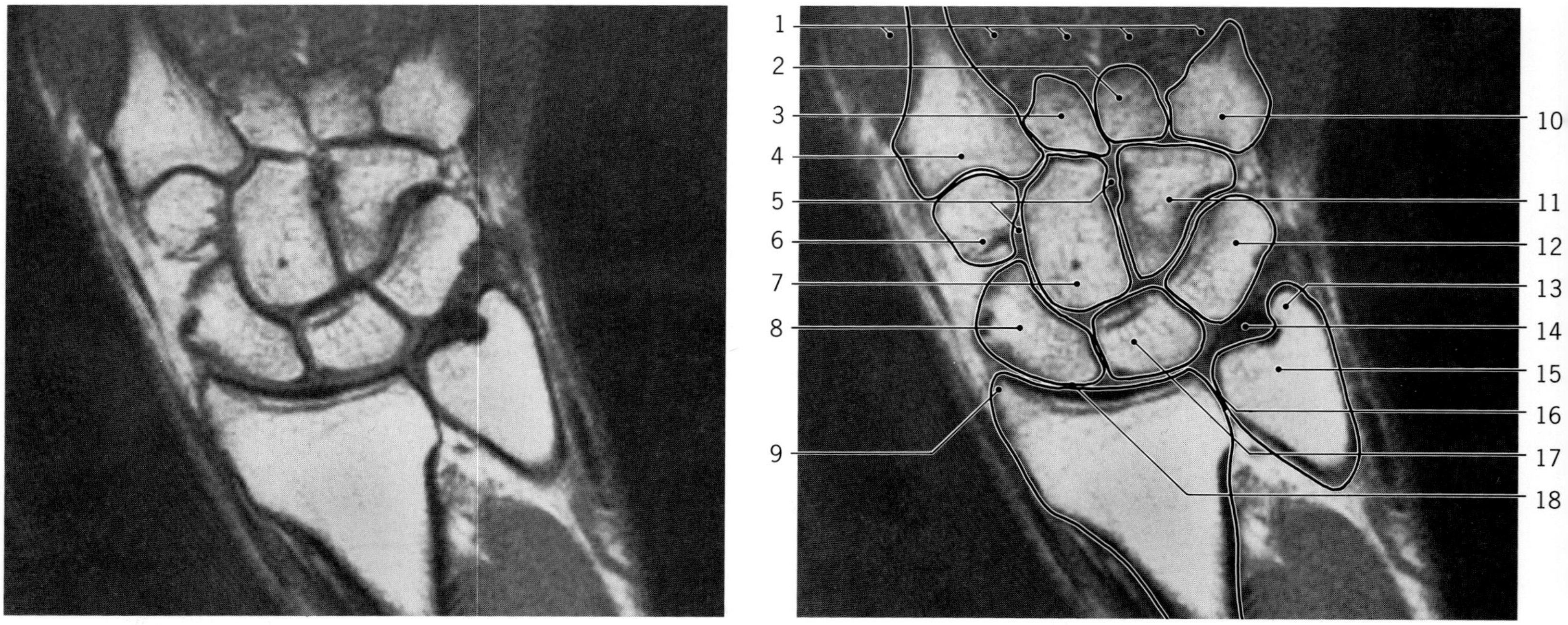

Wrist, coronal MR

1: Interossei muscles
2: Base of fourth metacarpal bone
3: Base of third metacarpal bone
4: Base of second metacarpal bone
5: Interosseous ligaments
6: Trapezoid bone
7: Capitate bone
8: Scaphoid bone
9: Styloid process of radius
10: Base of fifth metacarpal bone
11: Hamate bone
12: Triquetral bone
13: Styloid process of ulna
14: Articular disc
15: Head of ulna
16: Distal radio-ulnar joint
17: Lunate bone
18: Radiocarpal joint

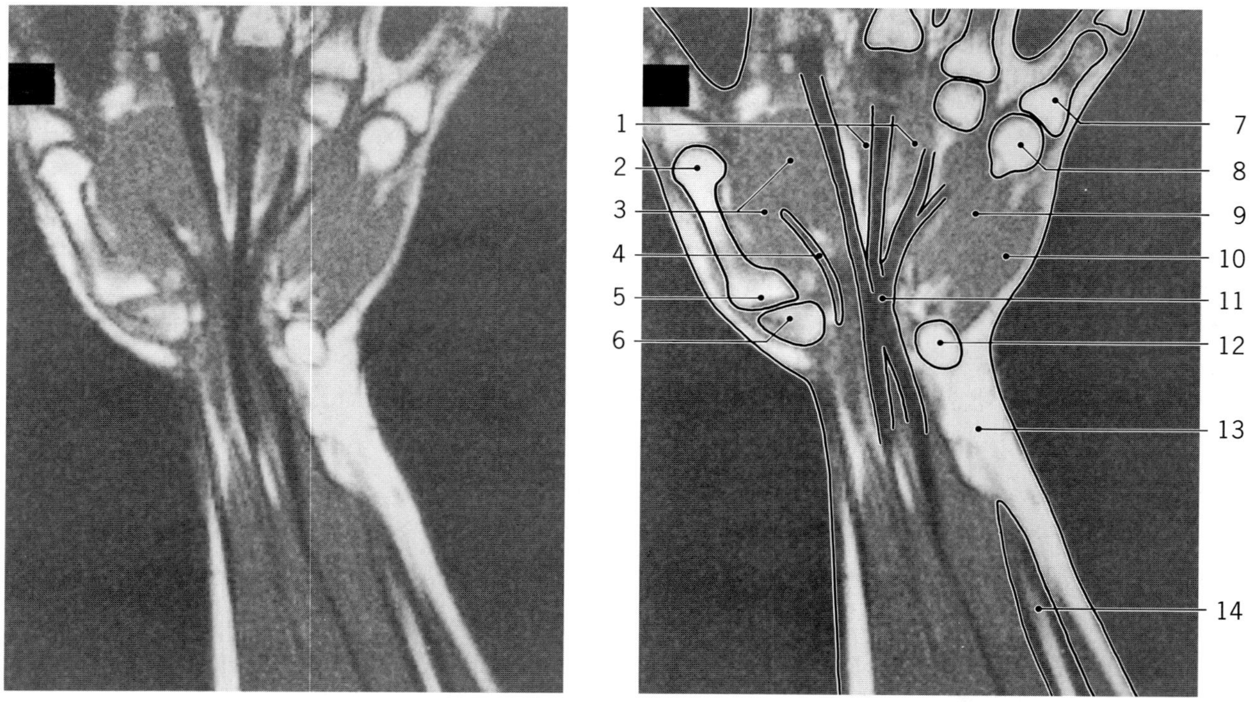

Carpal tunnel, coronal MR

1: Lumbricals
2: Head of first metacarpal bone
3: Flexor pollicis brevis, and adductor pollicis
4: Flexor pollicis longus (tendon)
5: Base of first metacarpal bone
6: Trapezium
7: Proximal phalanx of fifth finger
8: Head of fifth metacarpal bone
9: Flexor digiti minimi
10: Abductor digiti minimi
11: Long flexor tendons in canalis carpi
12: Pisiform bone
13: Subcutaneous fat
14: Shaft of ulna

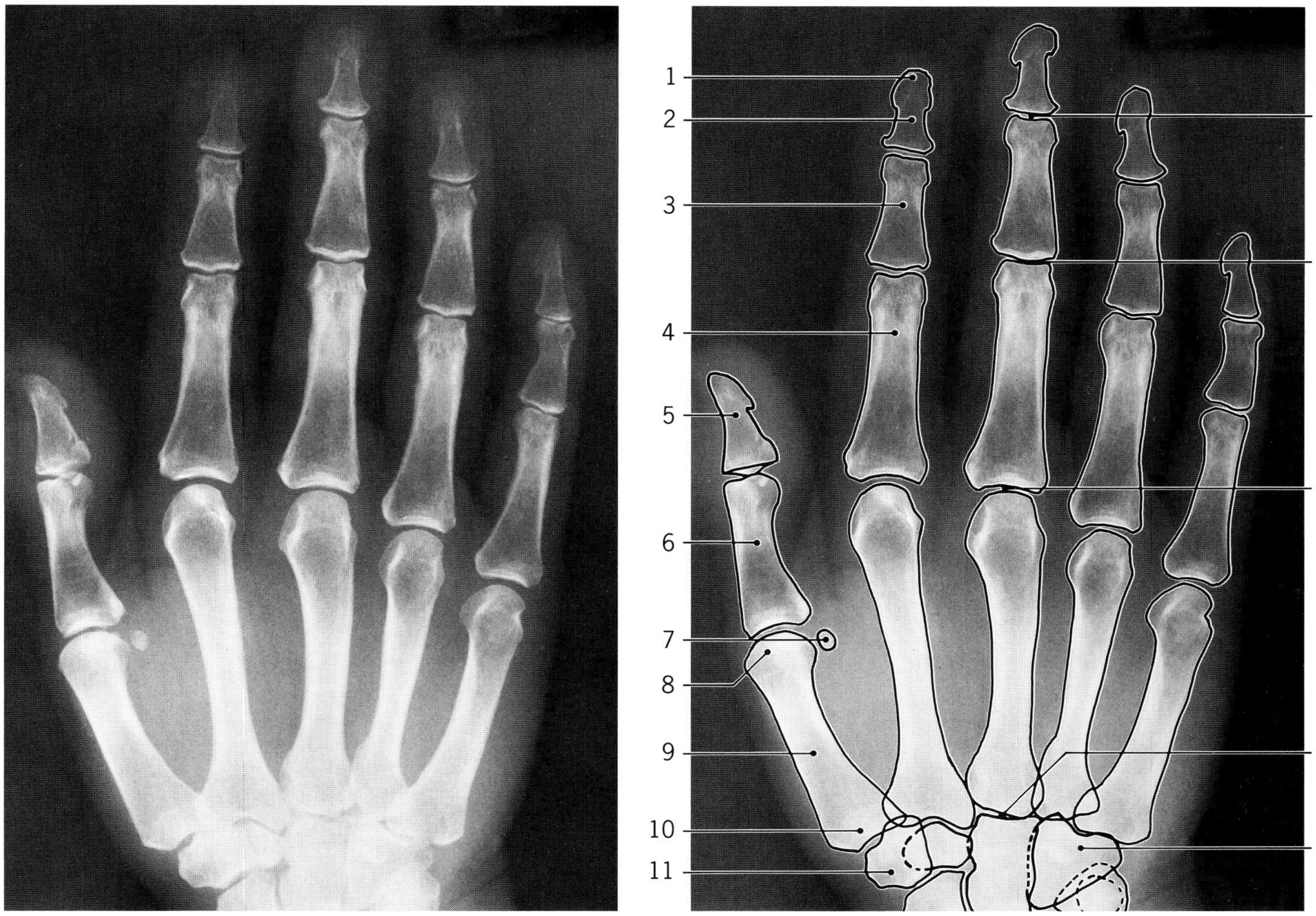

Hand, dorso-volar X-ray

1: Tuberosity of distal phalanx
2: Distal phalanx
3: Middle phalanx
4: Proximal phalanx
5: Distal phalanx of thumb
6: Proximal phalanx of thumb
7: Sesamoid bone
8: Head of first metacarpal bone
9: Shaft of first metacarpal bone
10: Base of first metacarpal bone
11: Trapezium
12: Distal interphalangeal joint ("DIP")
13: Proximal interphalangeal joint ("PIP")
14: Metacarpophalangeal joint ("MP")
15: Carpometacarpeal joint
16: Hamate bone

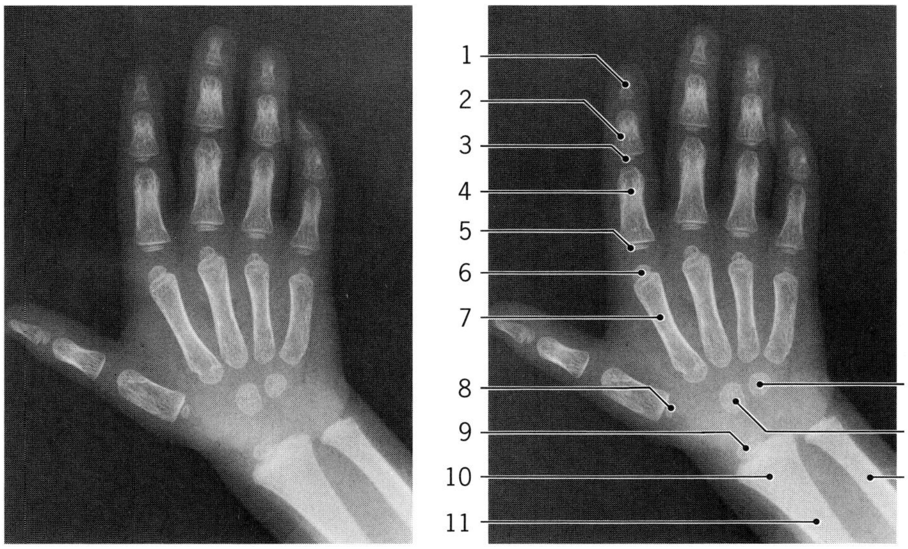

Hand, dorso-volar X-ray, child 1 year

1: Distal phalanx (diaphysis)
2: Middle phalanx (diaphysis)
3: Epiphysis of middle phalanx
4: Proximal phalanx (diaphysis)
5: Epiphysis of proximal phalanx
6: Epiphysis of second metacarpal bone
7: Second metacarpal bone (diaphysis)
8: Epiphysis of first metacarpal bone
9: Epiphysis of radius
10: Metaphysis of radius
11: Diaphysis of radius
12: Hamate bone (ossification center)
13: Capitate bone (ossification center)
14: Ulna (diaphysis)

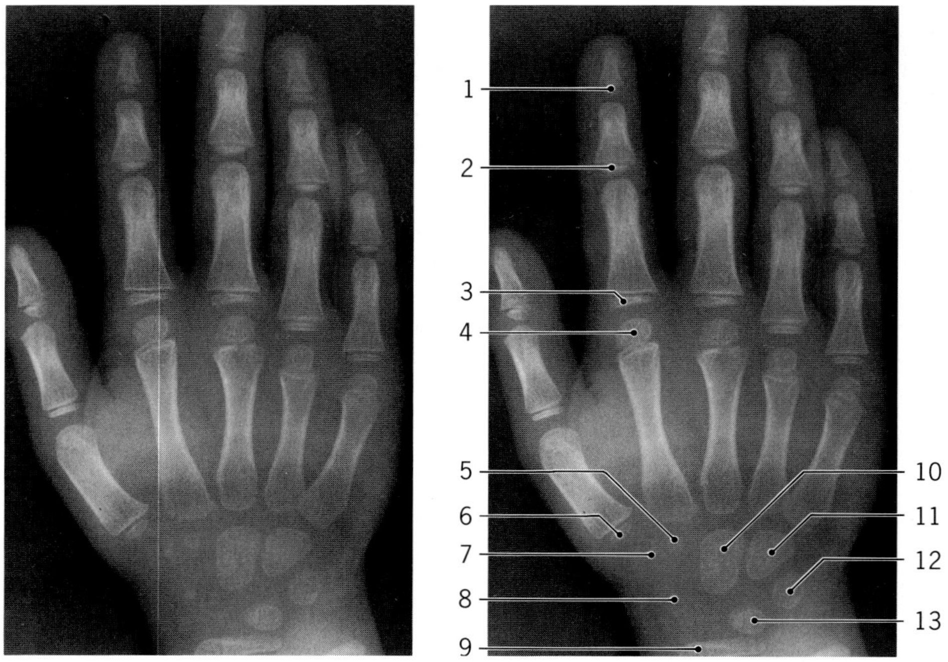

Hand, dorso-volar X-ray, child 6 years

1: Epiphysis of distal phalanx
2: Epiphysis of middle phalanx
3: Epiphysis of proximal phalanx
4: Epiphysis of second metacarpal bone
5: Trapezoid bone (ossification center)
6: Epiphysis of first metacarpal bone
7: Trapezium (ossification center)
8: Scaphoid bone (ossification center)
9: Epiphysis of radius
10: Capitate bone (ossification center)
11: Hamate bone (ossification center)
12: Triquetral bone (ossification center)
13: Lunate bone (ossification center)

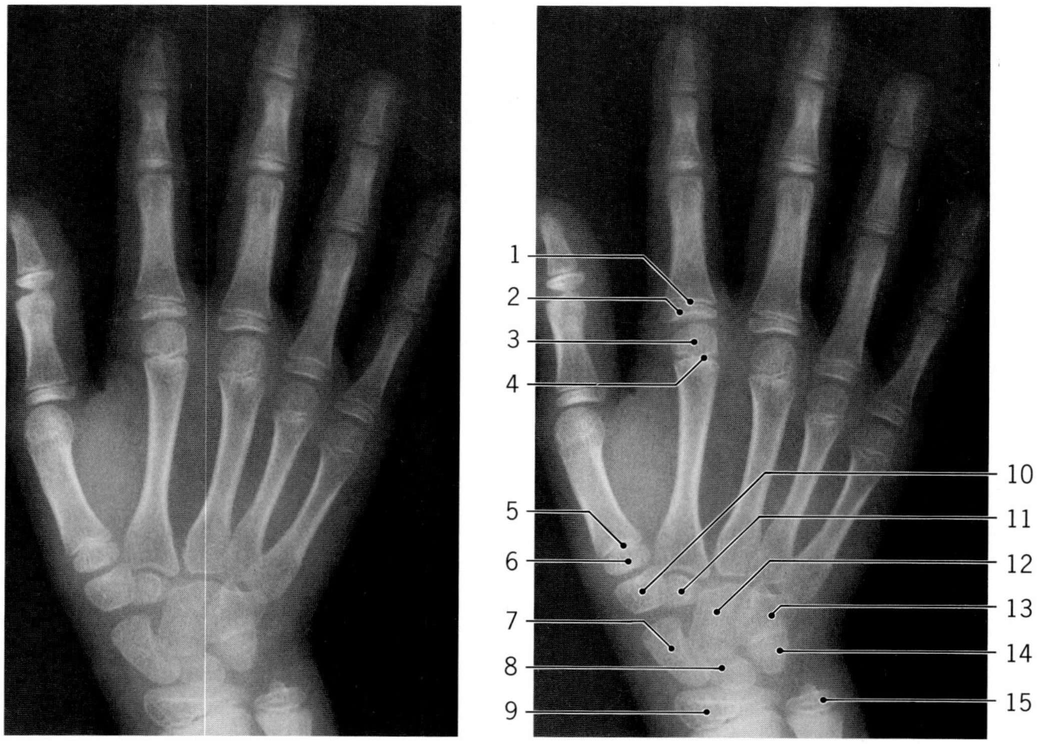

Hand, dorso-volar X-ray, child 10 years

1: Growth plate of proximal phalanx
2: Epiphysis of proximal phalanx
3: Epiphysis of second metacarpal bone
4: Growth plate of second metacarpal bone
5: Growth plate of first metacarpal bone
6: Epiphysis of first metacarpal bone
7: Scaphoid bone
8: Lunate bone
9: Epiphysis of radius
10: Trapezium
11: Trapezoid bone
12: Capitate bone
13: Hamate bone
14: Triquetral bone
15: Epiphysis of ulna

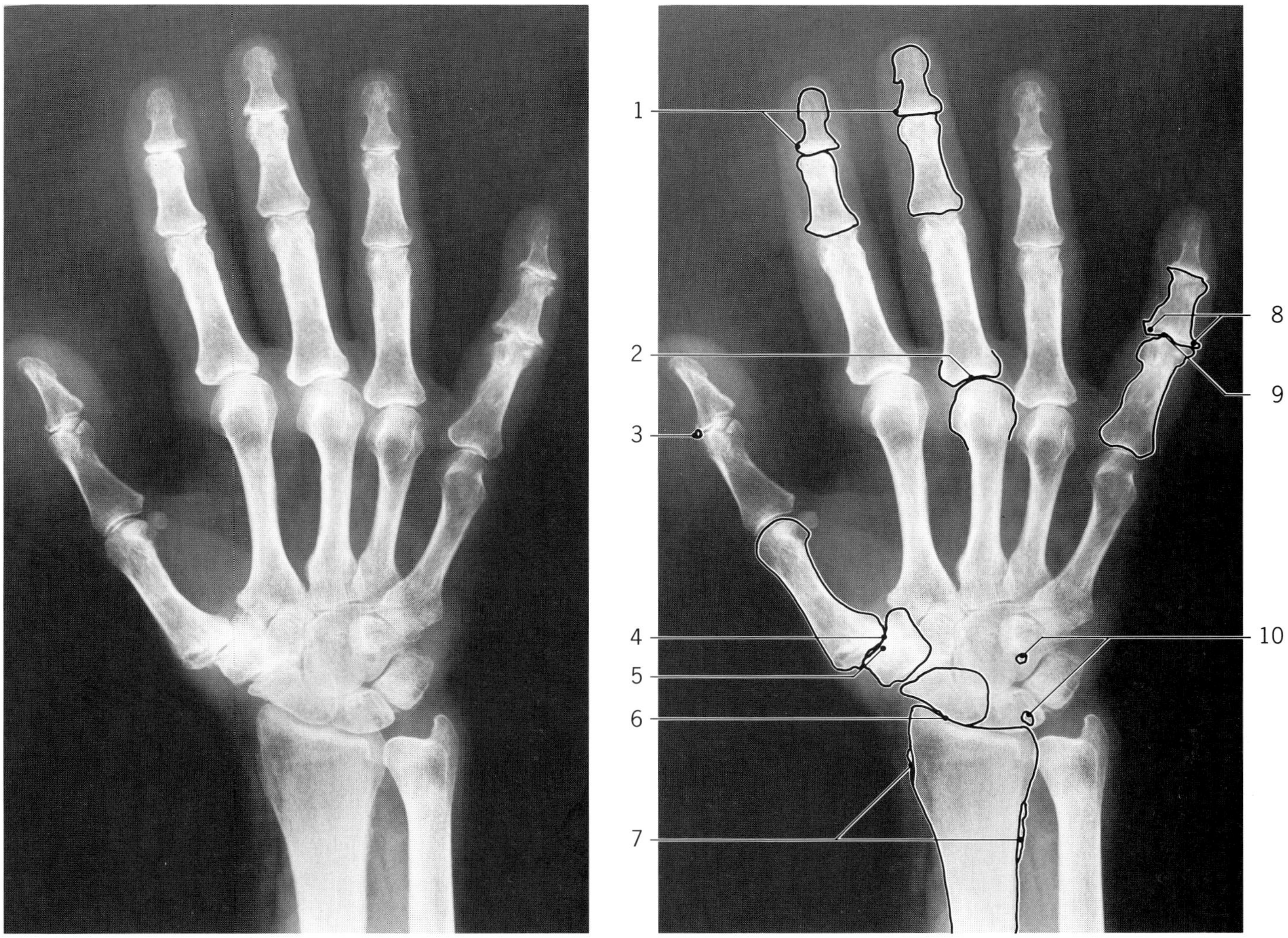

Hand, senescent, dorso-volar X-ray

1: Osteophytes
2: Subluxation of metacarpophalangeal joint
3: Soft tissue calcification
4: First carpometacarpeal joint (narrowed)
5: Subchondral sclerosis (sign of arthrosis)
6: Radiocarpal joint (narrowed)
7: Periosteal calcifications
8: Osteophytes
9: Interphalangeal joint (arthrosis)
10: Cysts in carpal bones

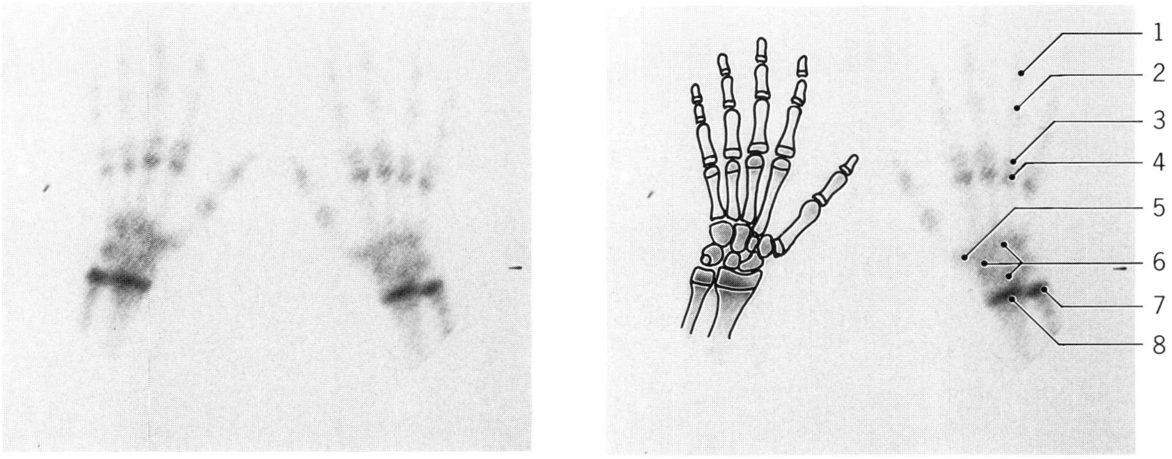

Hand, dorso-volar, ^{99m}Tc-DMP, scintigraphy, child 12 years

1: Growth plate of distal phalanx IV
2: Growth plate of middle phalanx IV
3: Growth plate of proximal phalanx IV
4: Growth plate of fourth metacarpal bone
5: Growth plate of first metacarpal bone
6: Carpal bones
7: Growth plate of distal epiphysis of ulna
8: Growth plate of distal epiphysis of radius

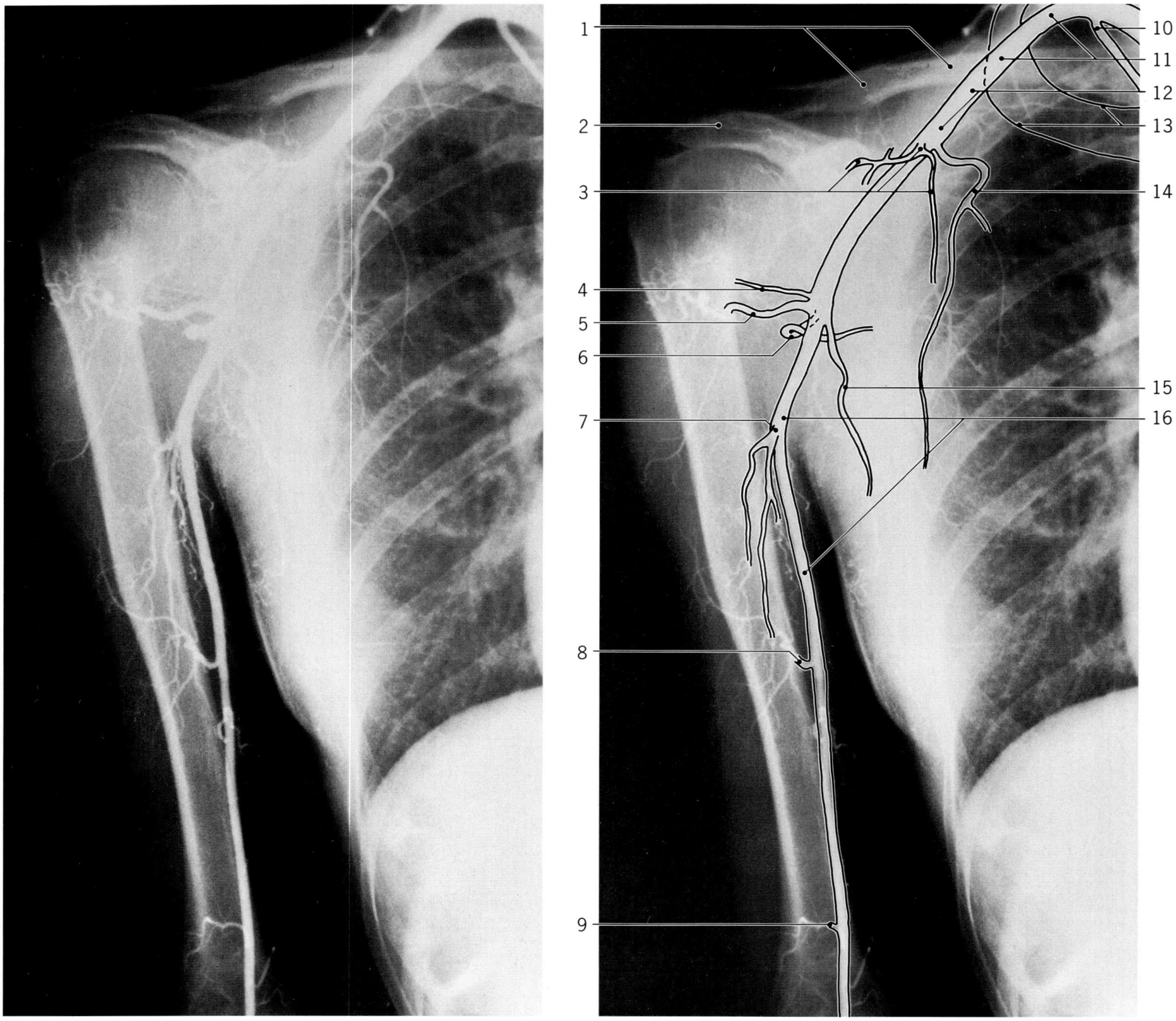

Shoulder, a-p X-ray, arteriography

1: Clavicula
2: Acromion
3: Thoraco-acromial artery
4: Anterior circumflex humeral artery
5: Posterior circumflex humeral artery
6: Circumflex scapular artery
7: Arteria profunda brachii
8: Branch to flexor muscles
9: Branch to rete cubiti
10: Internal thoracic artery
11: Subclavian artery
12: Axillary artery
13: First rib
14: Lateral thoracic artery
15: Thoracodorsal artery
16: Brachial artery

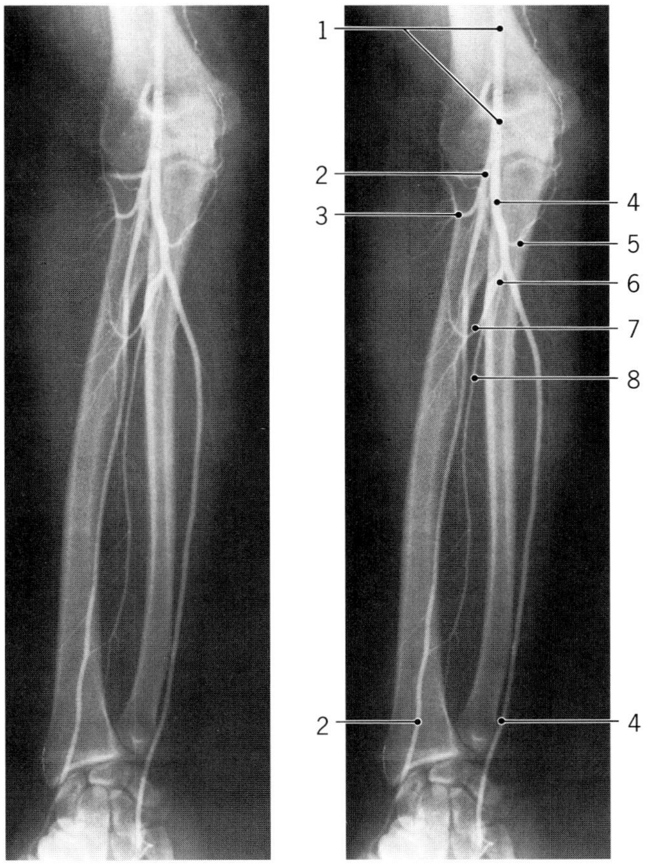

Lower arm, a-p X-ray, arteriography

1: Brachial artery
2: Radial artery
3: Recurrent radial artery
4: Ulnar artery
5: Recurrent ulnar artery
6: Common interosseous artery
7: Posterior interosseous artery
8: Anterior interosseous artery

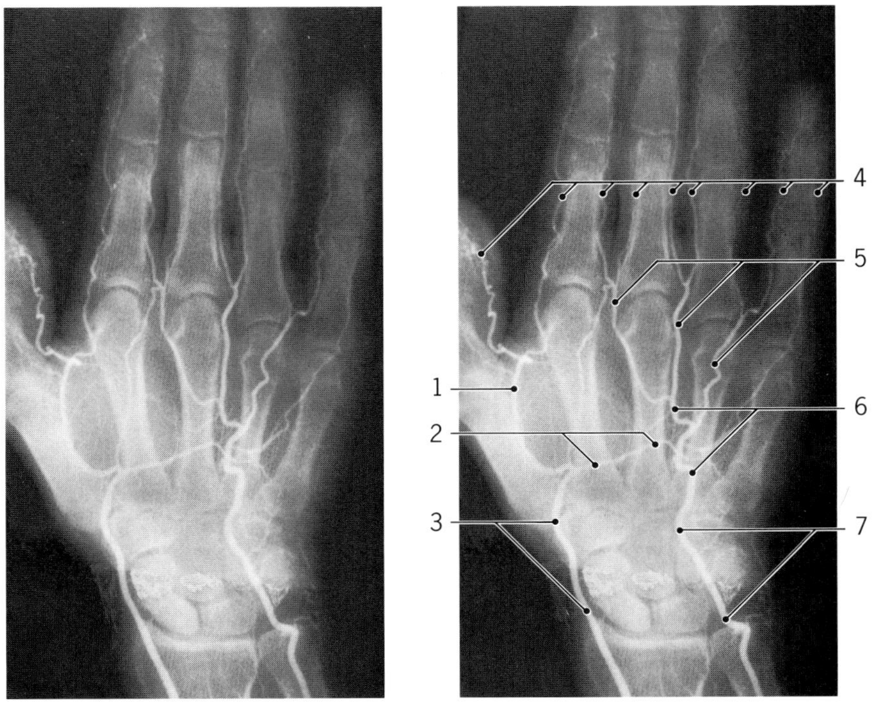

Hand, dorso-volar X-ray, arteriography

1: Arteria princeps pollicis
2: Deep palmar arch
3: Radial artery
4: Palmar digital arteries proper
5: Common palmar digital arteries
6: Superficial palmar arch (incomplete)
7: Ulnar artery

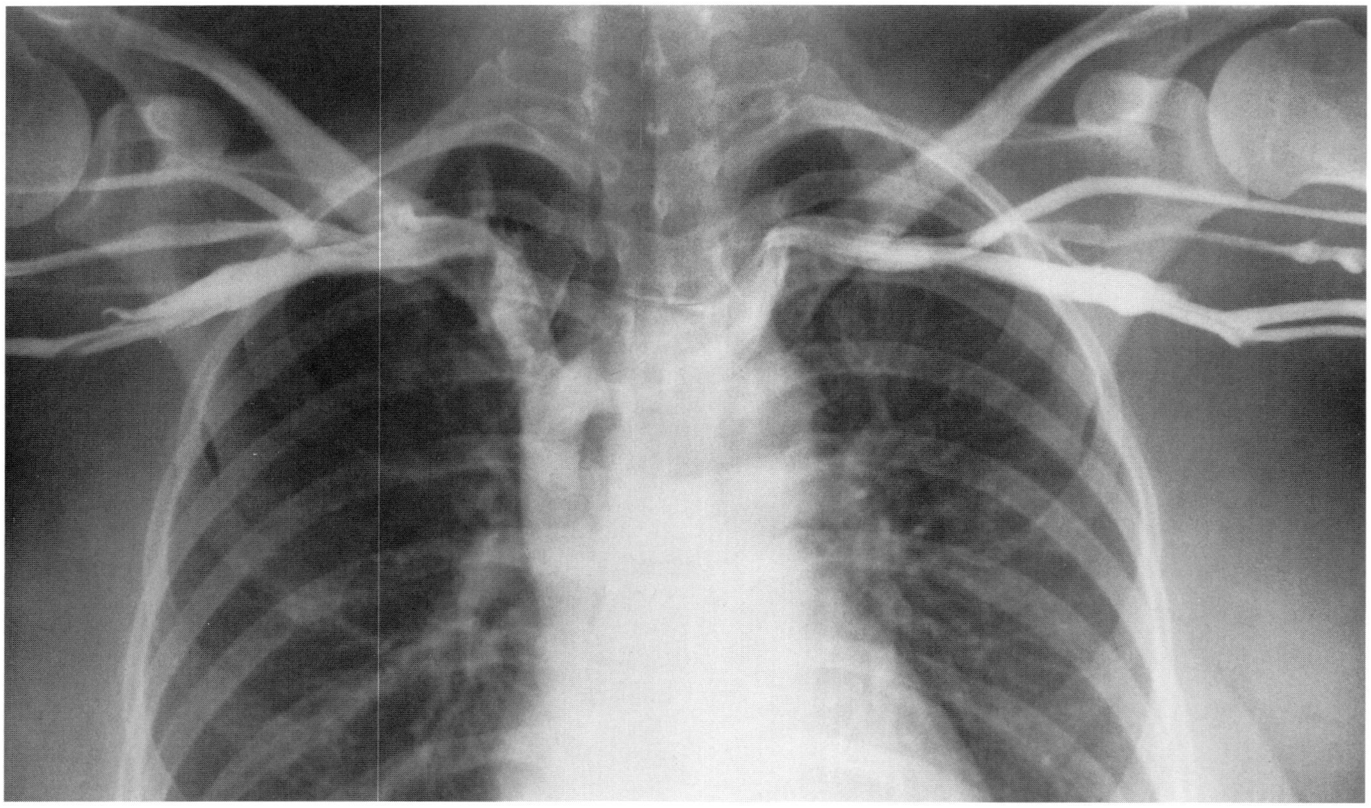

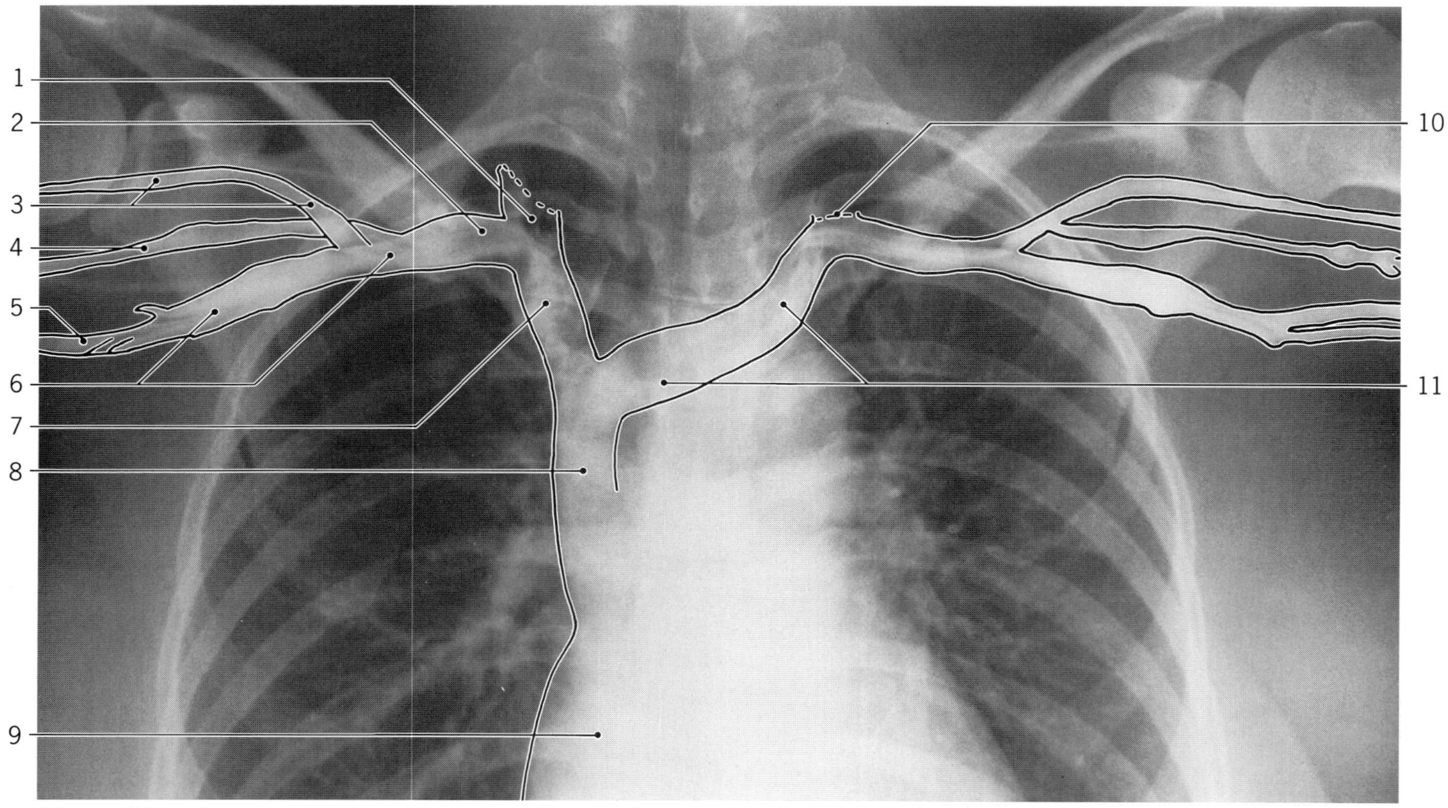

Shoulder, a-p X-ray, phlebography

1: Right internal jugular vein, (termination)
2: Subclavian vein
3: Cephalic vein
4: Brachial vein
5: Basilic vein
6: Axillary vein
7: Right brachiocephalic vein
8: Superior caval vein
9: Right atrium
10: Left internal jugular vein (termination)
11: Left brachiocephalic vein

Lower Limb

Pelvis

Hip and thigh

Knee

Lower leg

Ankle and foot

Arteries and veins

Lymphatics

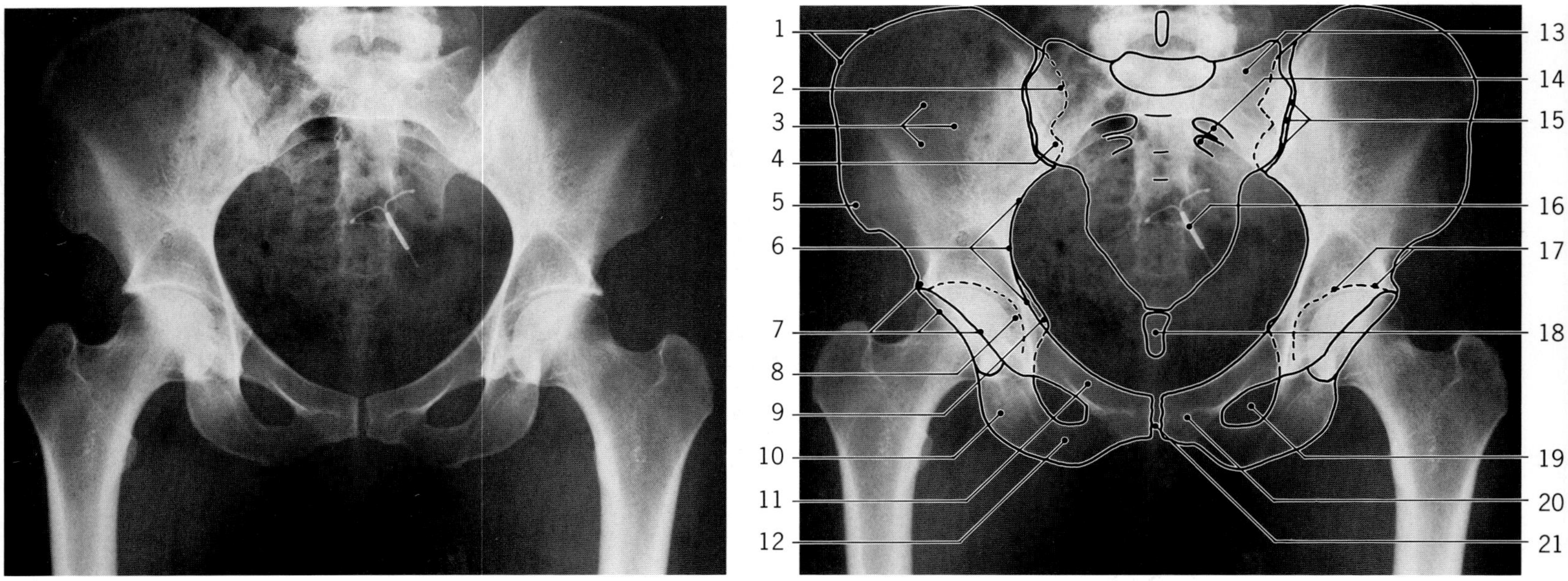

Pelvis, female, a-p X-ray, tilted

1: Iliac crest
2: Posterior superior iliac spine
3: Wing of ilium
4: Posterior inferior iliac spine
5: Anterior superior iliac spine
6: Arcuate line of ilium
7: Acetabular rim
8: Acetabular fossa
9: Ischial spine
10: Ischial tuberosity
11: Superior ramus of pubis
12: Inferior ramus of pubis
13: Ala of sacrum
14: Pelvic sacral foramina
15: Sacro-iliac joint
16: Intrauterine contraceptive device (IUD)
17: Lunate surface of acetabulum
18: Coccyx
19: Obturator foramen
20: Body of pubis
21: Pubic symphysis

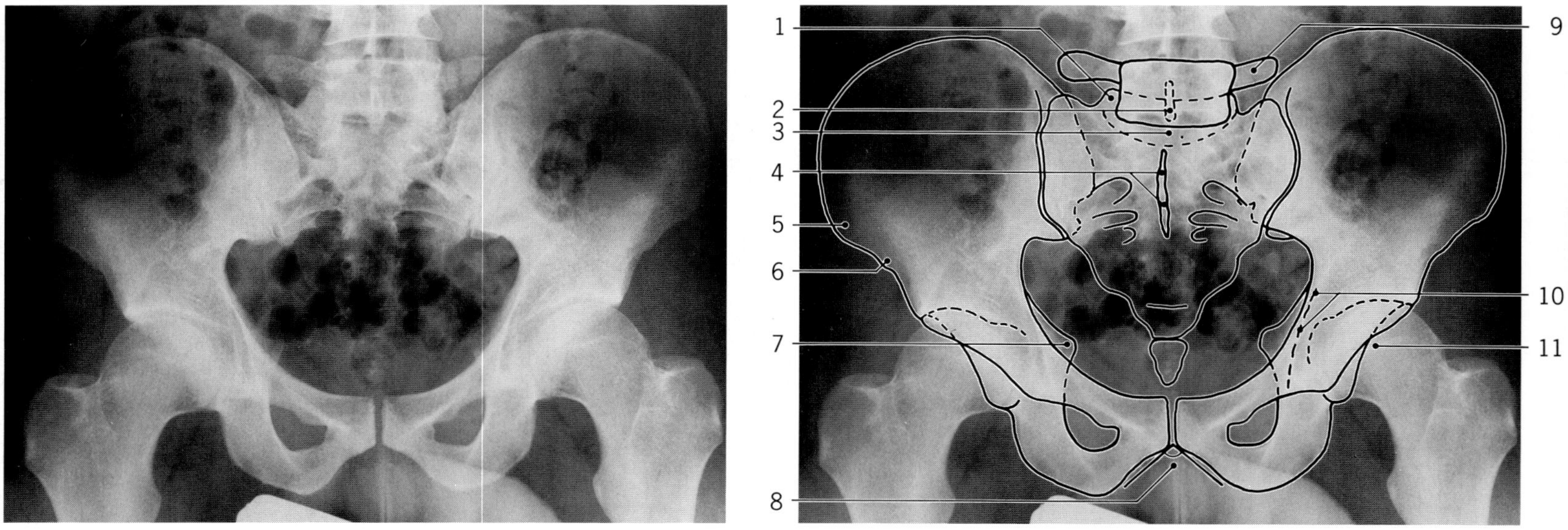

Pelvis, male, a-p X-ray, tilted

1: Zygapophyseal (facet) joint L V-S I
2: Spinous process of L V
3: Promontory
4: Median sacral crest
5: Anterior superior iliac spine
6: Anterior inferior iliac spine
7: Ischial spine
8: Subpubic angle
9: Transverse process of L V
10: Iliopectineal line (radiology term)
11: Femoral head

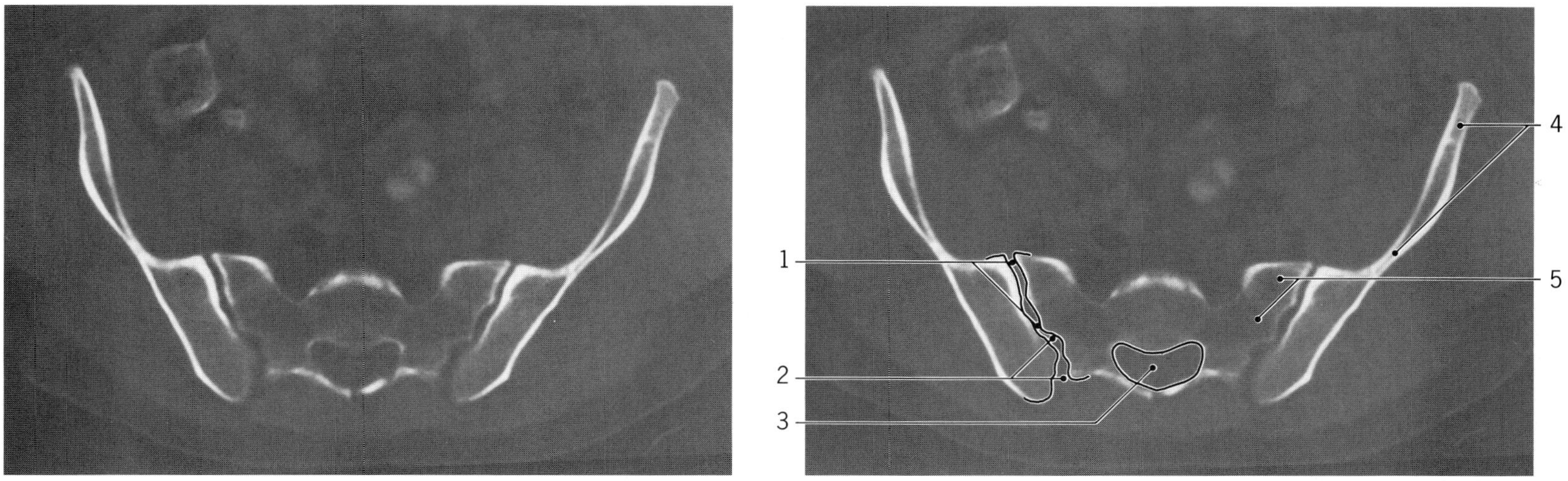

Sacro-iliac joints, axial CT (bone settings)

1: Sacro-iliac joint
2: Interosseous sacro-iliac ligament
3: Sacral canal
4: Ala of ilium
5: Ala of sacrum

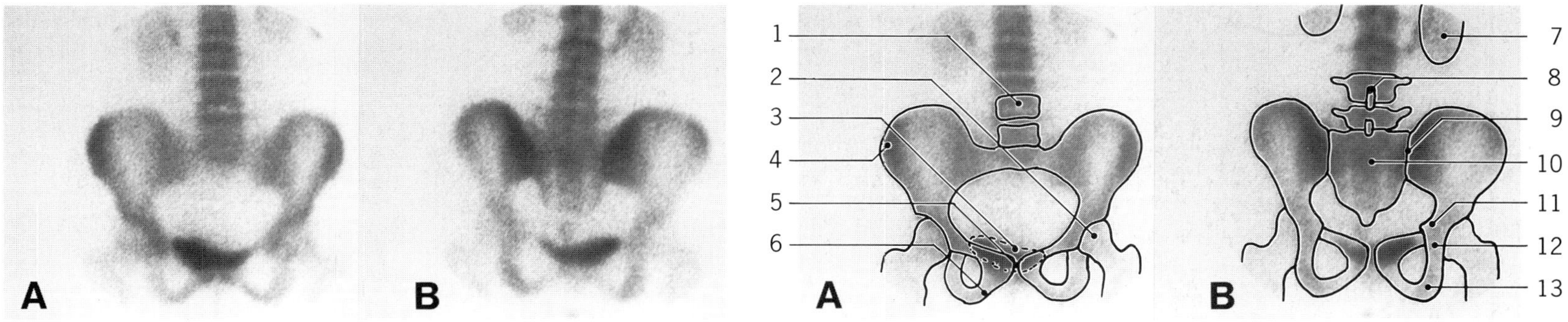

Pelvis, ^{99m}Tc-MDP scintigraphy

A: Anterior view. B: Posterior view

1: Body of fourth lumbar vertebra
2: Femoral head
3: Urinary bladder
4: Tubercle of ilium
5: Pubic symphysis
6: Inferior ramus of pubis
7: Right kidney
8: Spinous process L IV
9: Sacroiliac joint
10: Sacrum
11: Ischial spine
12: Body of ischium
13: Ischial tuberosity

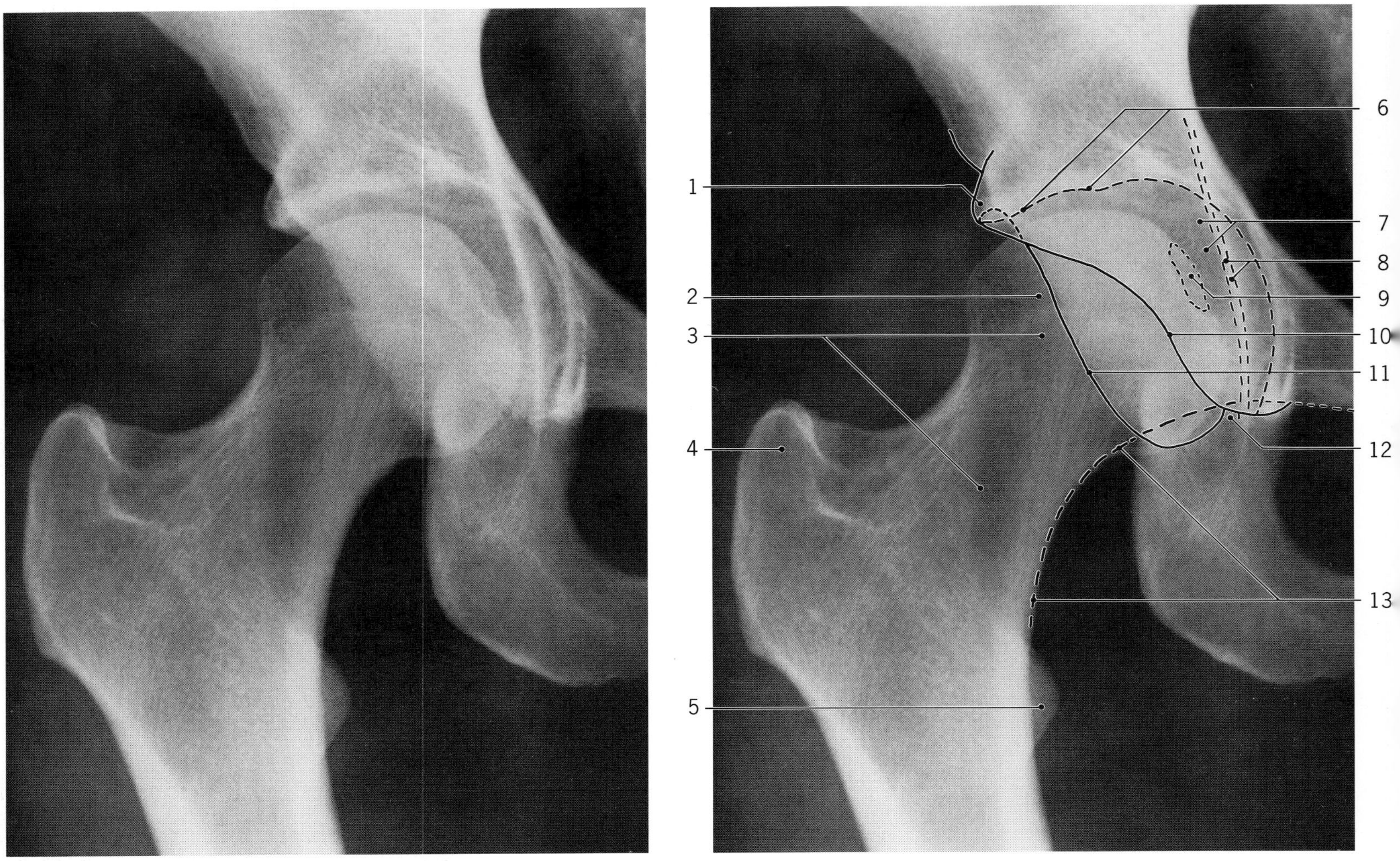

Hip, a-p X-ray

1: Acetabular rim
2: Femoral head
3: Femoral neck
4: Greater trochanter
5: Lesser trochanter
6: Lunate surface
7: Acetabular fossa
8: Iliopectineal line (radiology term)
9: Fovea of femoral head
10: Acetabular rim (anterior)
11: Acetabular rim (posterior)
12: Acetabular notch
13: Shenton's line (radiology term)

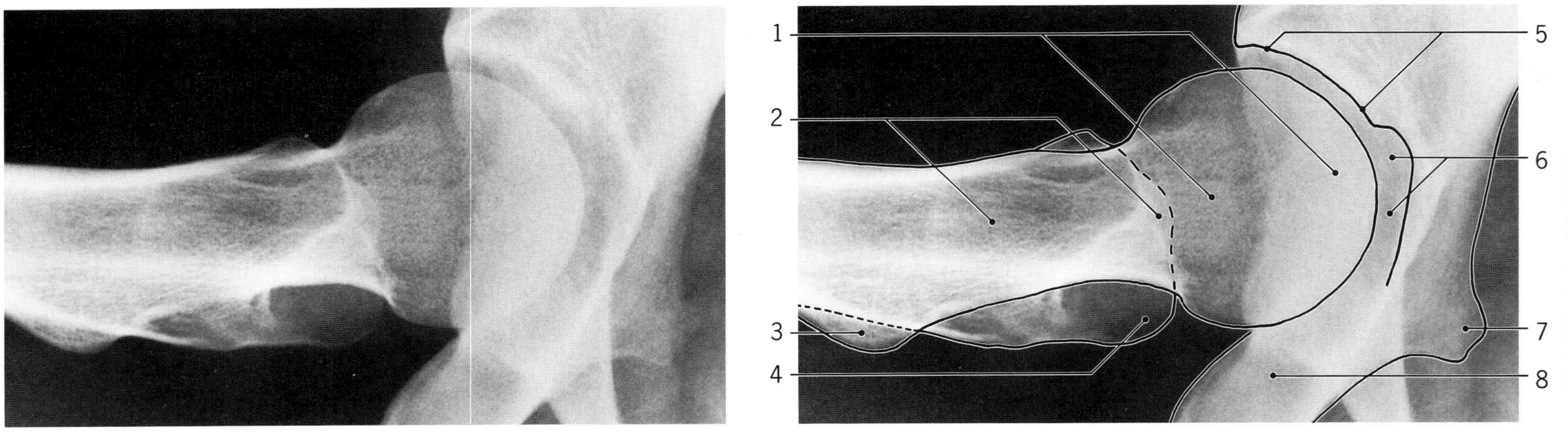

Hip, X-ray

Lauenstein projection (abduced, outward rotated hip joint)

1: Femoral head
2: Femoral neck
3: Lesser trochanter
4: Greater trochanter
5: Lunate surface of acetabulum
6: Acetabular fossa
7: Ischial spine
8: Body of ischium

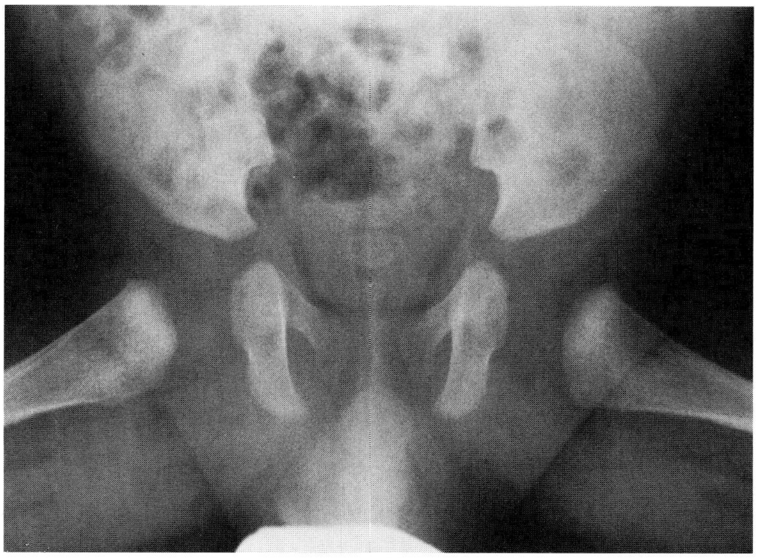

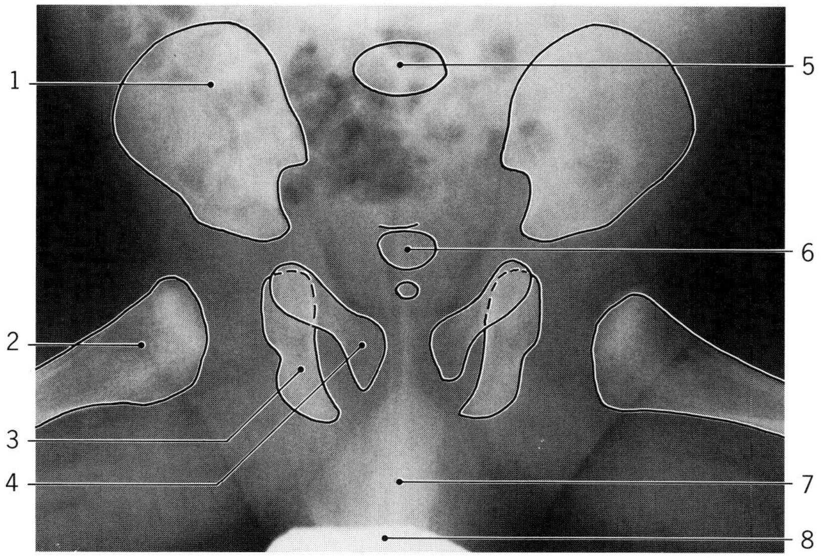

Pelvis, a-p X-ray, child 3 months

Lauenstein projection

1: Ilium
2: Metaphysis of femur
3: Ischium
4: Pubis
5: Sacral vertebra I
6: Sacral vertebra V
7: Penis
8: Gonadal lead shield

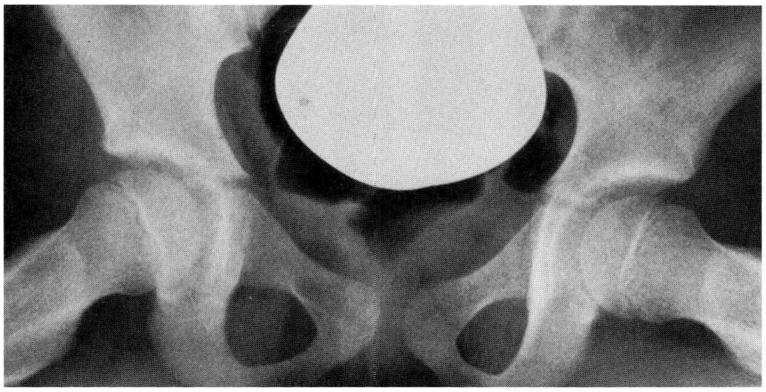

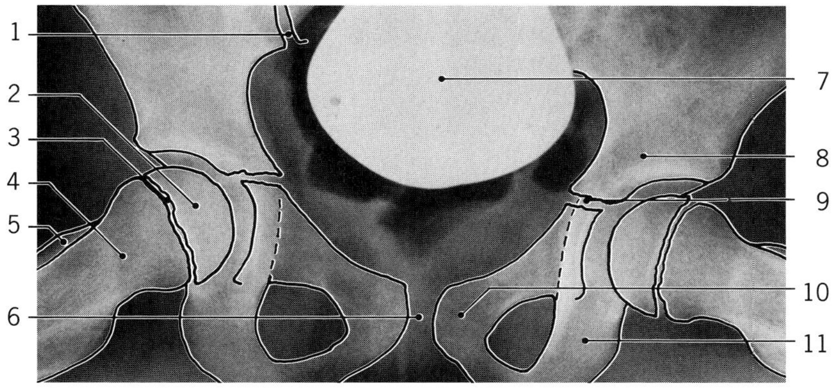

Pelvis, X-ray, child 7 years

Lauenstein projection

1: Sacro-iliac joint
2: Femoral head (epiphysis)
3: Epiphyseal growth plate
4: Femoral neck
5: Greater trochanter
6: Pubic symphysis
7: Gonadal lead shield
8: Body of ilium
9: Synchondrosis of acetabulum
10: Body of pubis
11: Body of ischium

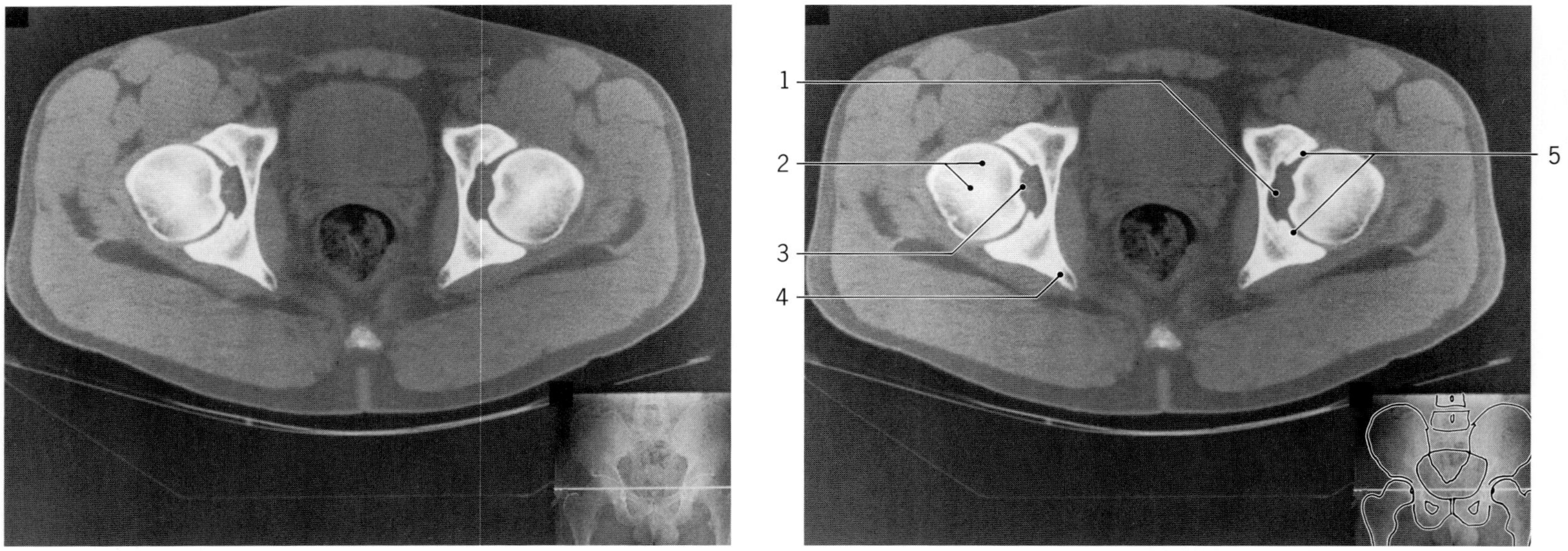

Hip, axial CT

1: Acetabular fossa
2: Femoral head
3: Fovea of femoral head
4: Ischial spine
5: Lunate surface of acetabulum

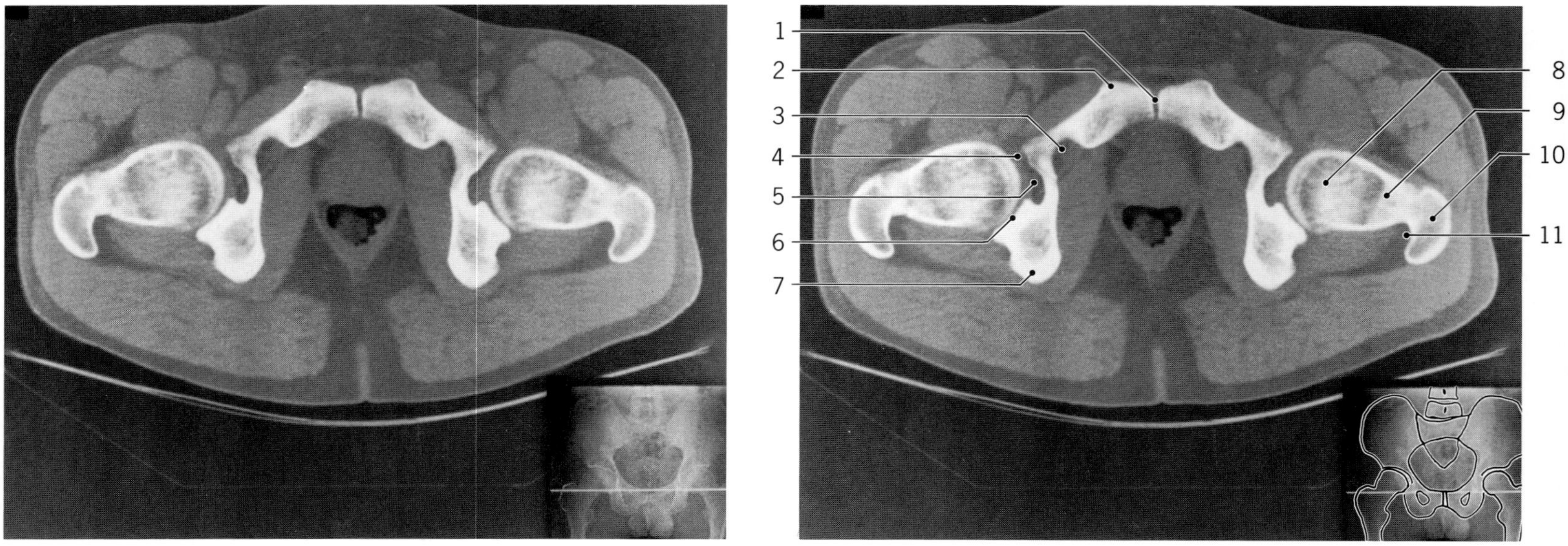

Hip, axial CT

1: Pubic symphysis
2: Pubic tubercle
3: Obturator canal
4: Acetabular notch
5: Acetabular fossa
6: Lunate surface
7: Body of ischium
8: Femoral head
9: Femoral neck
10: Greater trochanter
11: Trochanteric fossa

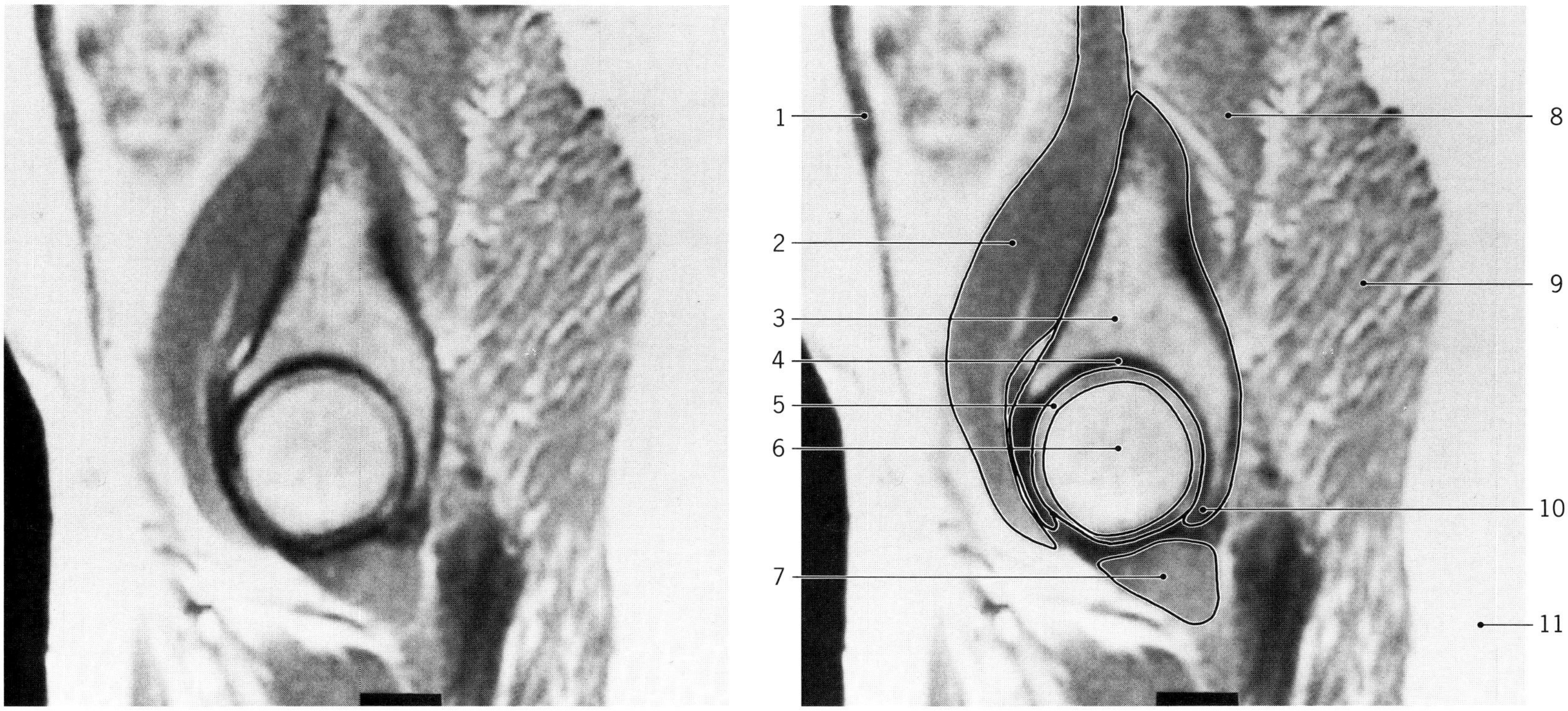

Hip, sagittal MR

1: Abdominal wall muscles
2: Iliopsoas
3: Ilium (red bone marrow)
4: Lunate surface
5: Articular cartilage
6: Femoral head
7: Obturatorius externus
8: Gluteus medius
9: Gluteus maximus
10: Acetabular rim (posteriorly)
11: Subcutaneous fat of nates

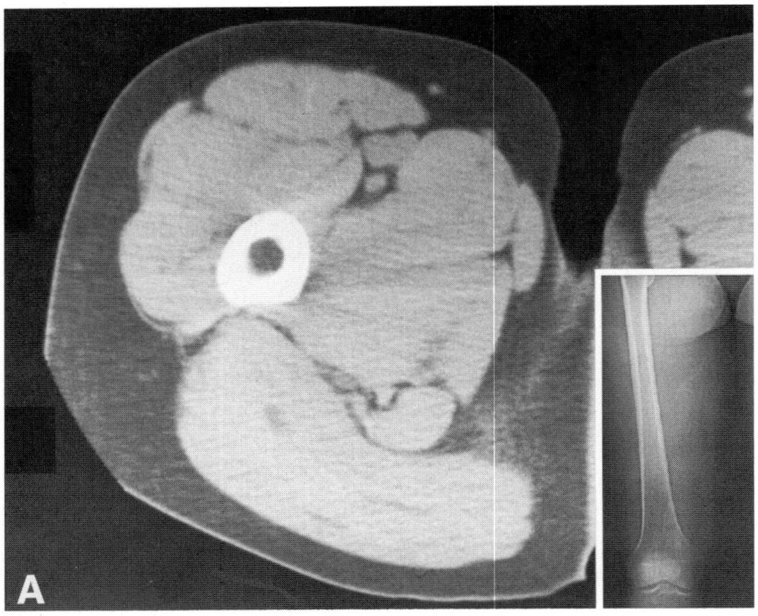

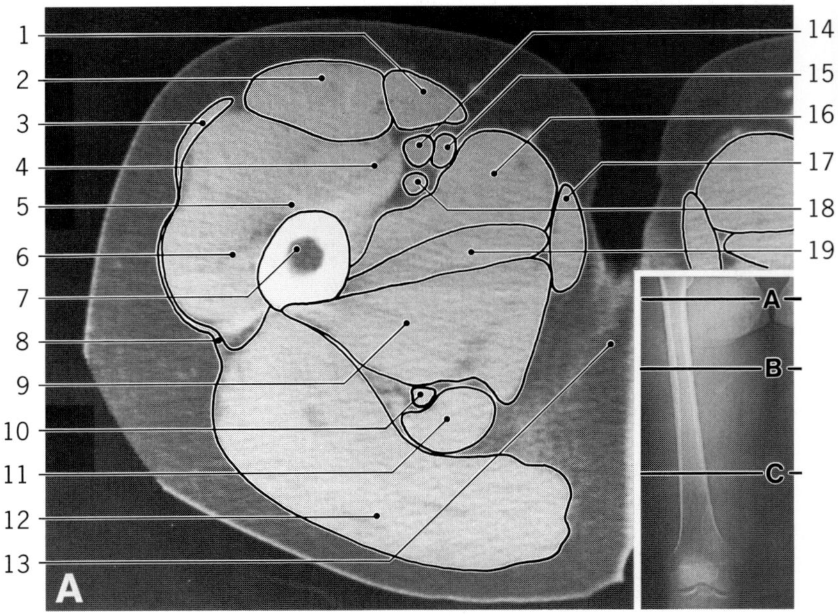

Thigh, proximal, axial CT

1: Sartorius
2: Rectus femoris
3: Tensor fasciae latae
4: Vastus medialis
5: Vastus intermedius
6: Vastus lateralis
7: Femoral shaft
8: Insertion of gluteus maximus in iliotibial tract
9: Adductor magnus
10: Sciatic nerve
11: Common origin of biceps femoris, semitendinosus and semimembranosus
12: Gluteus maximus
13: Perineum
14: Femoral artery
15: Femoral vein
16: Adductor longus
17: Gracilis
18: Profunda femoris artery
19: Adductor brevis

Sections B and C shown on next page

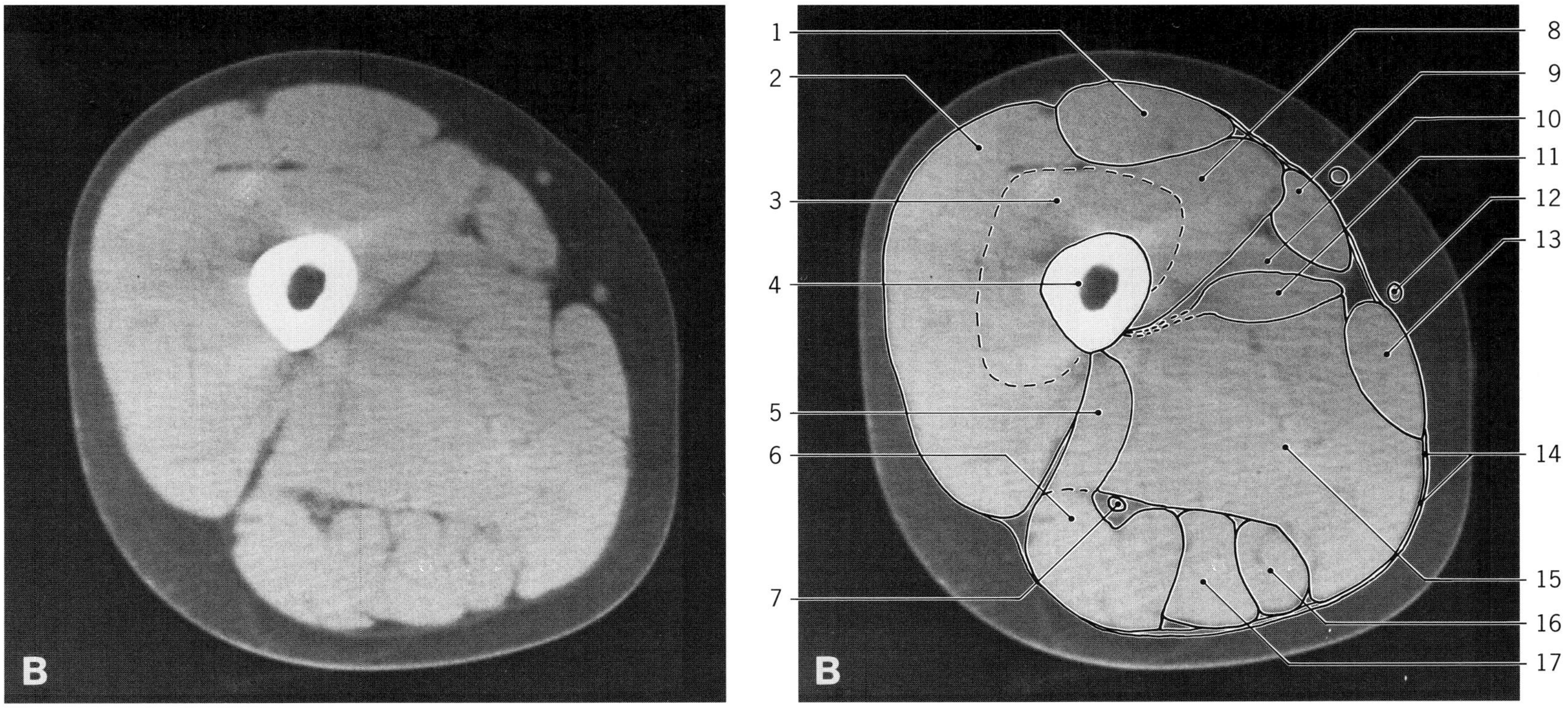

Thigh, middle, axial CT

Scout on previous page

1: Rectus femoris
2: Vastus lateralis
3: Vastus intermedius
4: Femoral shaft
5: Biceps femoris, short head
6: Biceps femoris, long head
7: Sciatic nerve
8: Vastus medialis
9: Sartorius
10: Femoral artery and vein in adductor canal
11: Adductor longus
12: Superficial vein
13: Gracilis
14: Fascia lata
15: Adductor magnus
16: Semimembranosus
17: Semitendinosus

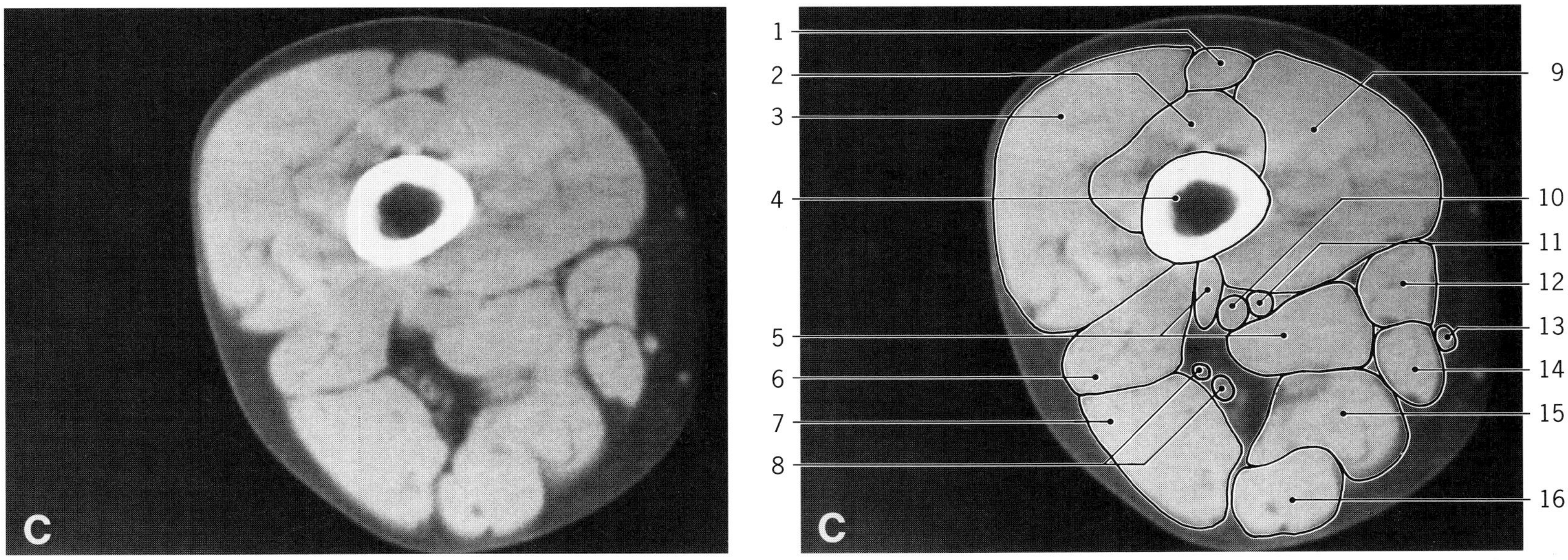

Thigh, distal, axial CT

Scout on previous page

1: Rectus femoris
2: Vastus intermedius
3: Vastus lateralis
4: Femoral shaft
5: Adductor magnus, on both sides of hiatus adductorius
6: Biceps femoris, short head
7: Biceps femoris, long head
8: Tibial and common peroneal nerve
9: Vastus medialis
10: Femoral vein (in hiatus adductorius)
11: Femoral artery
12: Sartorius
13: Great saphenous vein
14: Gracilis
15: Semimembranosus
16: Semitendinosus

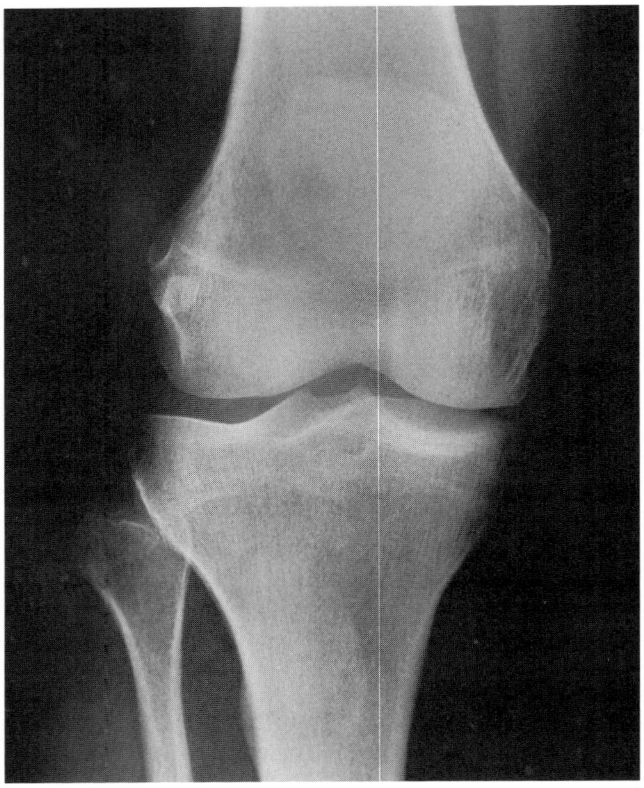

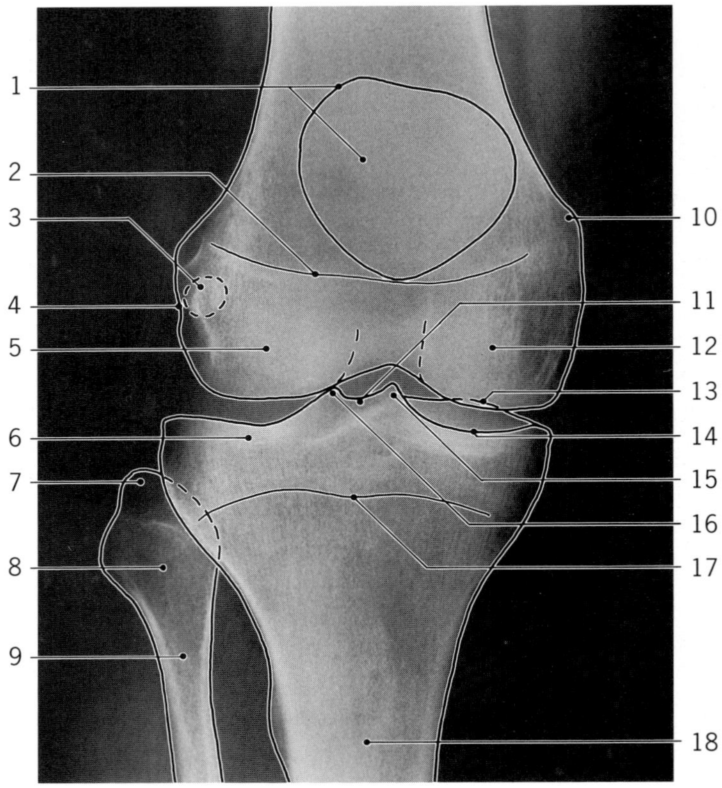

Knee, a-p X-ray

1: Patella
2: Epiphyseal scar
3: Fabella
4: Insertion of popliteus tendon
5: Lateral condyle of femur
6: Lateral condyle of tibia
7: Apex of fibula
8: Head of fibula
9: Neck of fibula
10: Adductor tubercle
11: Intercondylar eminence
12: Medial condyle of femur
13: Medial condyle of tibia (anterior margin)
14: Medial condyle of tibia (posterior margin)
15: Medial intercondylar tubercle
16: Lateral intercondylar tubercle
17: Epiphyseal scar
18: Body of tibia

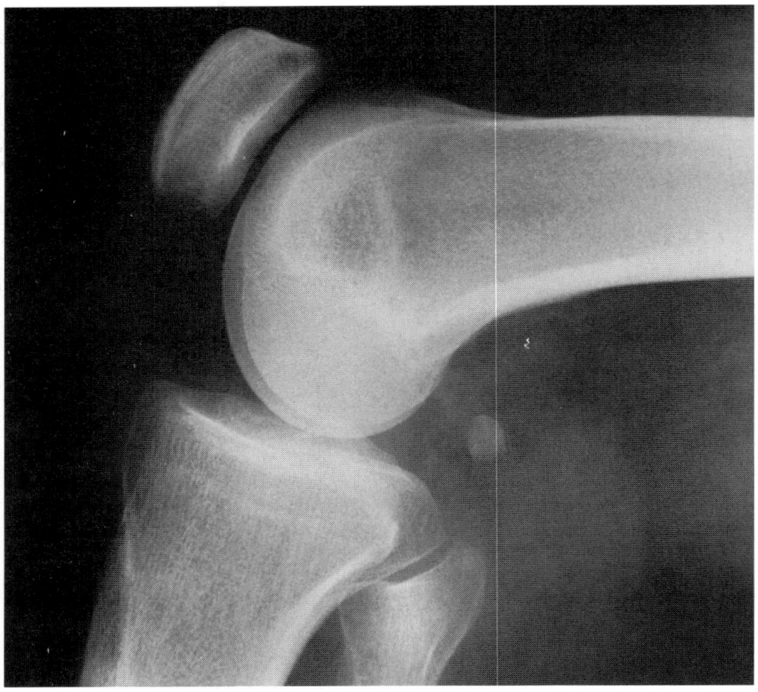

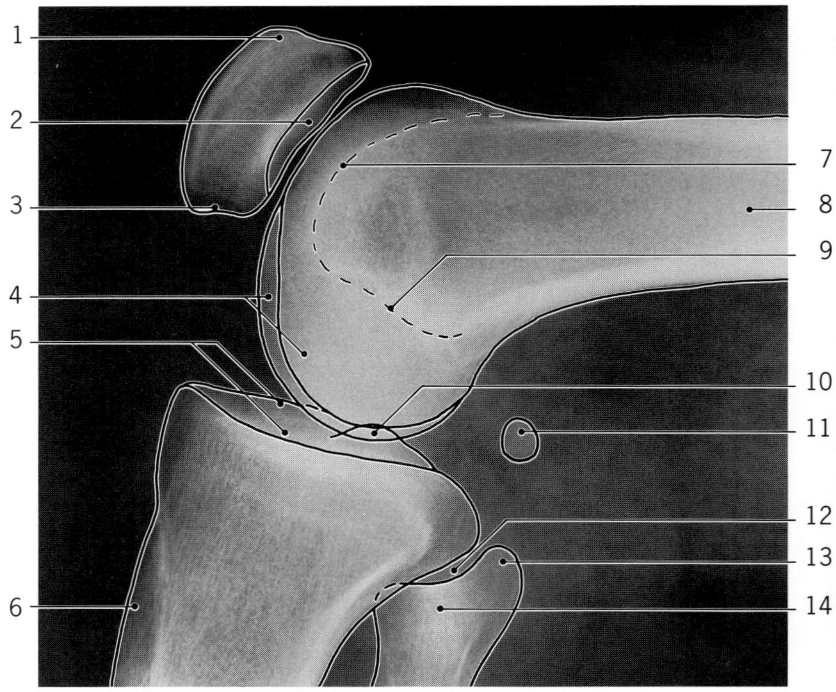

Knee, flexed, lateral X-ray

1: Base of patella
2: Articular surface of patella
3: Apex of patella
4: Femoral condyles
5: Superior articular surface of tibia
6: Tibial tuberosity
7: Patellar surface of femur
8: Shaft of femur
9: Intercondylar fossa (bottom)
10: Intercondylar eminence
11: Fabella
12: Tibiofibular joint
13: Apex of fibula
14: Head of fibula

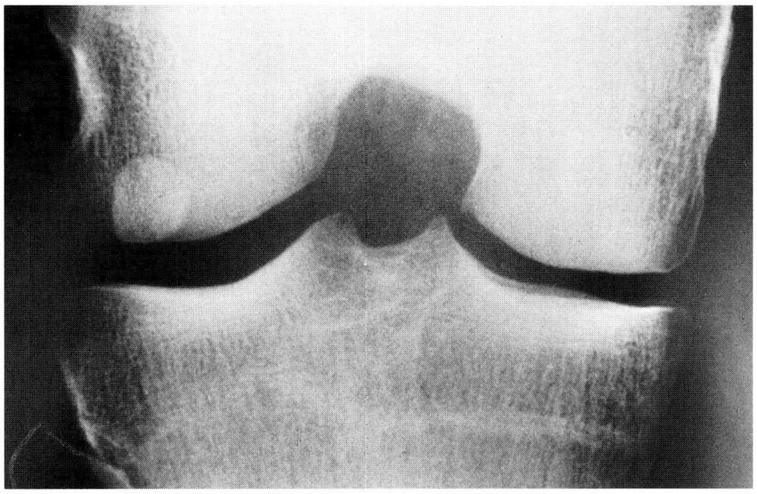

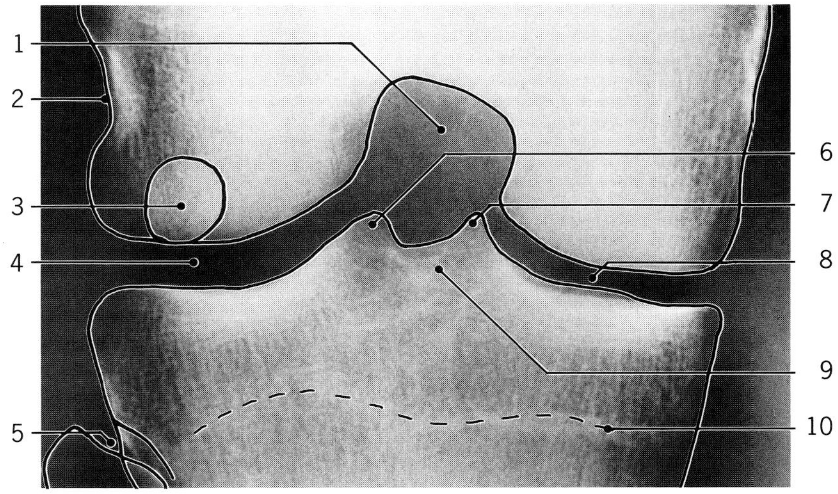

Knee, half flexed, tilted X-ray ("intercondylar notch projection")

1: Intercondylar fossa
2: Insertion of popliteus tendon
3: Fabella
4: Lateral femurotibial joint
5: Tibiofibular joint
6: Lateral intercondylar tubercle
7: Medial intercondylar tubercle
8: Medial femurotibial joint
9: Intercondylar eminence
10: Epiphyseal scar

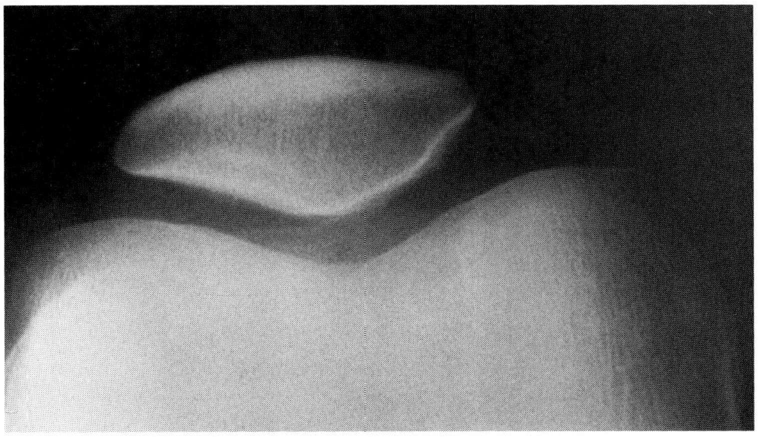

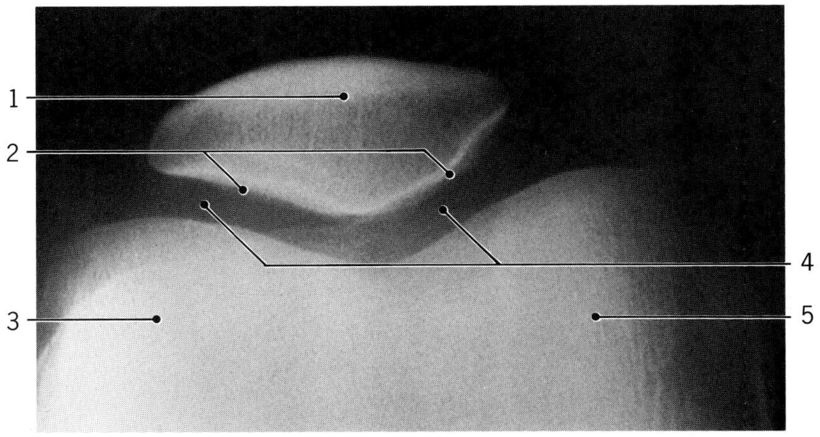

Knee, flexed, axial X-ray

"Sunrise" view of patella

1: Patella
2: Articular surface of patella
3: Lateral condyle of femur
4: Femuropatellar joint
5: Medial condyle of femur

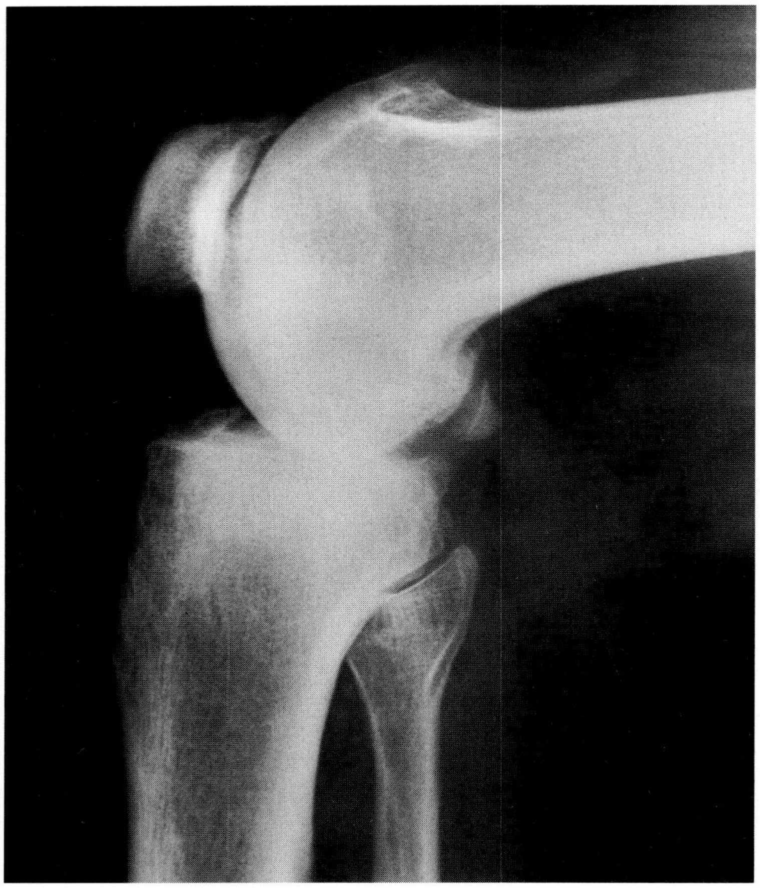

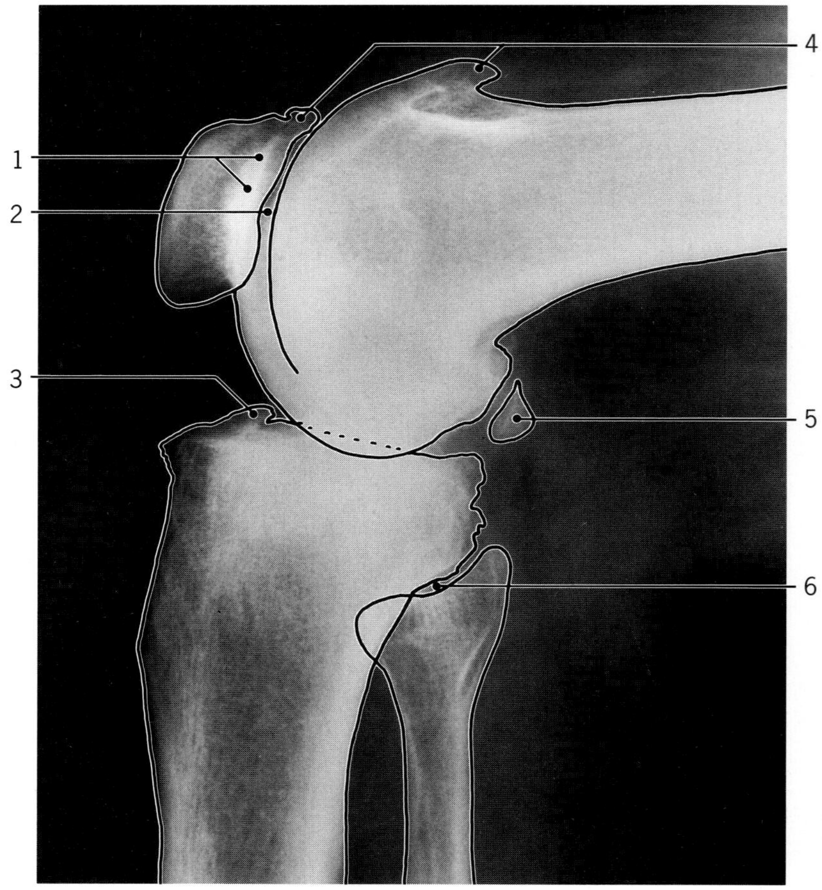

Knee, flexed, lateral X-ray, old age

With signs of arthrosis

1: Subchondral sclerosis of patella
2: Femuropatellar joint (narrow)
3: Osteophytes in anterior intercondylar area
4: Osteophytes
5: Fabella
6: Tibiofibular joint

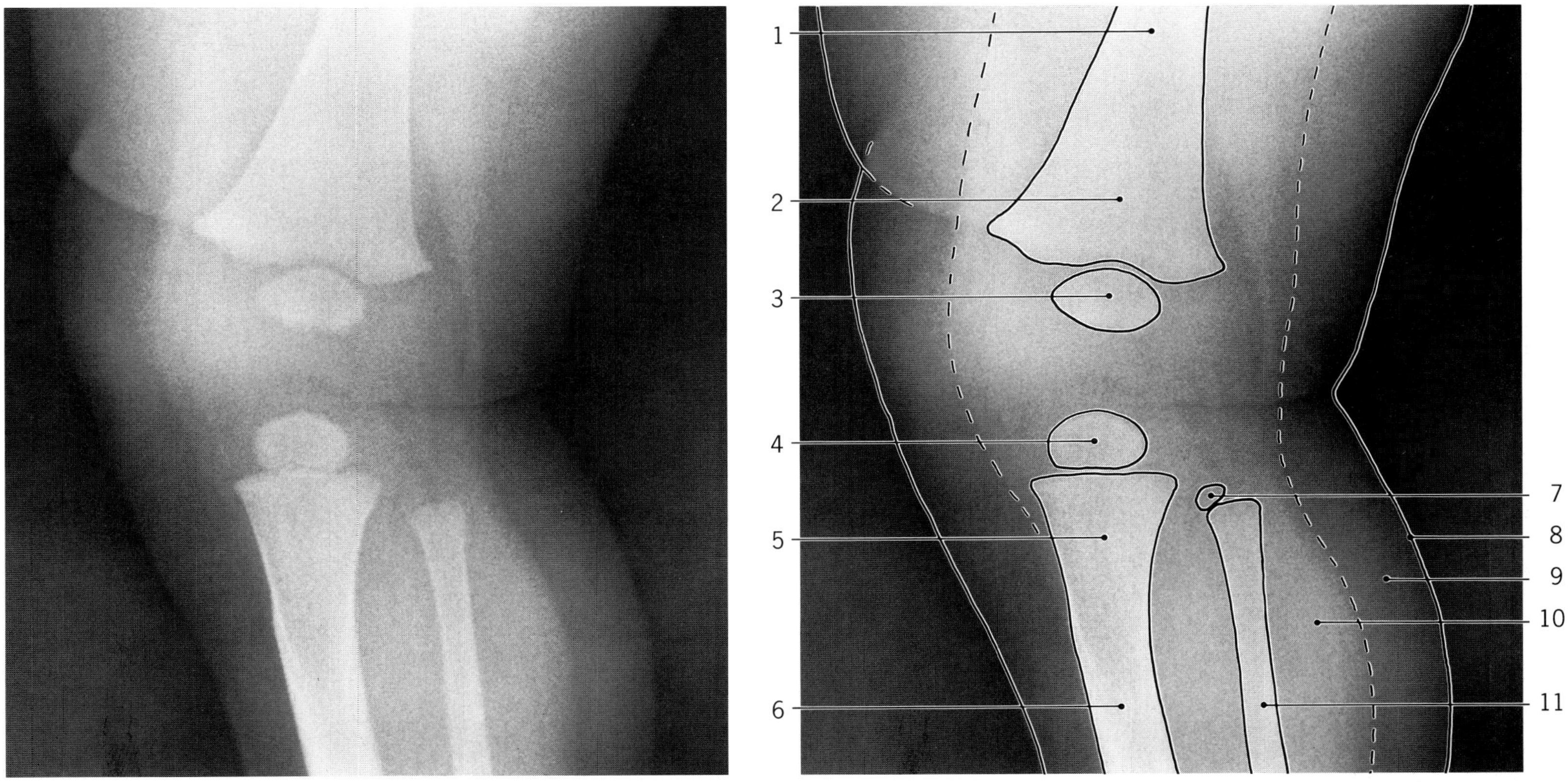

Knee, lateral X-ray, child 3 months

1: Diaphysis of femur
2: Metaphysis of femur
3: Distal epiphysis of femur (Béclard's nucleus)
4: Proximal epiphysis of tibia
5: Metaphysis of tibia
6: Diaphysis of tibia
7: Proximal epiphysis of fibula
8: Skin
9: Subcutis
10: Leg muscles
11: Diaphysis of fibula

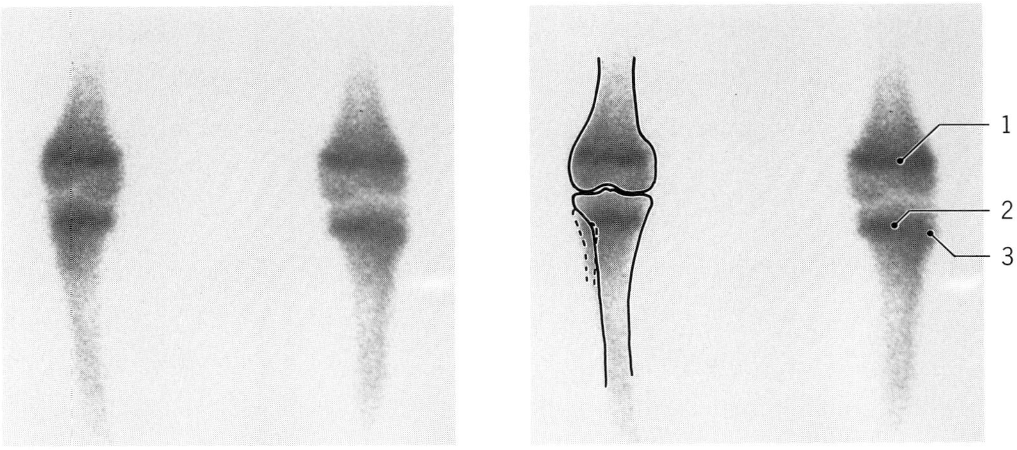

Knee, ^{99m}Tc-MDP, scintigraphy, child 12 years

1: Growth plate of distal epiphysis of femur
2: Growth plate of proximal epiphysis of tibia
3: Growth plate of proximal epiphysis of fibula

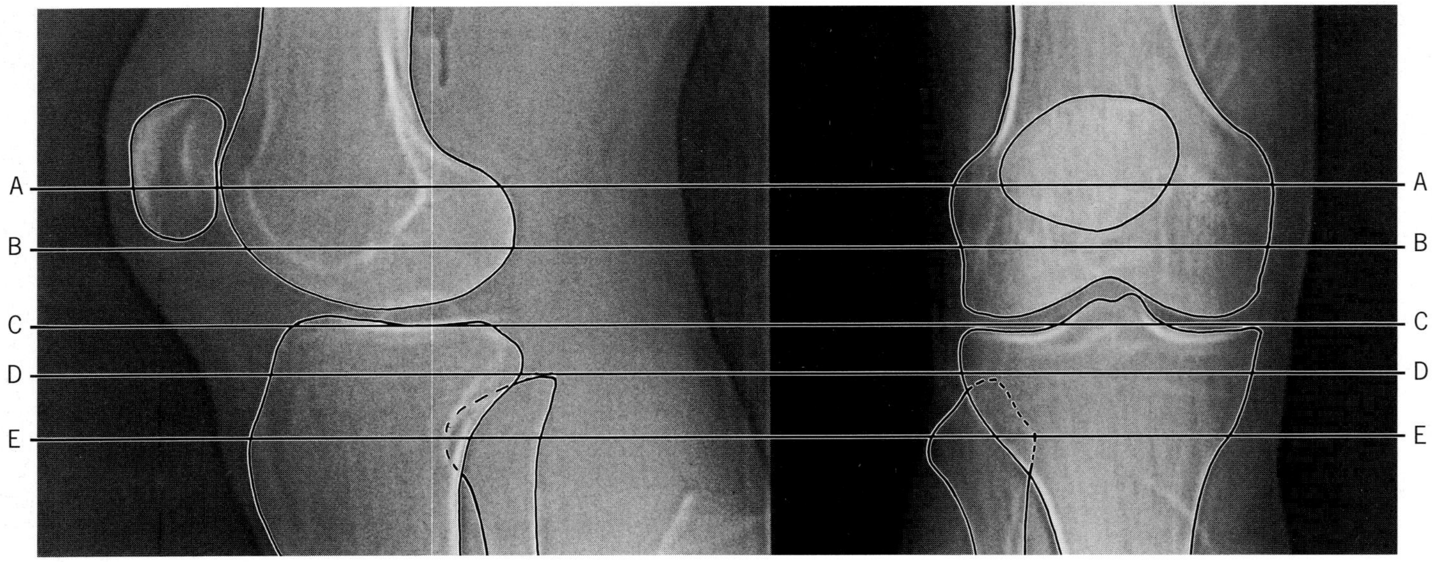

Knee, scout views

A to E indicate planes of sectioning for the following five tomograms.

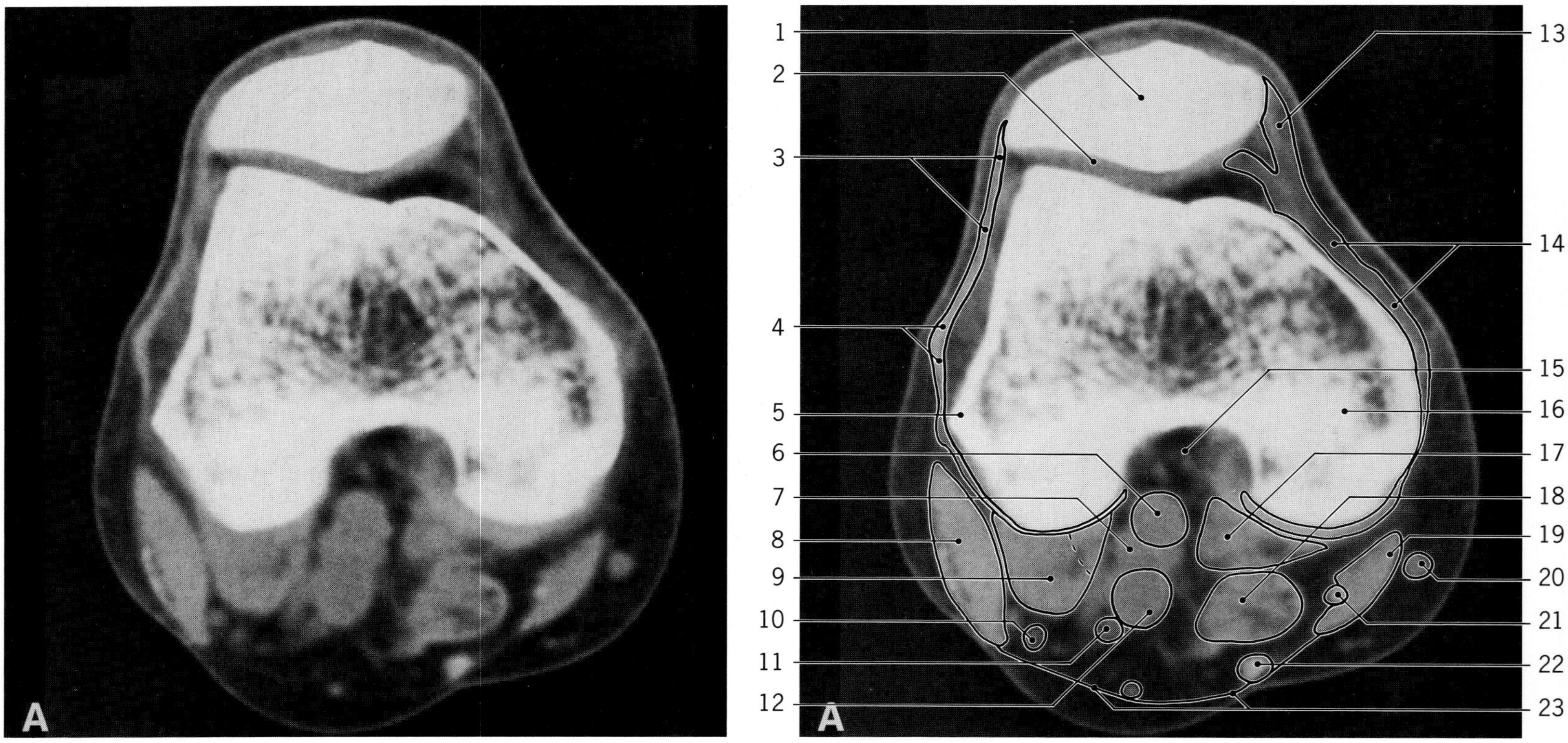

Knee, axial CT

Level of section indicated on scout view

1: Patella
2: Articular cartilage of femuropatellar joint
3: Articular capsule with lateral patellar retinaculum
4: Iliotibial tract
5: Lateral epicondyle of femur
6: Popliteal artery
7: Comitant veins
8: Biceps femoris
9: Gastrocnemius, lateral head, and plantaris
10: Common peroneal nerve
11: Tibial nerve
12: Popliteal vein
13: Vastus medialis (insertion)
14: Articular capsule
15: Intercondylar fossa
16: Medial condyle of femur
17: Gastrocnemius, medial head
18: Semimembranosus
19: Sartorius
20: Great saphenous vein
21: Gracilis (tendon)
22: Semitendinosus (tendon)
23: Fascia poplitea

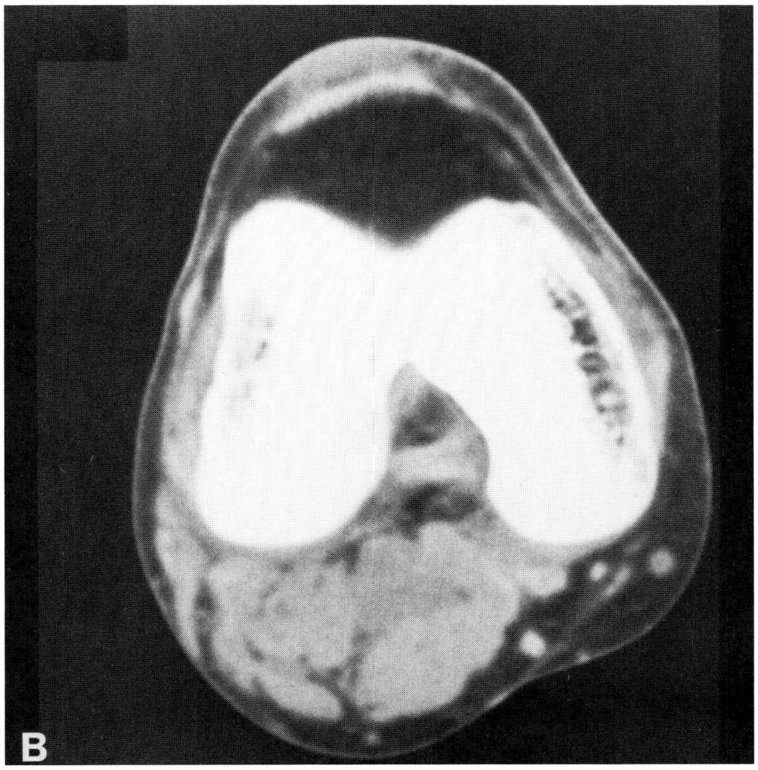

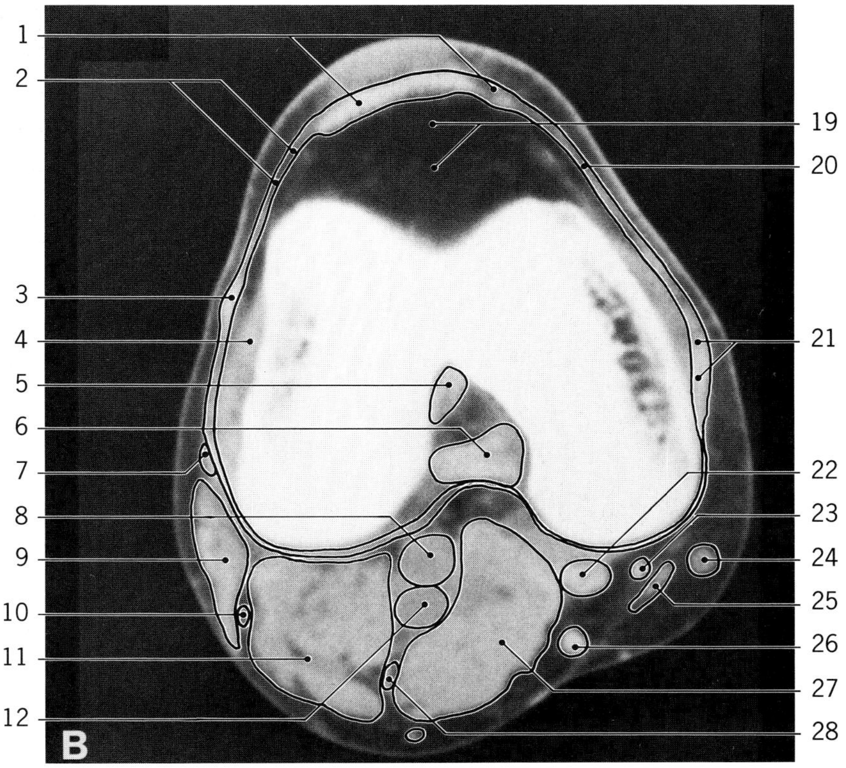

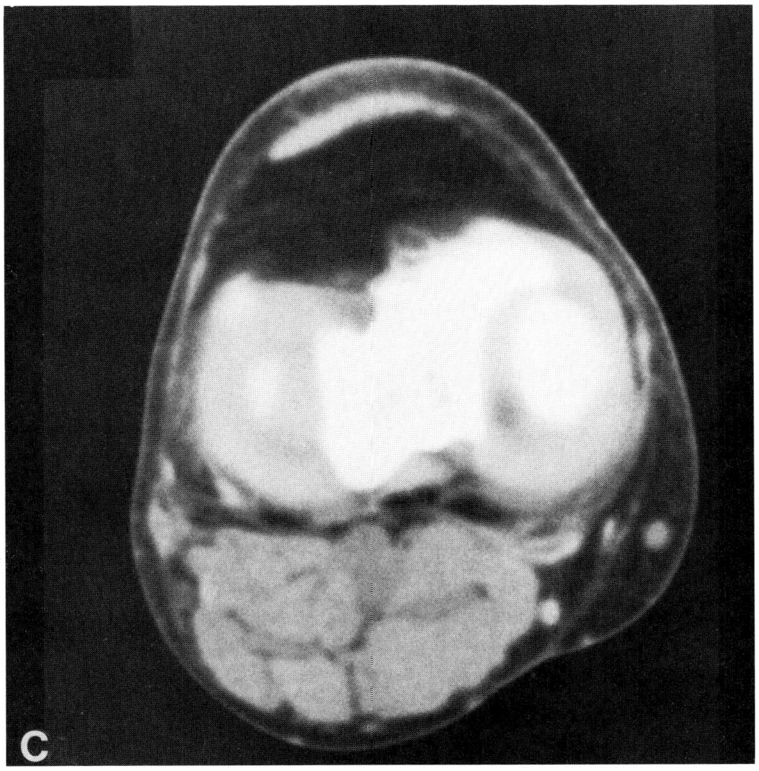

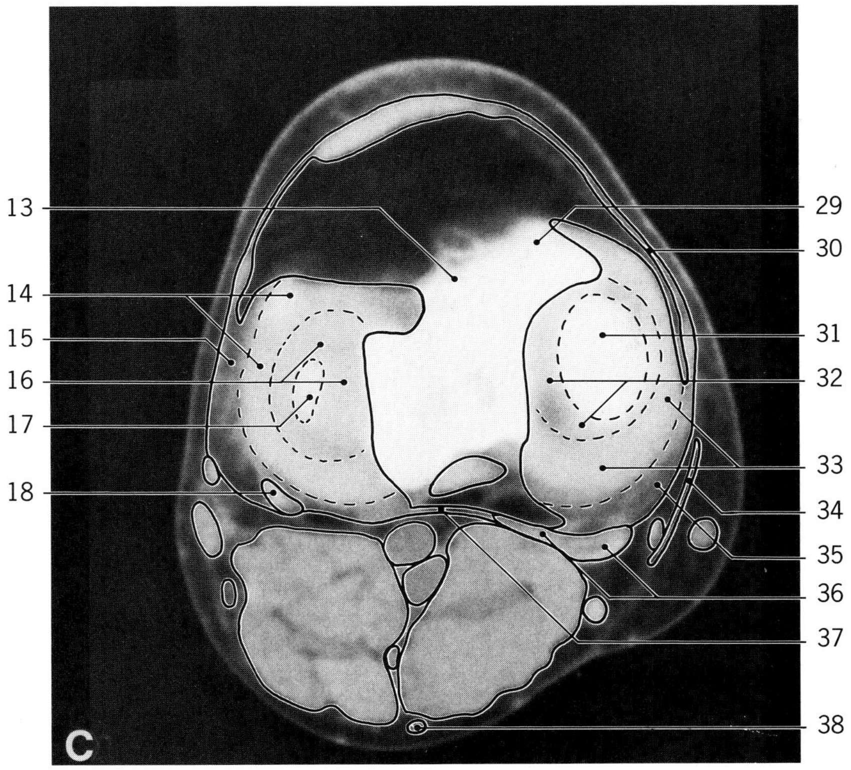

Knee, axial CT

Level of sections indicated on scout view

1: Lig. patellae
2: Lateral patellar retinaculum
3: Iliotibial tract
4: Popliteus (insertion)
5: Anterior cruciate ligament
6: Posterior cruciate ligament
7: Fibular collateral ligament
8: Popliteal artery
9: Biceps femoris
10: Common peroneal nerve
11: Gastrocnemius, lateral head
12: Popliteal vein
13: Anterior intercondylar area
14: Lateral meniscus
15: Connection of meniscus with capsule
16: Articular cartilage of femural condyle
17: Bone of femural condyle
18: Popliteus (tendon)
19: Infrapatellar fat pad
20: Medial patellar retinaculum
21: Tibial collateral ligament
22: Semimembranosus
23: Gracilis (tendon)
24: Great saphenous vein
25: Sartorius
26: Semitendinosus (tendon)
27: Gastrocnemius, medial head
28: Tibial nerve
29: Medial condyle of tibia, anterior rim
30: Articular capsule
31: Bone of femural condyle
32: Articular cartilage of femural condyle
33: Medial meniscus
34: Pes anserinus
35: Connection of meniscus with capsule
36: Semimembranosus, and oblique popliteal ligament
37: Articular capsule
38: Small saphenous vein

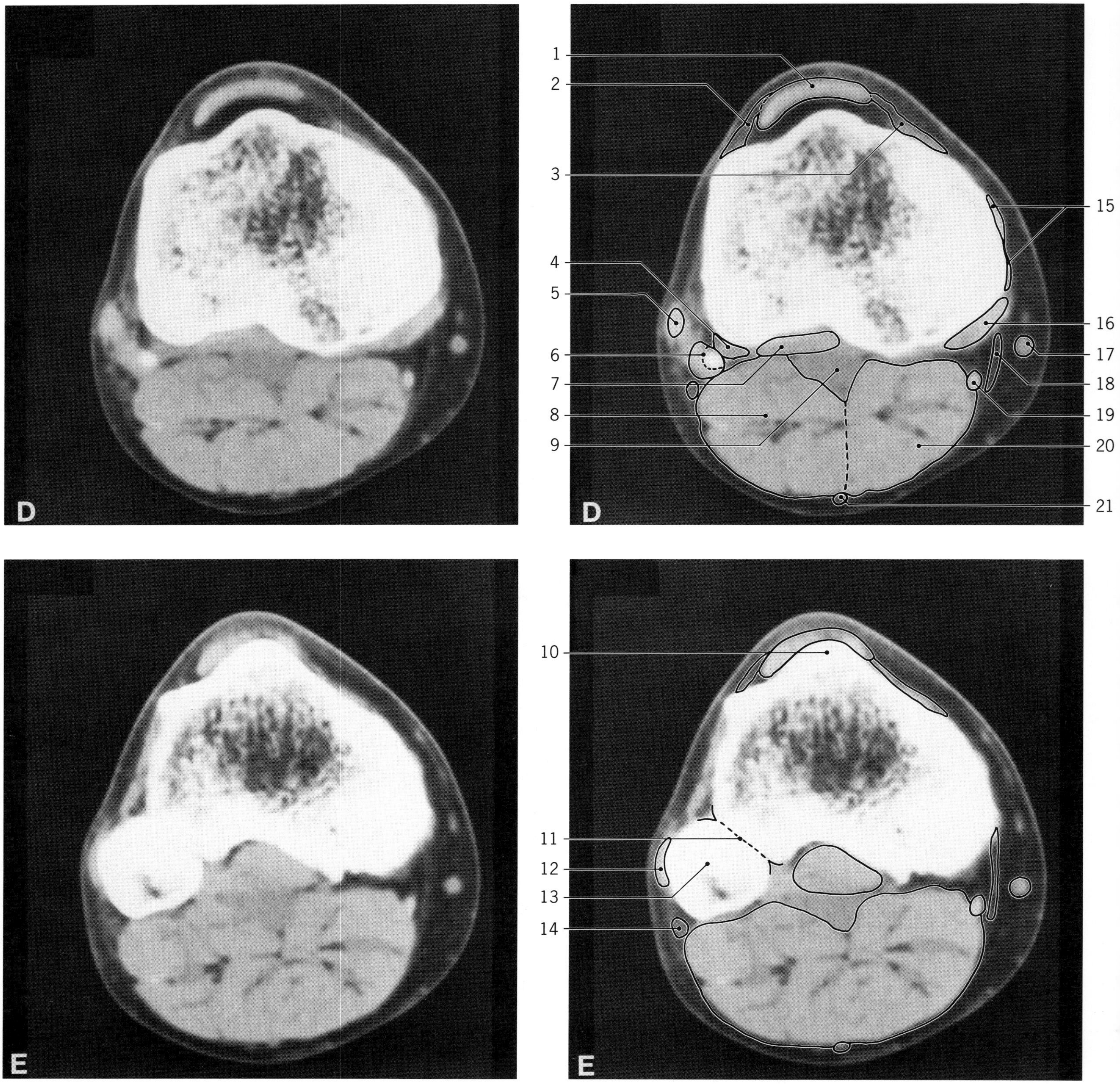

Knee, axial CT

Level of sections indicated on scout view p.92.

1: Ligamentum patellae
2: Lateral patellar retinaculum
3: Medial patellar retinaculum
4: Arcuate popliteal ligament
5: Fibular collateral ligament
6: Biceps femoris (insertion)
7: Popliteus
8: Gastrocnemius, lateral head
9: Popliteal artery and vein
10: Tibial tuberosity
11: Tibiofibular joint
12: Fibular collateral ligament (insertion)
13: Head of fibula
14: Common peroneal nerve
15: Tibial collateral ligament
16: Semimembranosus (insertion)
17: Great saphenous vein
18: Pes anserinus
19: Semitendinosus (tendon)
20: Gastrocnemius, medial head
21: Small saphenous vein

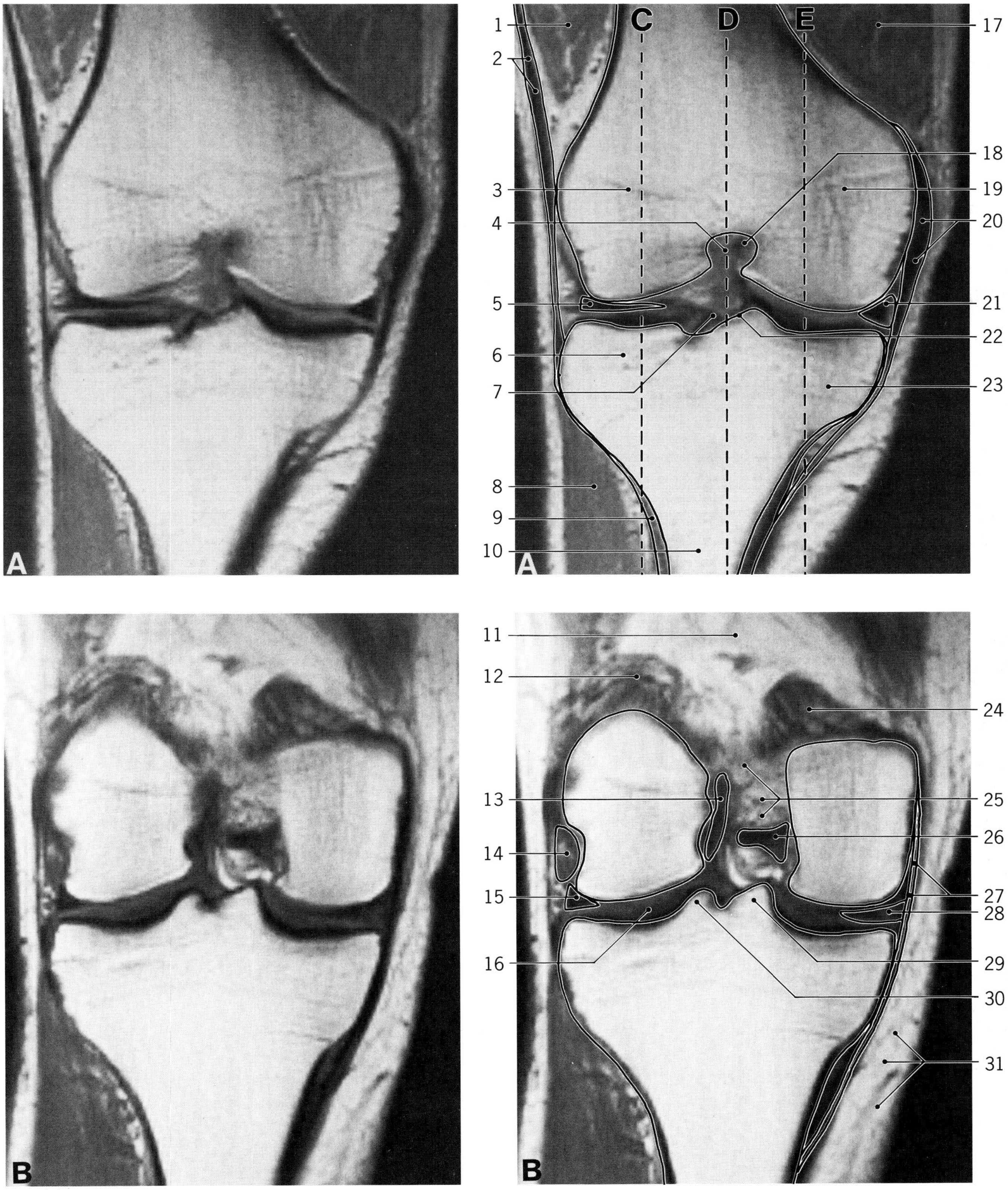

Knee, coronal MR

Plane of sectioning is indicated on section C (next page)

1: Vastus lateralis
2: Iliotibial tract
3: Lateral condyle of femur
4: Intercondylar fossa
5: Lateral meniscus
6: Lateral condyle of tibia
7: Anterior cruciate ligament
8: Tibialis anterior
9: Compact bone of tibia
10: Cancellous bone and bone marrow
11: Fat in popliteal fossa
12: Gastrocnemius, lateral head
13: Anterior cruciate ligament
14: Popliteus (tendon)
15: Lateral meniscus
16: Articular cartilage
17: Vastus medialis
18: Posterior cruciate ligament (origin)
19: Medial condyle of femur
20: Tibial collateral ligament
21: Medial meniscus
22: Anterior intercondylar area
23: Medial condyle of tibia
24: Gastrocnemius, medial head
25: Fat in intercondylar fossa
26: Posterior cruciate ligament
27: Articular capsule
28: Medial meniscus
29: Medial intercondylar tubercle
30: Lateral intercondylar tubercle
31: Subcutaneous fat

Stippled lines C, D and E mark position of sections on following pages.

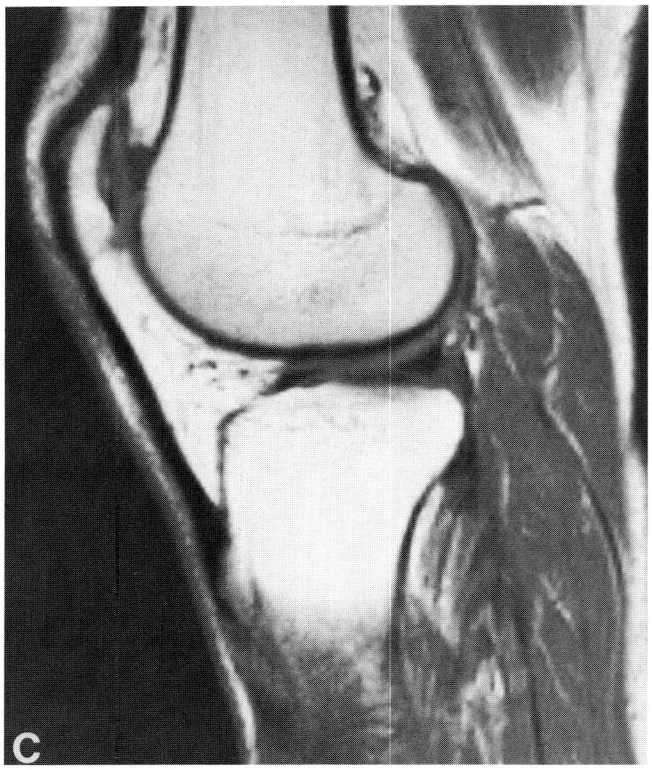

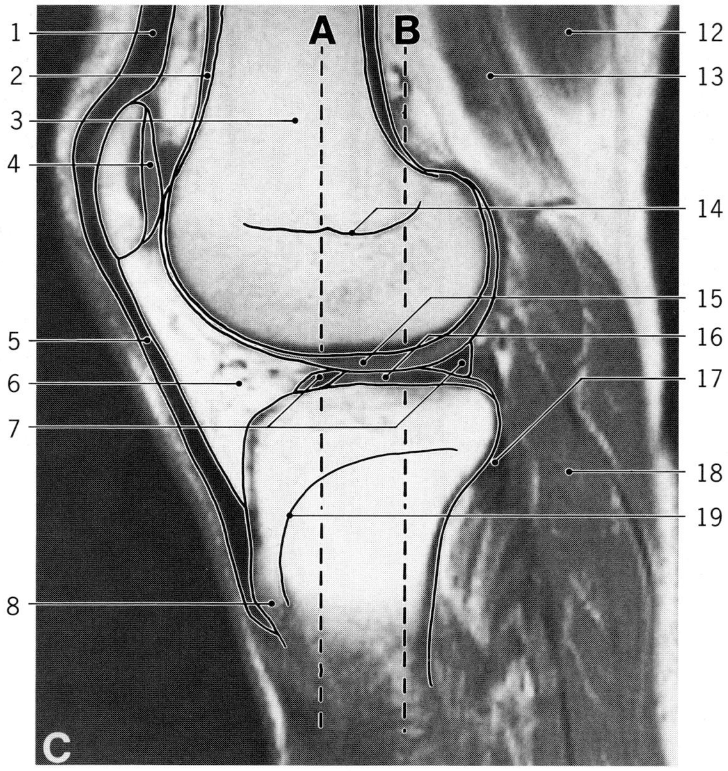

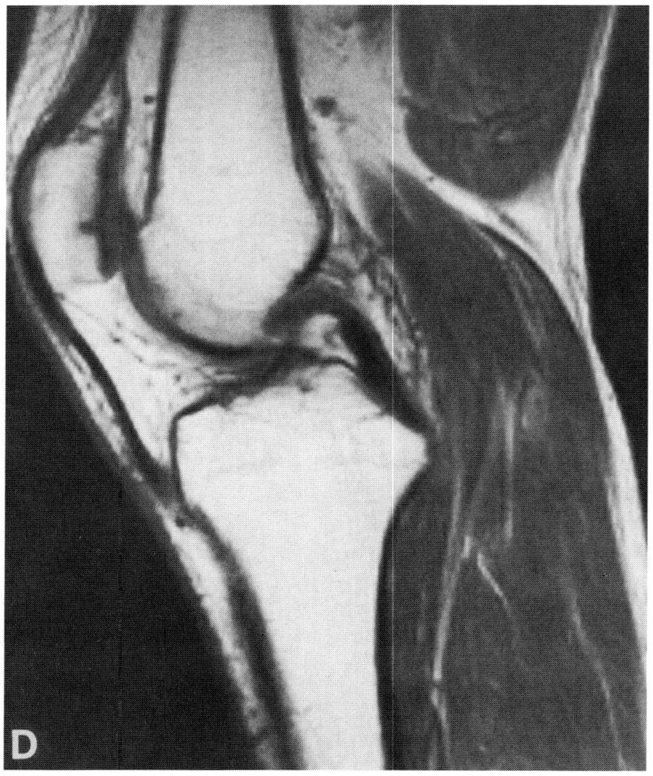

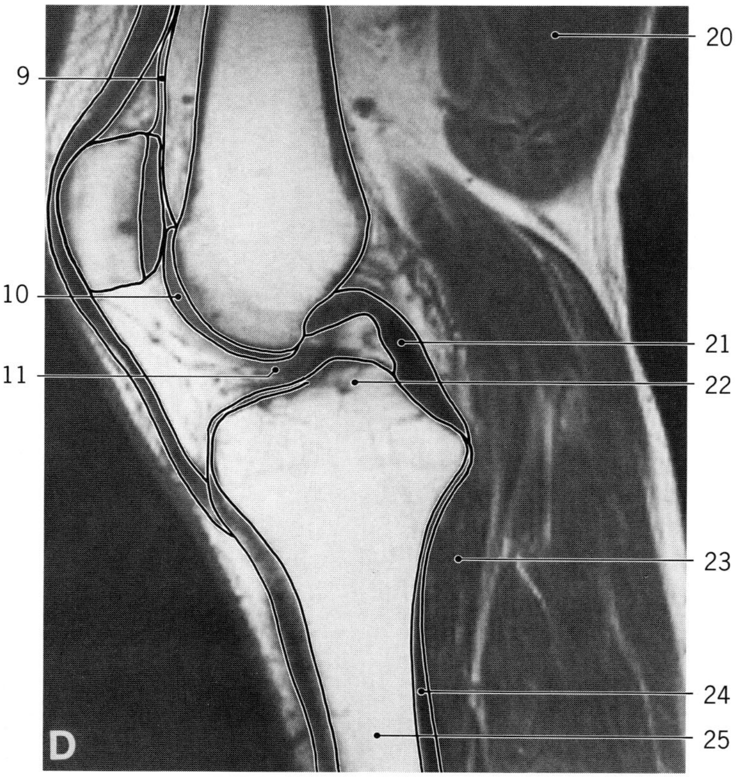

Knee, sagittal MR

C: Through lateral condyles. D: Through intercondylar fossa. Plane of sectioning indicated on section A (previous page)

1: Quadriceps femoris
2: Compact bone of femur
3: Cancellous bone and bone marrow
4: Articular cartilage of patella
5: Ligamentum patellae
6: Infrapatellar fat pad
7: Lateral meniscus
8: Tibial tuberosity
9: Suprapatellar bursa
10: Articular cartilage of femur
11: Infrapatellar synovial fold
12: Biceps femoris, long head
13: Biceps femoris, short head
14: Epiphyseal scar
15: Articular cartilage of lateral condyle of femur
16: Articular cartilage of lateral condyle of tibia
17: Popliteus (tendon)
18: Gastrocnemius, lateral head
19: Epiphyseal scar
20: Semimembranosus
21: Posterior cruciate ligament
22: Intercondylar eminence
23: Popliteus
24: Compact bone of tibia
25: Bone marrow of tibia

Stippled lines A and B mark position of sections on previous page.

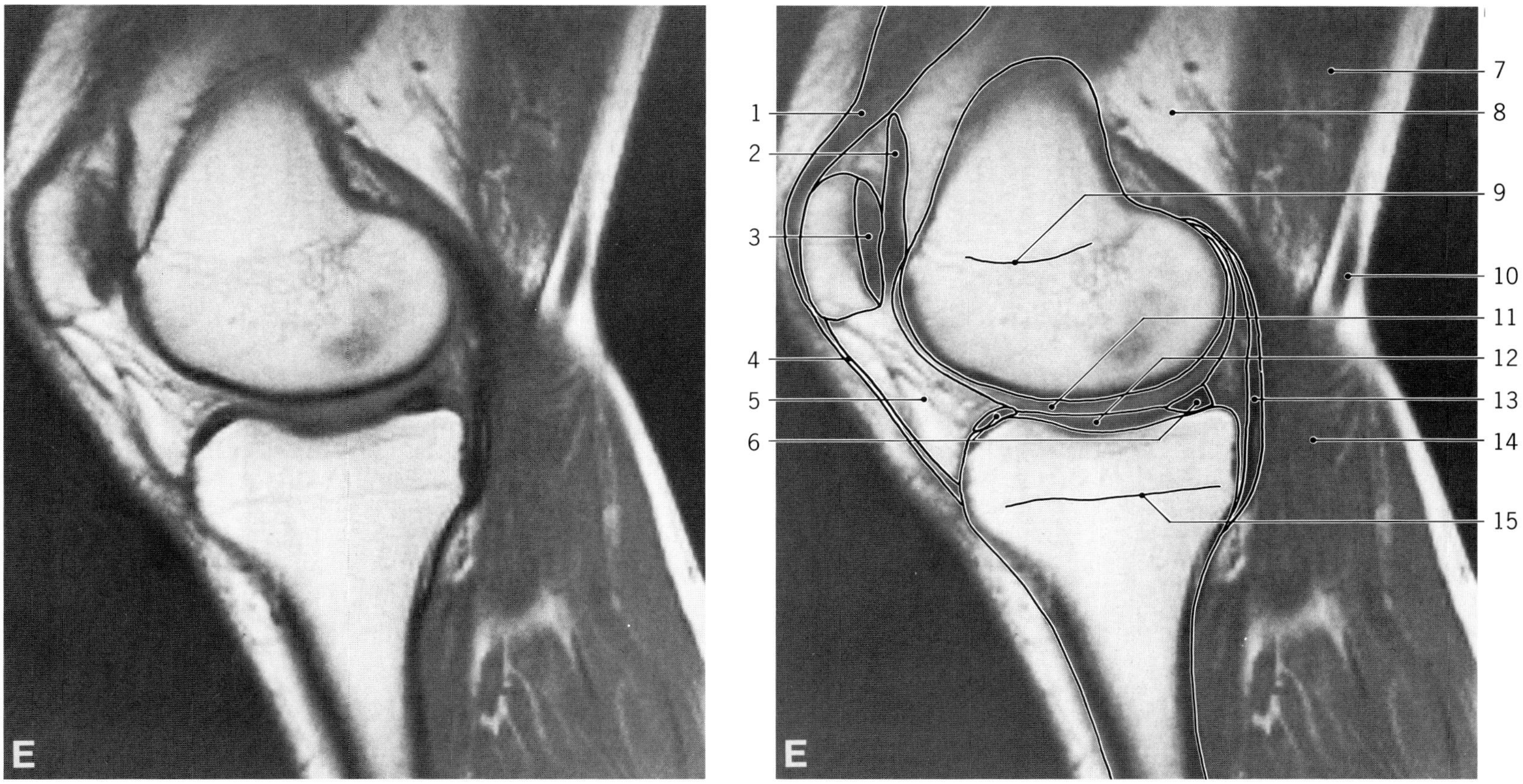

Knee, sagittal MR

E: Through medial condyles. Plane of section indicated on section A (p. 95)

1: Quadriceps femoris
2: Suprapatellar bursa
3: Articular cartilage of patella
4: Medial patellar retinaculum
5: Infrapatellar fat pad
6: Medial meniscus
7: Semimembranosus
8: Fat in popliteal fossa
9: Epiphyseal scar
10: Semitendinosus (tendon)
11: Articular cartilage of femur
12: Articular cartilage of tibia
13: Fibrous articular capsule
14: Gastrocnemius, medial head
15: Epiphyseal scar

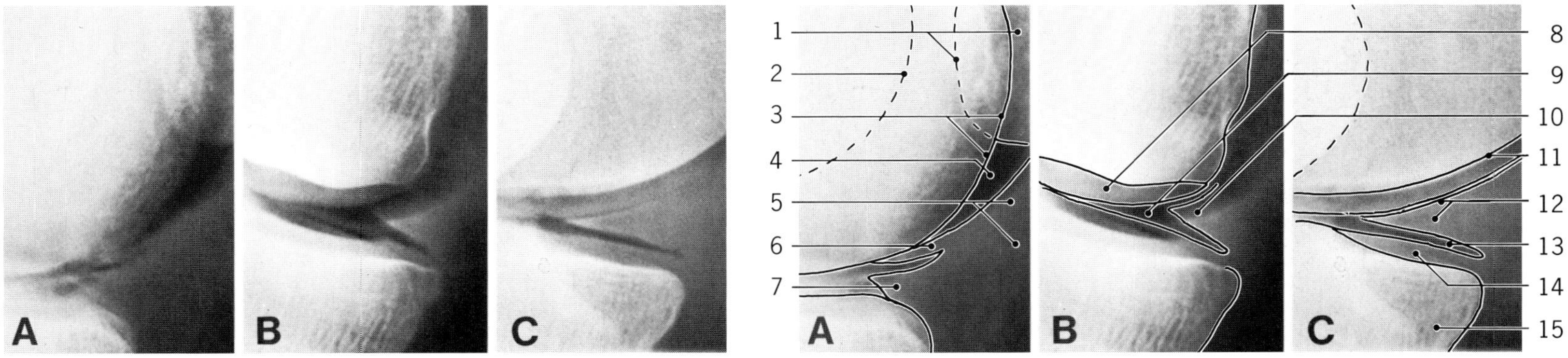

Knee, medial meniscus, X-ray, arthrography, rotational sequence

A: anterior, B: middle, C: posterior

1: Patella
2: Lateral condyle of femur
3: Medial condyle of femur
4: Femuropatellar joint cavity with air
5: Infrapatellar fat pad
6: Infrapatellar synovial fold
7: Medial meniscus (anterior horn)
8: Articular cartilage of medial femural condyle
9: Femurotibial joint cavity with air
10: Medial meniscus (middle section)
11: Medial condyle of femur
12: Medial meniscus (posterior horn)
13: Meniscotibial joint cavity
14: Articular cartilage
15: Medial condyle of tibia

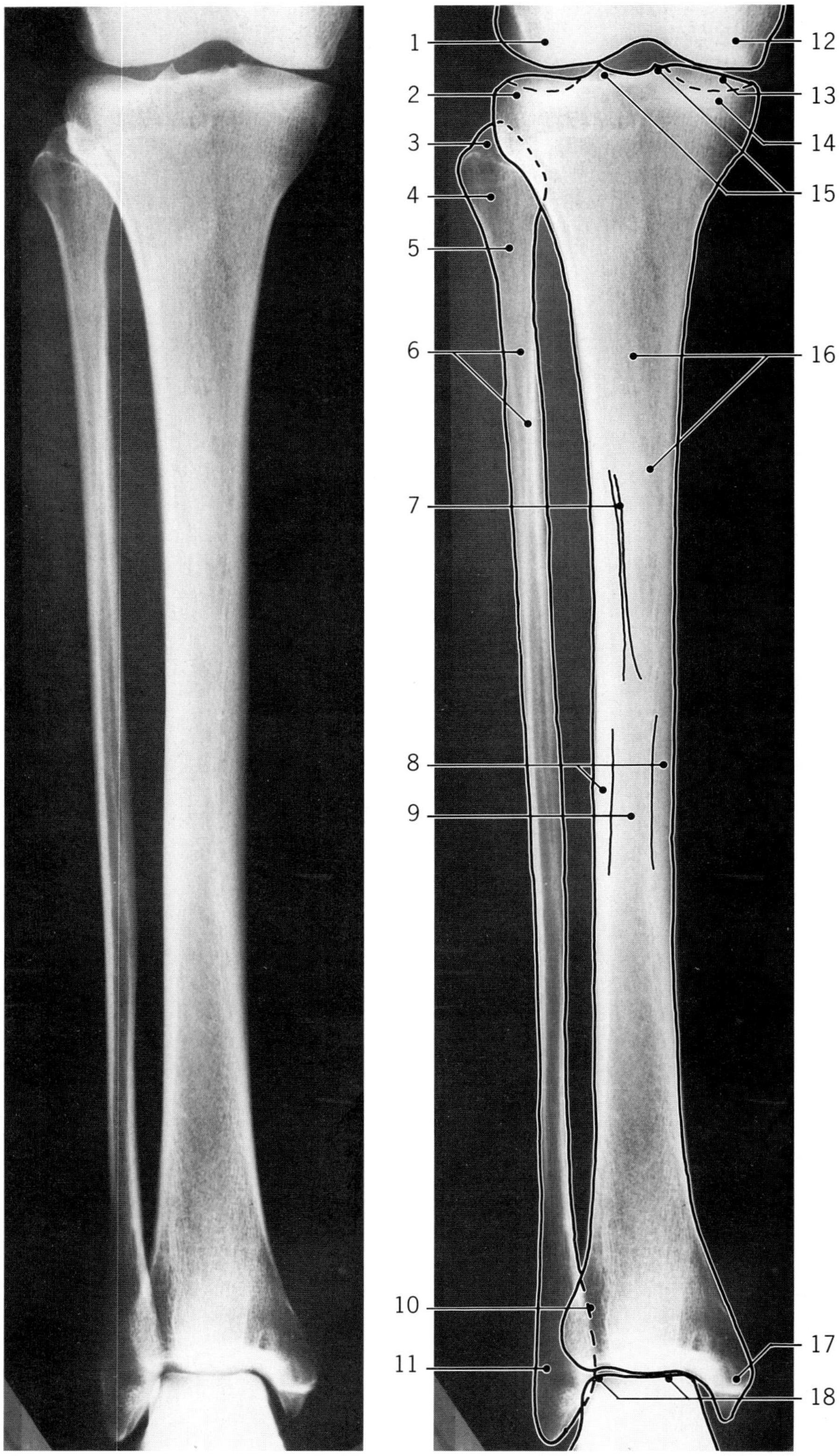

Lower leg, a-p X-ray

1: Lateral condyle of femur
2: Lateral condyle of tibia
3: Apex of fibula
4: Head of fibula
5: Neck of fibula
6: Shaft of fibula
7: Nutrient canal
8: Compact bone of tibial shaft
9: Medullary cavity of tibia
10: Fibular notch of tibia (syndesmosis)
11: Lateral malleolus
12: Medial condyle of femur
13: Superior articular surface of tibia
14: Medial condyle of tibia
15: Medial and lateral tubercle
16: Shaft of tibia
17: Medial malleolus
18: Trochlea of talus

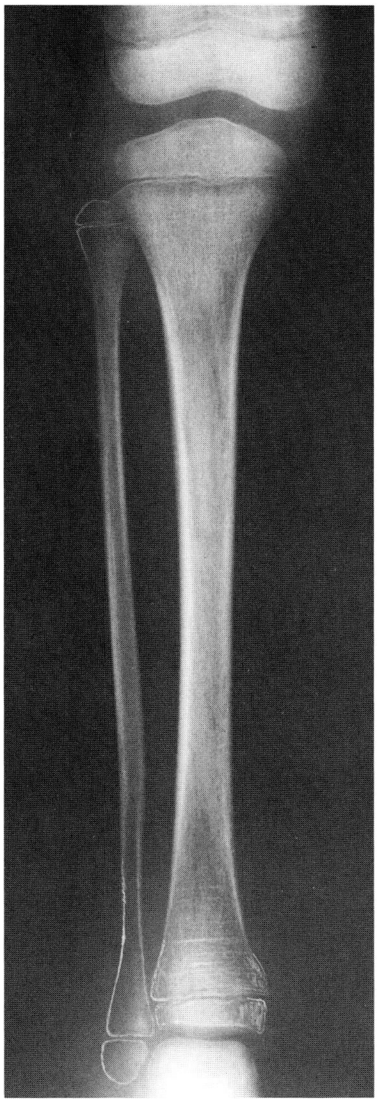

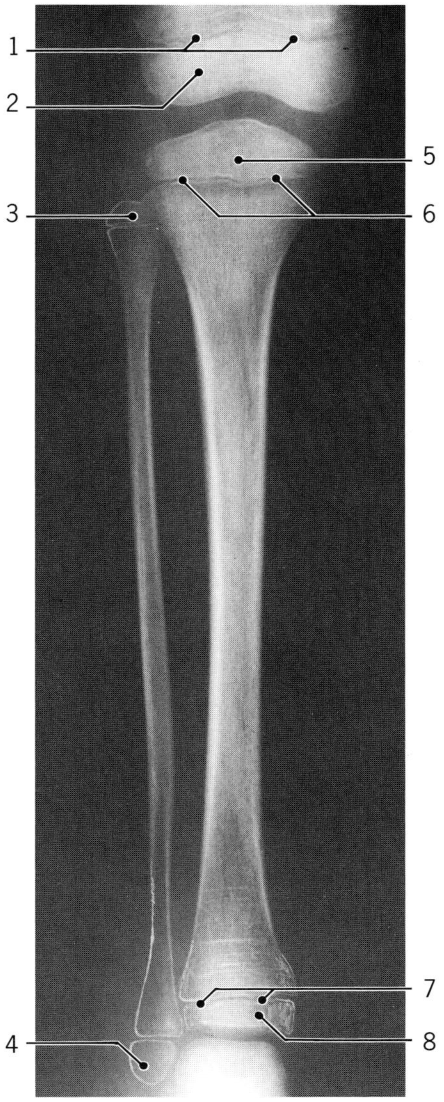

Lower leg, a-p X-ray, child 6 years

1: Growth plate
2: Distal epiphysis of femur
3: Proximal epiphysis of fibula
4: Distal epiphysis of fibula
5: Proximal epiphysis of tibia
6: Growth plate
7: Growth plate
8: Distal epiphysis of tibia

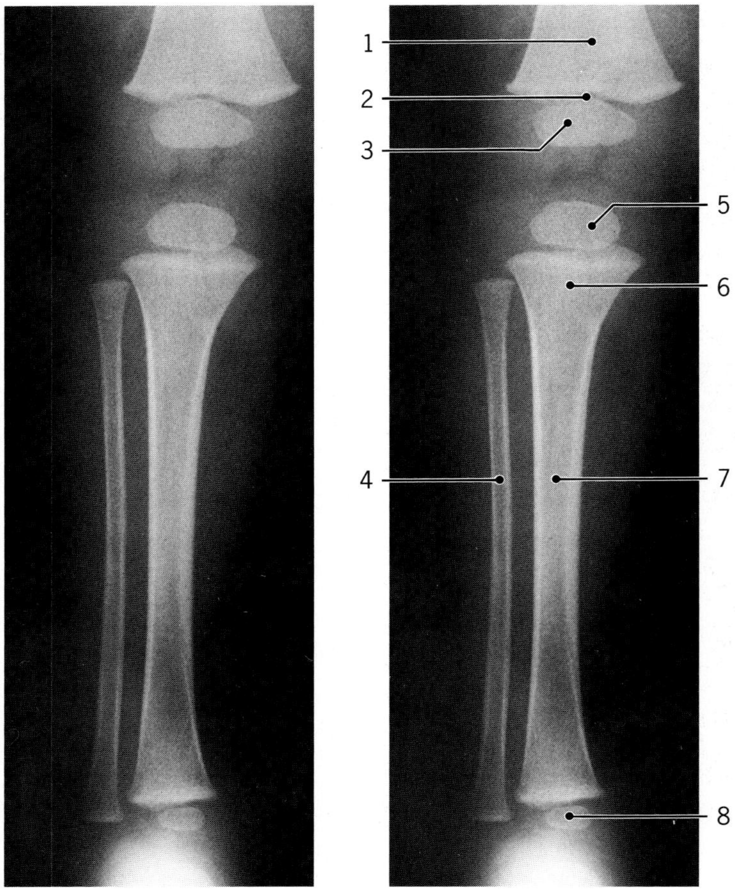

Lower leg, a-p X-ray, child 1 year

1: Metaphysis of femur
2: Growth plate
3: Distal epiphysis of femur
4: Diaphysis of fibula
5: Proximal epiphysis of tibia
6: Metaphysis of tibia
7: Diaphysis of tibia
8: Distal epiphysis of tibia

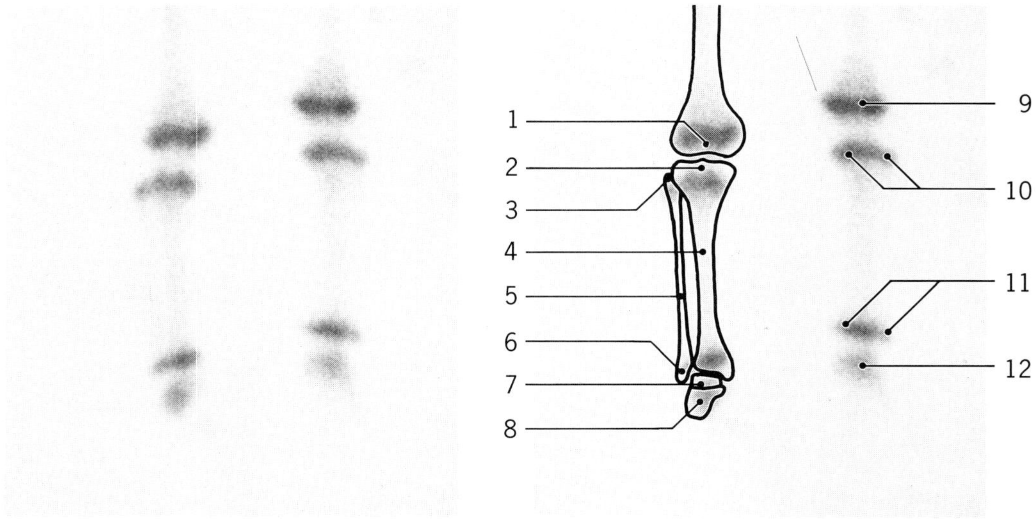

Lower leg, ^{99m}Tc- MDP, scintigraphy, child 12 years

1: Distal epiphysis of femur
2: Proximal epiphysis of tibia
3: Proximal epiphysis of fibula
4: Diaphysis of tibia
5: Diaphysis of fibula
6: Distal epiphysis of fibula
7: Talus
8: Calcaneus
9: Distal growth plate of femur
10: Proximal growth plates of tibia and fibula
11: Distal growth plates of tibia and fibula
12: Tarsal bones

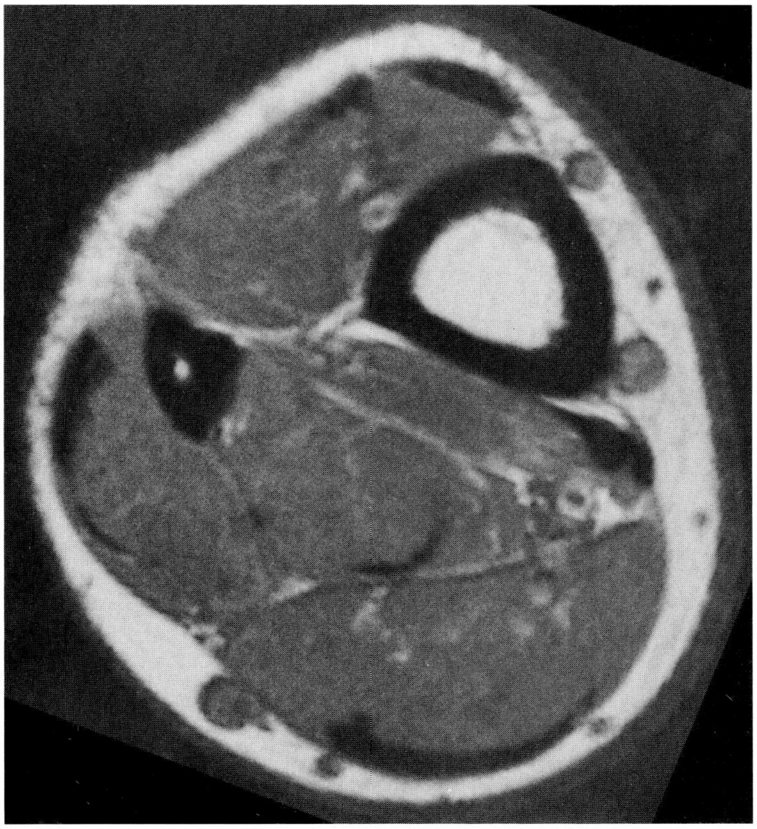

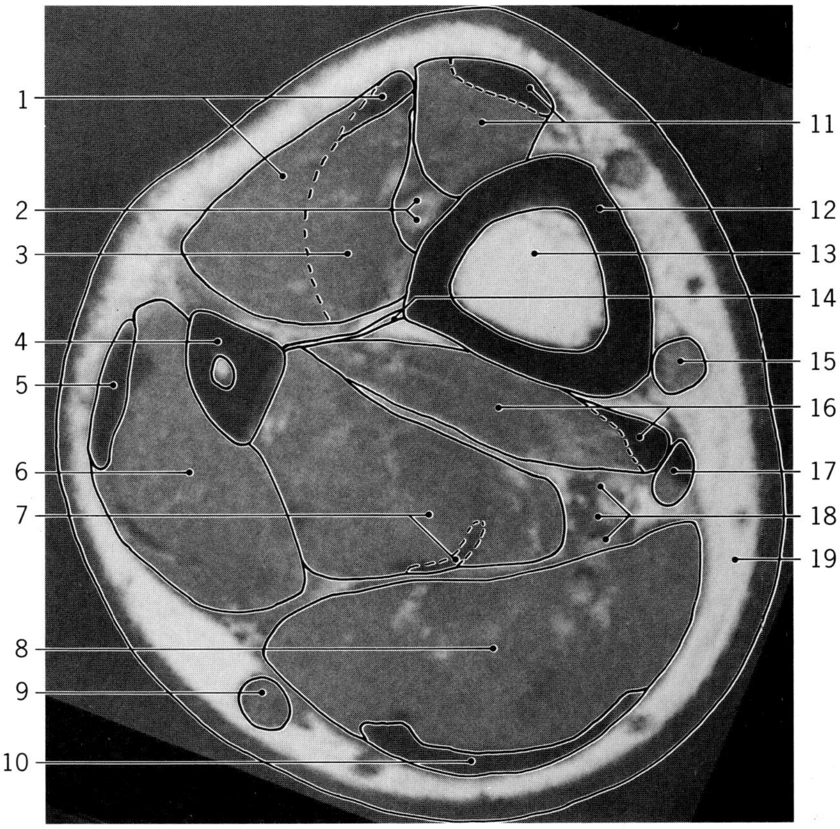

Lower leg, middle, axial MR

1: Extensor digitorum longus with tendon
2: Anterior tibial artery, and deep peroneal nerve
3: Extensor hallucis longus
4: Fibula
5: Peroneus longus (tendon)
6: Peroneus brevis
7: Flexor hallucis longus with tendon
8: Soleus
9: Small saphenous vein
10: Gastrocnemius (tendon)
11: Tibialis anterior (with tendon)
12: Compact bone of tibia
13: Bone marrow (yellow)
14: Interosseus membrane
15: Great saphenous vein
16: Tibialis posterior (with tendon)
17: Flexor digitorum longus (with tendon)
18: Posterior tibial artery, tibial nerve, and veins
19: Subcutaneous fat

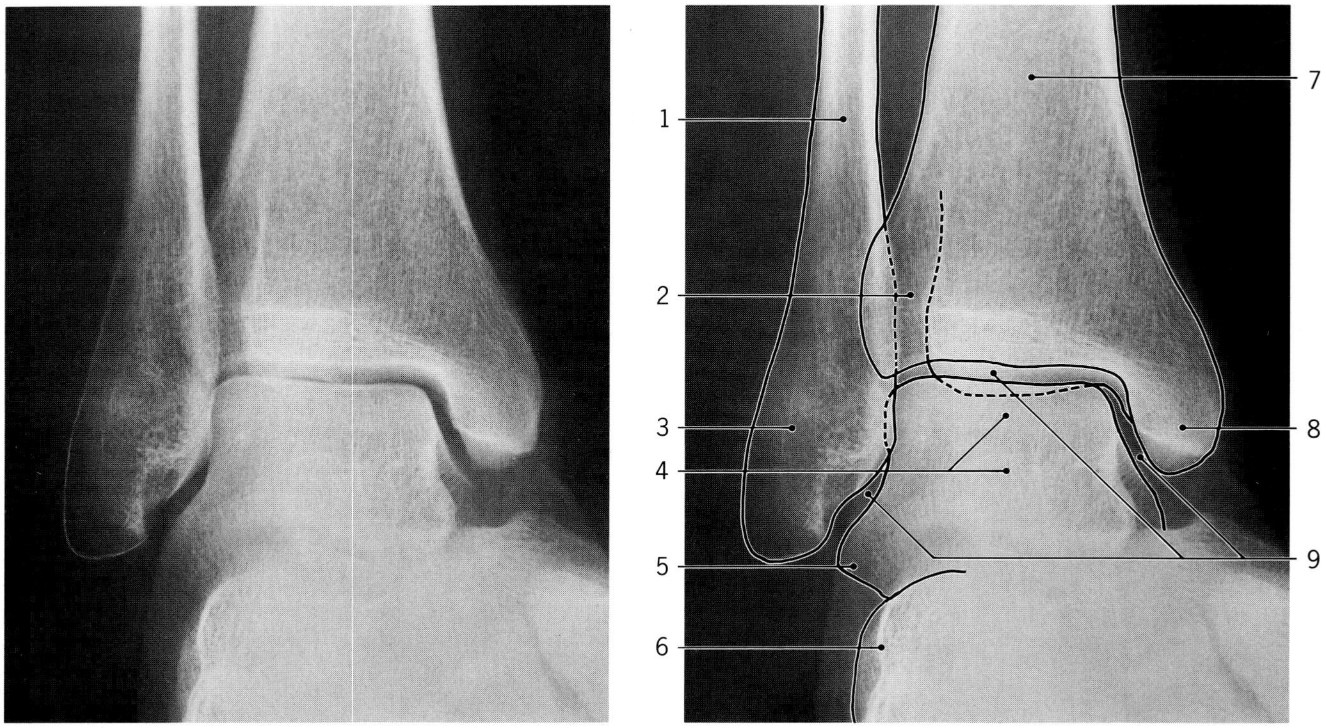

Ankle, a-p X-ray

1: Fibula
2: Tibiofibular syndesmosis
3: Lateral malleolus
4: Trochlea of talus
5: Lateral process of talus
6: Calcaneus
7: Tibia
8: Medial malleolus
9: Talocrural joint

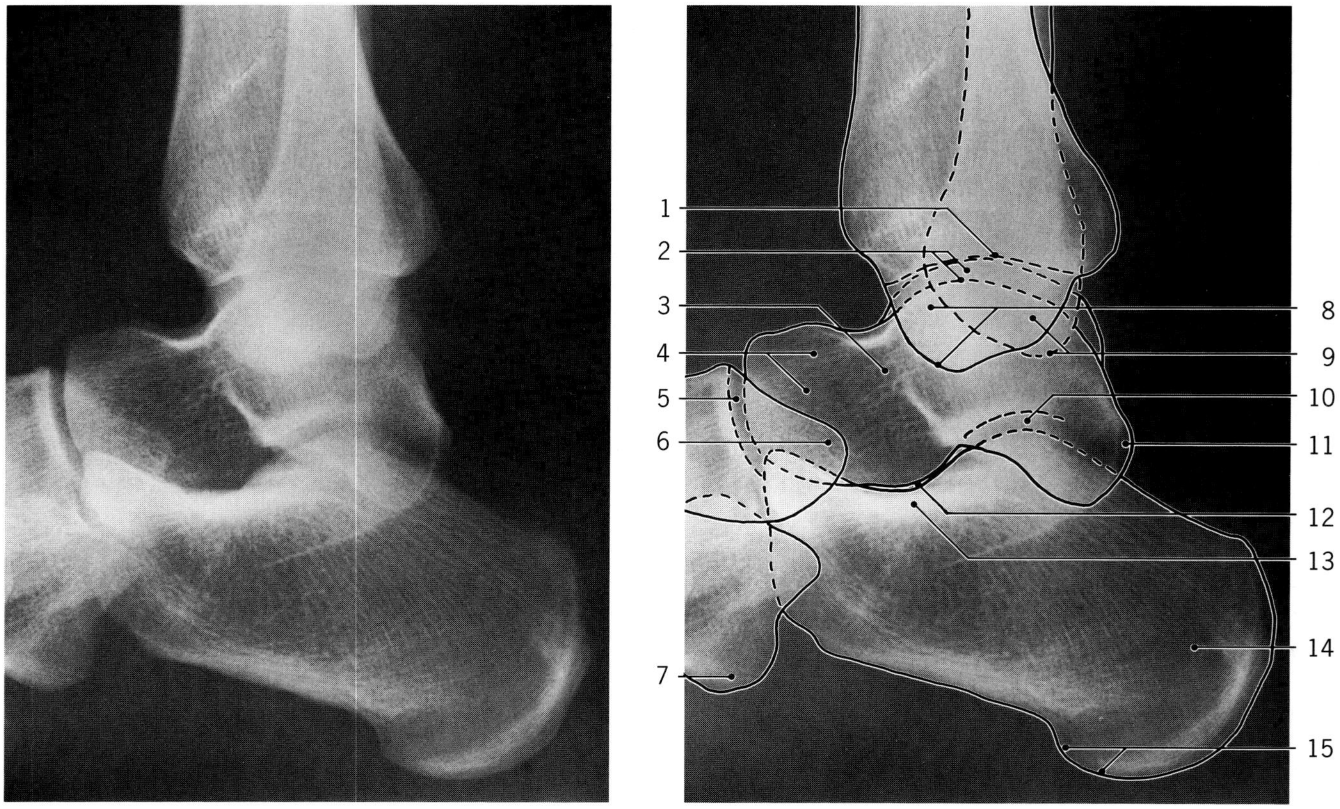

Ankle, lateral X-ray

1: Inferior articular surface of tibia
2: Trochlea of talus
3: Neck of talus
4: Head of talus
5: Talonavicular joint
6: Tuberosity of navicular bone
7: Tuberosity of cuboid bone
8: Medial malleolus
9: Lateral malleolus
10: Subtalar joint
11: Posterior process of talus
12: Middle talocalcanean joint
13: Sustentaculum tali
14: Tuber calcanei
15: Calcaneal tuberosity

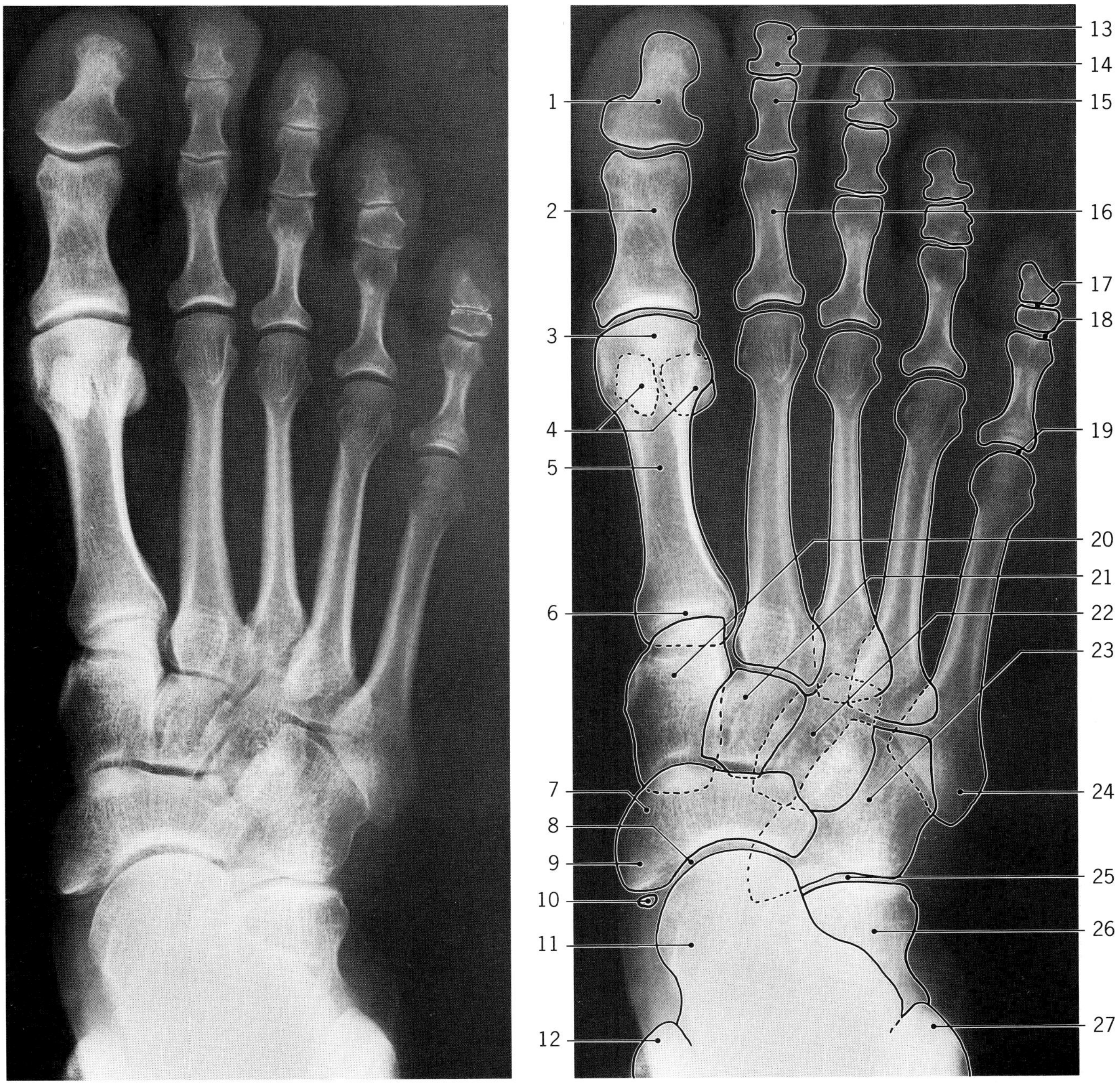

Foot, dorso-plantar X-ray

1: Distal phalanx of hallux
2: Proximal phalanx of hallux
3: Head of first metatarsal bone
4: Sesamoid bones
5: Shaft of first metatarsal bone
6: Base of first metatarsal bone
7: Navicular bone
8: Talonavicular joint
9: Tuberosity of navicular bone
10: Sesamoid bone in tendon of flexor digitorum longus
11: Head of talus
12: Medial malleolus
13: Tuberosity of distal phalanx
14: Distal phalanx
15: Middle phalanx
16: Proximal phalanx
17: Distal interphalangeal joint ("DIP")
18: Proximal interphalangeal joint ("PIP")
19: Metatarsophalangeal joint ("MTP")
20: Medial cuneiform bone
21: Intermediate cuneiform bone
22: Lateral cuneiform bone
23: Cuboid bone
24: Tuberosity of fifth metatarsal
25: Calcaneocuboideal joint
26: Calcaneus
27: Lateral malleolus

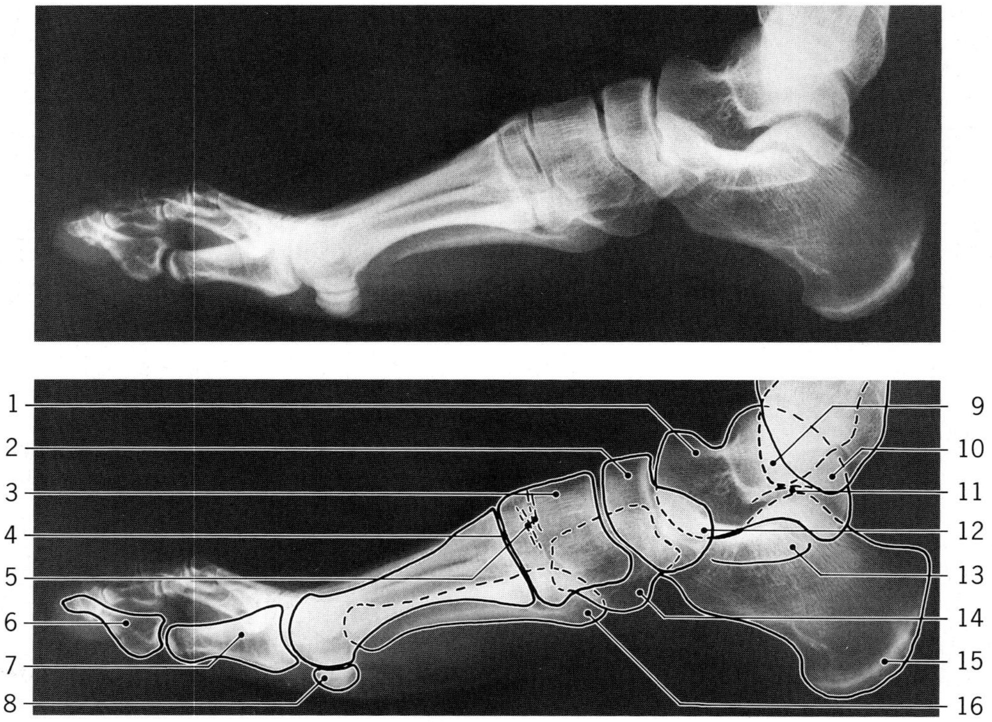

Foot, lateral X-ray

1: Head of talus
2: Navicular bone
3: Medial cuneiform bone
4: First tarsometatarseal joint
5: Second and third tarsometatarseal joints
6: Distal phalanx of hallux
7: Proximal phalanx of hallux
8: Sesamoid bones
9: Lateral malleolus
10: Medial malleolus
11: Subtalar joint
12: Tuberosity of navicular bone
13: Sustentaculum tali
14: Tuberosity of cuboid bone
15: Tuber calcanei
16: Tuberosity of fifth metatarseal

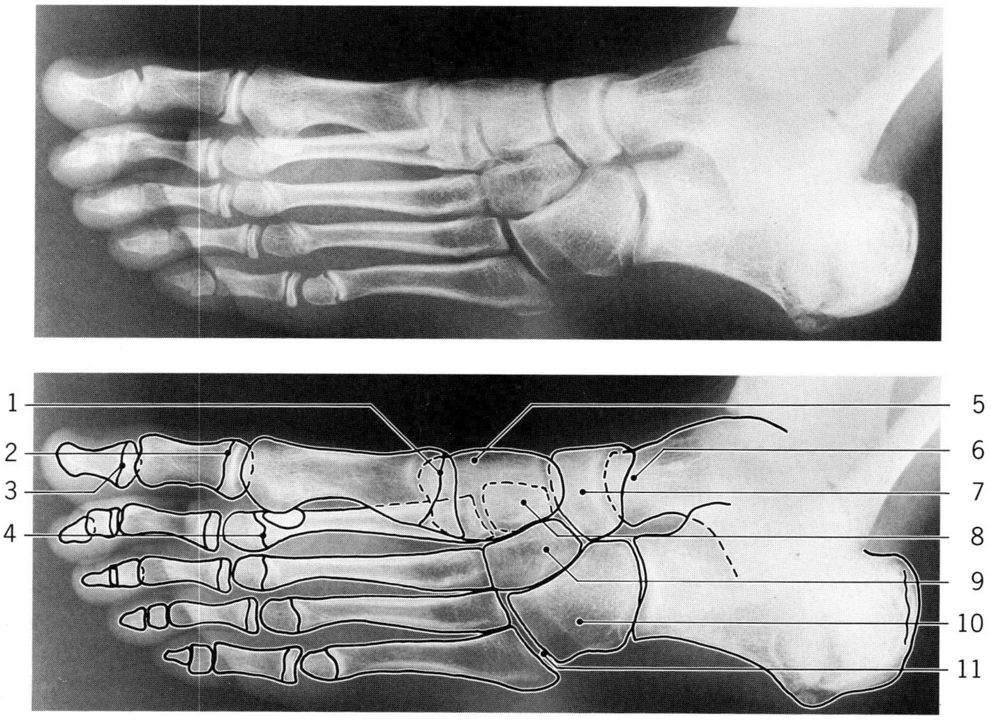

Foot, oblique X-ray

1: Growth plate of first metatarseal
2: Growth plate of proximal phalanx of hallux
3: Growth plate of distal phalanx of hallux
4: Growth plate of second metatarsal bone
5: Medial cuneiform bone
6: Head of talus
7: Navicular bone
8: Intermediate cuneiform bone
9: Lateral cuneiform bone
10: Cuboid bone
11: Fifth tarsometatarseal joint

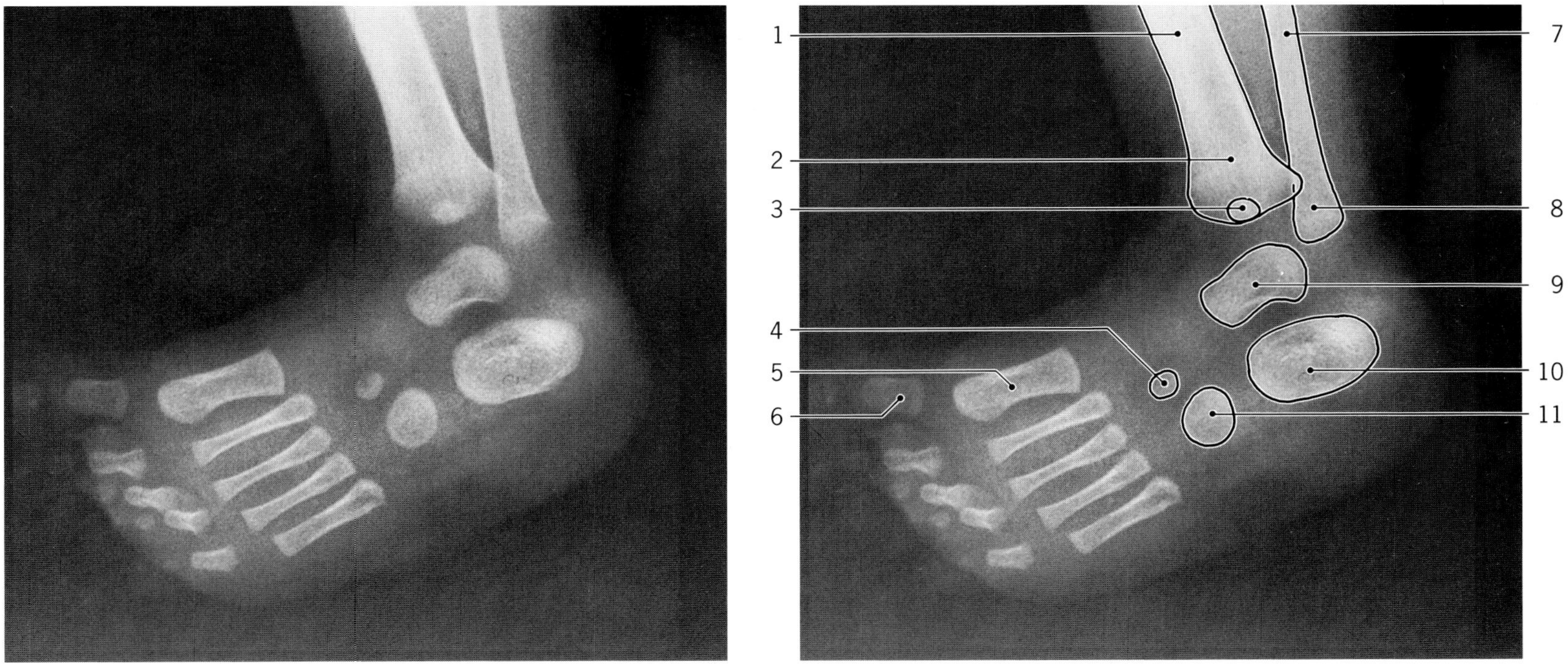

Foot, oblique X-ray, child 3 months

1: Diaphysis of tibia
2: Distal metaphysis of tibia
3: Distal epiphysis of tibia (ossification center)
4: Lateral cuneiform bone (ossification center)
5: Diaphysis of first metatarsal bone
6: Diaphysis of proximal phalanx of hallux
7: Diaphysis of fibula
8: Distal metaphysis of fibula
9: Talus (ossification center)
10: Calcaneus (ossification center)
11: Cuboid bone (ossification center)

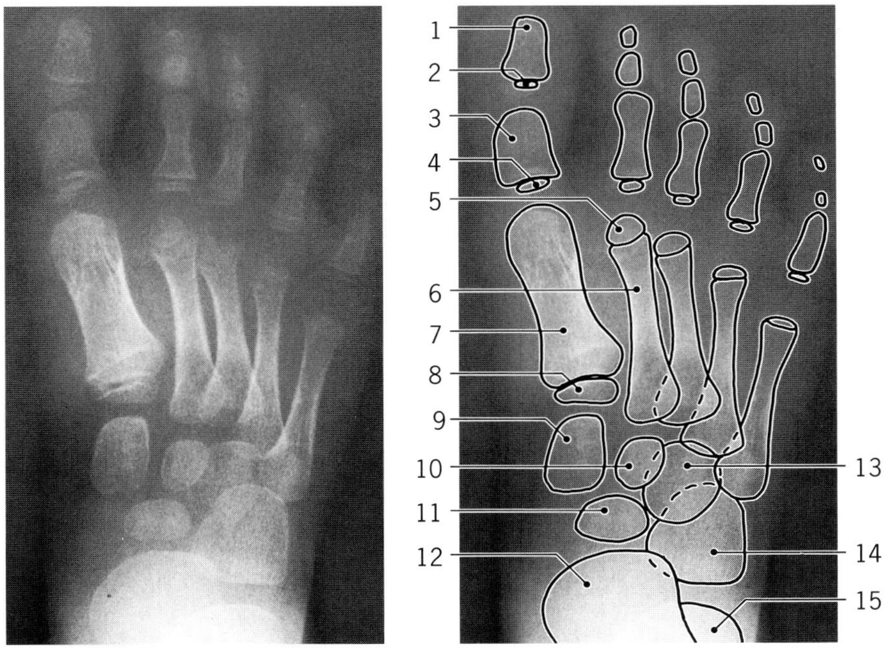

Foot, dorso-plantar X-ray, child 5 years

1: Diaphysis of distal phalanx of hallux
2: Epiphysis of distal phalanx of hallux
3: Diaphysis of proximal phalanx of hallux
4: Epiphysis of proximal phalanx of hallux
5: Epiphysis of second metatarsal bone
6: Diaphysis of second metatarsal bone
7: Diaphysis of first metatarsal bone
8: Epiphysis of first metatarsal bone
9: Medial cuneiforme bone
10: Intermediate cuneiforme bone
11: Navicular bone
12: Head of talus
13: Lateral cuneiforme bone
14: Cuboid bone
15: Calcaneus

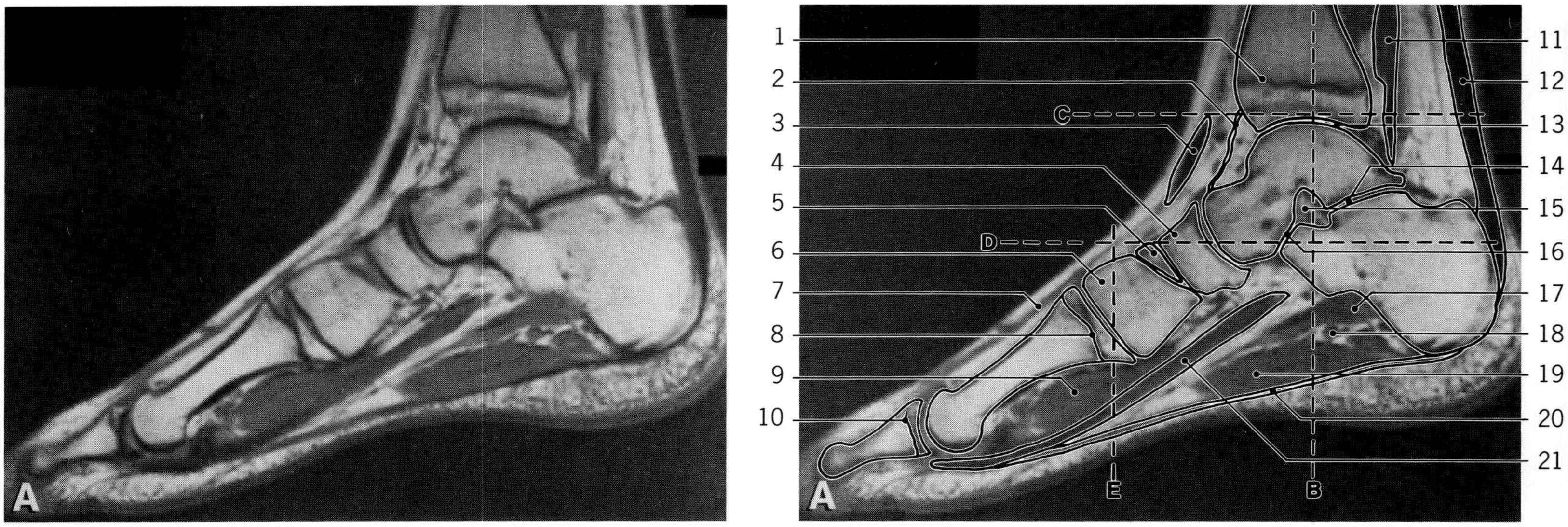

Ankle and foot, sagittal MR

1: Growth plate of tibia
2: Articular capsule
3: Tibialis anterior (tendon)
4: Navicular bone
5: Intermediate cuneiform bone
6: Medial cuneiform bone
7: Extensor hallucis longus (tendon)
8: Growth plate of first metatarsal bone
9: Flexor hallucis brevis
10: Growth plate of proximal phalanx of hallux
11: Flexor hallucis longus
12: Calcanean tendon (Achillis)
13: Talocrural joint
14: Subtalar joint
15: Sinus tarsi
16: Anterior talocalcanean joint
17: Quadratus plantae
18: Lateral plantar artery
19: Flexor digitorum brevis
20: Plantar aponeurosis
21: Flexor hallucis longus (tendon)

Dotted lines B, C, D and E indicate positions of following sections.

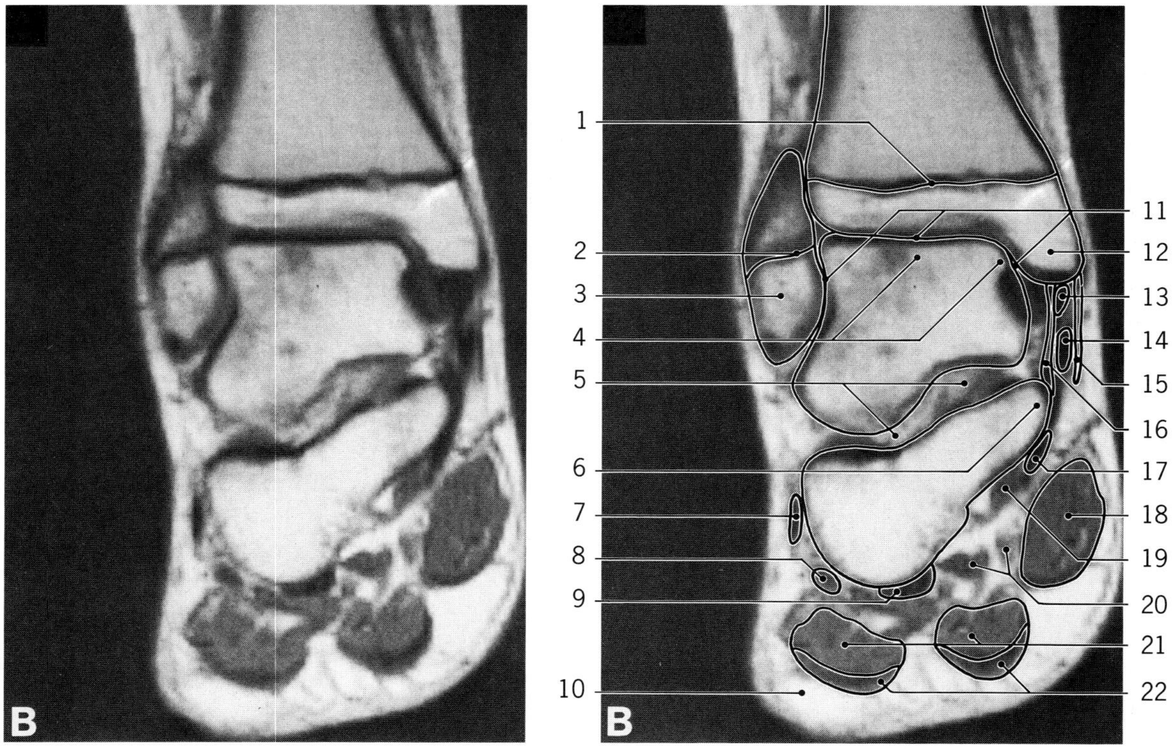

Ankle, coronal MR

Plane of section B indicated on section A (above).

1: Growth plate of tibia
2: Growth plate of fibula
3: Lateral malleolus
4: Trochlea of talus
5: Sinus tarsi
6: Sustentaculum tali
7: Peroneus brevis (tendon)
8: Peroneus longus (tendon)
9: Long plantar ligament
10: Subcutis of heel
11: Talocrural joint
12: Medial malleolus
13: Tibialis posterior (tendon)
14: Flexor digitorum longus (tendon)
15: Flexor retinacle
16: Deltoid ligament
17: Flexor hallucis longus
18: Abductor hallucis
19: Quadratus plantae
20: Plantar vessels and nerves
21: Flexor digitorum brevis
22: Plantar aponeurosis

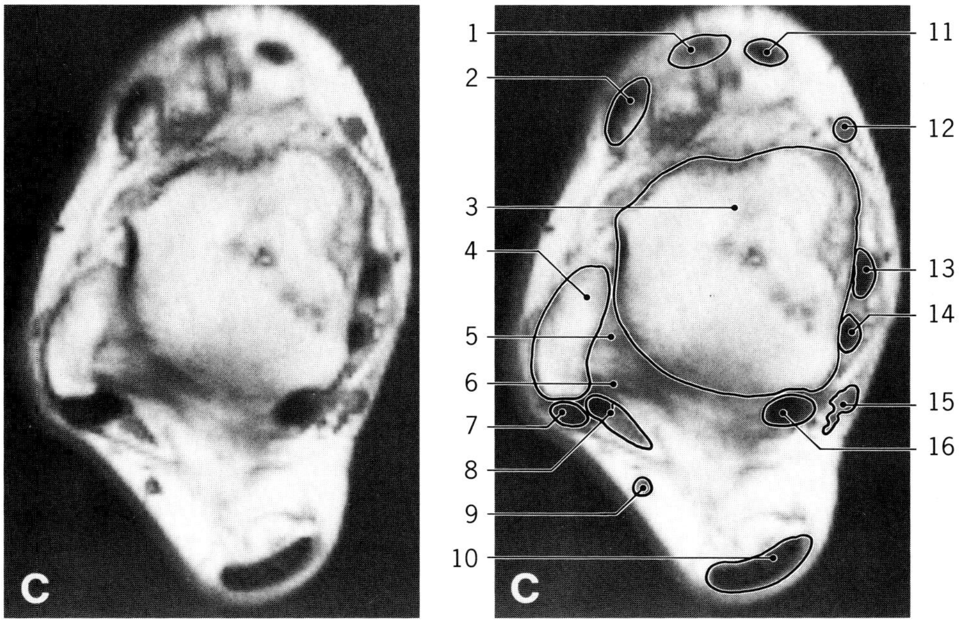

Ankle, axial MR

Plane of section C indicated on section A (opposite page).

1: Extensor hallucis longus (tendon)
2: Extensor digitorum longus (tendon)
3: Tibia
4: Lateral malleolus
5: Tibiofibular syndesmosis
6: Posterior talofibular ligament
7: Peroneus longus (tendon)
8: Peroneus brevis (muscle and tendon)
9: Small saphenous vein
10: Tendo calcanei
11: Tibialis anterior (tendon)
12: Great saphenous vein
13: Tibialis posterior (tendon)
14: Flexor digitorum longus (tendon)
15: Posterior tibial vessels and nerve
16: Flexor hallucis longus (tendon)

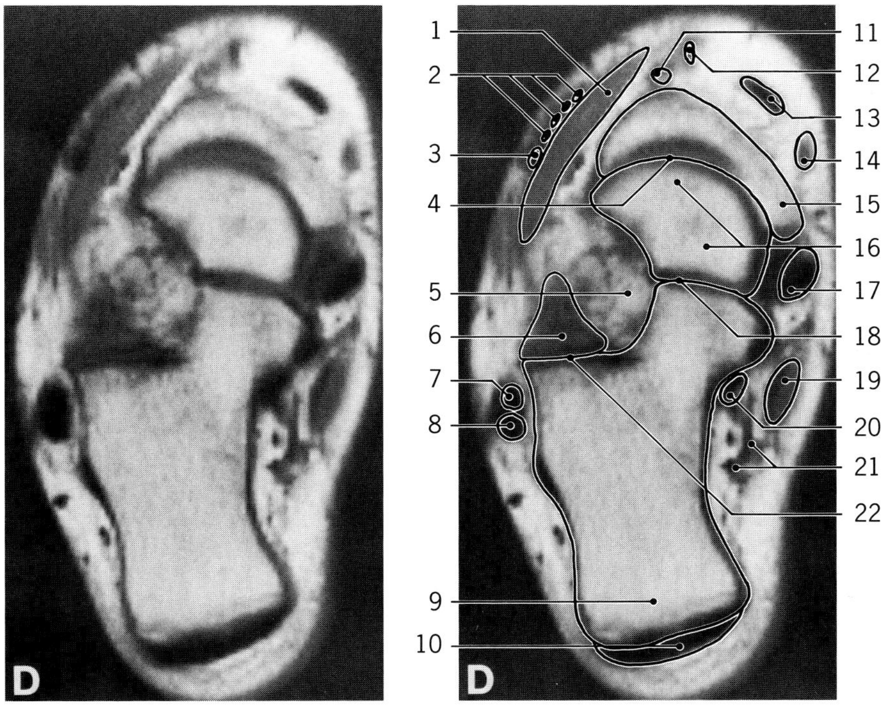

Tarsus, axial MR

Plane of section D indicated on section A (opposite page).

1: Extensor digitorum brevis
2: Extensor digitorum longus (tendons)
3: Peroneus tertius
4: Talonavicular joint
5: Sinus tarsi
6: Cuboid bone
7: Peroneus brevis (tendon)
8: Peroneus longus (tendon)
9: Tuber calcanei
10: Tendo calcanei
11: A. dorsalis pedis
12: Extensor hallucis longus (tendon)
13: Tibialis anterior (tendon)
14: Great saphenous vein
15: Tuberosity of navicular bone
16: Head of talus
17: Tibialis posterior (tendon)
18: Anterior talocalcanean joint
19: Flexor digitorum longus (tendon)
20: Flexor hallucis longus (tendon)
21: Posterior tibial vessels and nerve
22: Calcaneocuboideal joint

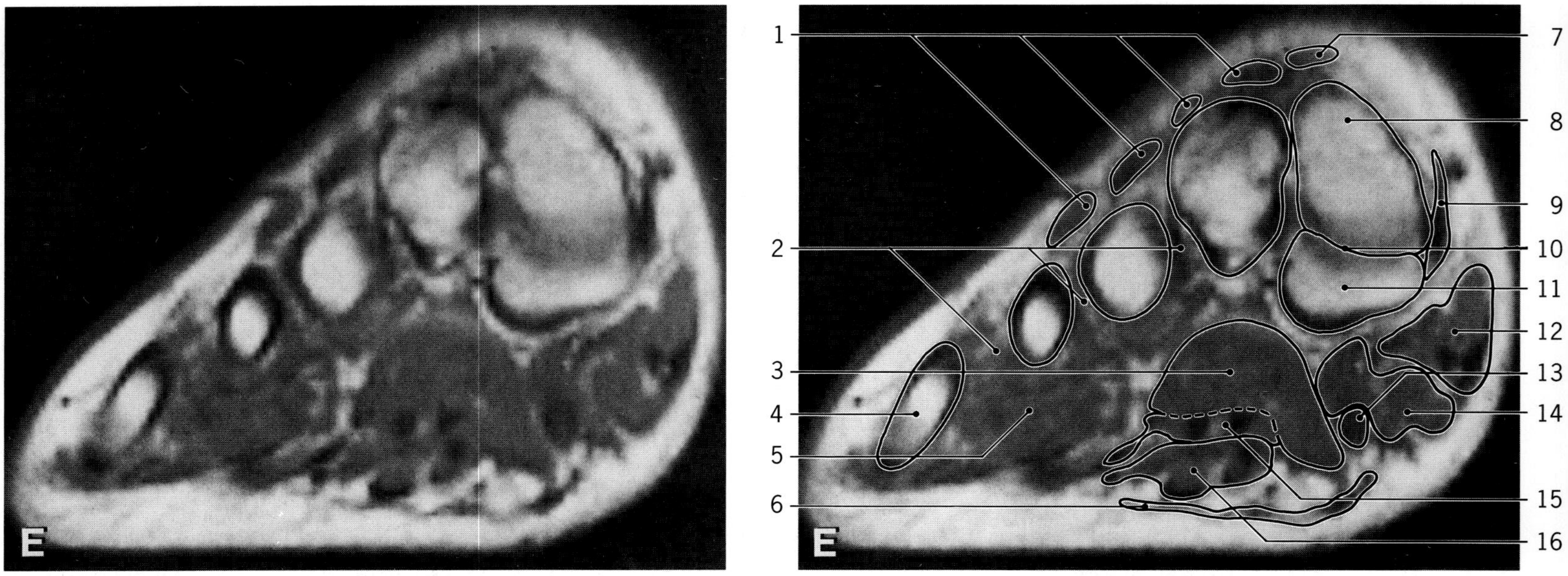

Metatarsus, cross section MR

Plane of section E indicated on section A (p. 106)

1: Extensor digitorum longus, and brevis (tendons)
2: Interossei muscles
3: Adductor hallucis, oblique head
4: Fifth metatarsal bone
5: Flexor digiti minimi
6: Plantar aponeurosis
7: Extensor hallucis longus (tendon)
8: Medial cuneiform bone
9: Tibialis anterior (insertion)
10: First tarsometatarsal joint
11: First metatarsal bone
12: Abductor hallucis
13: Flexor hallucis longus (tendon)
14: Flexor hallucis brevis
15: Flexor digitorum longus, and lumbricals
16: Flexor digitorum brevis

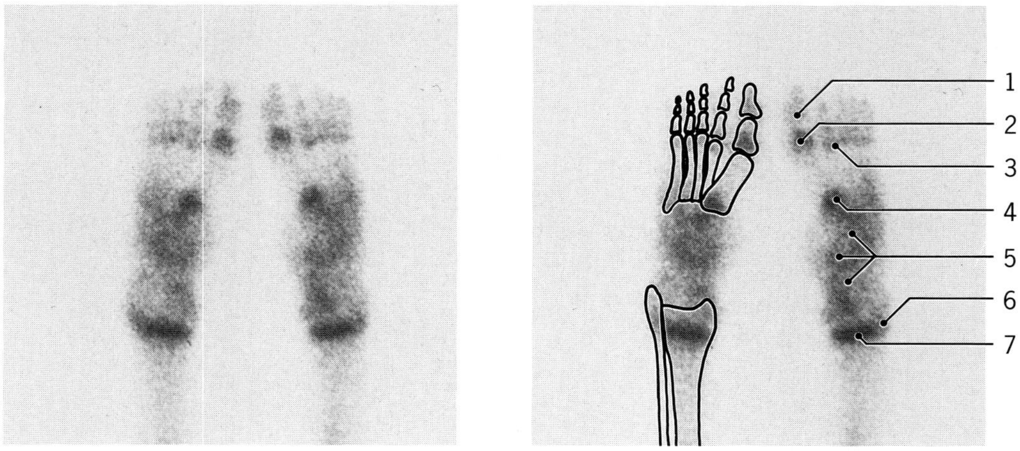

Foot, ^{99m}Tc- MDP, scintigraphy, child 14 years

1: Growth plate of distal phalanx of hallux
2: Growth plate of proximal phalanx of hallux
3: Growth plate of second metatarsal bone
4: Growth plate of first metatarsal bone
5: Tarsal bones
6: Growth plate of distal epiphysis of fibula
7: Growth plate of distal epiphysis of tibia

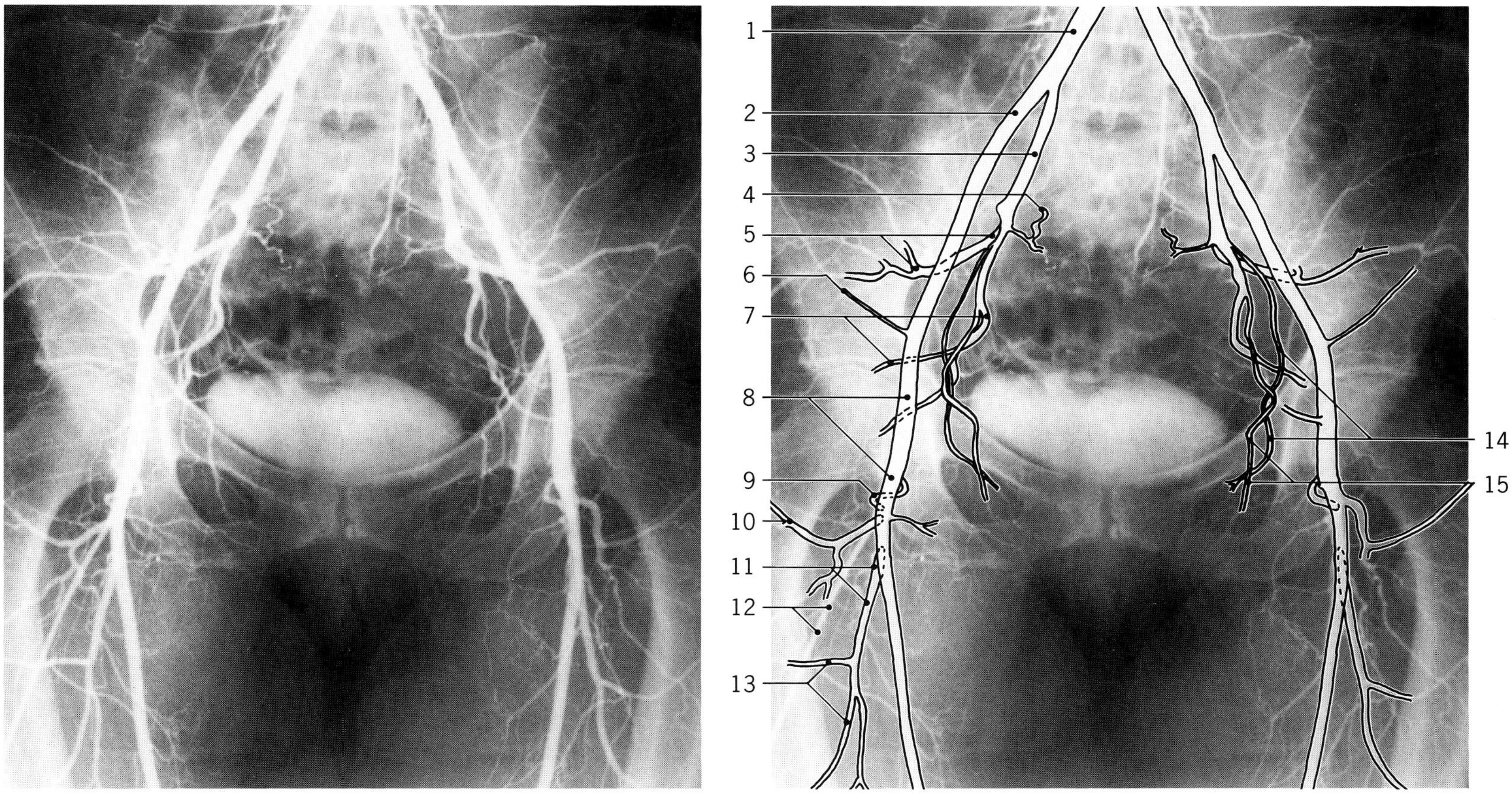

Iliac and femoral arteries, a-p X-ray, arteriography

1: Common iliac artery
2: External iliac artery
3: Internal iliac artery
4: Lateral sacral artery
5: Superior gluteal artery
6: Deep circumflex iliac artery
7: Inferior gluteal artery
8: Femoral artery
9: Medial circumflex femoral artery
10: Lateral circumflex femoral artery
11: A. profunda femoris
12: Catheter
13: Perforating arteries
14: Internal pudendal artery
15: Obturator artery

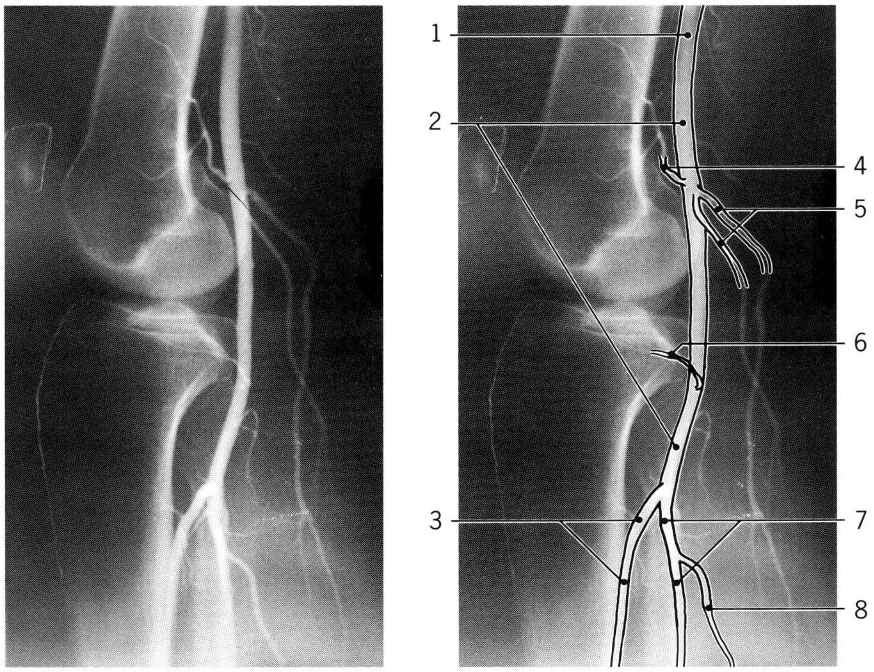

Popliteal artery, lateral X-ray, arteriography

1: Femoral artery
2: Popliteal artery
3: Anterior tibial artery
4: Superior genicular artery
5: Muscular branches to gastrochnemius
6: Inferior genicular artery
7: Posterior tibial artery
8: Muscular branch
(Peroneal artery not visible)

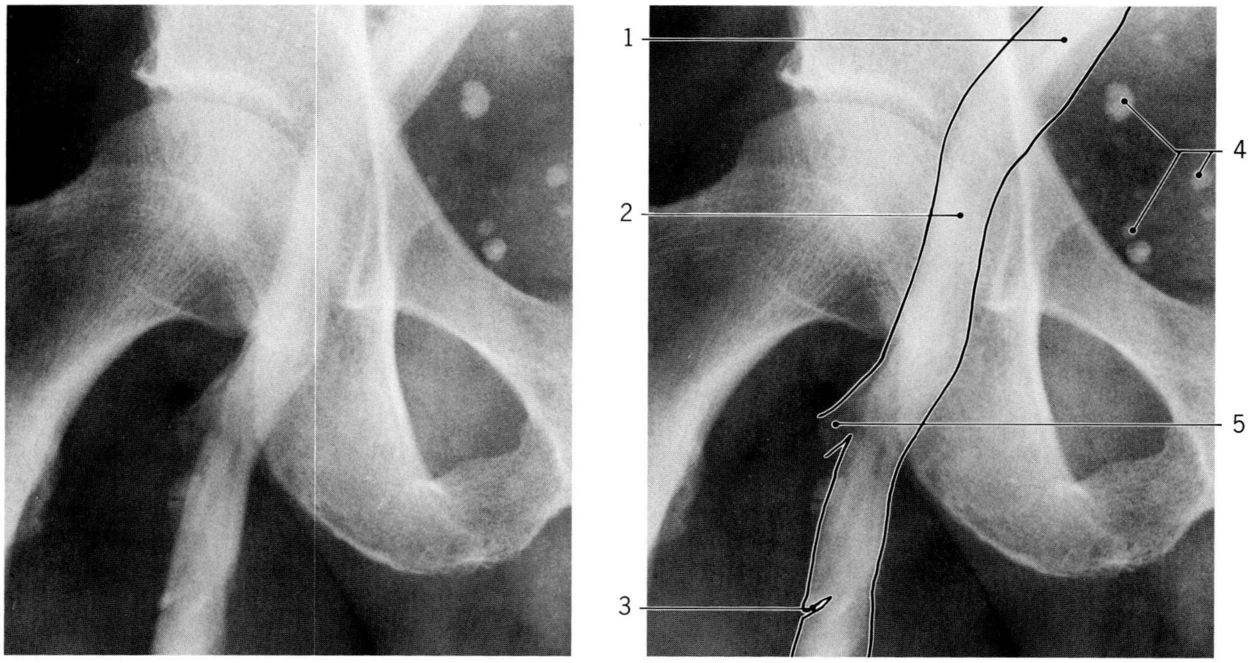

Femoral vein, a-p X-ray, phlebography

1: External iliac vein
2: Femoral vein
3: Venous valve
4: Calcifications in pelvic veins (phlebolites)
5: V. profunda femoris

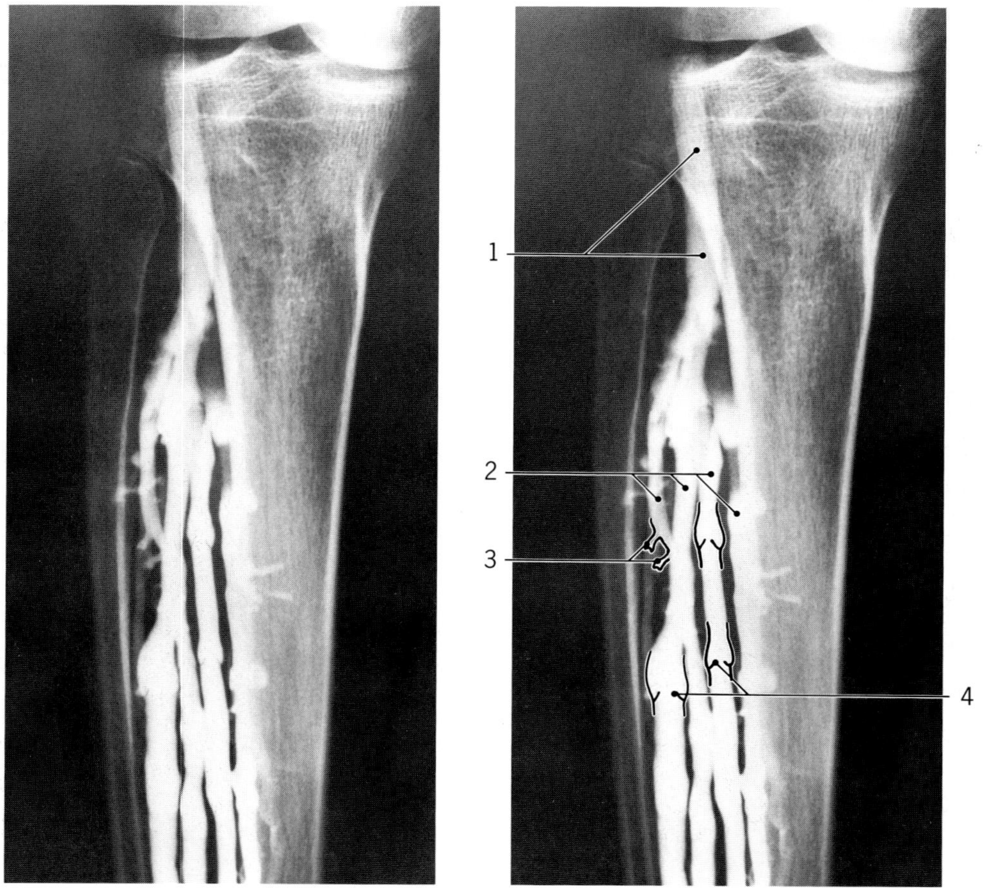

Deep veins of lower leg, oblique X-ray, phlebography

1: Popliteal vein
2: Deep crural veins
3: Perforating veins
4: Venous valves

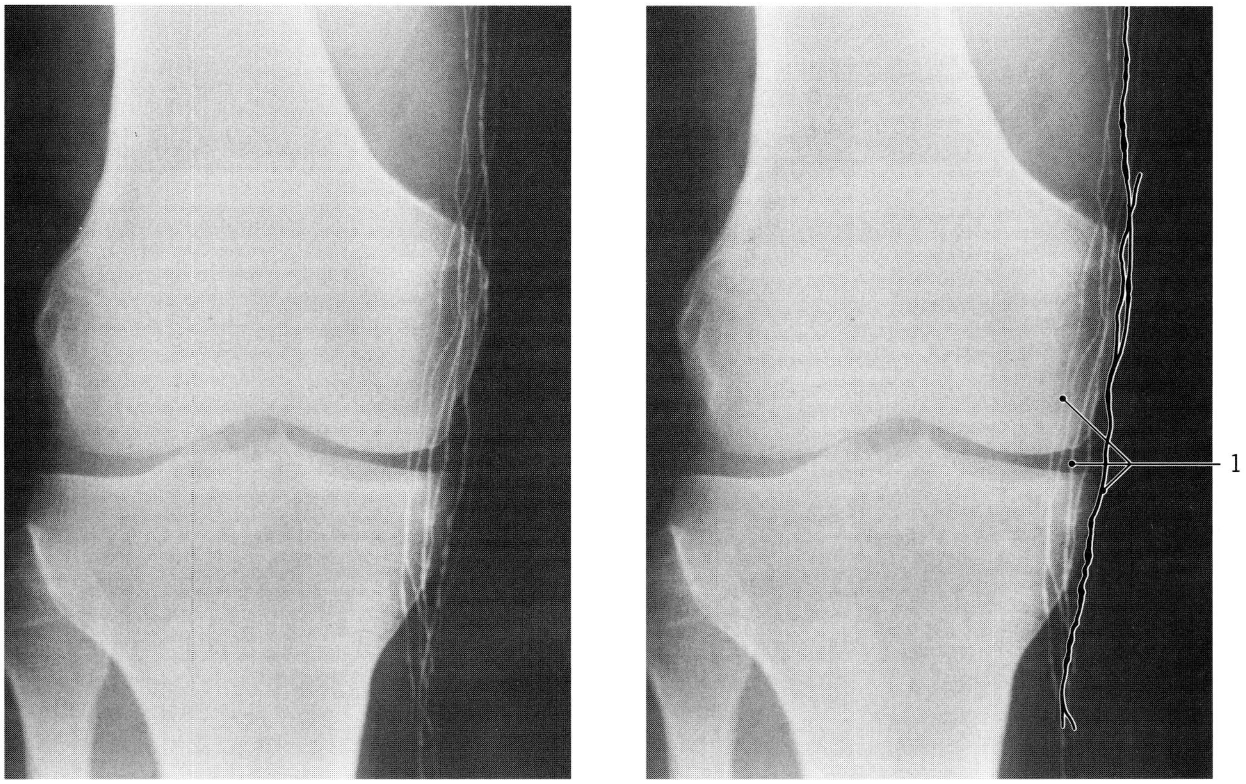

Knee, a-p X-ray, lymphography

1: Lymphatic vessels along great saphenous vein

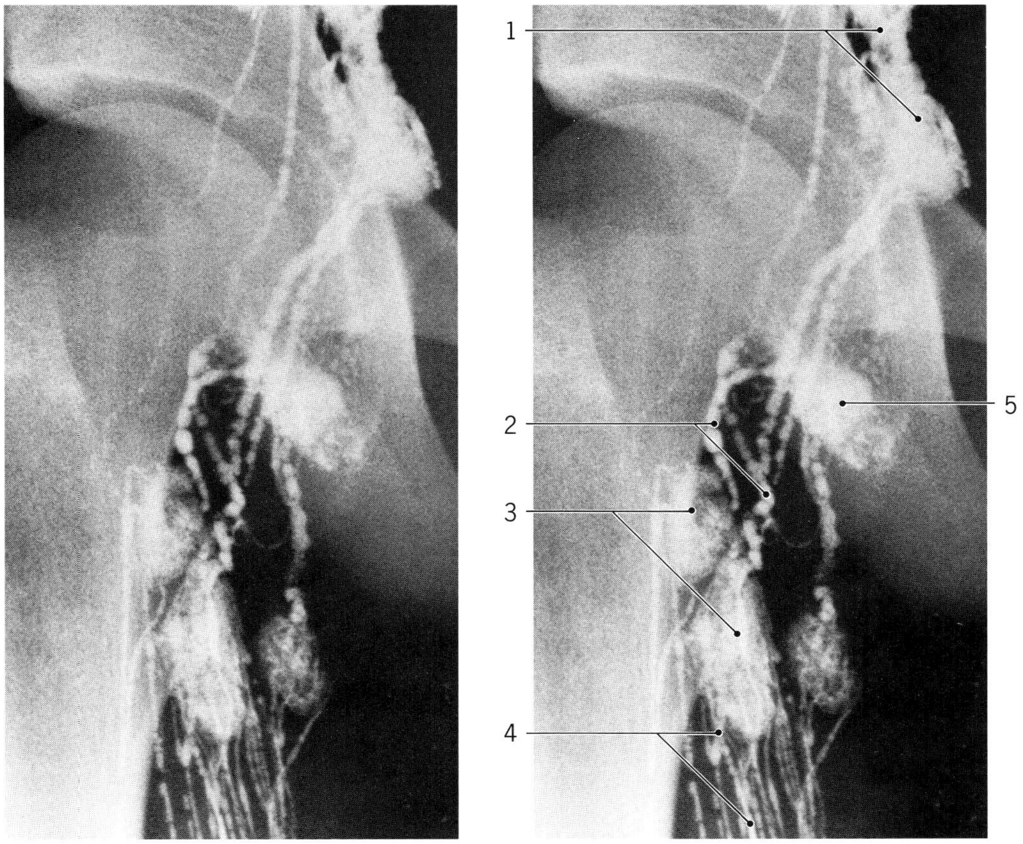

Groin, a-p X-ray, lymphography

1: External iliac lymph nodes
2: Efferent lymphatic vessels
3: Superficial inguinal lymph nodes
4: Afferent lymphatic vessels
5: Deep inguinal lymph node

SPINE

Cervical spine
Thoracic spine
Lumbar spine

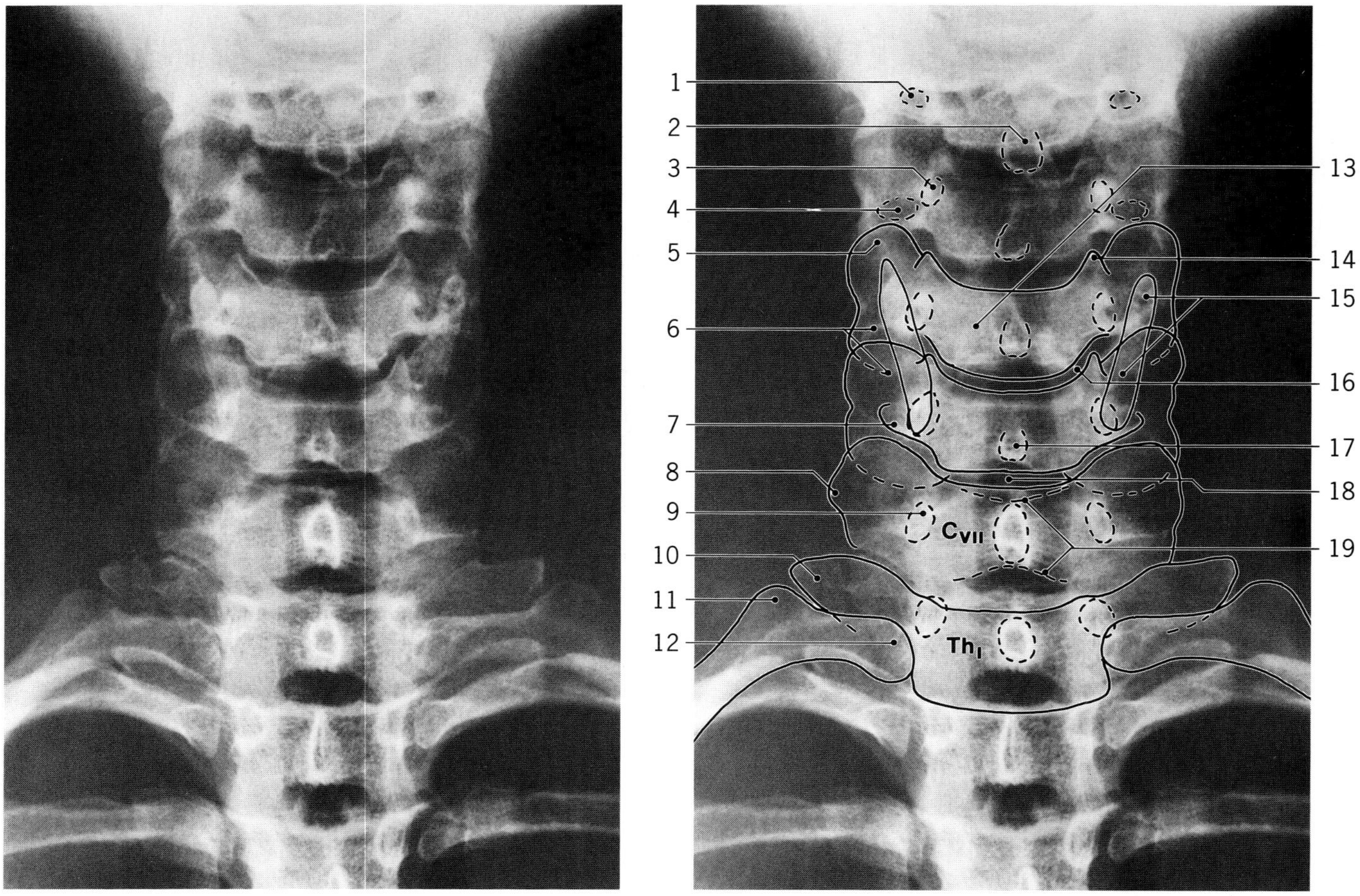

Cervical spine, a-p X-ray

1: Foramen transversarium of C III
2: Spinous process of C III
3: Pedicle of vertebral arch
4: Foramen transversarium of C IV
5: Superior articular process of C V
6: Inferior articular process of C V
7: Anterior tubercle of C VI
8: Transverse process of C VII
9: Pedicle of C VII
10: Transverse process of Th I
11: Tubercle of first rib
12: Head of first rib
13: Body of vertebra C V
14: Uncus (lip) of C V
15: Lamina of thyroid cartilage (calcified)
16: Uncovertebral joint (Luschka)
17: Spinous process of C VI
18: Intervertebral disc C VI - C VII
19: Lamina of vertebral arch C VII

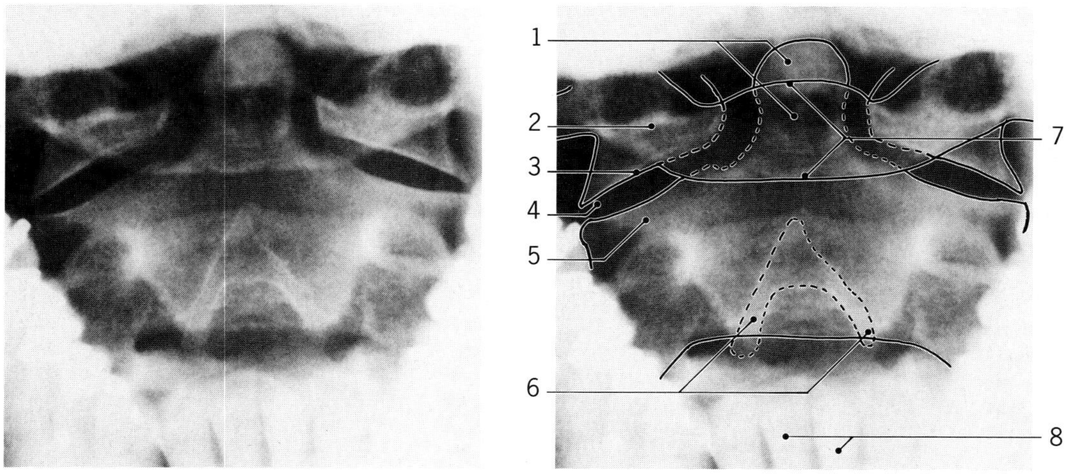

Atlas and axis, a-p X-ray, through open mouth

1: Dens axis
2: Lateral mass of atlas
3: Inferior articular facet of atlas
4: Lateral atlanto-axial joint
5: Superior articular process of axis
6: Spinous process of axis (bifid)
7: Anterior and posterior arch of atlas
8: Lower incisor teeth

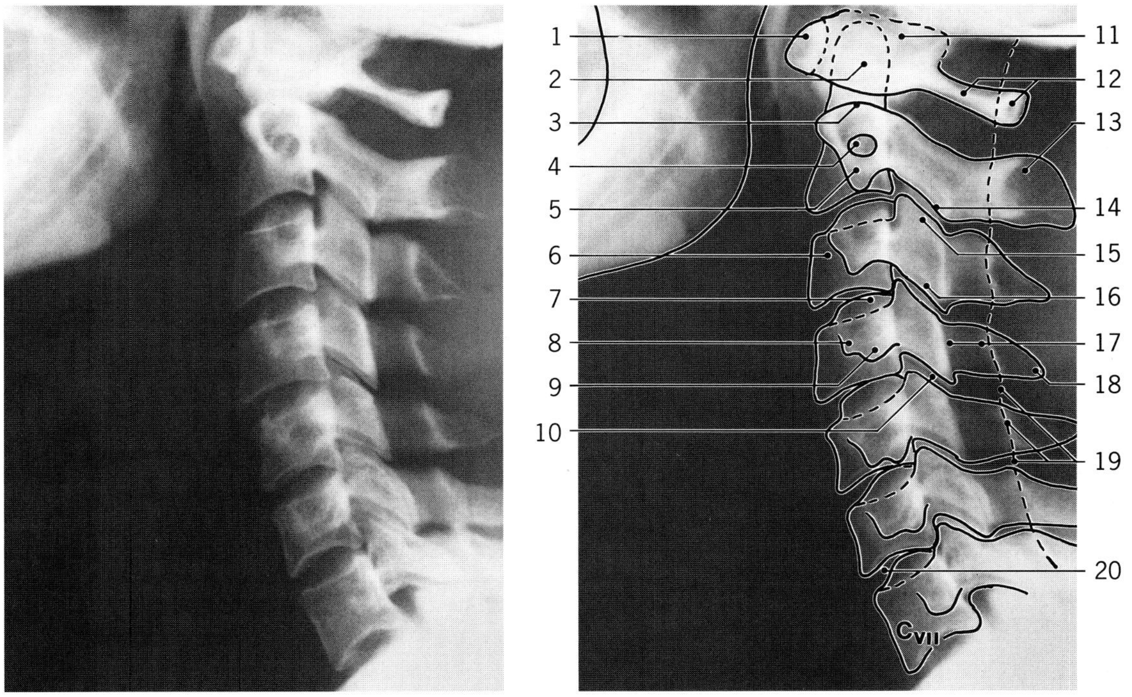

Cervical spine, lateral X-ray

1: Anterior arch of atlas
2: Dens axis
3: Superior articular facet of axis
4: Foramen transversarium of axis
5: Transverse process of axis
6: Body of C III
7: Uncus of C IV
8: Anterior tubercle
9: Posterior tubercle
10: Zygapophyseal (facet) joint C IV - C V
11: Lateral mass of atlas
12: Posterior arch of atlas
13: Spinous process of axis
14: Inferior articular process of axis
15: Superior articular process of C III
16: Inferior articular process of C III
17: Lamina of vertebral arch C IV
18: Spinous process of C IV
19: Posterior wall of vertebral canal
20: Intervertebral disc C VI - C VII

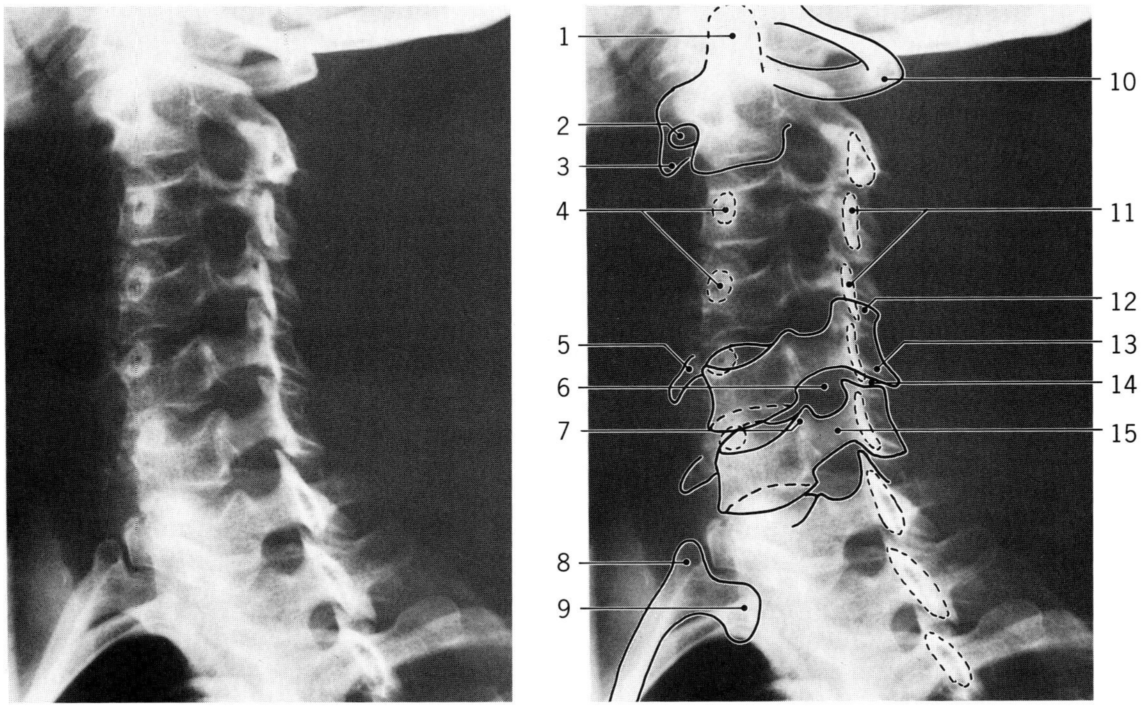

Cervical spine, oblique X-ray

1: Dens axis
2: Foramen transversarium of axis
3: Transverse process of axis
4: Pedicles of vertebral arches C III and C IV
5: Transverse process of C V
6: Intervertebral foramen for sixth cervical spinal nerve
7: Uncus (lip) of vertebral body
8: Tubercle of first rib
9: Head of first rib
10: Posterior arch of atlas
11: Laminae of vertebral arches C III and C IV
12: Superior articular process C V
13: Inferior articular process C V
14: Zygapophyseal (facet) joint C V - C VI
15: Pedicle of vertebral arch C VI

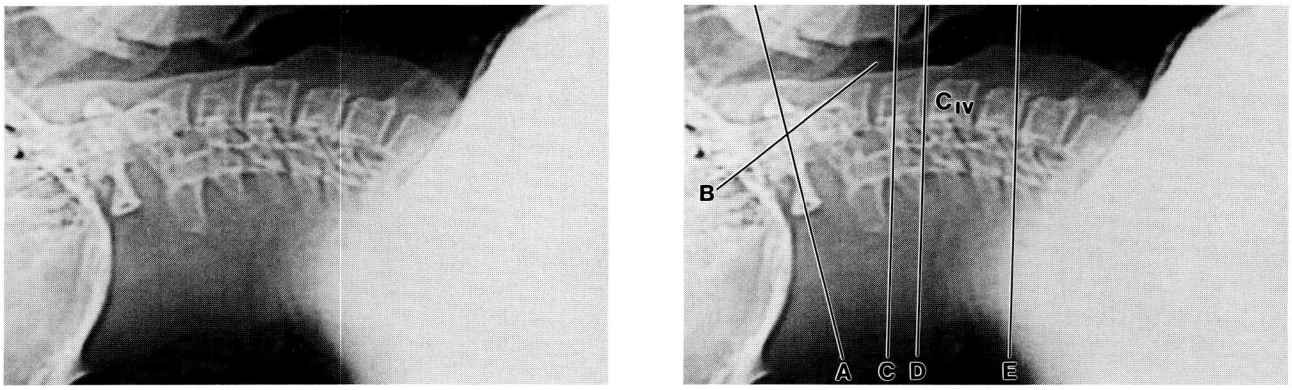

Scout view

Lines A to E indicate position of following sections

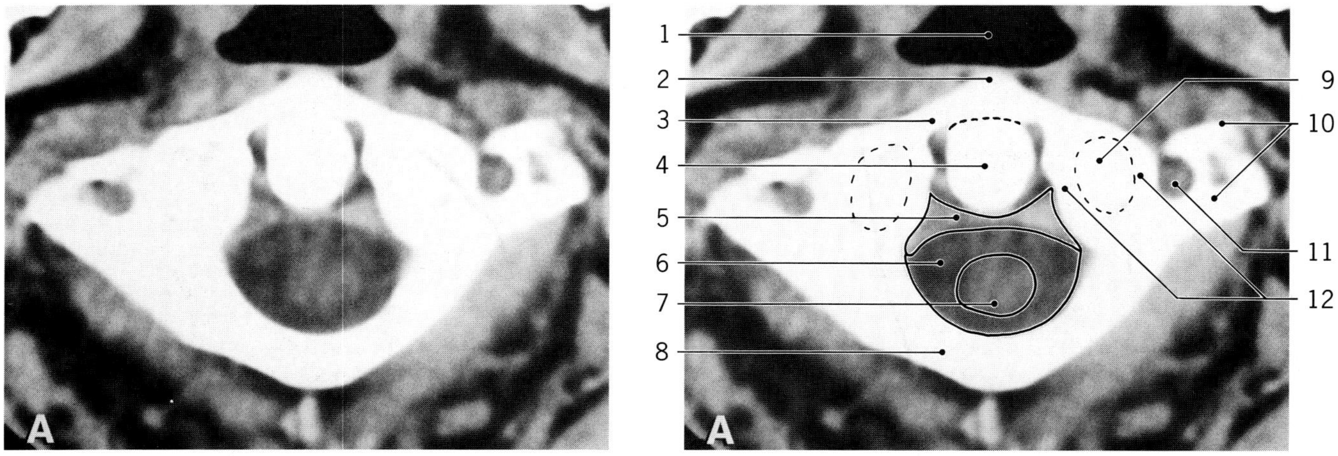

Atlas and axis, axial CT

Position of section A indicated on scout view

1: Pharynx, nasal part
2: Anterior tubercle of atlas
3: Anterior arch of atlas
4: Dens axis
5: Transverse ligament of atlas
6: Subarachnoid space
7: Spinal cord
8: Posterior arch of atlas
9: Occipital condyle
10: Transverse process of atlas
11: Foramen transversarium of atlas
12: Lateral mass of atlas

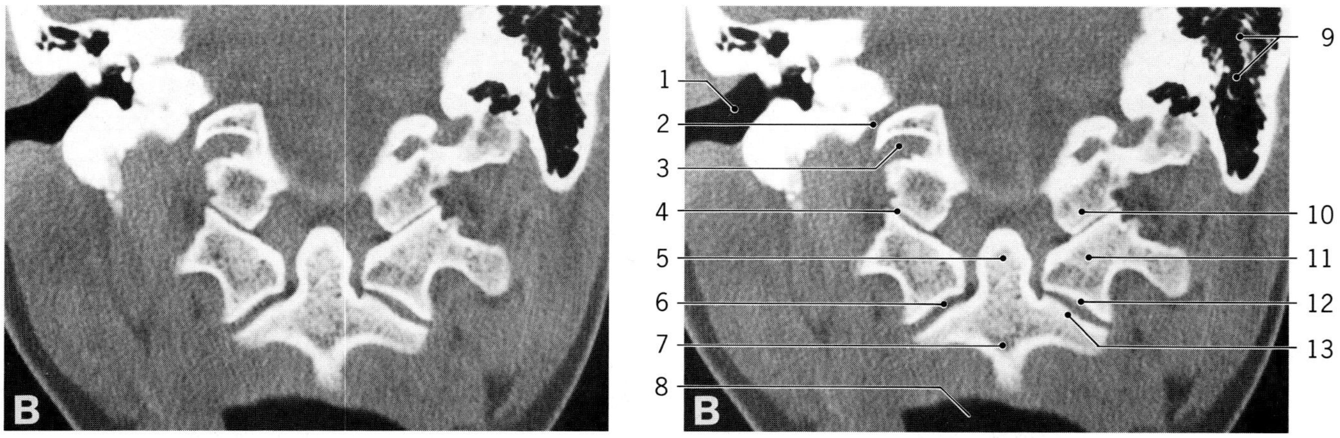

Atlas and axis, coronal CT

Position of section B indicated on scout view

1: External acoustic meatus
2: Jugular foramen
3: Hypoglossal canal
4: Atlanto-occipital joint
5: Dens axis
6: Lateral atlanto-axial joint
7: Body of axis
8: Pharynx
9: Mastoid process
10: Occipital condyle
11: Lateral mass of atlas
12: Inferior articular facet of atlas
13: Superior articular facet of axis

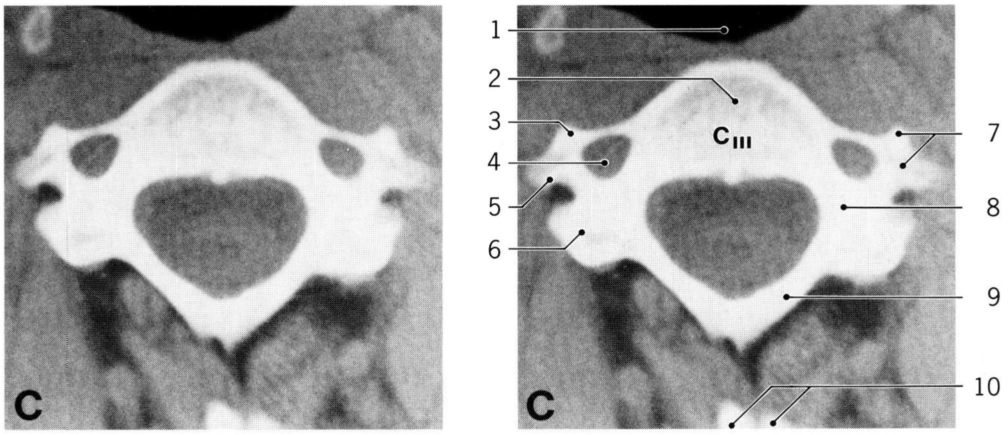

Cervical spine, axial CT

Position of section C indicated on scout view

1: Pharynx
2: Body of vertebra
3: Anterior tubercle
4: Foramen transversarium
5: Posterior tubercle
6: Superior articular process
7: Transverse process
8: Pedicle of vertebral arch
9: Lamina of vertebral arch
10: Spinous process of axis

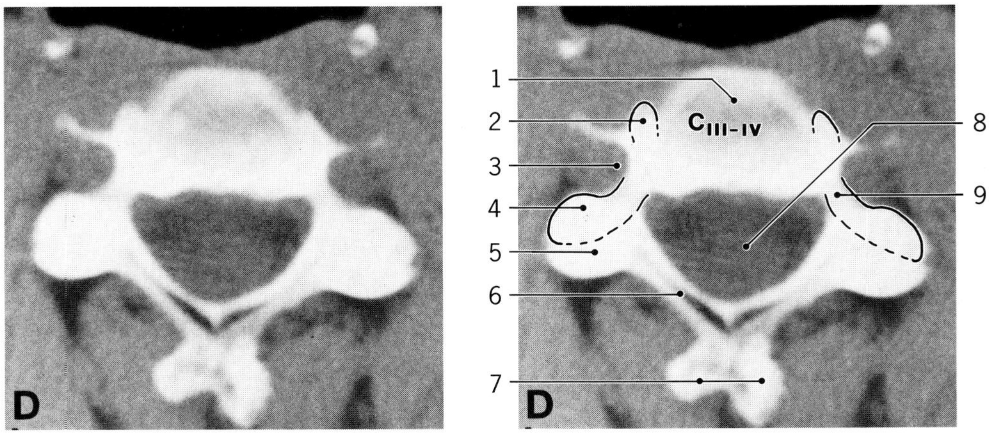

Cervical spine, axial CT

Position of section D indicated on scout view

1: Intervertebral disc
2: Uncus (lip) of body of C IV
3: Groove for spinal nerve
4: Superior articular process of C IV
5: Inferior articular process of C III
6: Lamina of vertebral arch C III
7: Spinous process of C III (bifid)
8: Vertebral canal
9: Pedicle of vertebral arch C IV

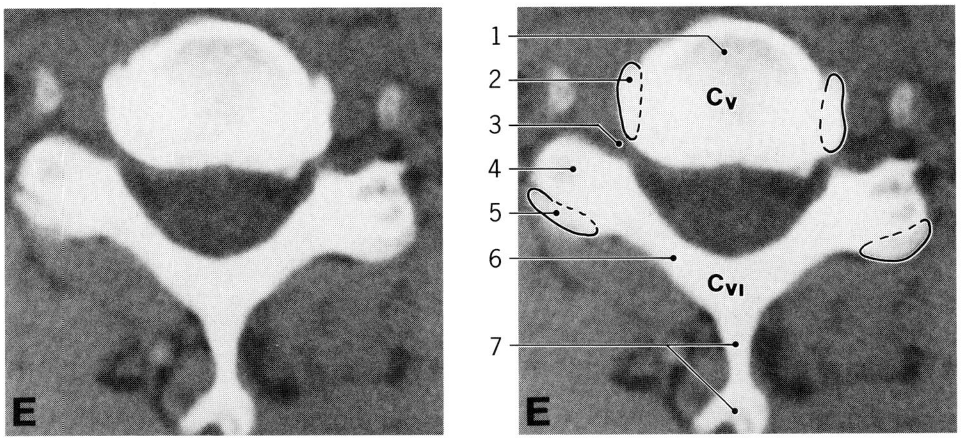

Cervical spine, axial CT

Position of section E indicated on scout view

1: Body of vertebra
2: Uncus (lip) of body of C VI
3: Intervertebral foramen for sixth cervical spinal nerve
4: Superior articular process of C VI
5: Inferior articular process of C V
6: Lamina of vertebral arch
7: Spinous process

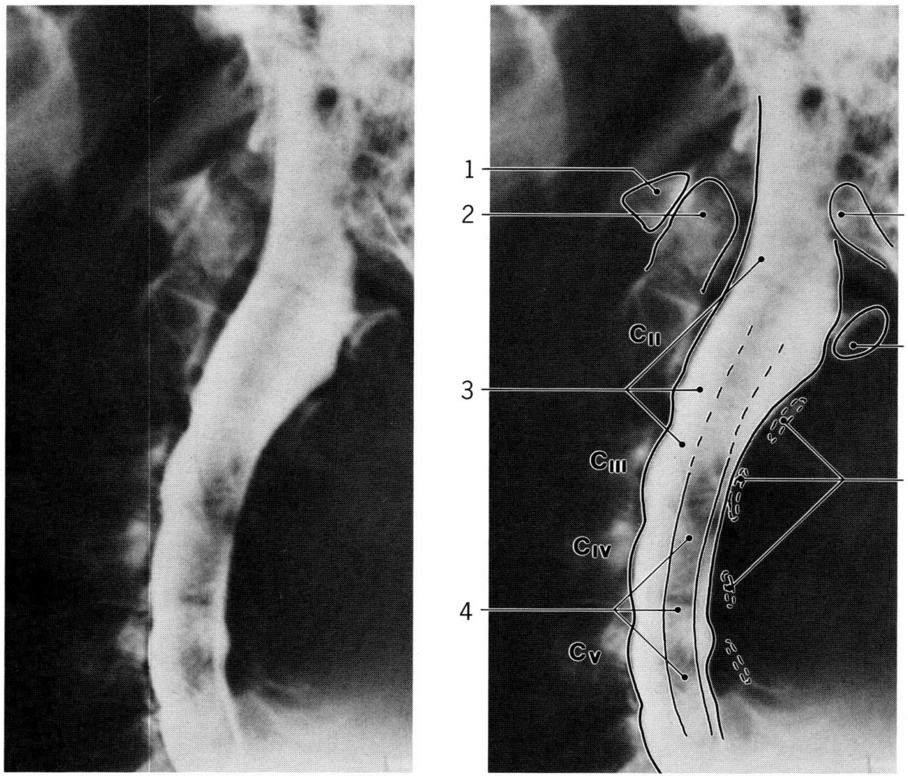

Cervical spine, lateral X-ray, myelography

1: Anterior arch of atlas
2: Dens axis
3: Subarachnoid space
4: Spinal cord
5: Posterior edge of foramen magnum
6: Posterior arch of atlas
7: Laminae of vertebral arches C III, C IV and C V

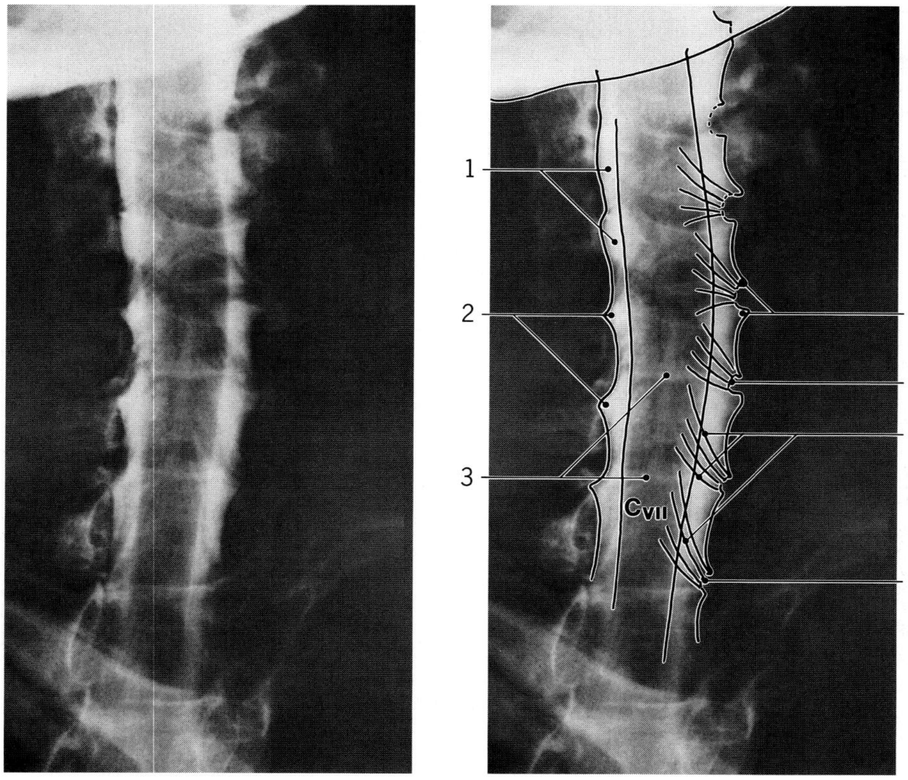

Cervical spine, oblique X-ray, myelography

1: Subarachnoid space
2: Root pouches of subarachnoid space
3: Spinal cord
4: Root pouch of fifth cervical spinal nerve
5: Sixth cervical spinal nerve
6: Spinal nerve rootlets
7: Eighth cervical spinal nerve

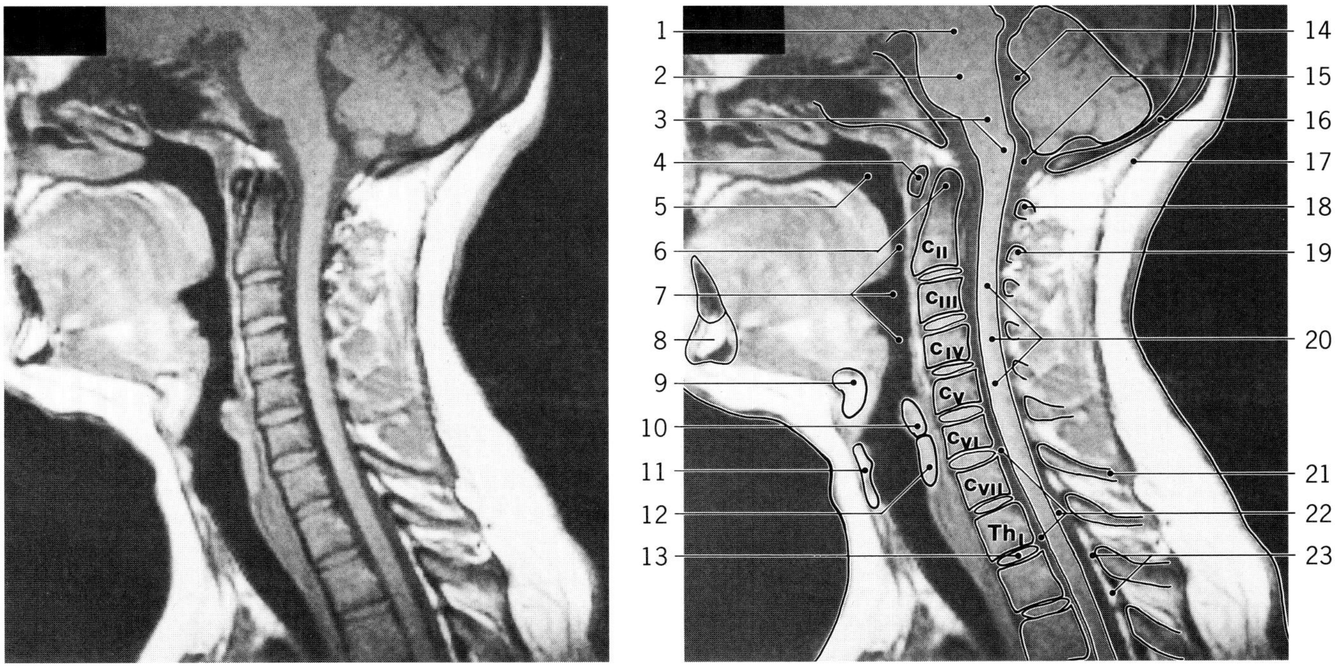

Cervical spine, median MR

1: Mesencephalon
2: Pons
3: Medulla oblongata
4: Anterior arch of atlas
5: Nasal part of pharynx
6: Dens axis
7: Oral part of pharynx
8: Mandible
9: Body of hyoid bone
10: Arythenoid cartilage
11: Thyroid cartilage
12: Lamina of cricoid cartilage
13: Intervertebral disc Th I - Th II
14: Fourth ventricle
15: Cerebello-medullary cistern
16: Squamous part of occipital bone
17: Lig. nuchae
18: Posterior arch of atlas
19: Lamina of vertebral arch C II
20: Spinal cord
21: Spinous process of C VII
22: Subarachnoid space
23: Fat in epidural space

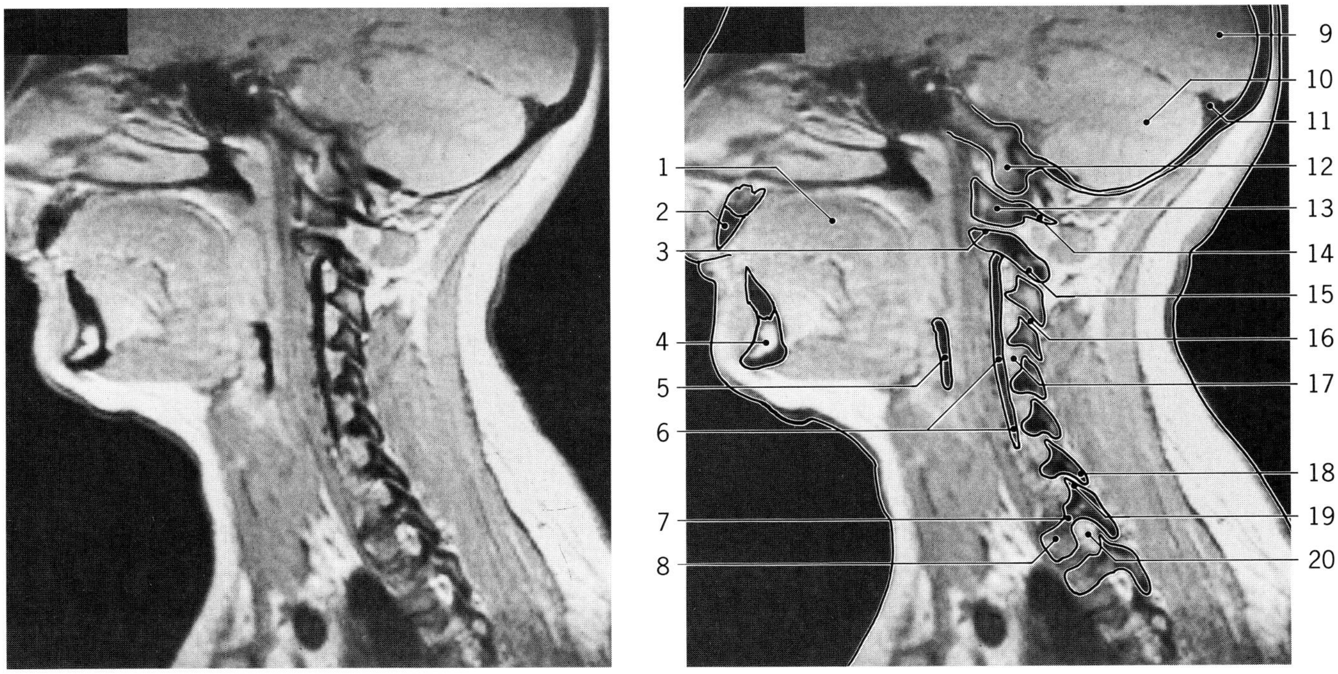

Cervical spine, para-median MR

1: Tongue
2: Upper incisive tooth
3: Superior articular facet of axis
4: Mandible
5: Piriform fossa
6: Vertebral artery
7: Pedicle of vertebral arch Th I
8: Body of vertebra Th I
9: Occipital lobe
10: Cerebellum
11: Transverse sinus
12: Occipital condyle
13: Lateral mass of atlas
14: Posterior arch of atlas
15: Inferior articular process of axis
16: Zygapophyseal (facet) joint C III - C IV
17: Intervertebral foramen with fifth cervical spinal nerve, vessels and fat
18: Inferior articular process of C VII
19: Superior articular process of Th I
20: Intervertebral foramen of first thoracic spinal nerve

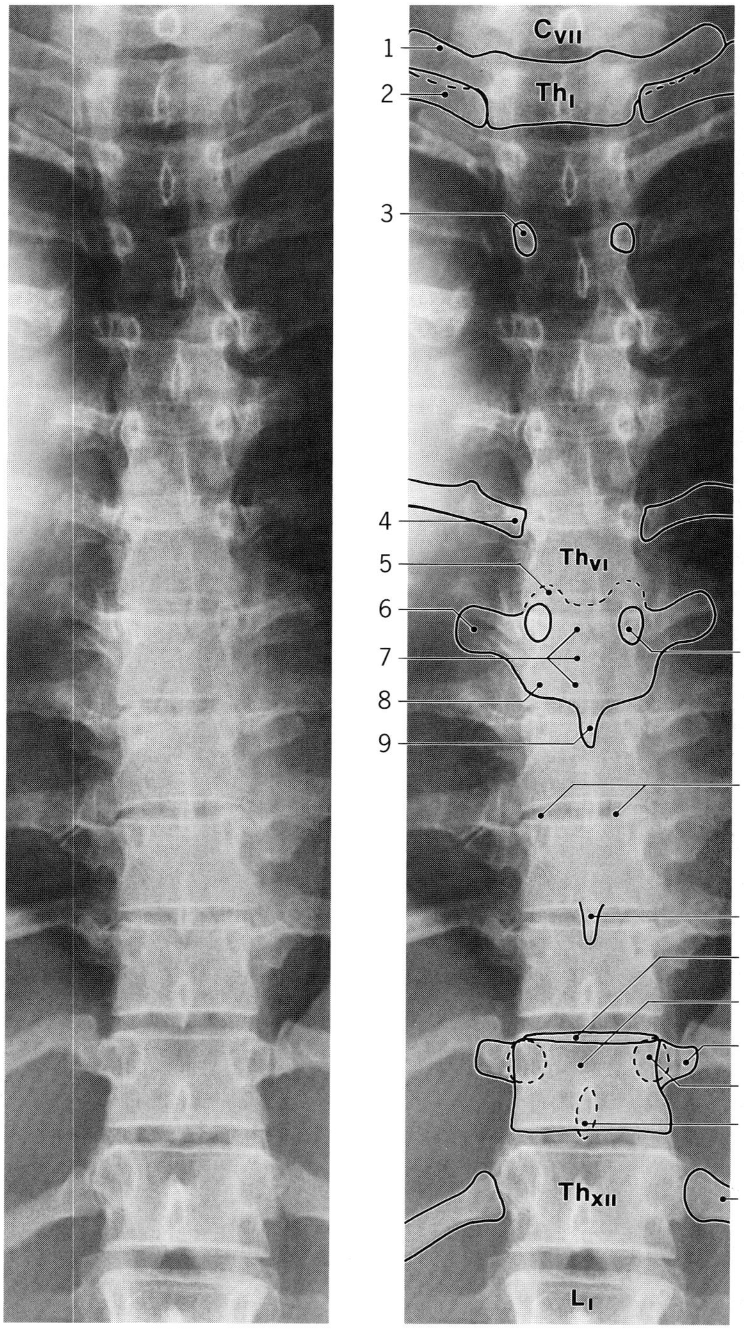

Thoracic spine, a-p X-ray

1: Transverse process
2: First rib
3: Pedicle of vertebral arch Th III
4: Head of sixth rib
5: Superior articular process of Th VII
6: Transverse process of Th VII
7: Lamina of vertebral arch Th VII
8: Inferior articular process of Th VII
9: Spinous process of Th VII
10: Pedicle of vertebral arch Th VII
11: Intervertebral disc Th VIII - Th IX
12: Spinous process of Th IX
13: End plate of vertebral body of Th XI
14: Body of vertebra Th XI
15: Transverse process of Th XI
16: Pedicle of vertebral arch Th XI
17: Spinous process of Th XI
18: 12th rib

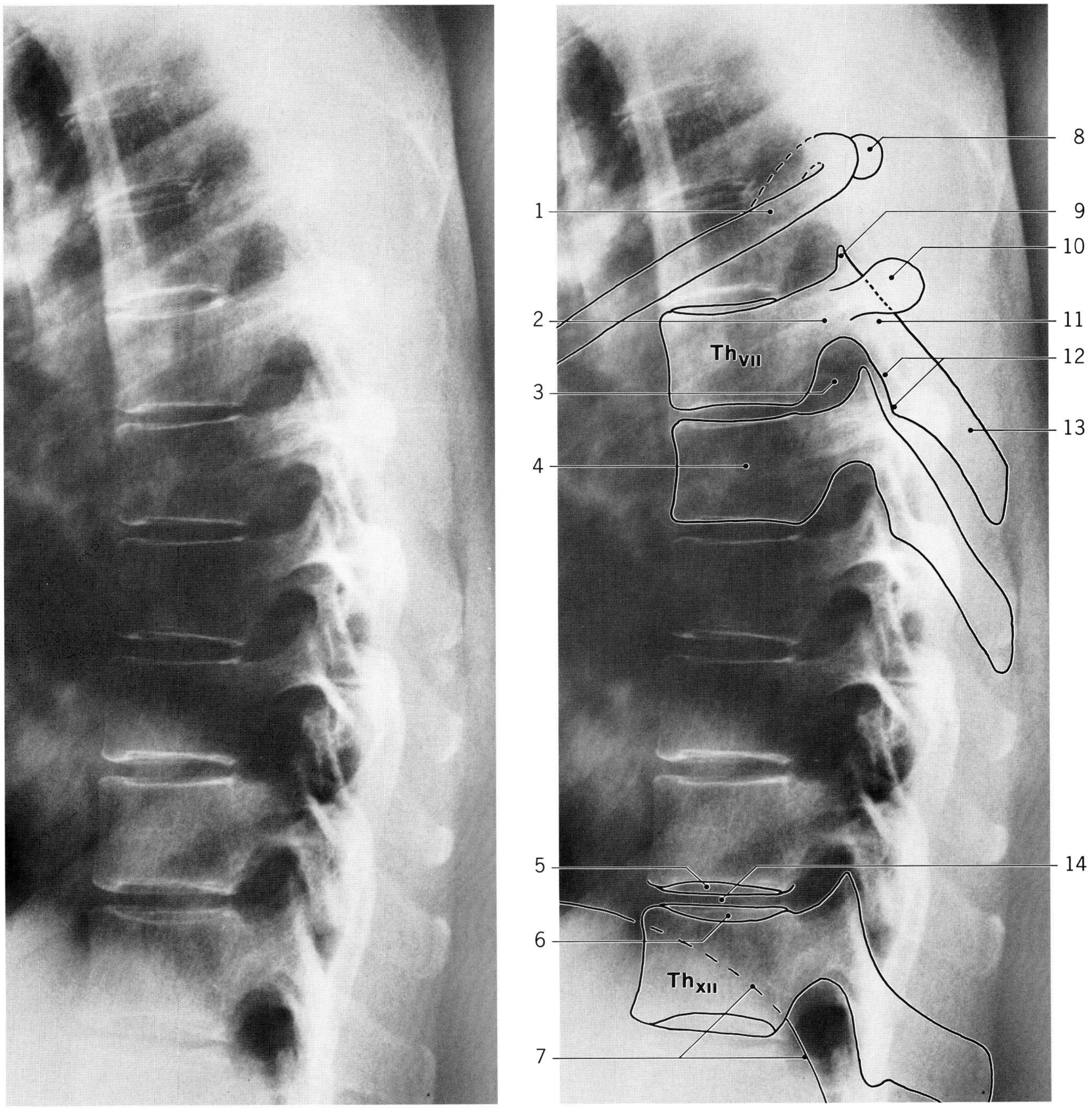

Thoracic spine, lateral X-ray

1: Sixth rib
2: Pedicle of vertebral arch
3: Intervertebral foramen
4: Body of vertebra
5: Lower end plate of Th XI
6: Upper end plate of Th XII
7: Diaphragm
8: Transverse process of Th VI
9: Superior articular process
10: Transverse process
11: Lamina of vertebral arch
12: Inferior articular process
13: Spinous process
14: Intervertebral disc Th XI - Th XII

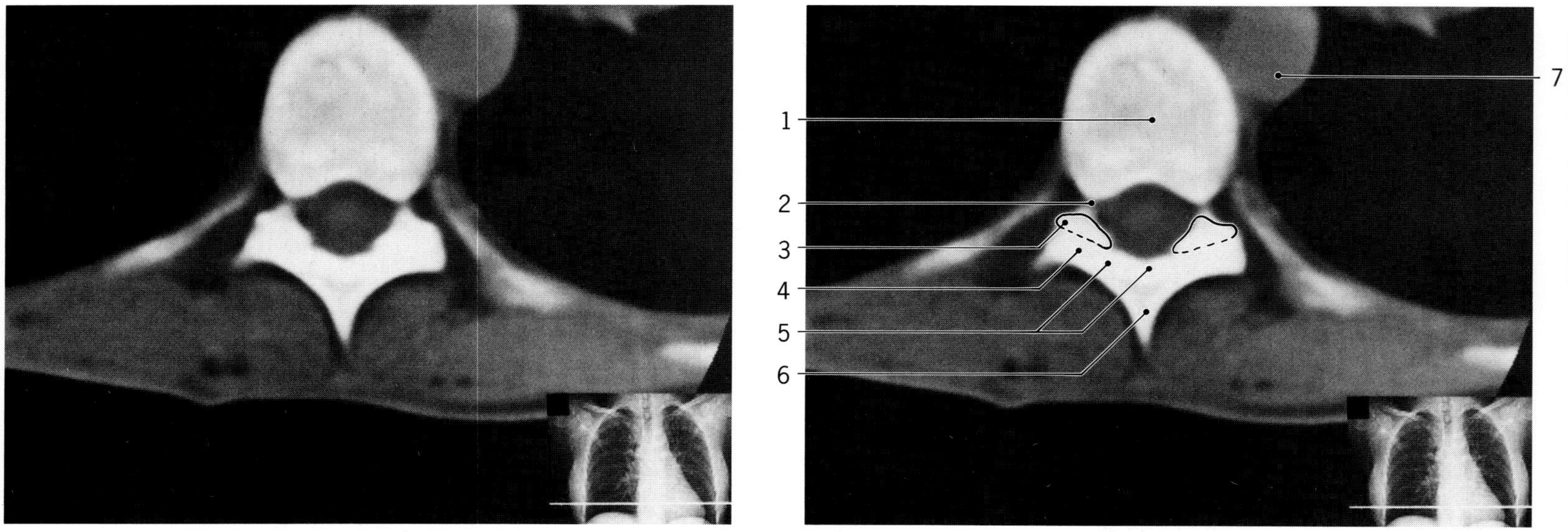

Thoracic spine, axial CT

Section at level of intervertebral disc Th X - Th XI

1: Intervertebral disc Th X - Th XI
2: Intervertebral foramen
3: Superior articular process Th XI
4: Inferior articular process Th X
5: Lamina of vertebral arch
6: Spinous process of Th X
7: Thoracic aorta

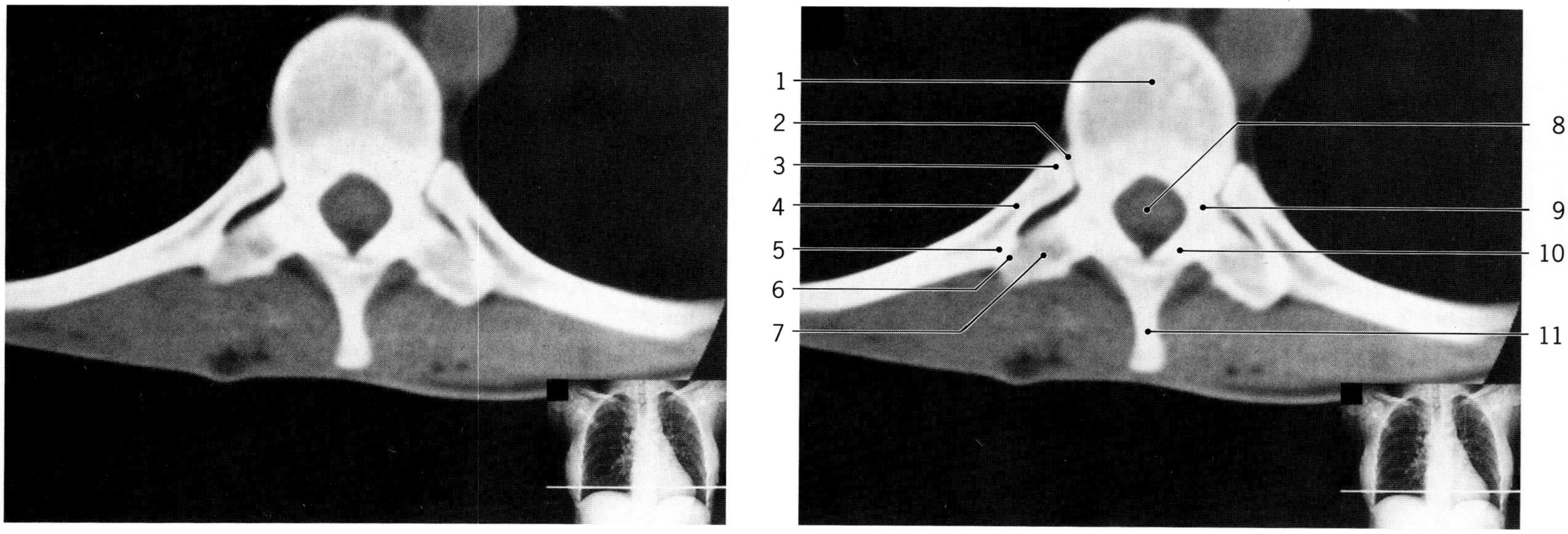

Thoracic spine, axial CT

Level of vertebral body Th XI

1: Body of vertebra Th XI
2: Costovertebral joint
3: Head of 11th rib
4: Neck of 11th rib
5: Tubercle of 11th rib
6: Costotransverse joint
7: Transverse process Th XI
8: Vertebral foramen
9: Pedicle of vertebral arch
10: Lamina of vertebral arch
11: Spinous process of Th XI

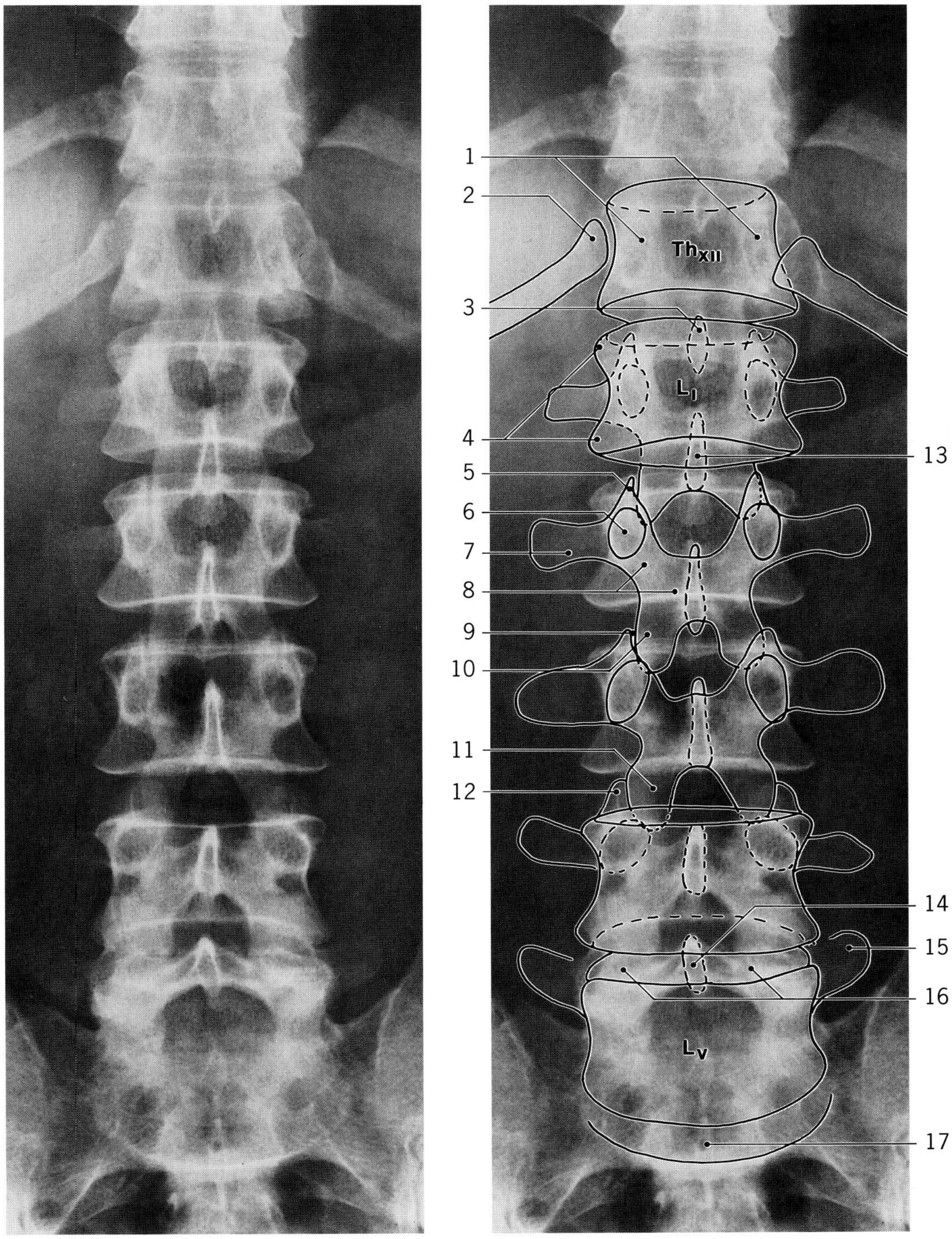

Lumbar spine, a-p X-ray

1: Body of vertebra Th XII
2: Head of 12th rib
3: Spinous process of Th XII
4: Upper and lower ambitus eminens of L I
5: Superior articular process of L II
6: Pedicle of vertebral arch L II
7: Transverse process L II
8: Lamina of vertebral arch L II
9: Zygapophyseal (facet) joint L II - L III
10: Inferior articular process of L II
11: Inferior articular process of L III
12: Superior articular process of L IV
13: Spinous process of L I
14: Spinous process of L V
15: Transverse process of L V
16: Intervertebral disc L IV - L V
17: Base of sacrum

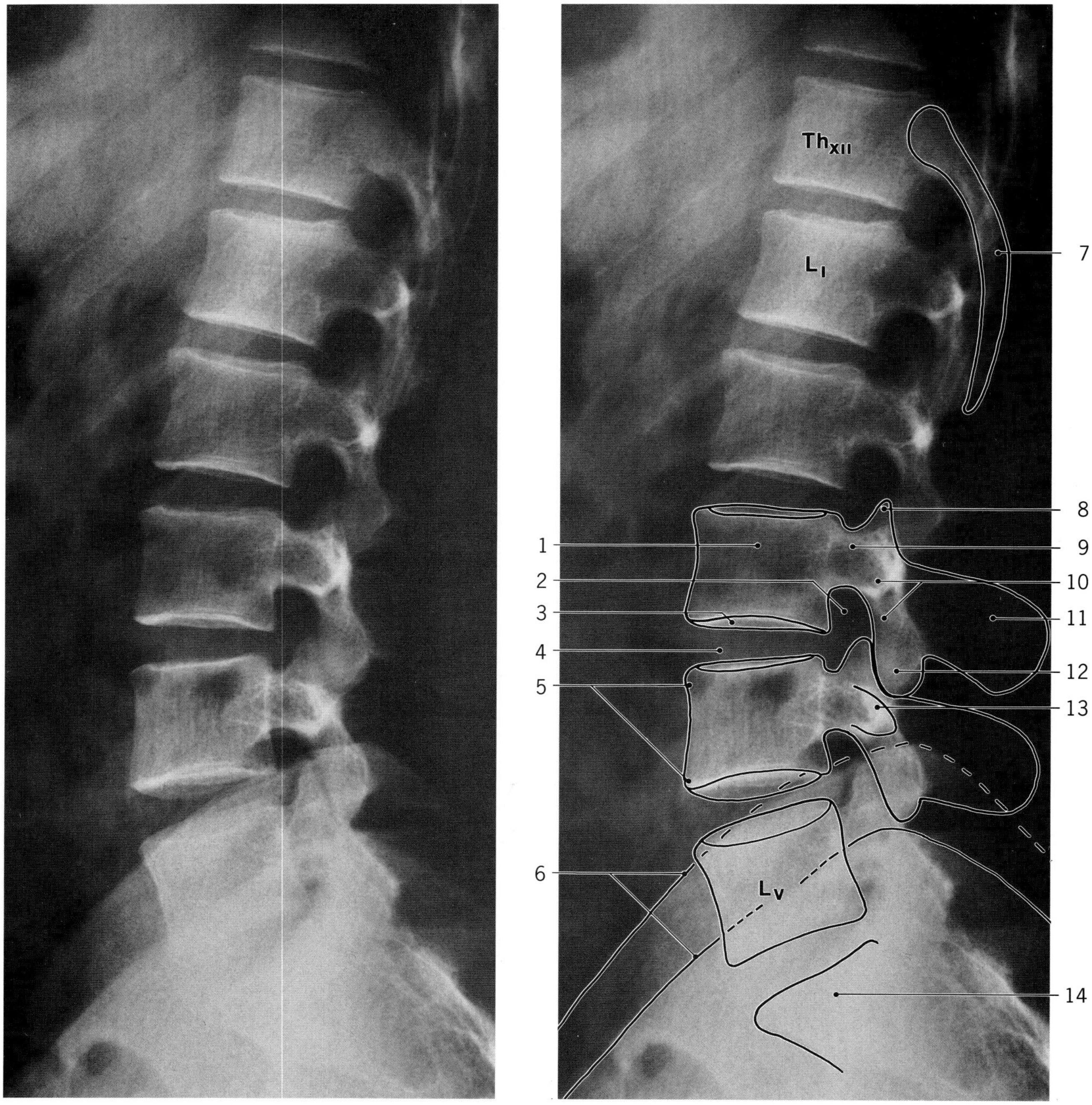

Lumbar spine, lateral X-ray

1: Body of vertebra
2: Intervertebral foramen
3: Lower end plate of L III
4: Intervertebral disc L III - L IV
5: Upper and lower ambitus eminens
6: Iliac crests
7: 12th rib
8: Superior articular process
9: Pedicle of vertebral arch
10: Lamina of vertebral arch
11: Spinous process
12: Inferior articular process
13: Transverse (costal) process
14: Sacrum

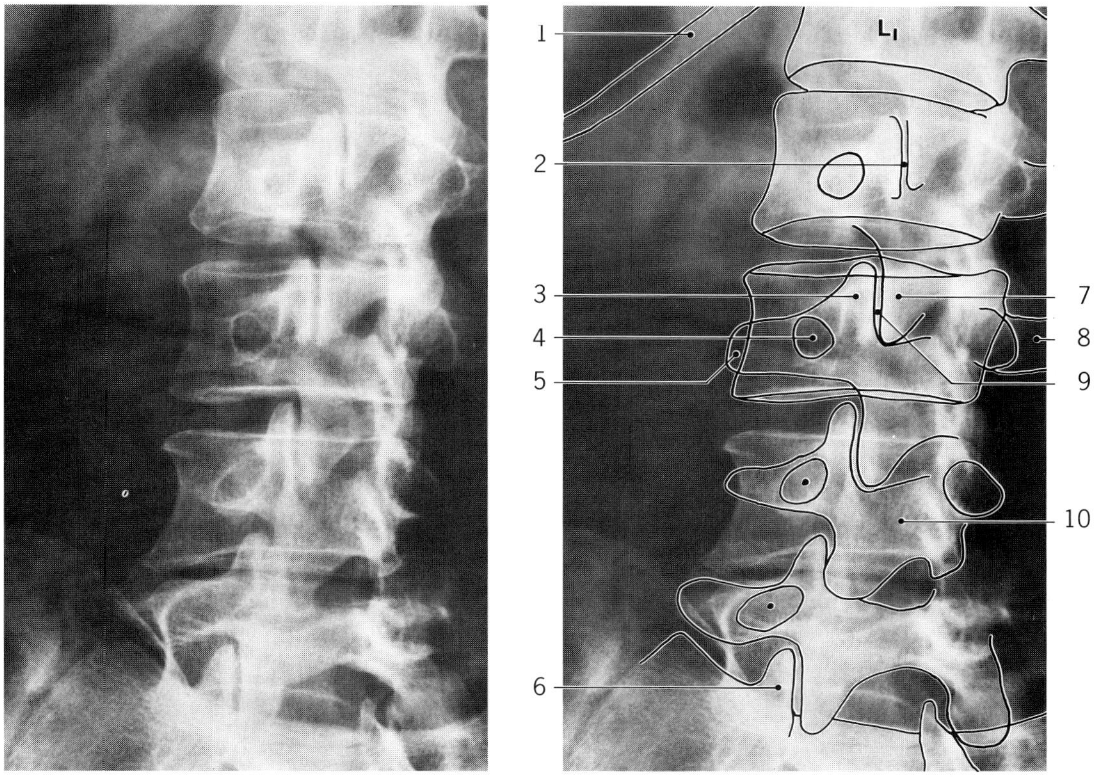

Lumbar spine, oblique X-ray

The "Scottie dog" projection

1: 12th rib
2: Zygapophyseal (facet) joint L I - L II
3: Superior articular process of L III
4: Pedicle of vertebral arch L III
(eye of "Scottie dog")
5: Transverse process of L III
(snout of "Scottie dog")
6: Superior articular process of sacrum
7: Inferior articular process of L II
8: Transverse process of L III
9: Zygapophyseal (facet) joint L II - L III
10: Lamina of vertebral arch L IV

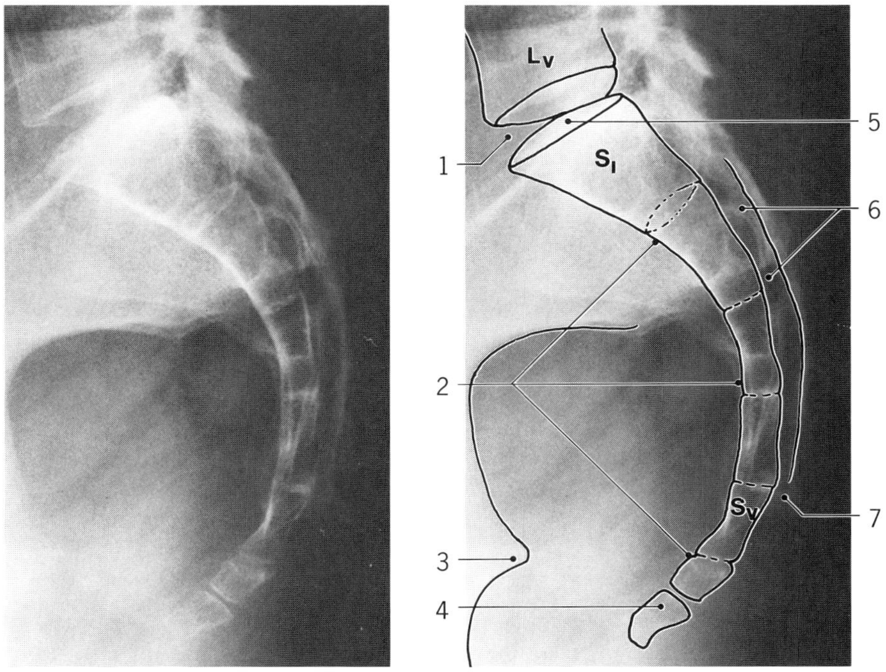

Sacrum, lateral X-ray

1: Intervertebral disc L V - S I
2: Pelvic surface of sacrum
3: Ischial spine
4: Coccyx
5: Base of sacrum
6: Sacral canal
7: Sacral hiatus

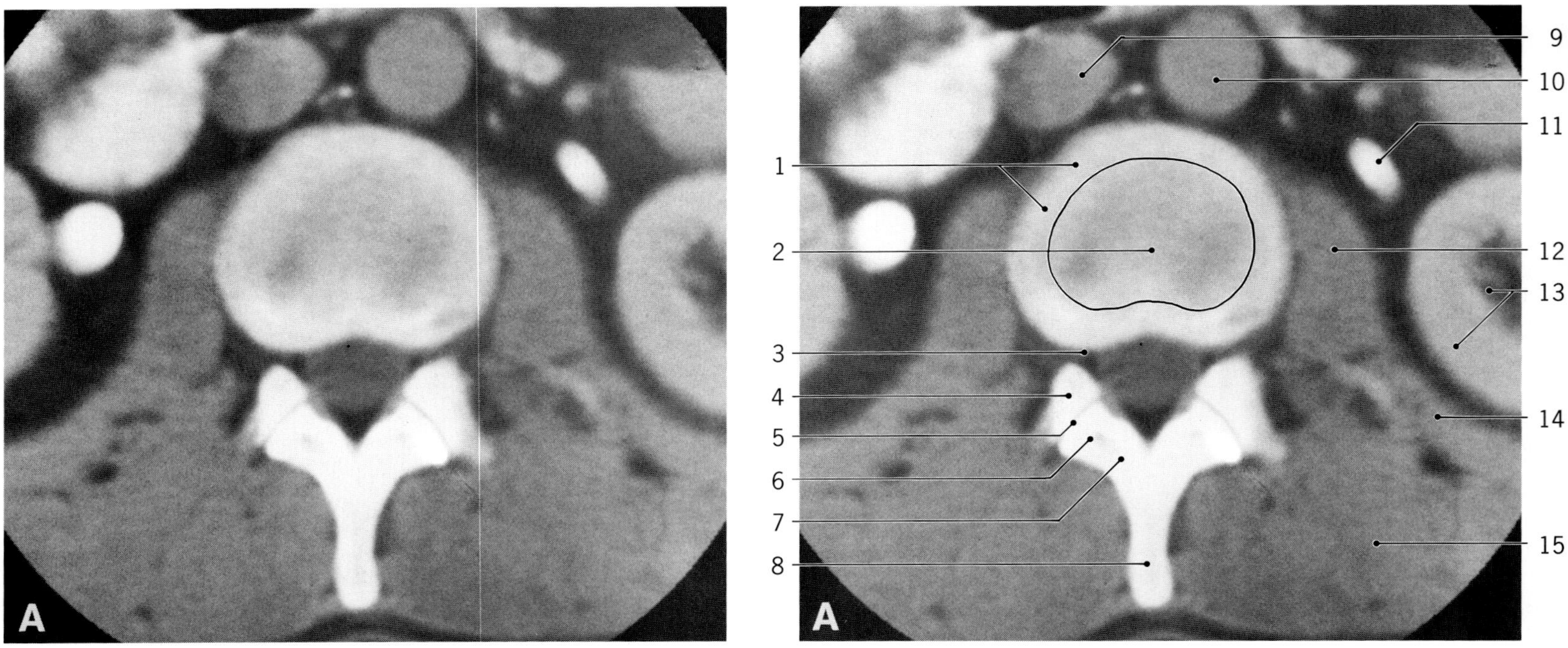

Lumbar spine, axial CT

Level of section A indicated on scout view on opposite page

1: Annulus fibrosus of intervertebral disc
2: Nucleus pulposus
3: Intervertebral foramen for spinal nerve L II
4: Superior articular process of L III
5: Zygapophyseal (facet) joint
6: Inferior articular process of L II
7: Lamina of vertebral arch
8: Spinous process of L II
9: Inferior caval vein
10: Abdominal aorta
11: Left ureter/pelvis (with contrast medium)
12: Psoas major
13: Left kidney
14: Quadratus lumborum
15: Erector spinae

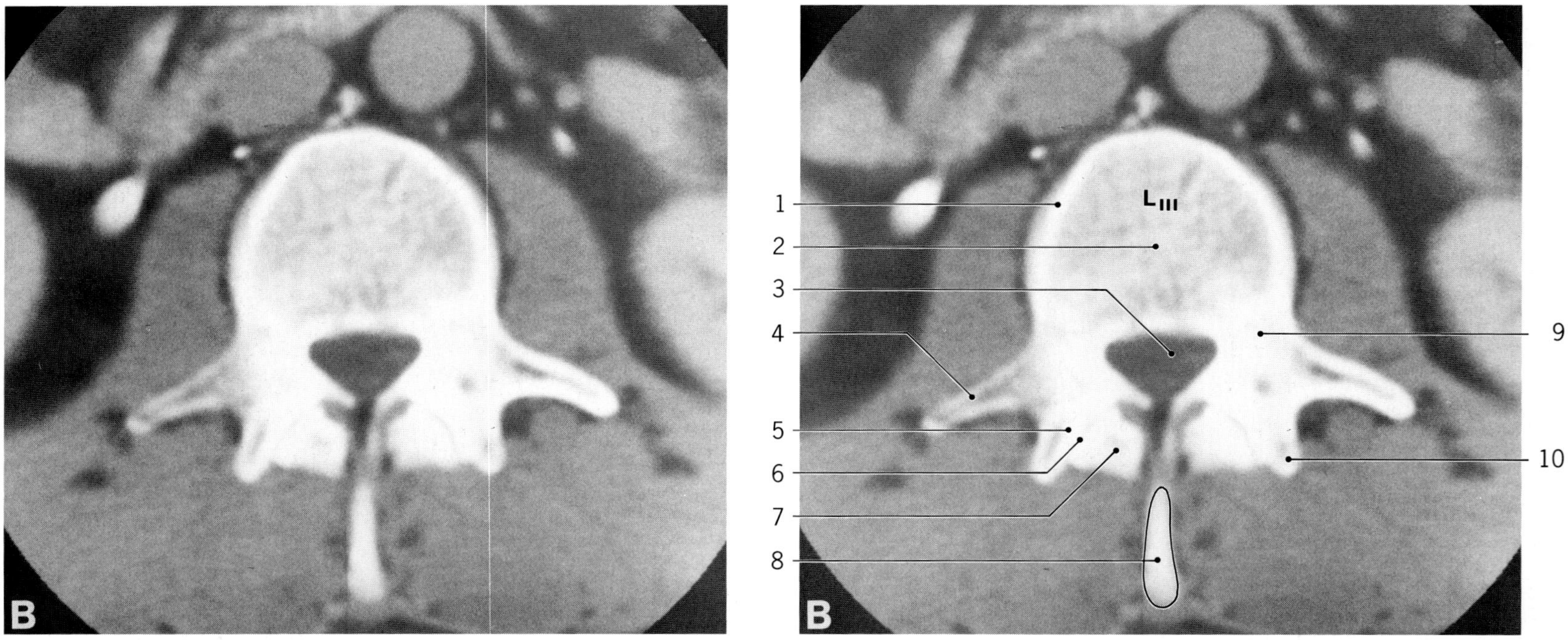

Lumbar spine, axial CT

Level of section B indicated on scout view on opposite page

1: Compact bone
2: Cancelleous bone
3: Vertebral foramen
4: Transverse (costal) process
5: Superior articular process
6: Zygapophyseal (facet) joint L II - L III
7: Inferior articular process of L II
8: Spinous process of L III
9: Pedicle of vertebral arch
10: Mammillary process

Lumbar spine, CT scout view

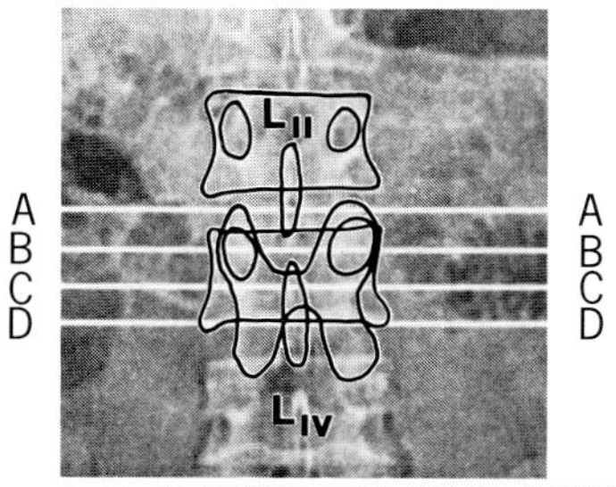

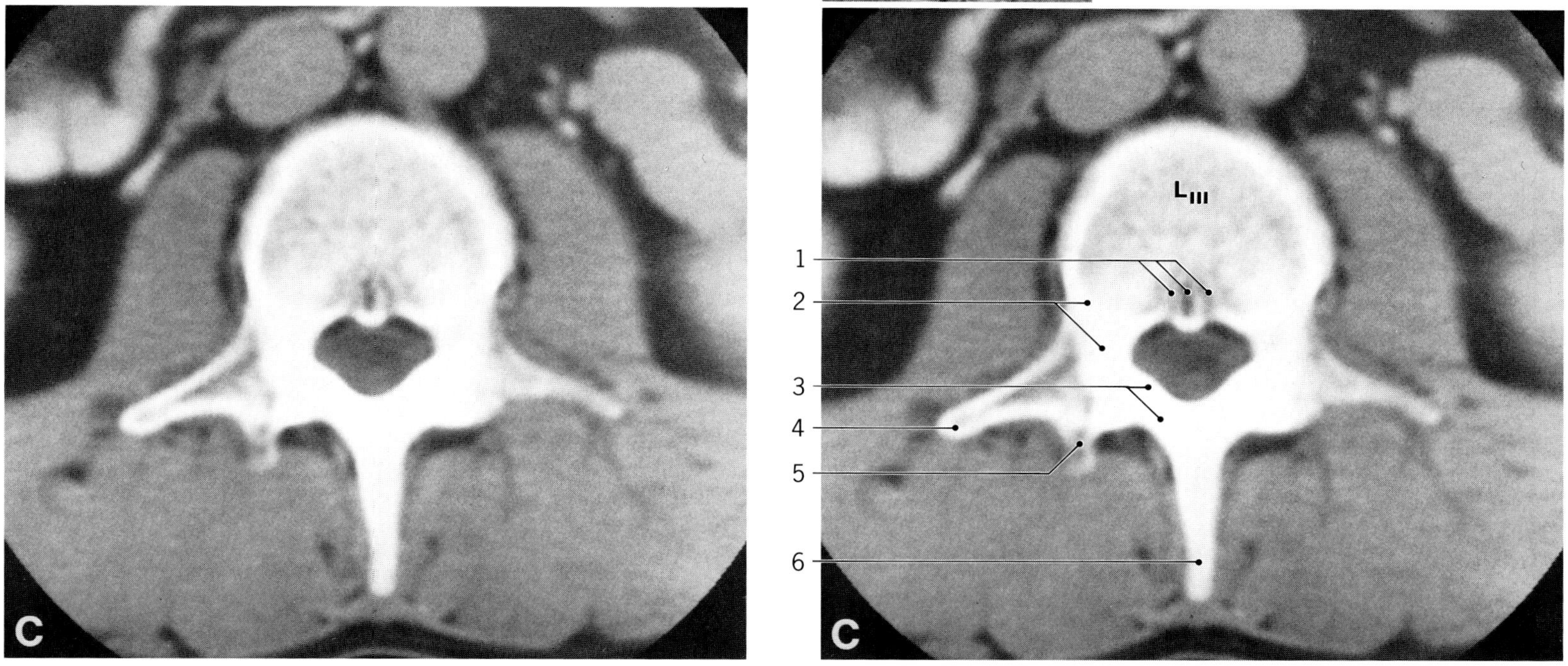

Lumbar spine, axial CT

Level of section C indicated on scout view

1: Basivertebral veins
2: Pedicle of vertebral arch
3: Lamina of vertebral arch
4: Transverse (costal) process
5: Accessory process
6: Spinous process

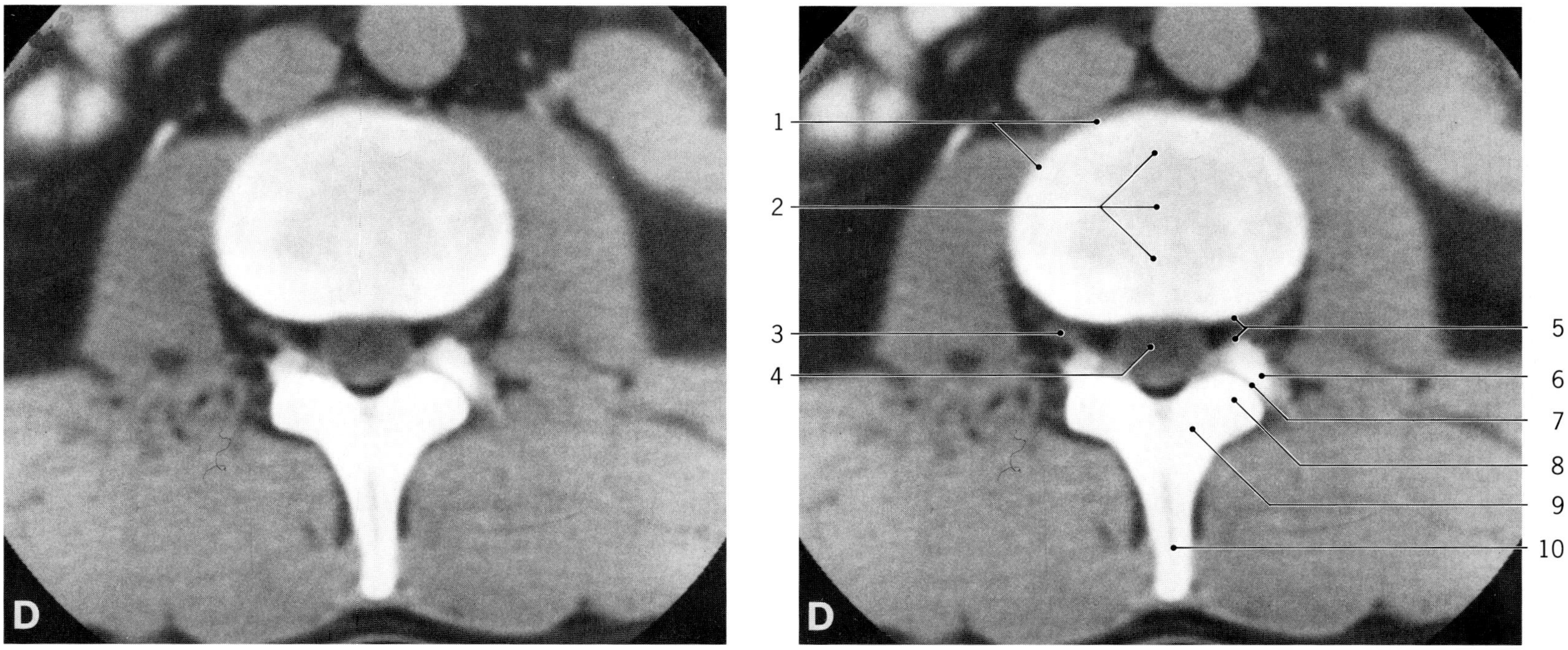

Lumbar spine, axial CT

Level of section D indicated on scout view

1: Ambitus eminens
2: Lower “end plate” of vertebral body L III
3: Third lumbar spinal nerve with ganglion
4: Cauda equina
5: Intervertebral foramen
6: Superior articular process of L IV
7: Zygapophyseal (facet) joint L III - L IV
8: Inferior articular process of L III
9: Lamina of vertebral arch
10: Spinous process of L III

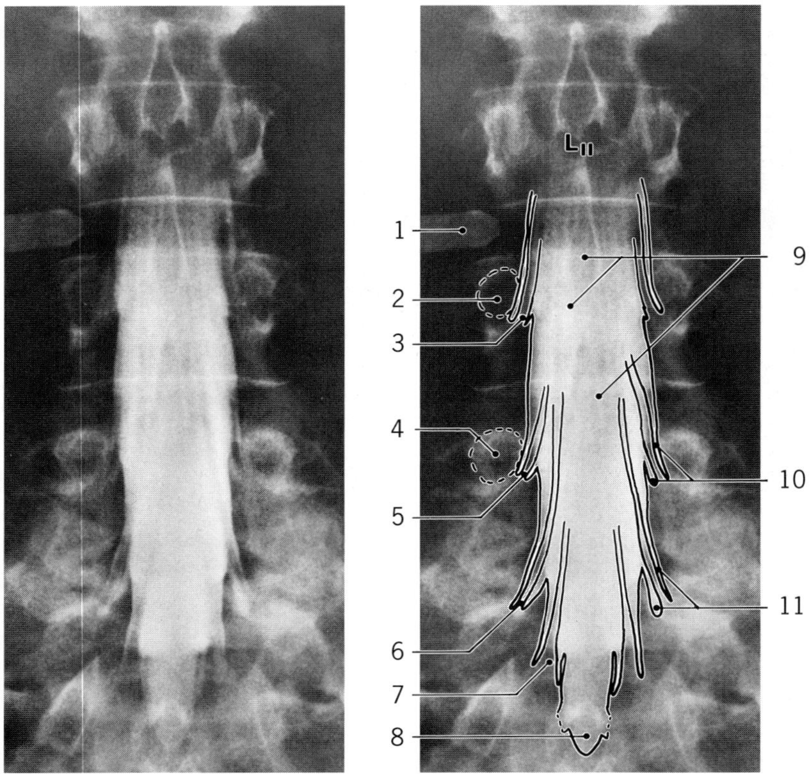

Lumbar spine, a-p X-ray, myelography

1: Marker of level of injection
2: Pedicle of vertebral arch L III
3: Spinal nerve L III
4: Pedicle of vertebral arch L IV
5: Spinal nerve L IV
6: Spinal nerve L V
7: Spinal nerve S I
8: Caudal termination of subarachnoid space
9: Cauda equina
10: Root pouch of spinal nerve L IV
11: Root pouch of spinal nerve L V

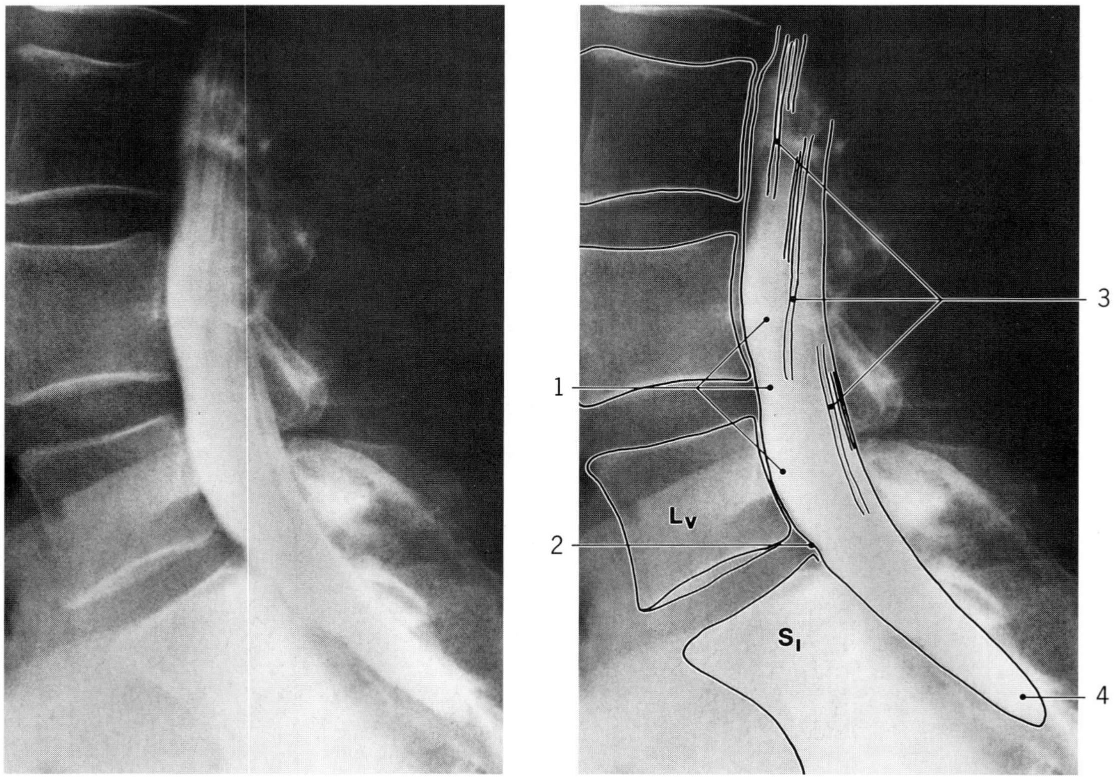

Lumbar spine, lateral X-ray, myelography

1: Subarachnoid space
2: Impression of intervertebral disc
3: Spinal nerve rootlets
4: Caudal termination of subarachnoid space

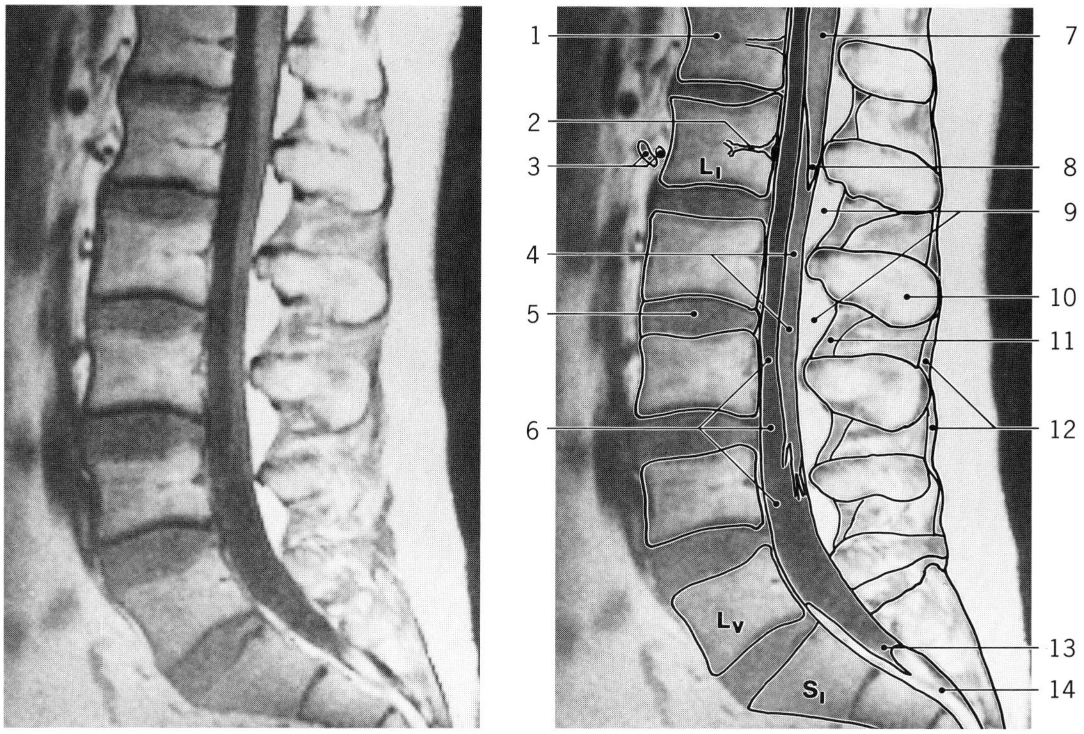

Lumbar spine, median MR

1: Body of 12th thoracic vertebra
2: Basivertebral vein
3: Lumbar artery and vein
4: Cauda equina
5: Intervertebral disc L II - L III
6: Subarachnoid space
7: Spinal cord
8: Conus medullaris
9: Epidural fat
10: Spinous process of L II
11: Lig. flavum
12: Supraspinous ligament
13: Caudal termination of subarachnoid space
14: Sacral canal

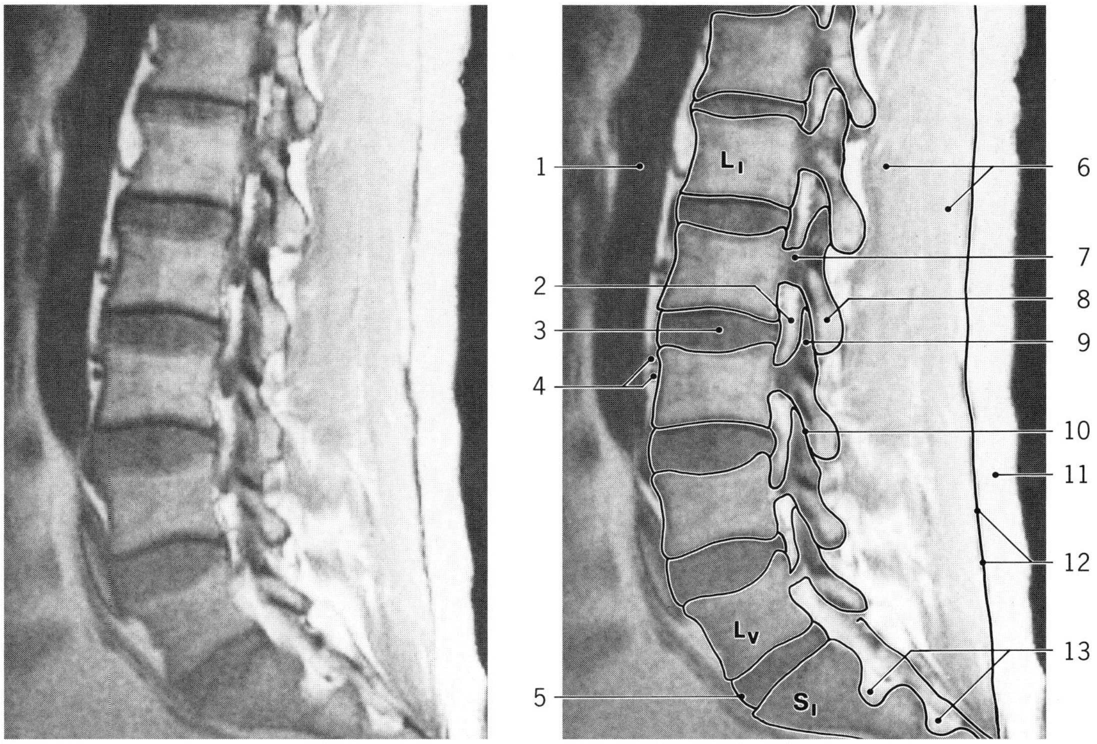

Lumbar spine, para-median MR

1: Abdominal aorta
2: Intervertebral foramen with spinal nerve L II
3: Intervertebral disc L II - L III
4: Lumbar artery and vein
5: Promontory
6: Erector spinae, and transversospinal muscles
7: Pedicle of vertebral arch
8: Inferior articular process L II
9: Superior articular process L III
10: Zygapophyseal (facet) joint L II - L III
11: Subcutaneous fat
12: Thoracolumbar fascia
13: Dorsal sacral foramina

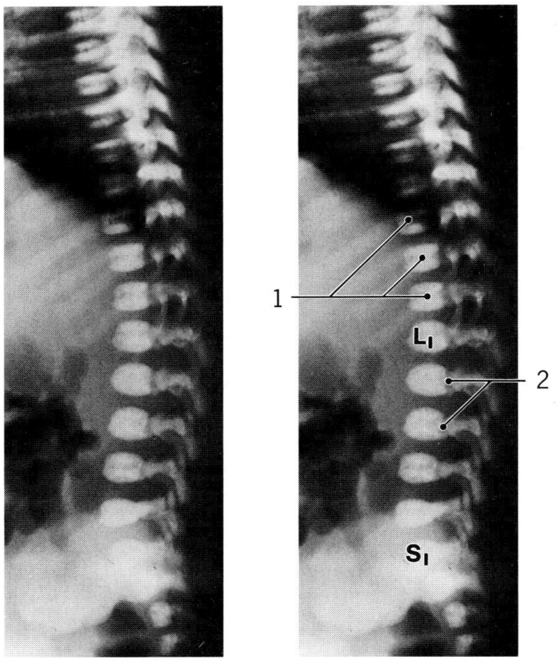

Thoracolumbar spine, lateral X-ray, newborn

1: Yet incomplete fusion of ossification centers in vertebral body

2: Synchondrosis between arch and body of vertebra (neurocentral synchondrosis)

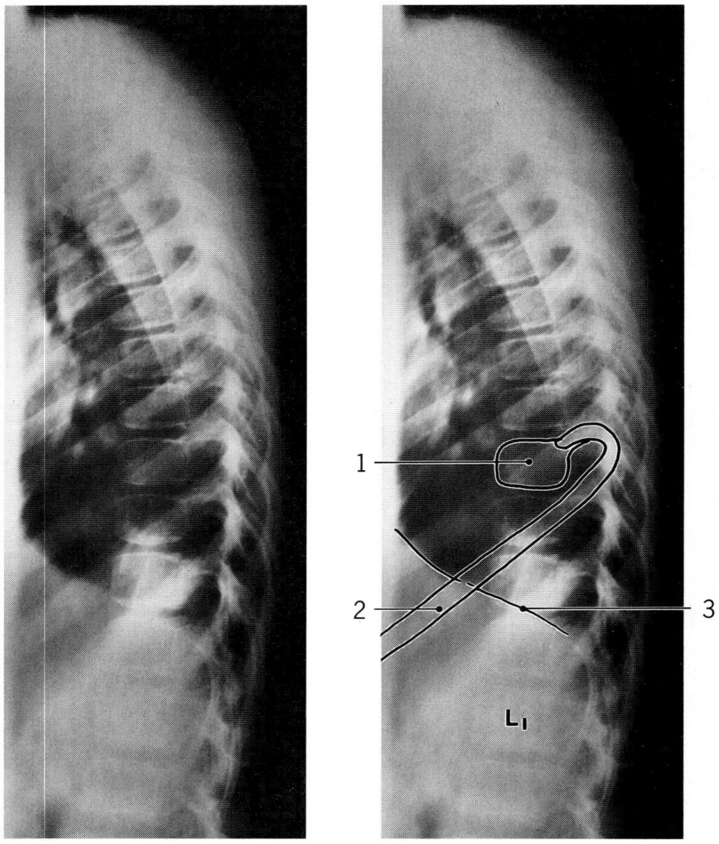

Thoracolumbar spine, lateral X-ray, child 12 years

1: Body of vertebra Th IX. Annular ossification center of end plate has not yet appeared.

2: Ninth rib

3: Diaphragm

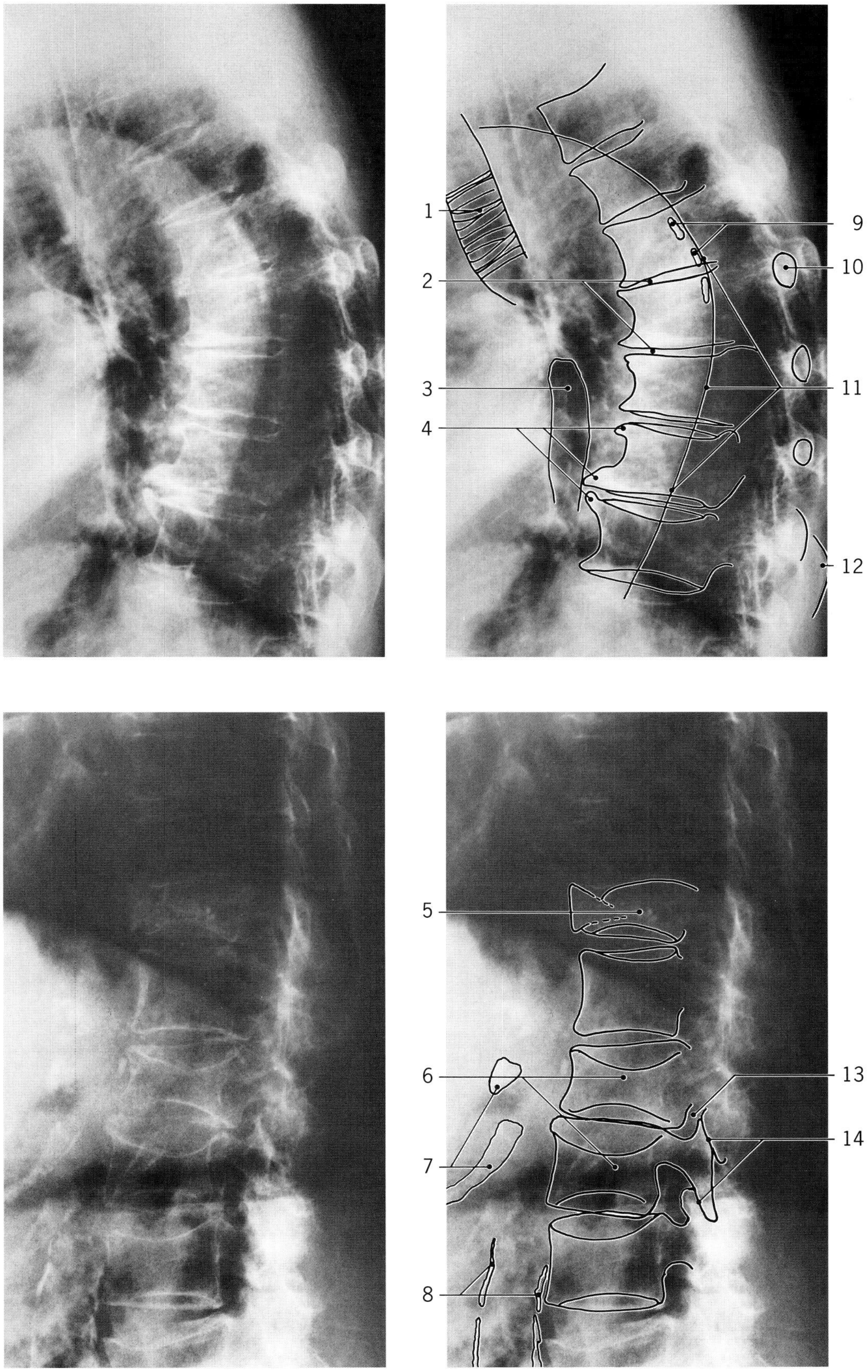

Thoracolumbar spine, lateral X-ray, old age

1: Trachea with calcified cartilages
2: Intervertebral disc (reduced thickness)
3: Esophagus with air
4: Osteophytes
5: Collapsed body of vertebra
6: Vertebral bodies with central compression/fracture
7: Calcified costal cartilage
8: Abdominal aorta (calcified)
9: Calcifications in thoracic aorta
10: Transverse process (tip)
11: Thoracic aorta (posterior wall), elongated
12: Rib
13: Intervertebral foramen (narrowed)
14: Zygapophyseal (facet) joints with subchondral sclerosis (sign of arthrosis)

HEAD

Skull

Ear

Orbita

Paranasal sinuses

Temporomandibular joint

Teeth

Salivary glands

Arteries of neck and face

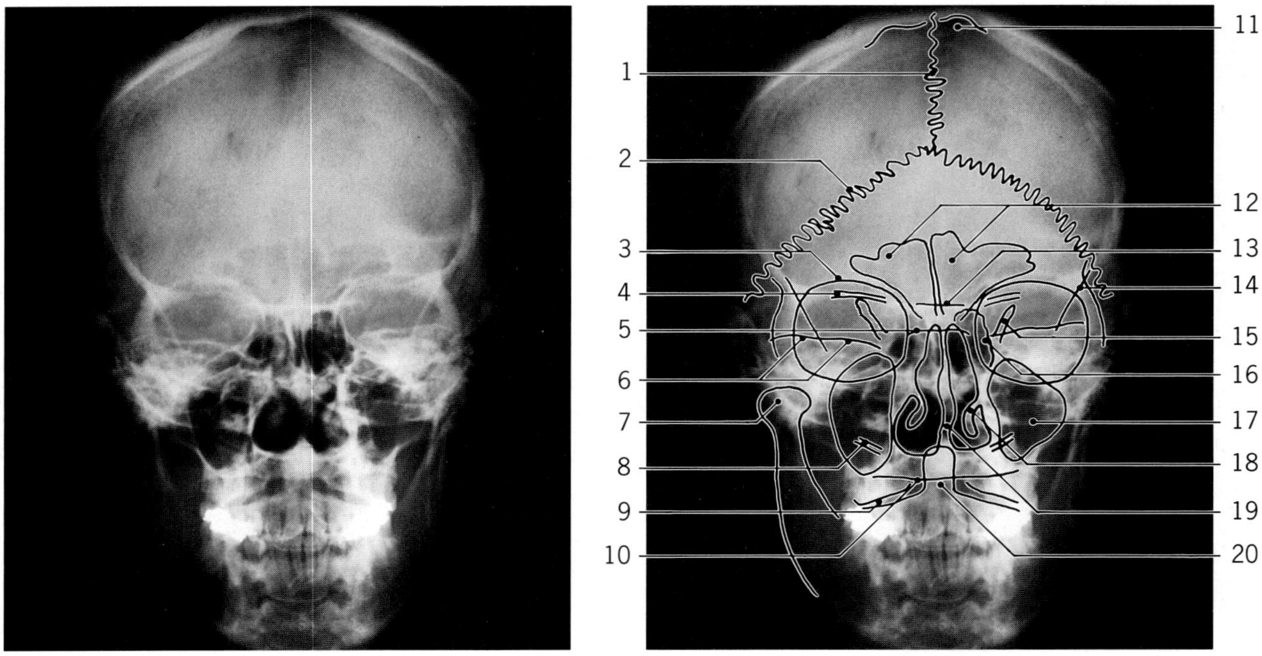

Skull, a-p X-ray

1: Sagittal suture
2: Lambdoid suture
3: Supra-orbital margin
4: Lesser wing of sphenoid bone
5: Hypophysial fossa
6: Crista pyramidis (upper edge of petrous bone)
7: Head of mandible
8: Atlanto-occipital joint
9: Lateral atlanto-axial joint
10: Squama occipitalis
11: Granular foveola
12: Frontal sinus
13: Jugum sphenoidale
14: Innominate line (radiology term) (tangential view of greater wing of sphenoid bone)
15: Superior orbital fissure
16: Ethmoidal air cells
17: Maxillary sinus
18: Inferior nasal concha
19: Nasal septum
20: Dens axis

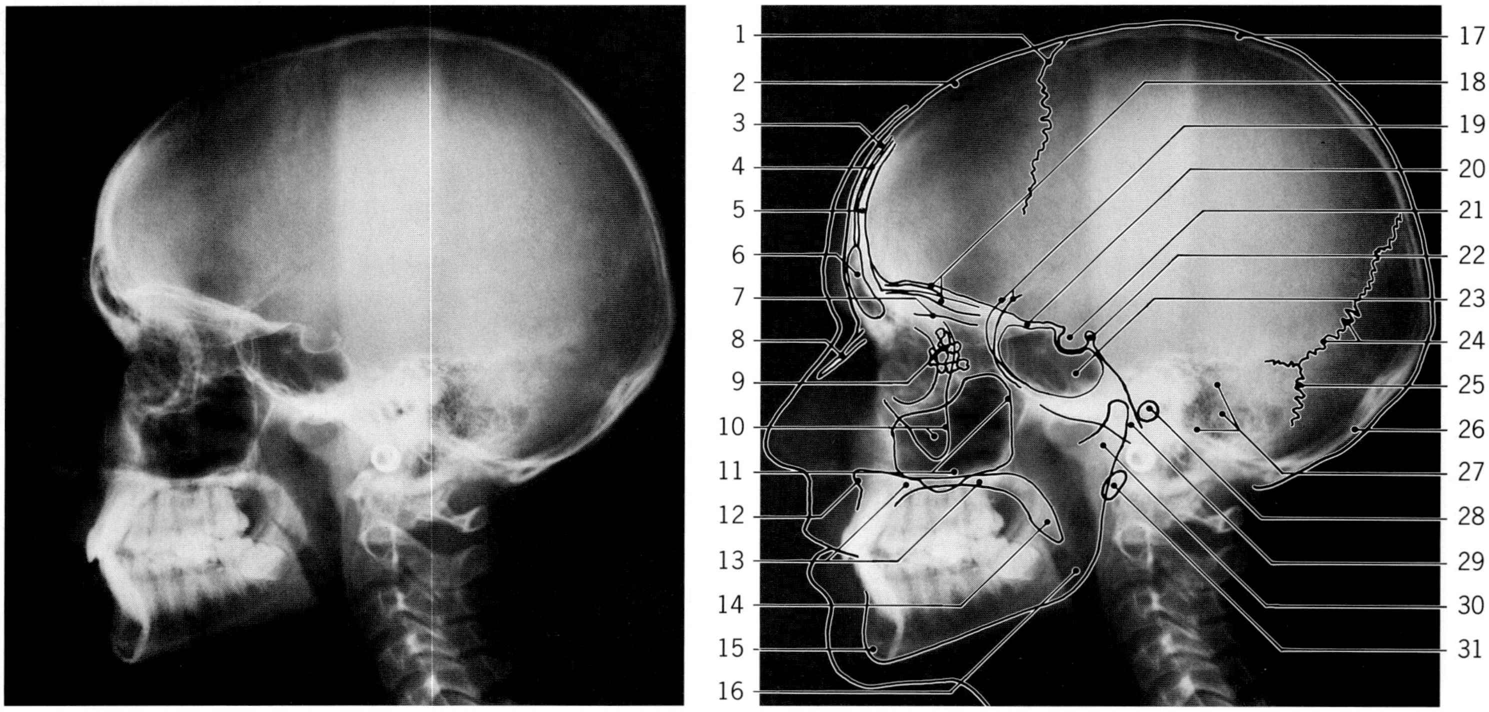

Skull, lateral X-ray

1: Coronal suture
2: Frontal bone
3: Outer table of calvaria
4: Diploë
5: Inner table of calvaria
6: Frontal sinus
7: Cribriform plate
8: Nasal bone
9: Ethmoidal air cells
10: Zygomatic process of maxilla
11: Maxillary sinus
12: Anterior nasal spine
13: Hard palate
14: Uvula
15: Mental protuberance
16: Angle of mandible
17: Parietal bone
18: Orbital plates of frontal bone
19: Greater wings of sphenoid bone
20: Jugum sphenoidale
21: Hypophyseal fossa
22: Dorsum sellae
23: Sphenoidal sinus
24: Lambdoid suture
25: Occipitomastoid suture
26: Squamous part of occipital bone
27: Mastoid air cells
28: External acoustic meatus
29: Clivus
30: Mandibular neck
31: Anterior arch of atlas

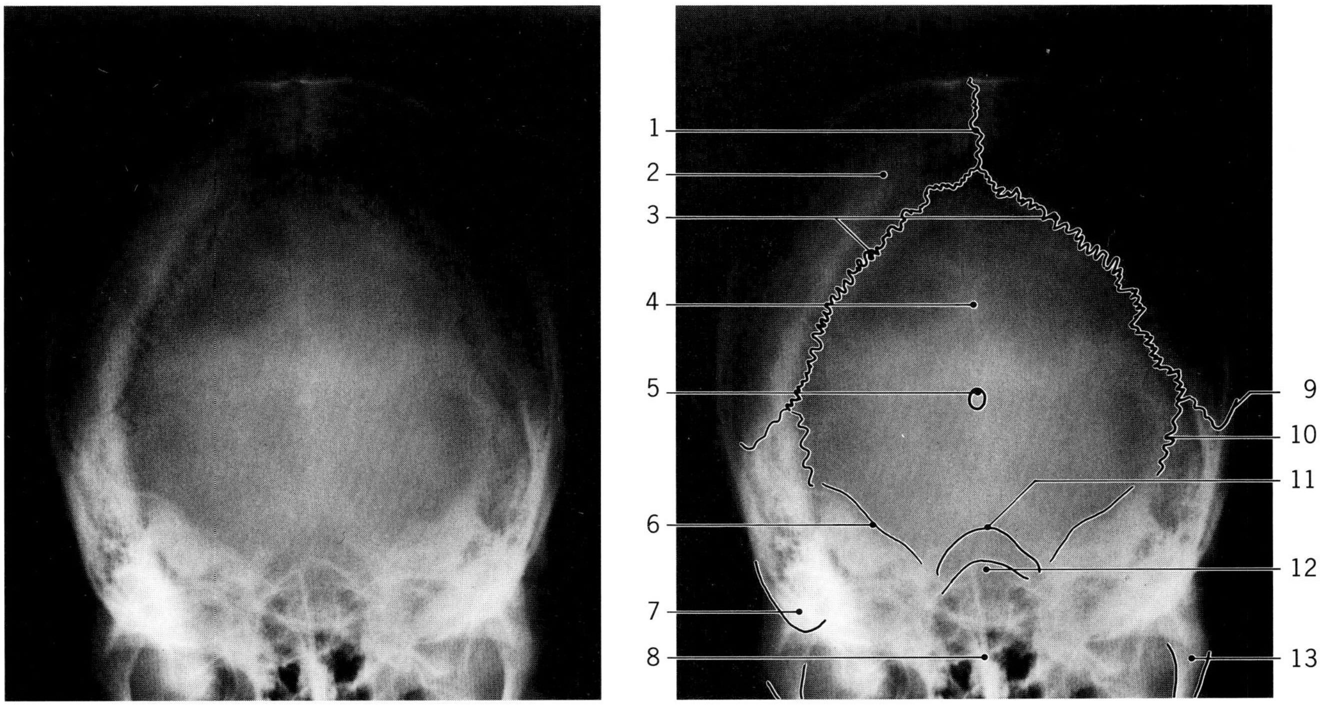

Skull, X-ray, Towne's projection

1: Sagittal suture
2: Parietal bone
3: Lambdoid suture
4: Squamous part of occipital bone
5: Pineal gland (calcified)
6: Petrous part of temporal bone
7: Mastoid process
8: Nasal septum
9: Squamosal suture
10: Occipitomastoid suture
11: Foramen magnum
12: Sphenoidal sinus
13: Mandibular neck

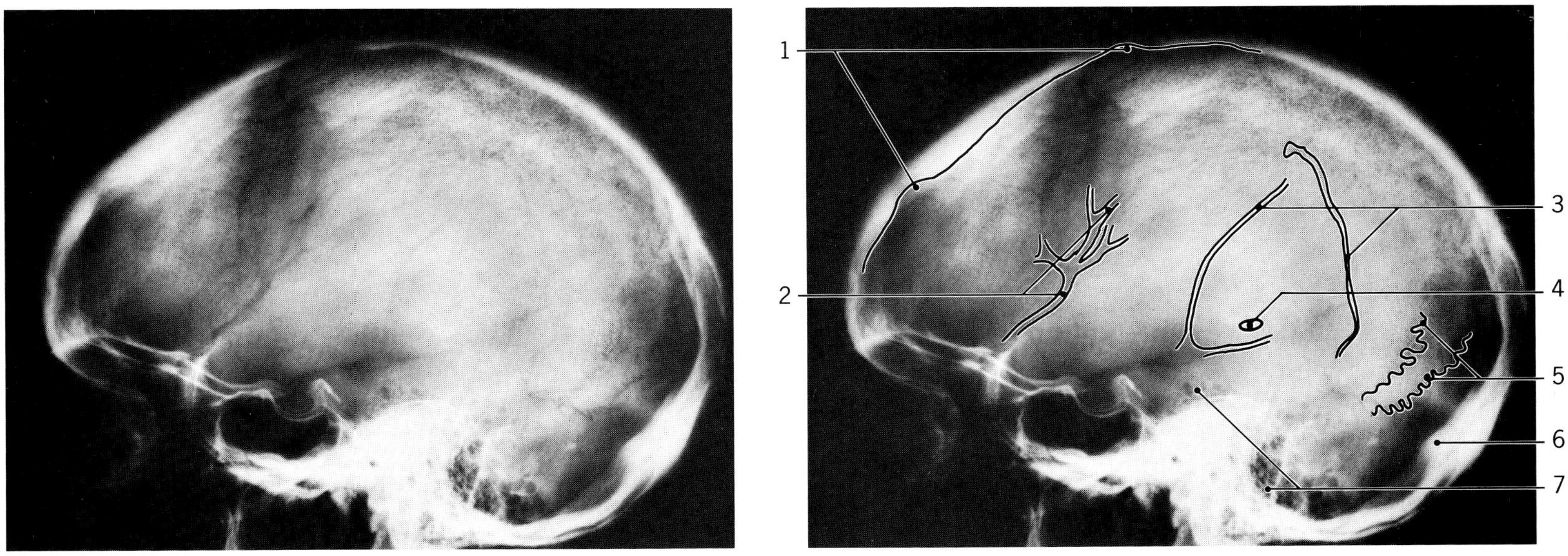

Skull, lateral X-ray, old age

1: Granular foveolae
2: Grooves for branches of middle meningeal artery
3: Diploic veins
4: Pineal gland (calcified)
5: Lambdoid suture
6: Internal occipital protuberance
7: Air cells in temporal bone

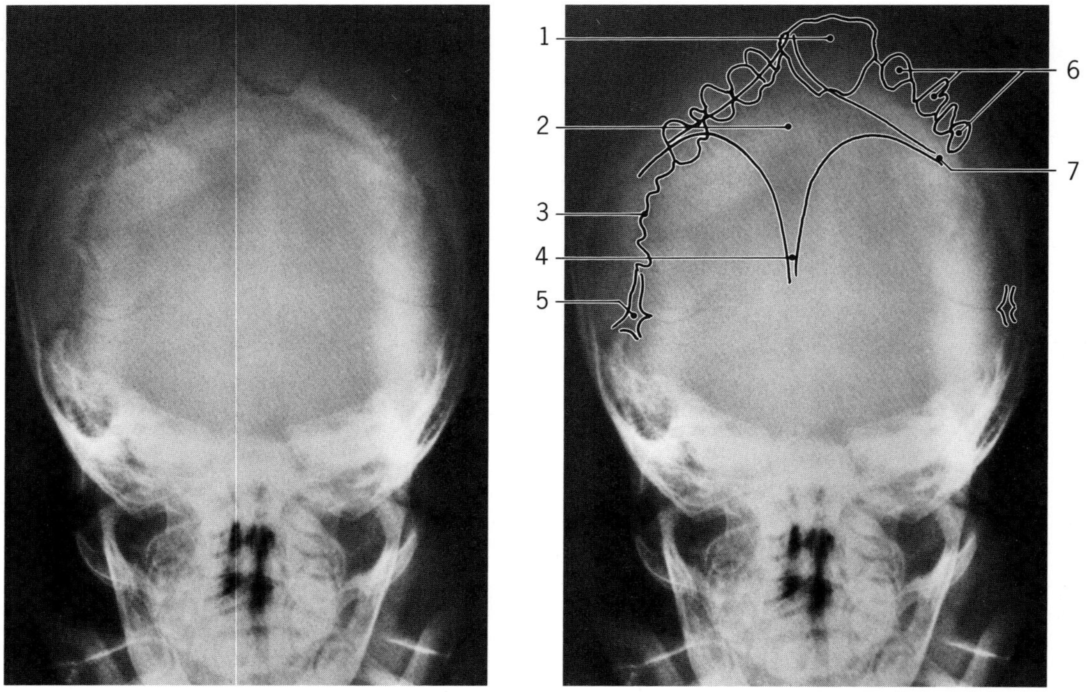

Skull, a-p, tilted X-ray, child 5 months

1: Interparietal bone (Inca bone)
2: Anterior fontanelle
3: Lambdoid suture
4: Sagittal suture
5: Mastoid fontanelle
6: Sutural (Wormian) bones
7: Coronal suture

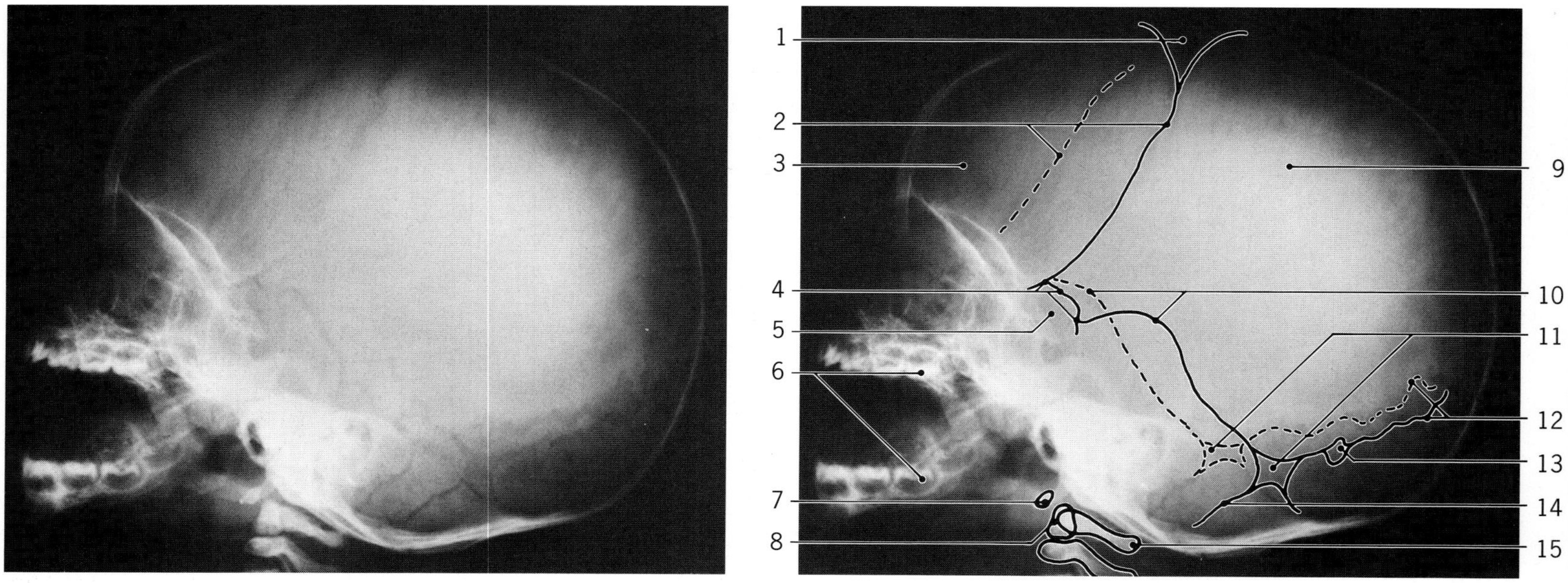

Skull, lateral X-ray, child 5 months

1: Anterior fontanelle
2: Coronal suture
3: Frontal bone
4: Pterion (sphenoidal fontanelle)
5: Greater wing of sphenoid bone
6: Deciduous teeth
7: Anterior arch of atlas
8: Dens axis
9: Parietal bone
10: Squamosal sutures
11: Mastoid fontanelles
12: Lambdoid suture
13: Sutural bone
14: Occipitomastoid suture
15: Posterior arch of atlas

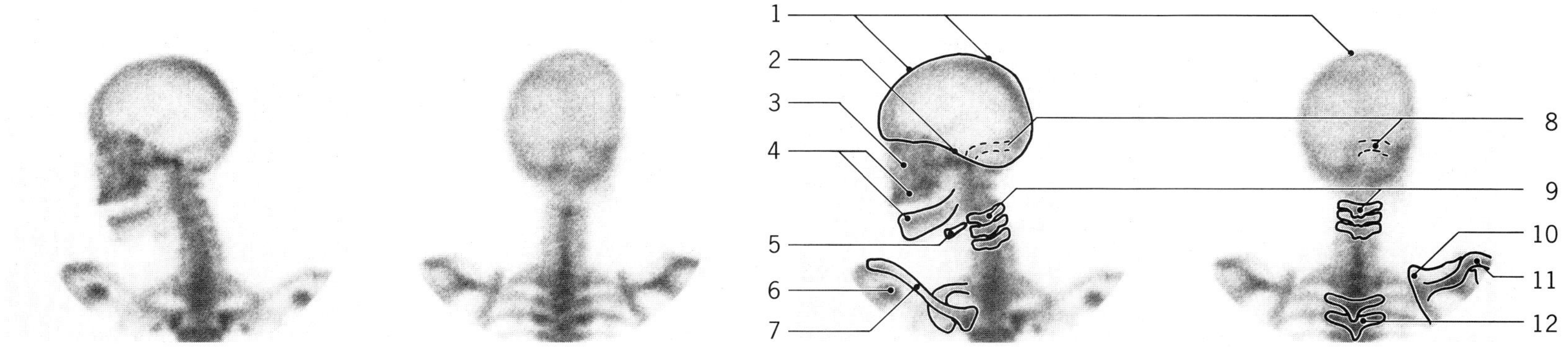

Skull, lateral and posterior view, ^{99m}MDP, scintigraphy

1: Calvaria
2: Base of skull
3: Facial skeleton
4: Alveolar process of maxilla and alveolar part of mandible
5: Hyoid bone
6: Coracoid process
7: Clavicle
8: Transverse and sigmoid sinus
9: Cervical vertebra
10: Superior angle of scapula
11: Acromion
12: Thoracic vertebra

Scout view

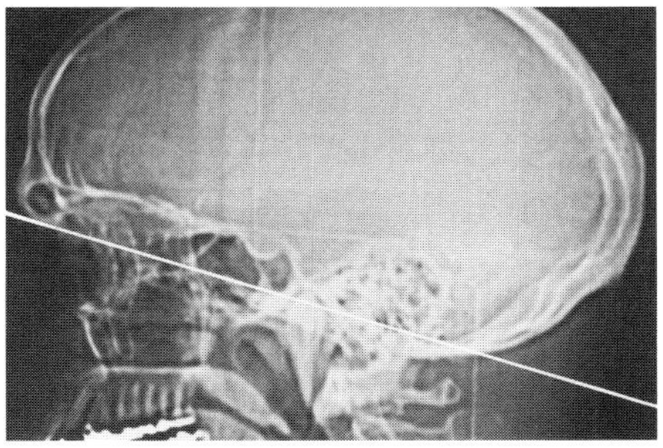

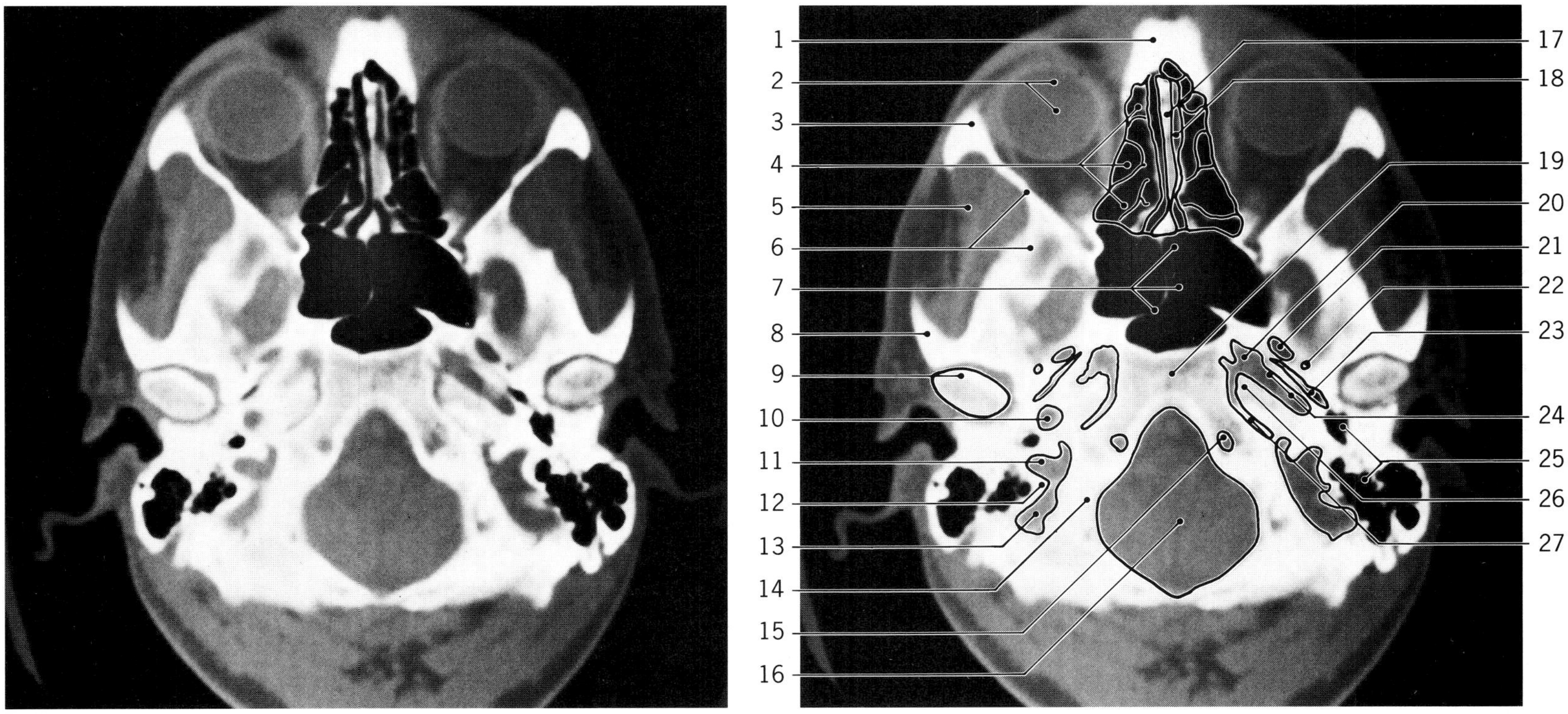

Base of skull, axial CT

1: Nasal spine of frontal bone
2: Eyeball
3: Frontal process of zygomatic bone
4: Ethmoidal air cells
5: Temporal fossa
6: Greater wing of sphenoid bone
7: Sphenoidal sinus
8: Zygomatic process of temporal bone
9: Head of mandible
10: Carotid canal, first part
11: Jugular foramen, anterior part
12: Intrajugular process
13: Jugular foramen, posterior part
14: Lateral part of occipital bone
15: Hypoglossal canal
16: Foramen magnum
17: Nasal septum
18: Nasal cavity
19: Body of sphenoid bone
20: Foramen lacerum
21: Foramen ovale
22: Foramen spinosum
23: Sphenopetrous fissure/ Eustachian tube
24: Carotid canal, second part
25: Air cells in temporal bone
26: Apex of petrous bone
27: Petro-occipital fissure

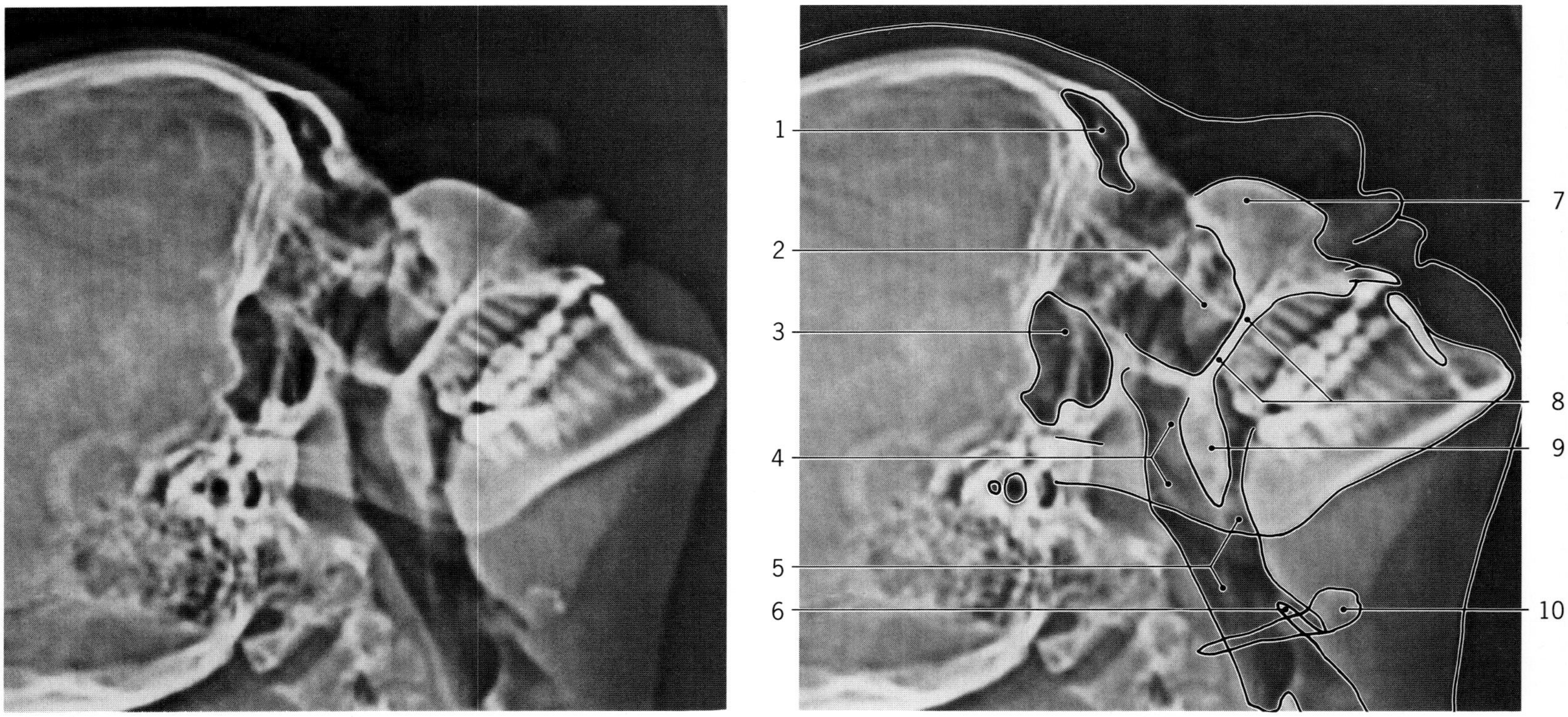

Scout view

1: Frontal sinus
2: Maxillary sinus
3: Sphenoidal sinus
4: Nasal part of pharynx
5: Oral part of pharynx
6: Epiglottis
7: Frontal process of maxilla
8: Hard palate
9: Soft palate
10: Hyoid bone

Scout view

Lines #1-10 indicate positions of sections in the following CT series.

Consecutive sections, 10 mm thick. Prone position with hyperextended neck.

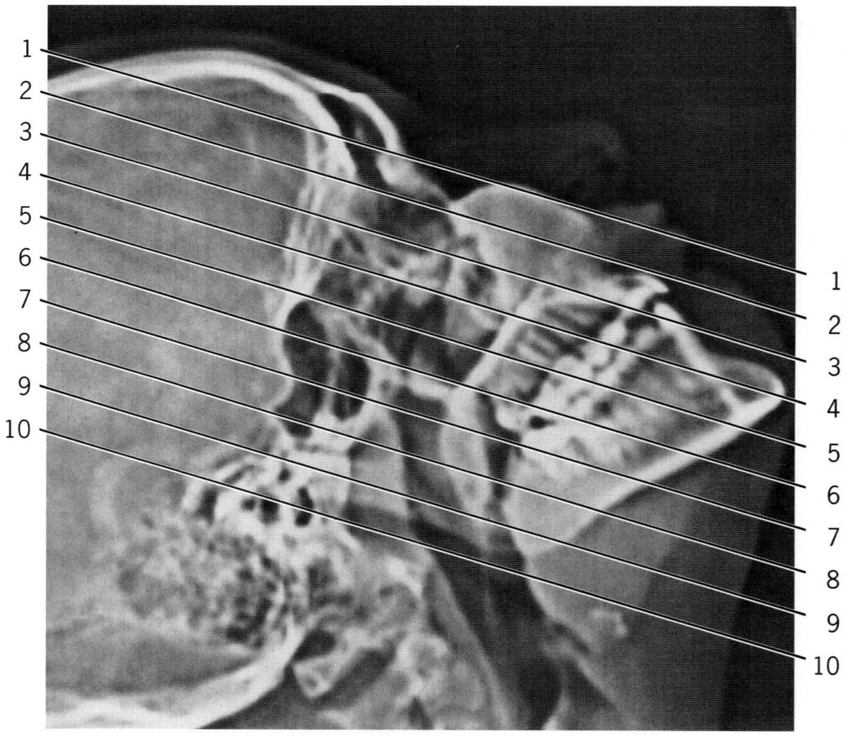

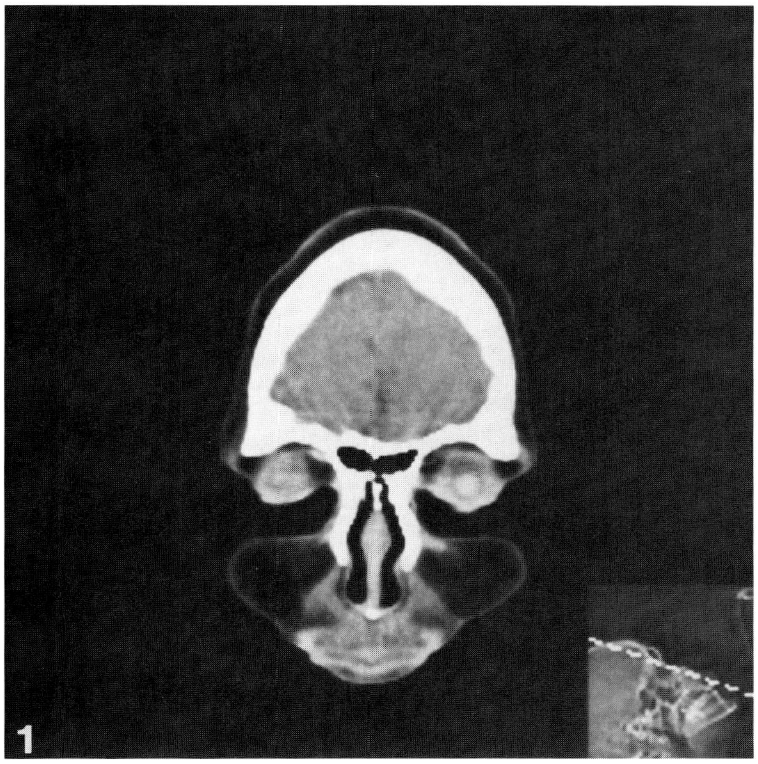

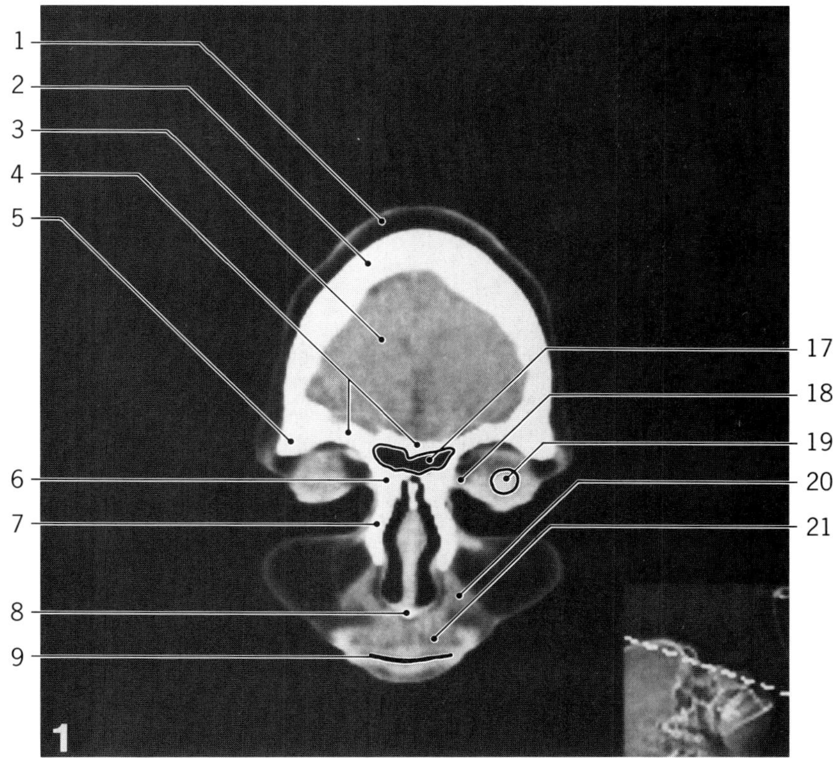

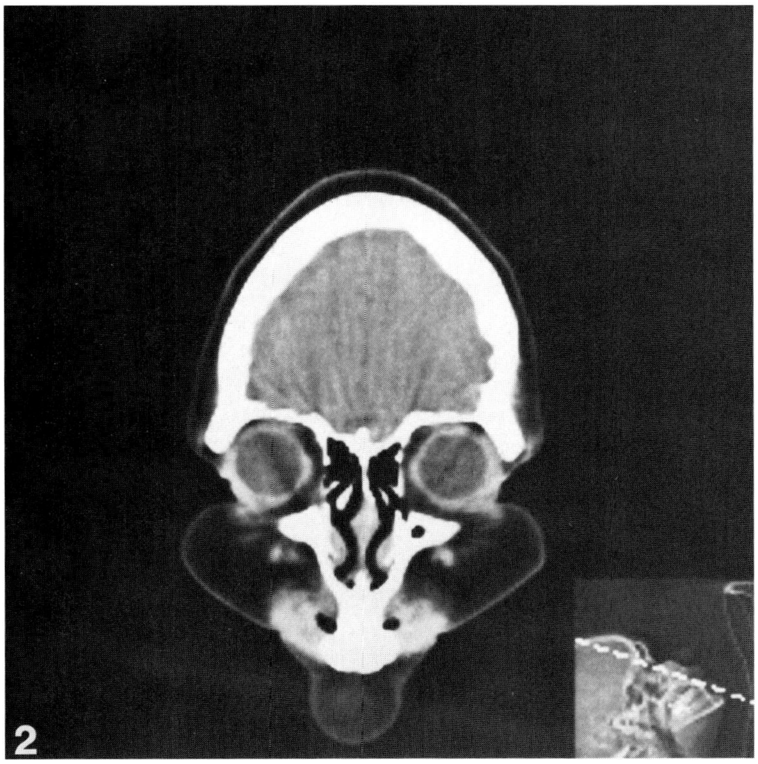

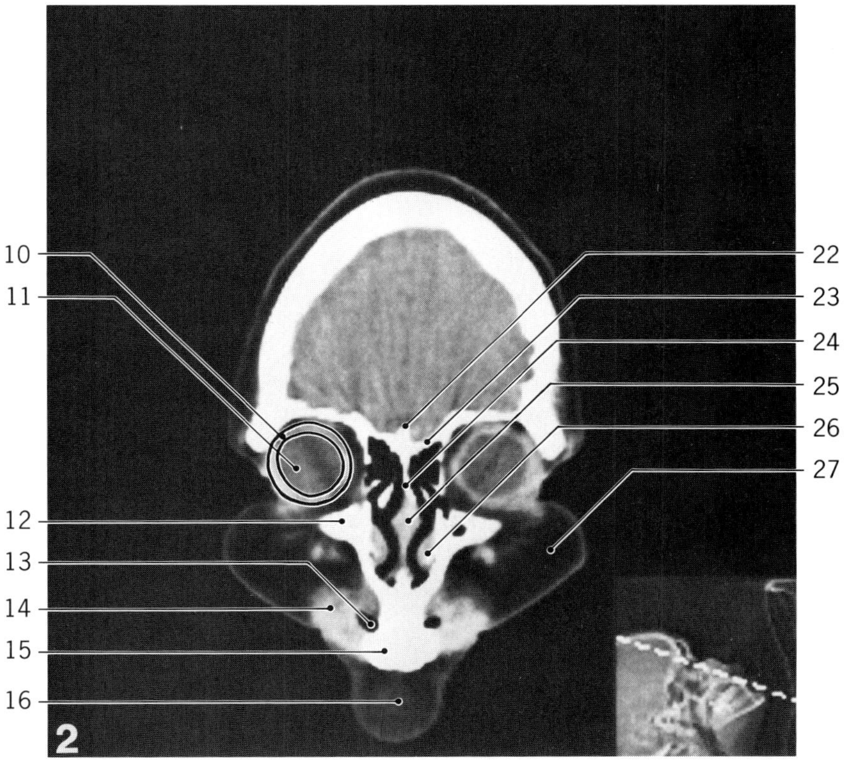

Head, coronal CT

Scout view on opposite page.

1: Scalp
2: Squamous part of frontal bone
3: Frontal lobe
4: Orbital plate of frontal bone
5: Zygomatic process of frontal bone
6: Nasal spine of frontal bone
7: Frontal process of maxilla
8: Anterior nasal spine
9: Oral fissure

10: Sclera
11: Vitreous body
12: Body of maxilla
13: Air in vestibule of mouth
14: Orbicularis oris
15: Upper incisor teeth
16: Chin
17: Frontal sinus
18: Medial palpebral ligament

19: Lens
20: Levator labii superioris
21: Upper lip
22: Crista galli
23: Cribriform plate
24: Perpendicular plate of ethmoid bone
25: Cartilage of nasal septum
26: Inferior nasal concha
27: Cheek

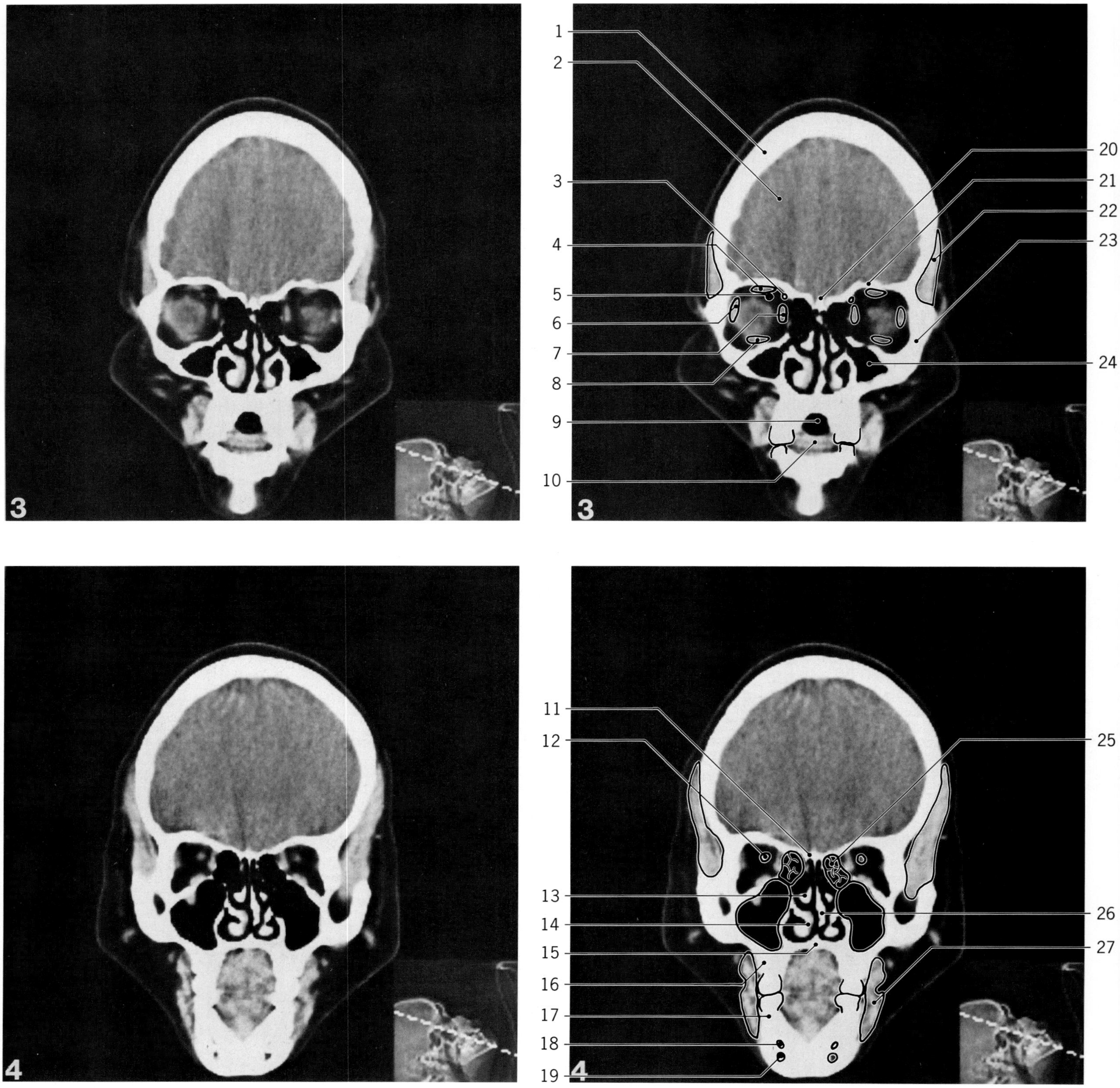

Head, coronal CT

Scout veiw on page 138

1: Squamous part of frontal bone
2: Frontal lobe
3: Obliquus superior
4: Rectus superior, and levator palpebrae
5: Ophthalmic artery, or superior orbital vein
6: Rectus lateralis
7: Rectus medialis
8: Rectus inferior
9: Air in oral cavity
10: Apex of tongue
11: Cribriform plate
12: Optic nerve
13: Middle nasal concha
14: Inferior nasal concha
15: Hard palate
16: Alveolar process of maxilla
17: Alveolar part of mandible
18: Mental foramen
19: Marrow cavity of mandible
20: Crista galli
21: Orbital plate of frontal bone
22: Temporalis muscle
23: Zygomatic bone
24: Maxillary sinus
25: Ethmoidal air cells
26: Nasal septum
27: Buccinator

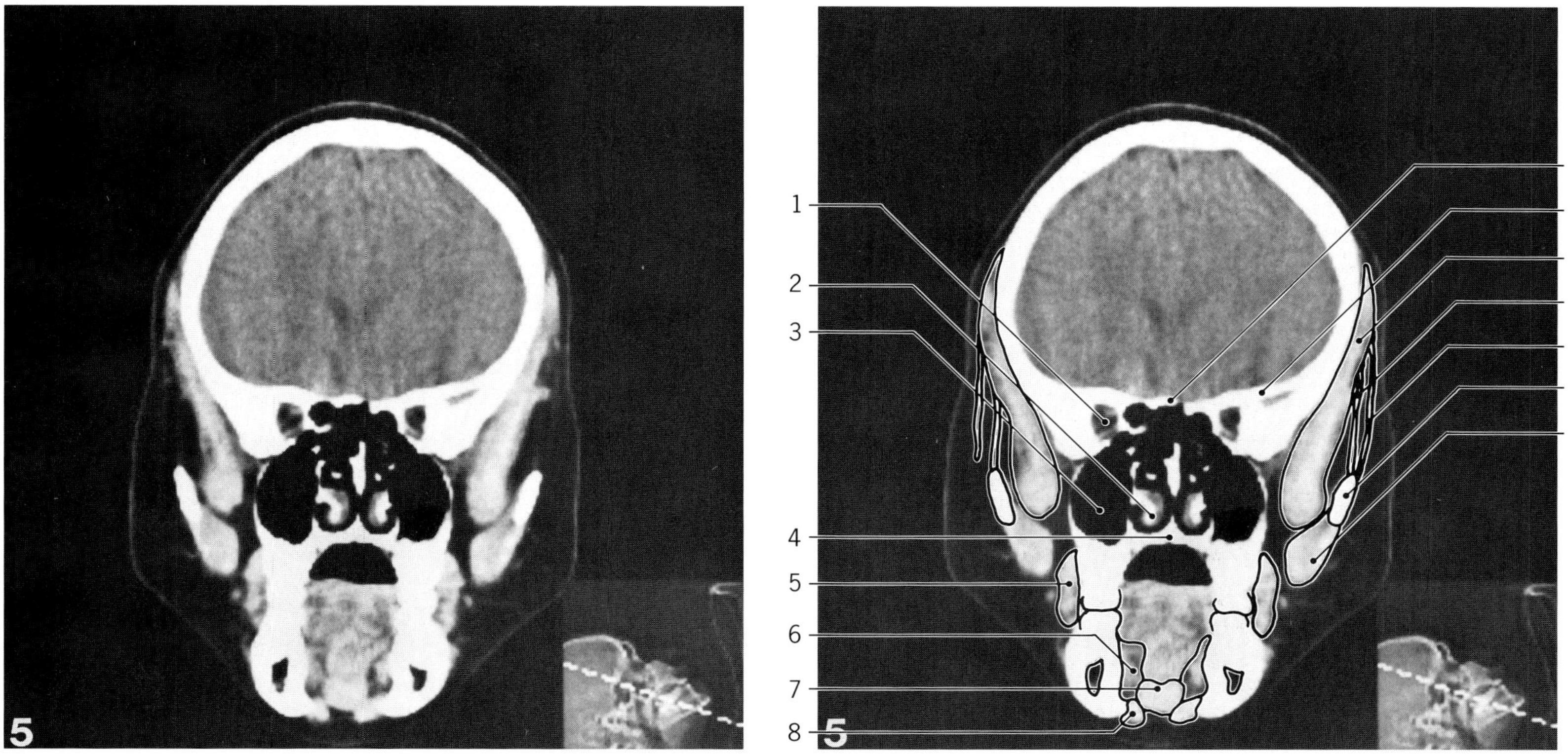

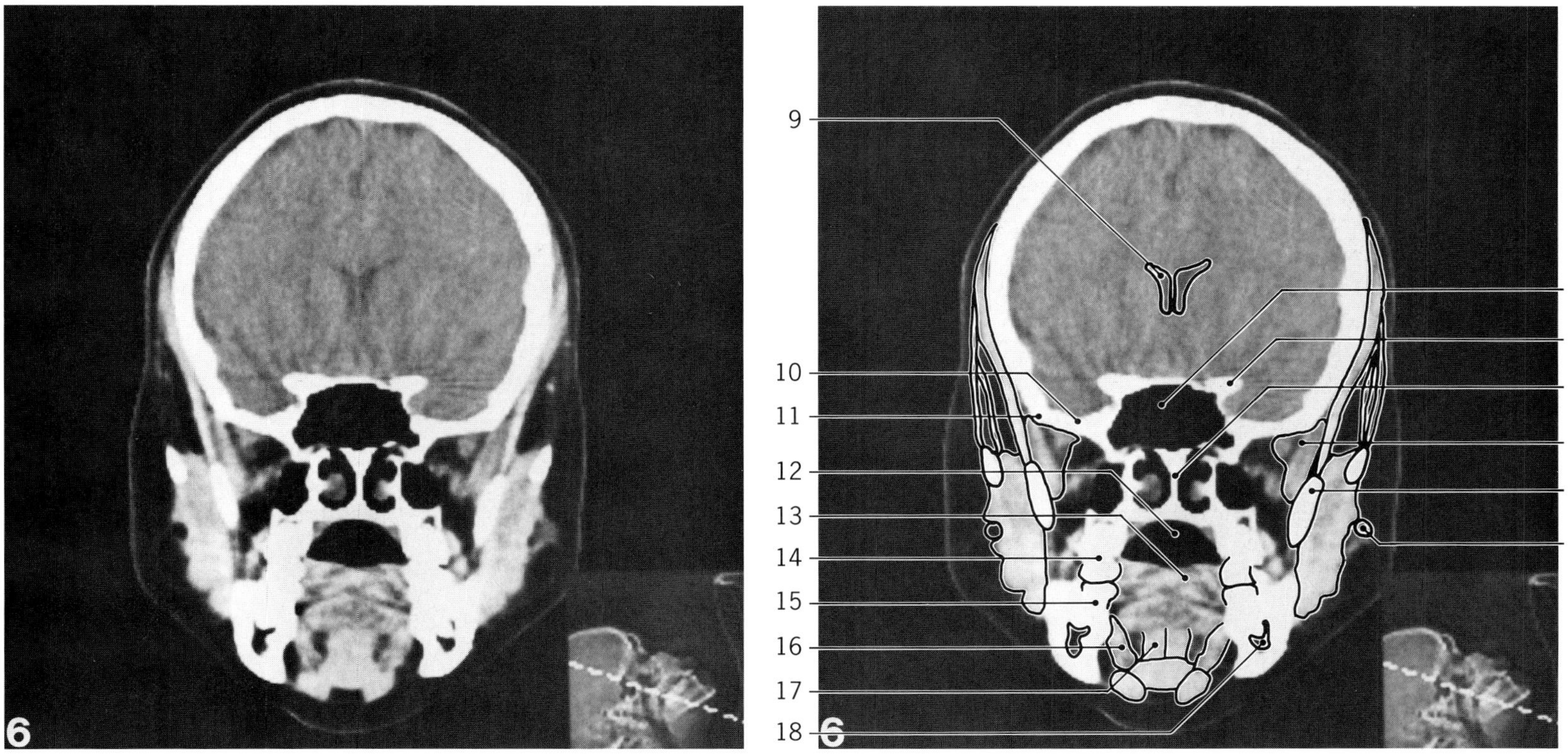

Head, coronal CT

Scout view on page 138

1: Apex of orbita
2: Inferior nasal concha
3: Maxillary sinus
4: Hard Palate
5: Buccinator
6: Sublingual region
7: Geniohyoideus
8: Digastricus, anterior belly
9: Lateral ventricle
10: Greater wing of sphenoid bone
11: Infratemporal crest
12: Oral cavity
13: Tongue
14: Upper molar tooth
15: Lower molar tooth
16: Mylohyoideus
17: Genioglossus
18: Marrow cavity of mandible/ mandibular canal
19: Jugum sphenoidale
20: Lesser wing of sphenoid bone
21: Temporalis muscle
22: Temporal fascia
23: Galea aponeurotica
24: Zygomatic arch
25: Masseter
26: Sphenoidal sinus
27: Anterior clinoid process
28: Vomer
29: Lateral pterygoid muscle
30: Coronoid process of mandible
31: Parotid duct

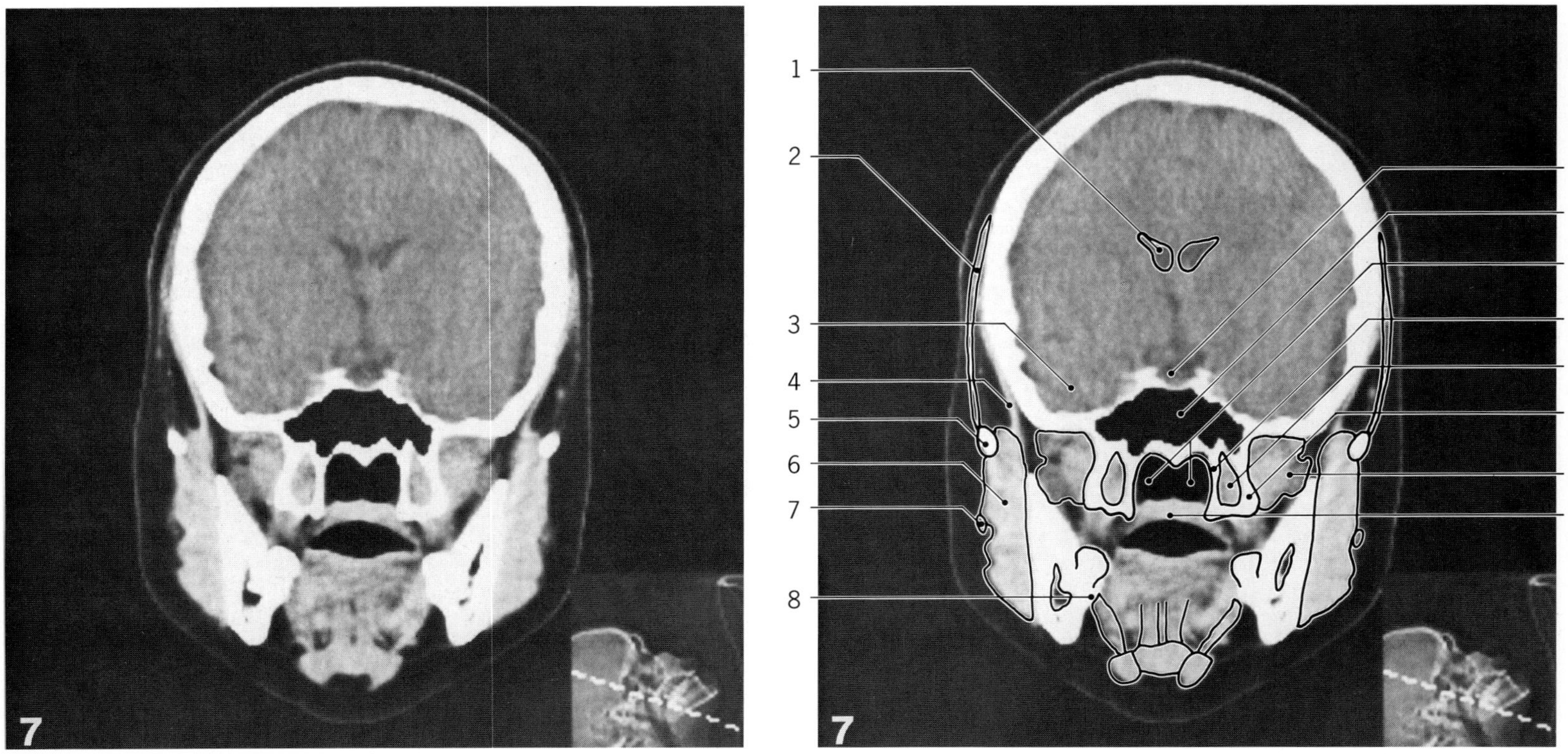

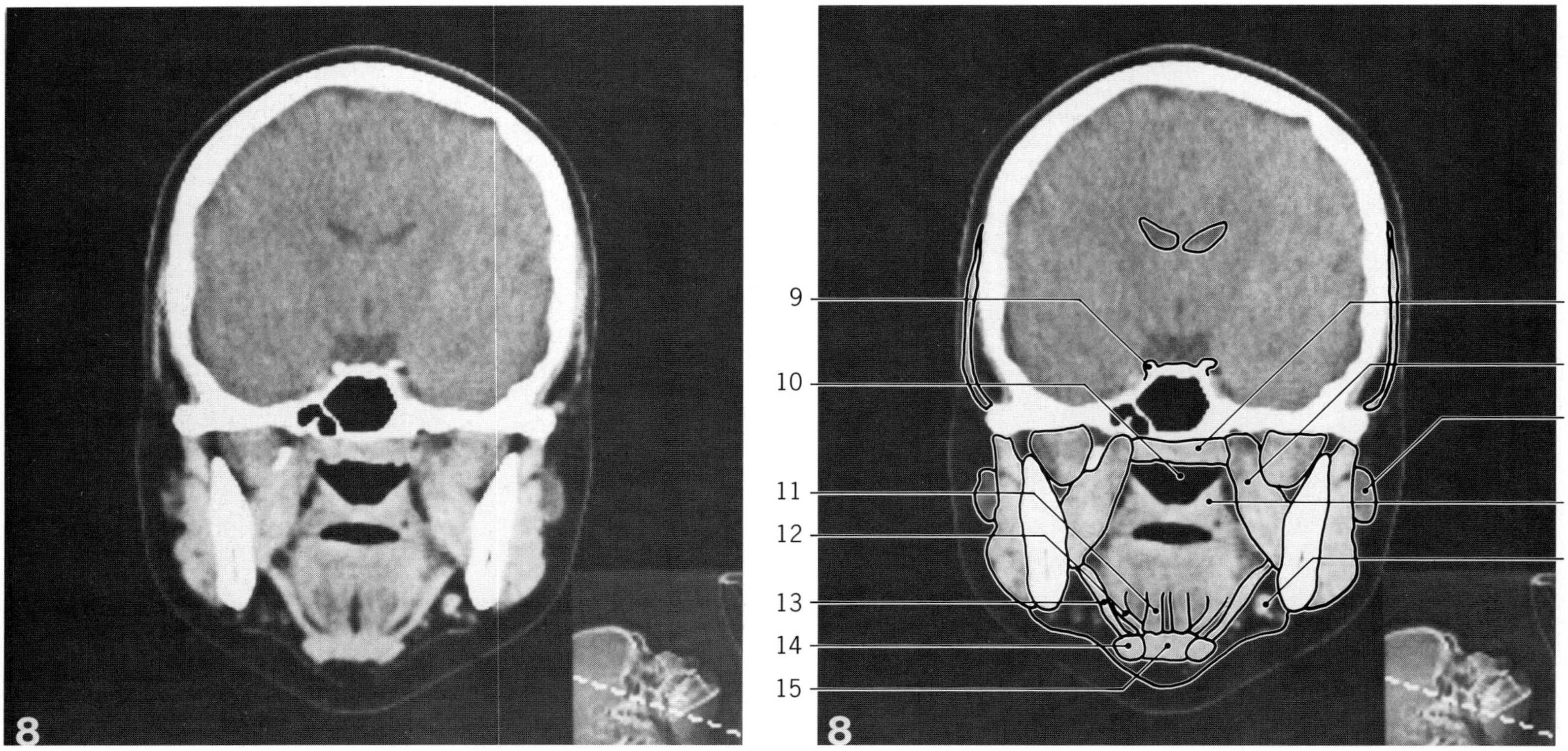

Head, coronal CT

Scout view on page 138

1: Lateral ventricle of brain
2: Galea aponeurotica
3: Temporal lobe
4: Temporalis (tendon)
5: Zygomatic arch
6: Masseter
7: Parotid duct
8: Mylohyoid line
9: Posterior clinoid process
10: Nasal part of pharynx
11: Genioglossus
12: Hyoglossus
13: Mylohyoideus
14: Digastricus, anterior belly
15: Geniohyoideus
16: Hypophyseal fossa
17: Sphenoidal sinus
18: Choanae
19: Medial pterygoid plate
20: Pterygoid fossa
21: Lateral pterygoid plate
22: Lateral pterygoid muscle
23: Soft palate
24: Longus capitis
25: Medial pterygoid muscle
26: Accessory parotid gland
27: Levator veli palatini
28: Submandibular lymph node

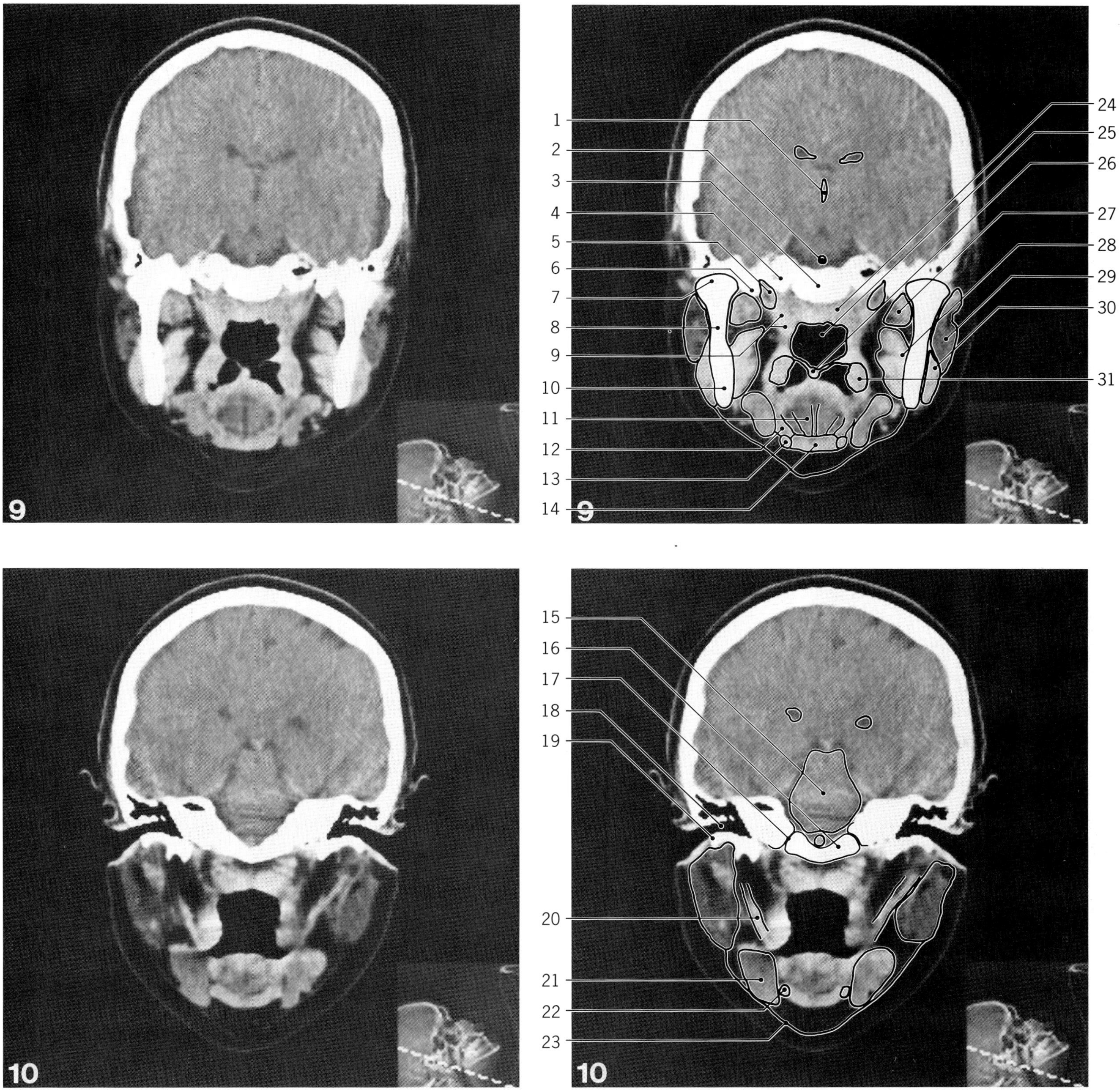

Head, coronal CT

Scout view on page 138

1: Third ventricle
2: Basilary artery
3: Body of sphenoid bone
4: Petrous part of temporal bone
5: Auditory tube
6: Spine of sphenoid bone
7: Head of mandible
8: Neck of mandible
9: Levator and tensor veli palatini
10: Angle of mandible
11: Genioglossus
12: Hyoglossus
13: Digastricus, anterior belly
14: Geniohyoideus
15: Brain stem
16: Basilar part of occipital bone
17: Petro-occipital fissure
18: External acoustic meatus
19: Tympanic part of temporal bone
20: Styloglossus
21: Submandibular gland
22: Digastricus (tendon)
23: Platysma
24: Longus capitis
25: Nasal part of pharynx
26: Uvula
27: Lateral pterygoid muscle
28: Medial pterygoid muscle
29: Parotid gland
30: Masseter
31: Palatine tonsil

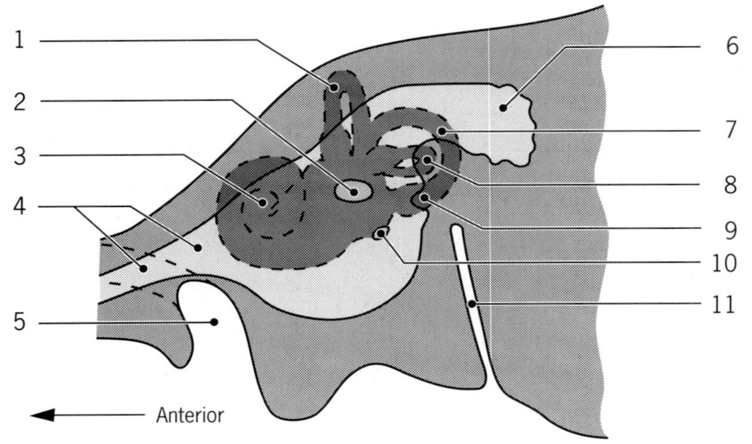

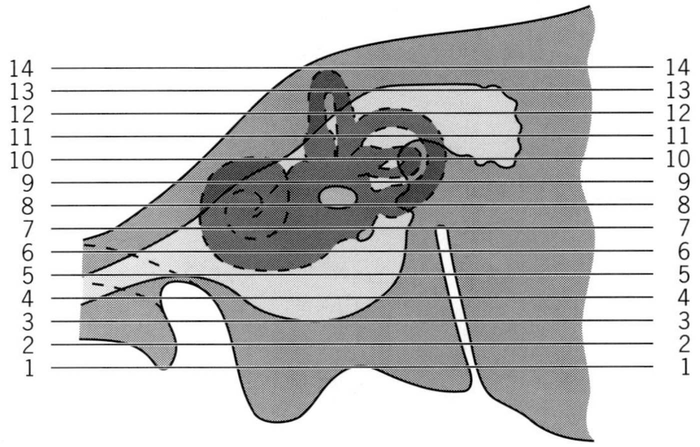

Petrous bone, CT series, diagrammatic scout view

Lines #1-14 indicate positions of sections in the following CT series. Consecutive sections, 3 mm thick

1: Anterior semicircular canal
2: Fenestra vestibuli
3: Cochlea
4: Auditory tube
5: Carotid canal
6: Mastoid antrum
7: Posterior semicircular canal
8: Lateral semicircular canal
9: Pyramidal process
10: Fenestra cochleae
11: Facial canal

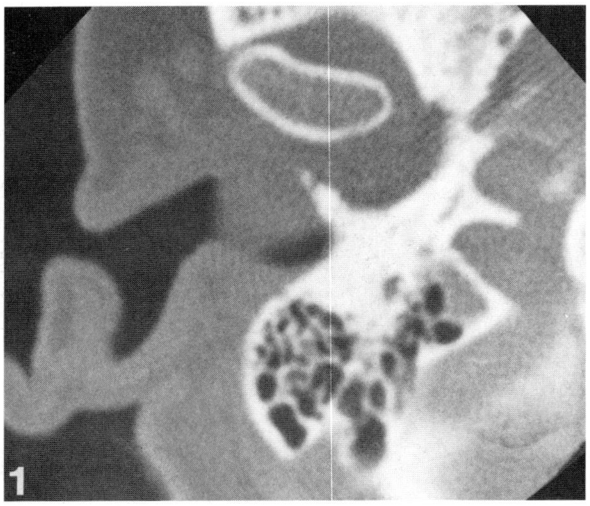

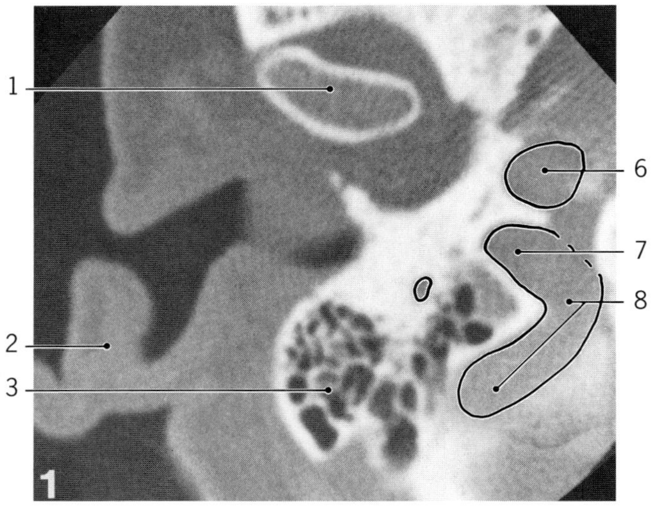

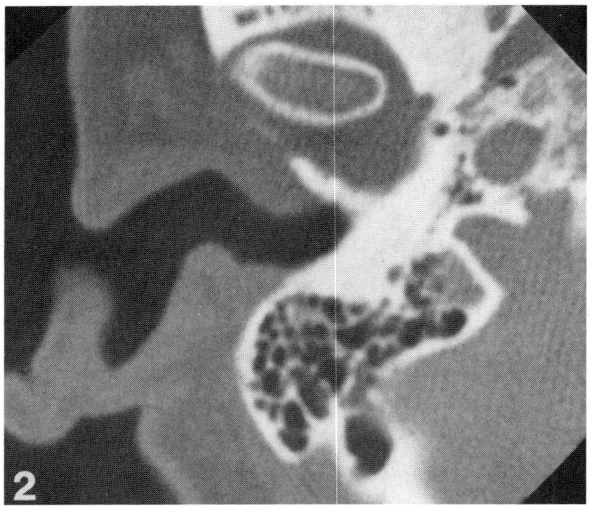

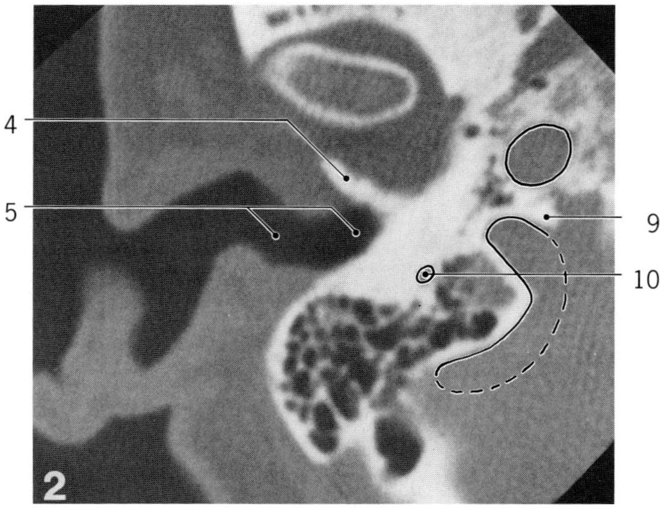

Ear, axial CT

Positions of sections #1-2 are indicated above

1: Head of mandible
2: Auricle
3: Mastoid process with air cells
4: Tympanic part of temporal bone
5: External acoustic meatus
6: Carotid canal
7: Bulb of internal jugular vein
8: Sigmoid sinus
9: Intrajugular process
10: Facial canal

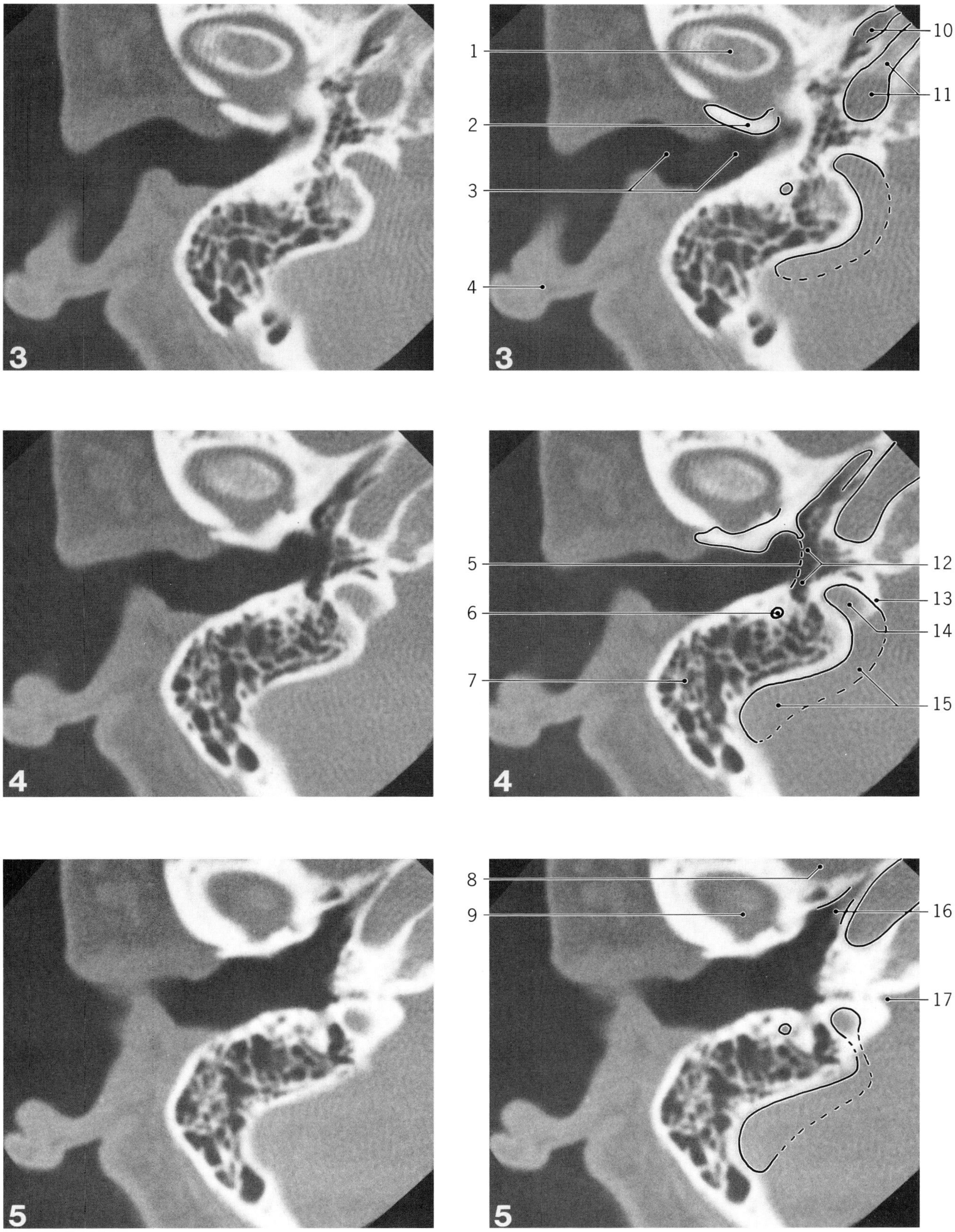

Ear, axial CT

Positions of section #3-5 are indicated on opposite page

1: Head of mandible
2: Tympanic part (plate) of temporal bone
3: External auditory meatus
4: Auricle
5: Tympanic membrane
6: Facial canal
7: Mastoid process with air cells
8: Middle cranial fossa
9: Articular disc of temporomandibular joint
10: Auditory tube
11: Carotid canal
12: Tympanic cavity
13: Intrajugular process
14: Bulb of internal jugular vein
15: Sigmoid sinus
16: Tympanic ostium of auditory tube
17: Aperture of cochlear canaliculus (perilymphatic duct)

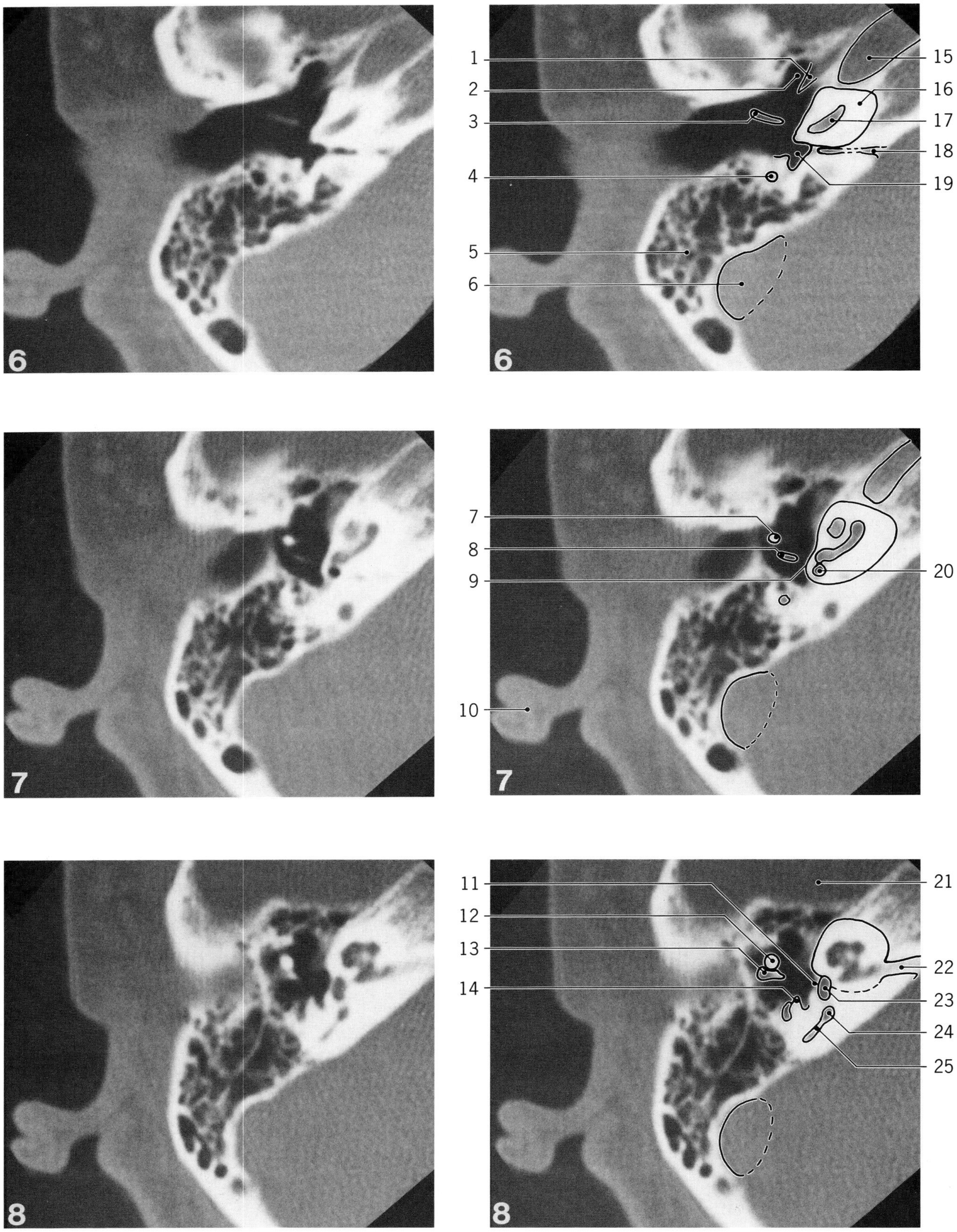

Ear, axial CT

Positions of section #6-8 are indicated on page 144

1: Tensor tympani muscle
2: Tympanic ostium of auditory tube
3: Manubrium of malleus
4: Facial canal
5: Air cells in mastoid process
6: Sigmoid sinus
7: Neck of malleus
8: Crus longum of incus
9: Promontory
10: Auricle
11: Base of stapes in fenestra vestibuli
12: Head of malleus
13: Body of incus
14: Pyramidal eminence
15: Carotid canal
16: Cochlea
17: Spiral canal
18: Canaliculus cochleae (perilymphatic duct)
19: Sinus tympani
20: Fenestra cochleae
21: Middle cranial fossa
22: Internal acoustic meatus
23: Vestibulum
24: Ampulla of posterior semicircular canal
25: Posterior semicircular canal

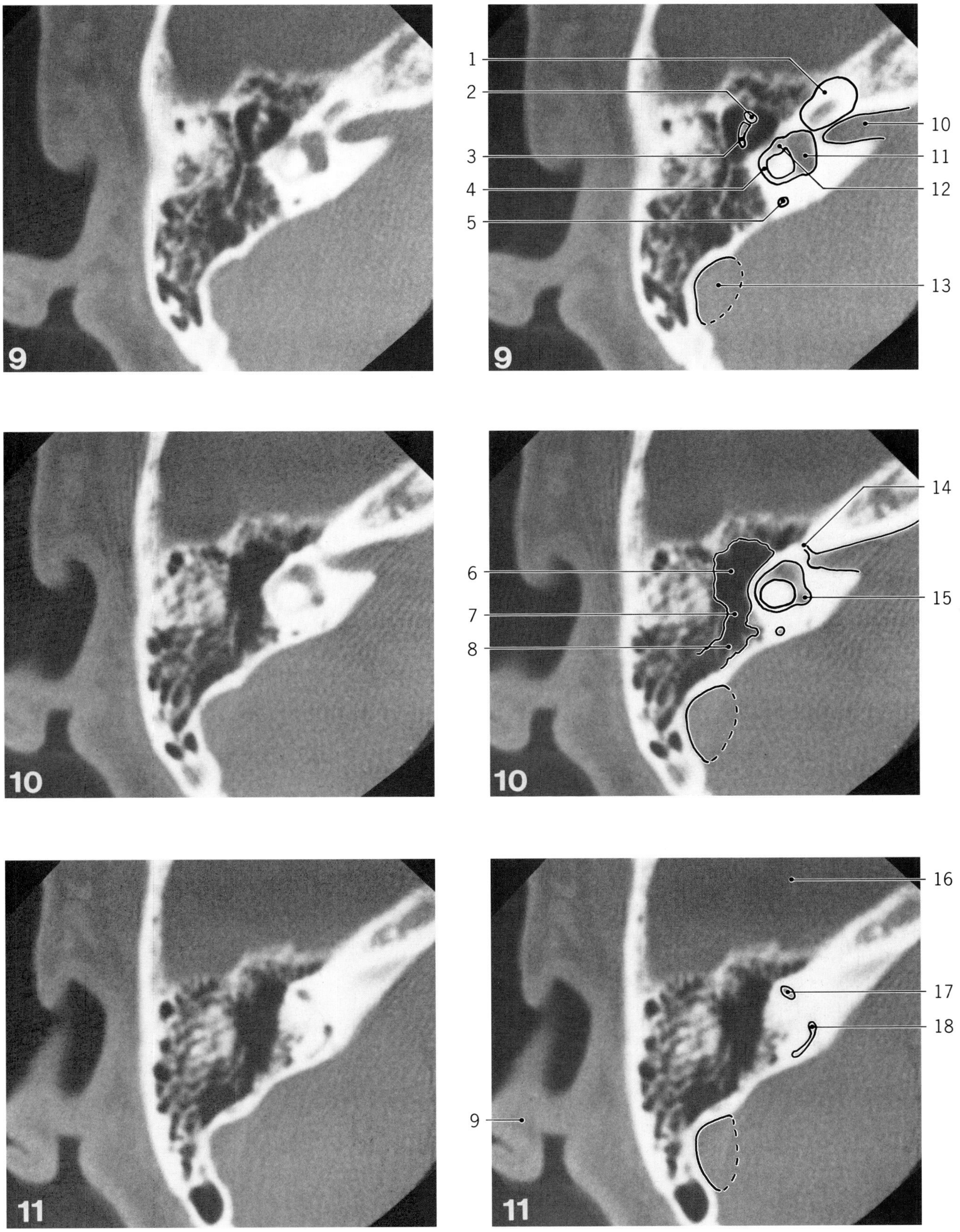

Ear, axial CT

Positions of section #9-11 are indicated on page 144

1: Cochlea
2: Head of malleus
3: Crus breve of incus
4: Lateral semicircular canal
5: Posterior semicircular canal
6: Epitympanic recess
7: Aditus ad antrum
8: Mastoid antrum
9: Auricle
10: Internal auditory meatus
11: Vestibulum
12: Ampulla of lateral semicircular canal
13: Sigmoid sinus
14: Facial canal
15: Elliptical recess
16: Middle cranial fossa
17: Ampulla of anterior semicircular canal
18: Crus commune of ant. and post. semicircular canals

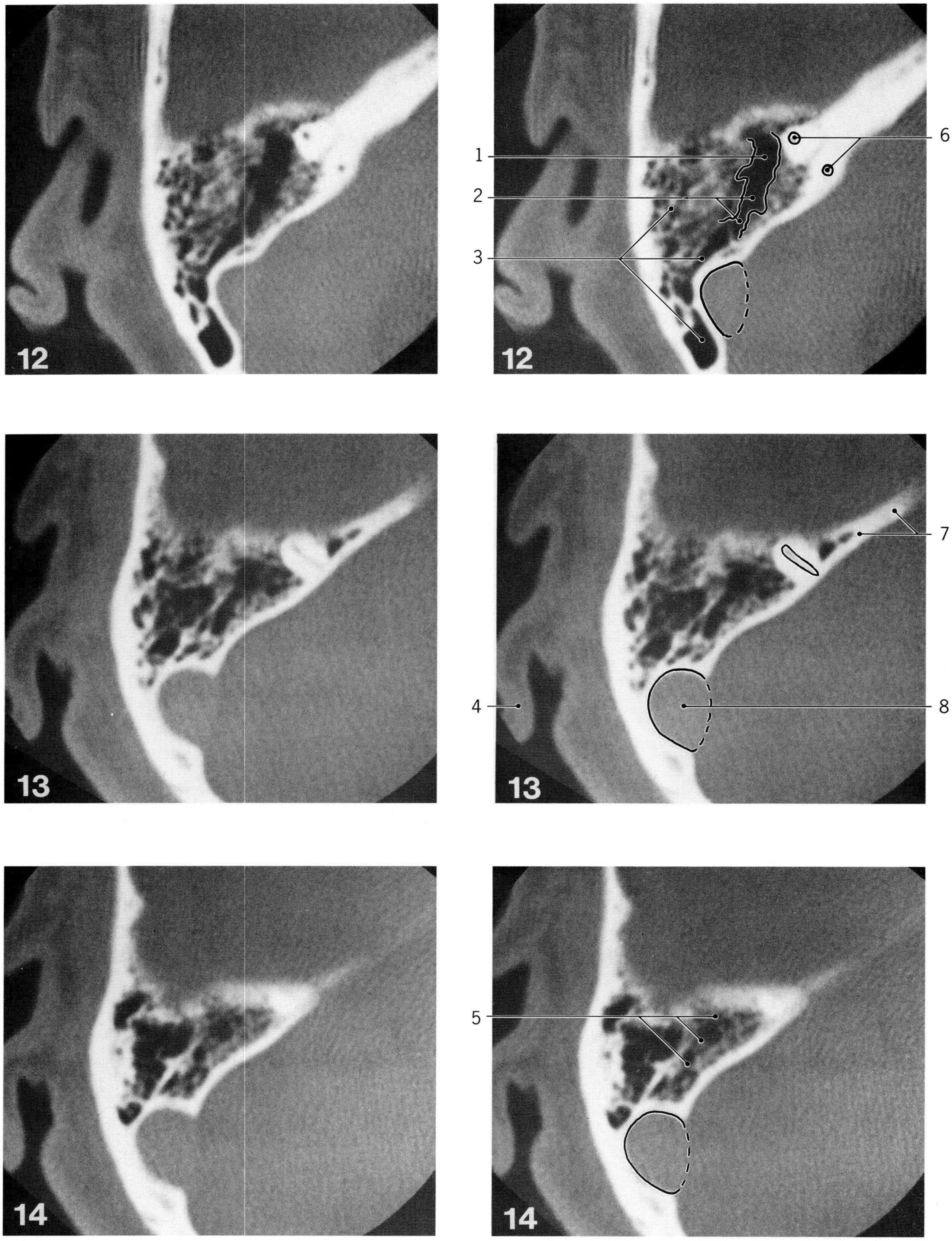

Ear, axial CT

Positions of section #12-14 are indicated on page 144

1: Epitympanic recess
2: Mastoid antrum
3: Air cells in mastoid process
4: Auricle
5: Tegmen tympani
6: Anterior semicircular canal
7: Superior margin of petrous bone
8: Sigmoid sinus

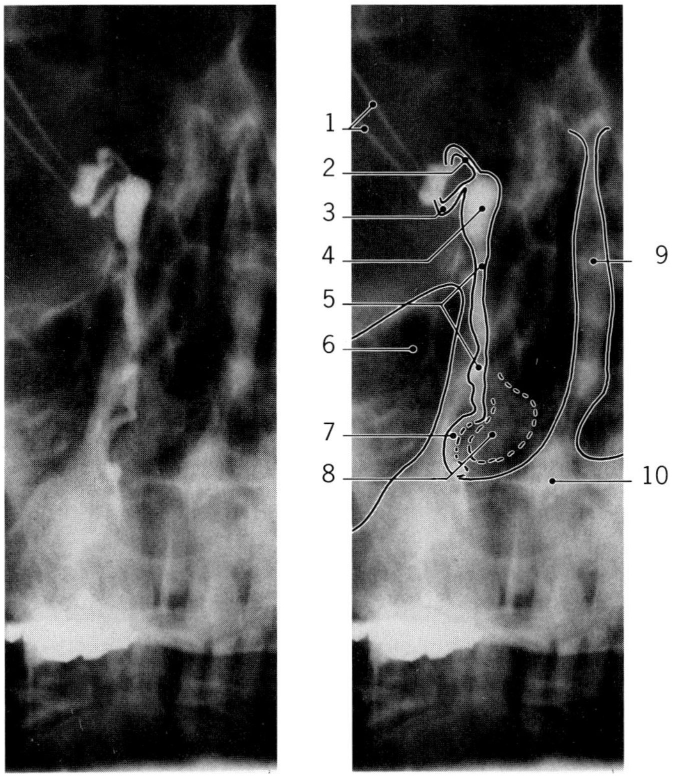

Lacrimal ducts, a-p X-ray, dacryography

1: Catheters inserted in puncta lacrimalia
2: Superior lacrimal canaliculus
3: Inferior lacrimal canaliculus
4: Lacrimal sac
5: Nasolacrimal duct
6: Maxillary sinus
7: Contrast medium flowing into nasal cavity
8: Inferior nasal concha
9: Nasal septum
10: Hard palate

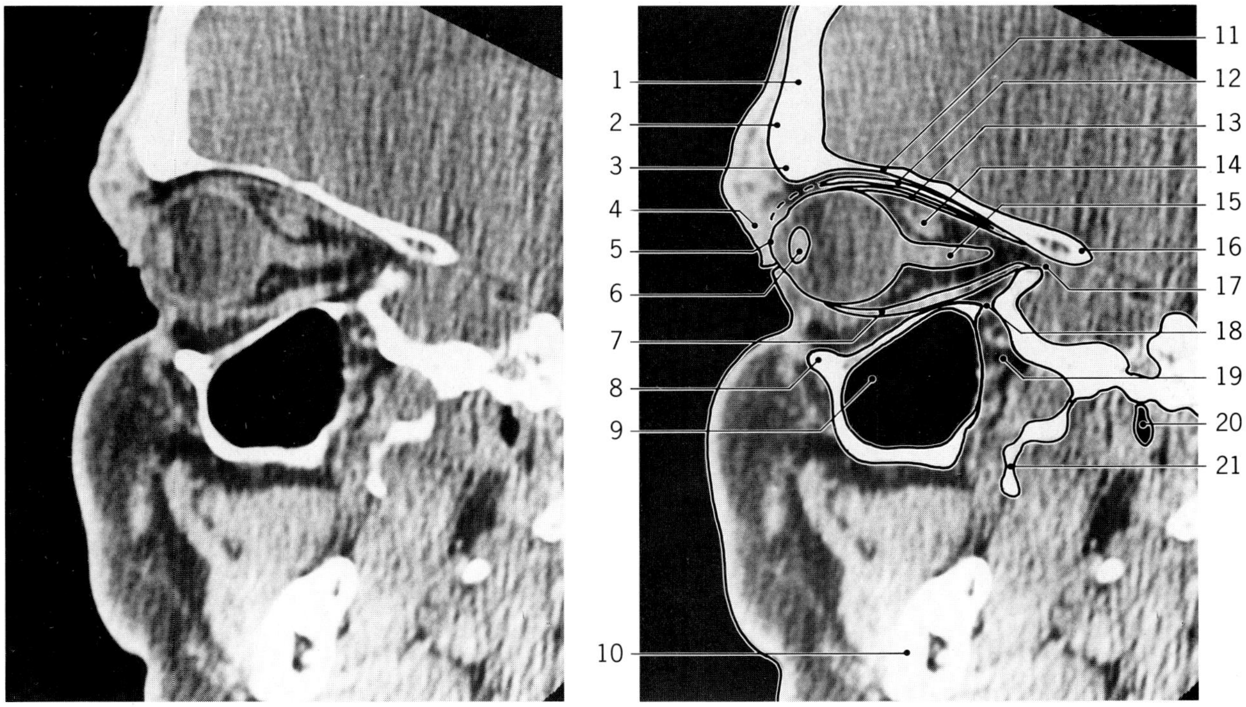

Orbita, longitudinal CT

1: Pars squamosa of frontal bone
2: Superciliary arch
3: Supra-orbital margin
4: Upper eyelid
5: Cornea
6: Lens
7: Rectus inferior
8: Infra-orbital margin
9: Maxillary sinus
10: Mandible
11: Orbital plate of frontal bone
12: Levator palpebrae
13: Rectus superior
14: Orbital veins
15: Optic nerve
16: Anterior clinoid process
17: Superior orbital fissure
18: Inferior orbital fissure
19: Pterygopalatine fossa
20: Auditory tube
21: Lateral plate of pterygoid process

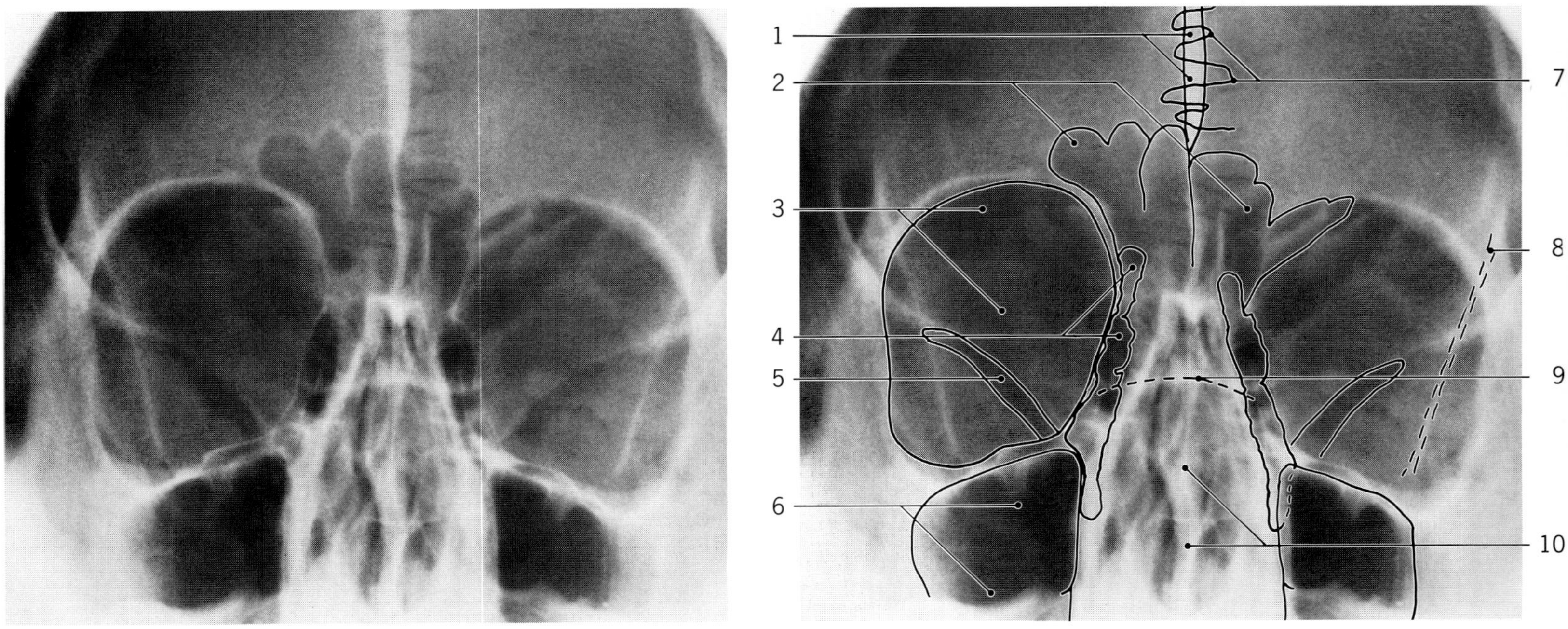

Paranasal sinuses, a-p X-ray

1: Falx cerebri (calcified)
2: Frontal sinus
3: Orbita
4: Ethmoidal air cells
5: Superior orbital fissure
6: Maxillary sinus
7: Sagittal suture
8: Innominate line (radiology term, tangential view of greater wing of sphenoid bone)
9: Hypophyseal fossa (bottom)
10: Nasal septum

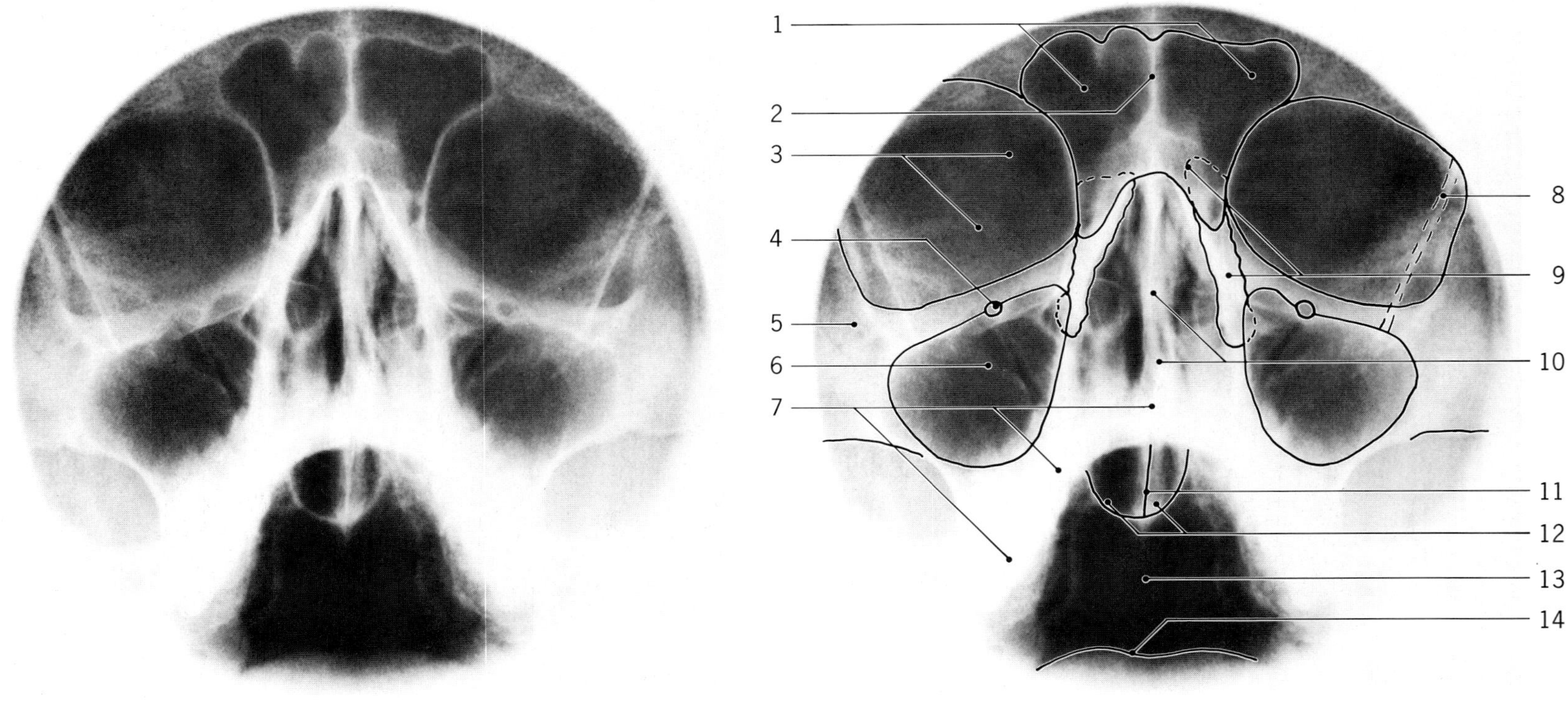

Paranasal sinuses, a-p, tilted X-ray

1: Frontal sinus
2: Septum of frontal sinus
3: Orbita
4: Infraorbital foramen
5: Zygomatic bone
6: Maxillary sinus
7: Superior dental arch
8: Innominate line (radiology term)
9: Ethmoidal air cells
10: Nasal septum
11: Septum of sphenoidal sinus
12: Sphenoidal sinus
13: Oral cavity
14: Dorsum of tongue

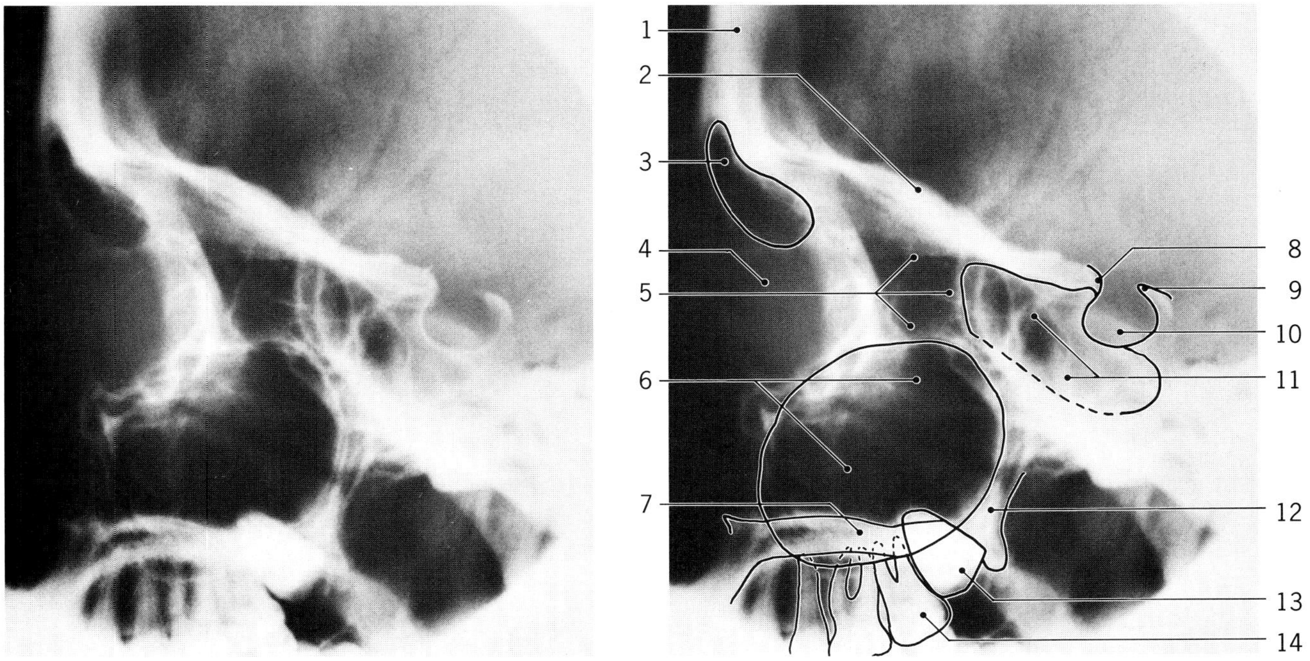

Paranasal sinuses, lateral X-ray

1: Frontal bone
2: Orbital plates of frontal bone
3: Frontal sinus
4: Orbita
5: Ethmoidal air cells
6: Maxillary sinus
7: Hard palate
8: Anterior clinoid process
9: Posterior clinoid process
10: Hypophyseal fossa
11: Sphenoidal sinus
12: Pterygoid process
13: Third upper molar (retended)
14: Second upper molar

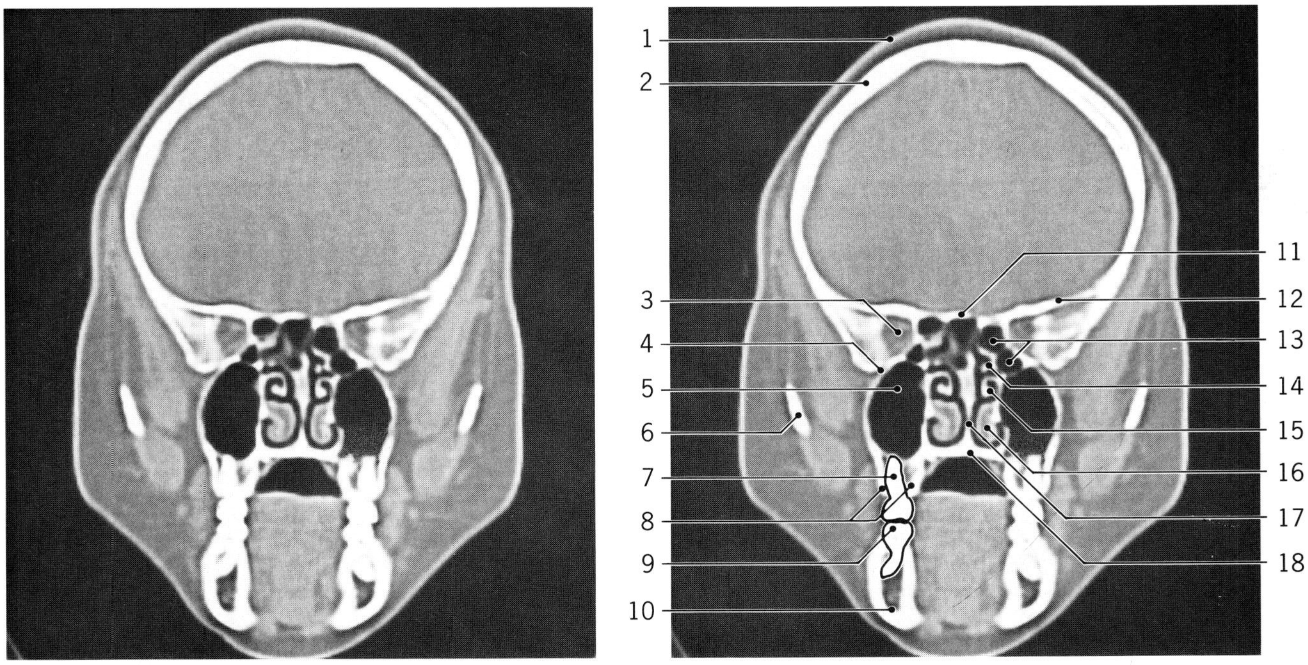

Maxillary sinus, coronal CT (bone settings)

1: Skin
2: Frontal bone
3: Apex of orbita
4: Inferior orbital fissure
5: Maxillary sinus
6: Zygomatic arch
7: Root of upper molar
8: Alveolar process of maxilla
9: Crown of lower molar
10: Body of mandible
11: Jugum sphenoidale
12: Lesser wing of sphenoid bone
13: Ethmoidal air cells
14: Superior nasal concha
15: Middle nasal concha
16: Inferior nasal concha
17: Nasal septum
18: Hard palate

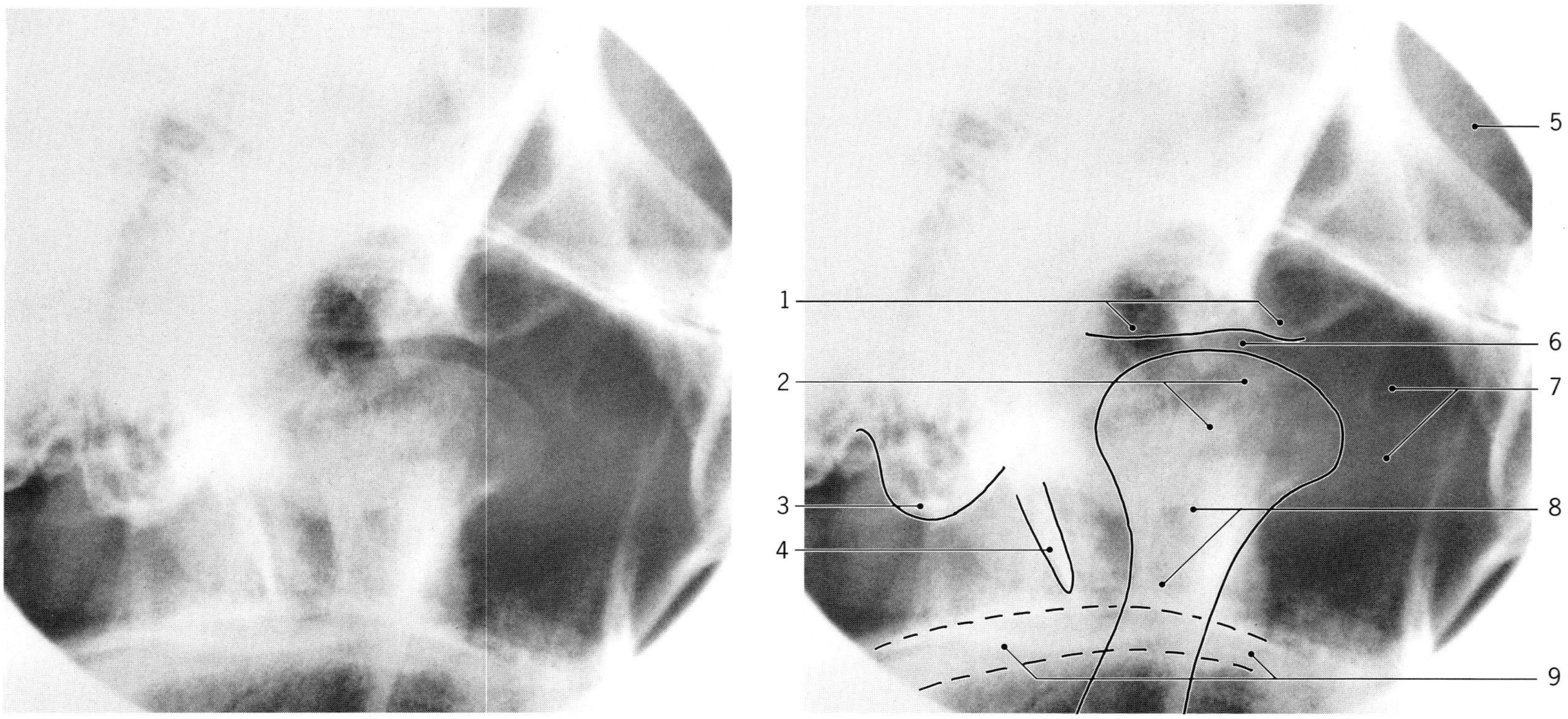

Temporomandibular joint, oblique X-ray, transmaxillary

1: Articular tubercle
2: Head of mandible
3: Mastoid process
4: Styloid process
5: Orbita
6: Temporomandibular joint (with disc)
7: Maxillary sinus
8: Neck of mandible
9: Hard palate

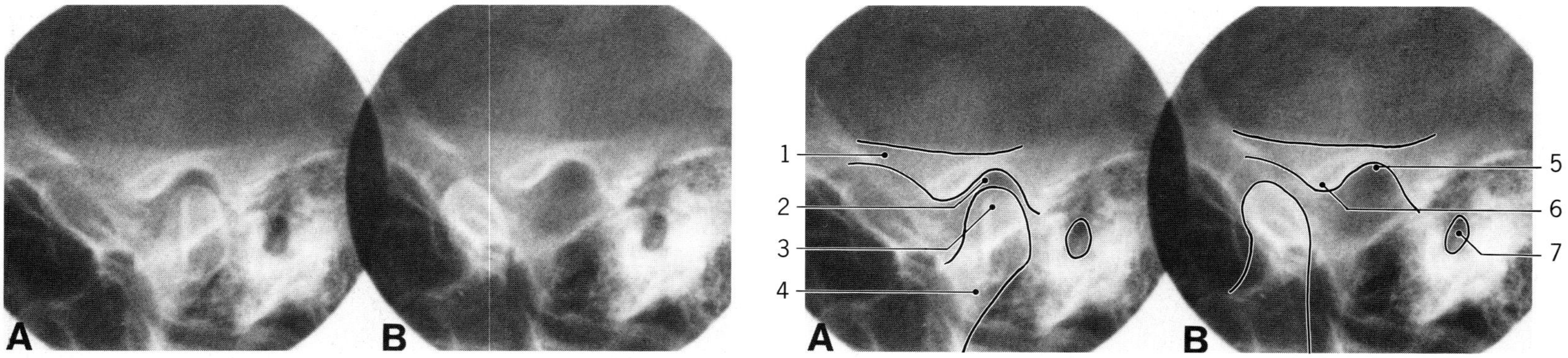

Temporomandibular joint, oblique X-ray

A: mouth closed, B: mouth open

1: Zygomatic arch
2: Temporomandibular joint (with disc)
3: Head of mandible
4: Neck of mandible
5: Mandibular fossa
6: Articular tubercle
7: External auditory meatus

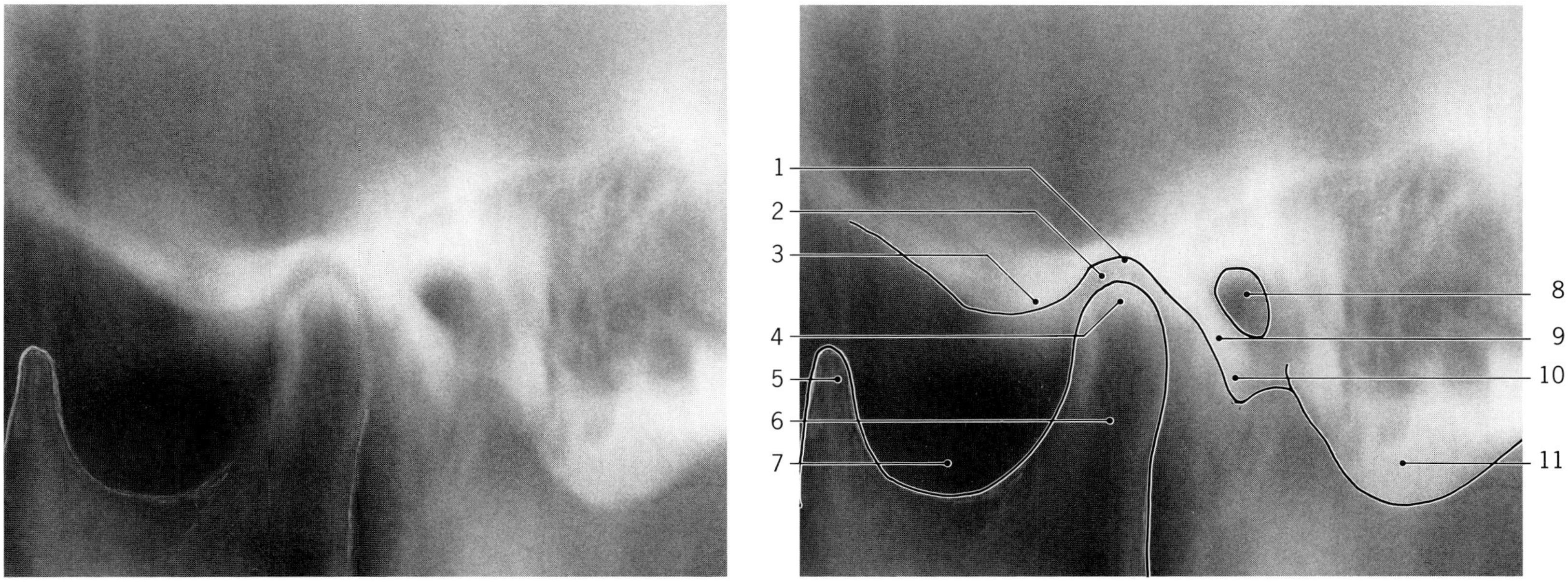

Temporomandibular joint, lateral X-ray, tomography

1: Mandibular fossa
2: Articular disc
3: Articular tubercle
4: Head of mandible
5: Coronoid process
6: Neck of mandible
7: Mandibular incisure
8: External acoustic meatus
9: Tympanic part (plate) of temporal bone
10: Styloid process (root)
11: Mastoid process

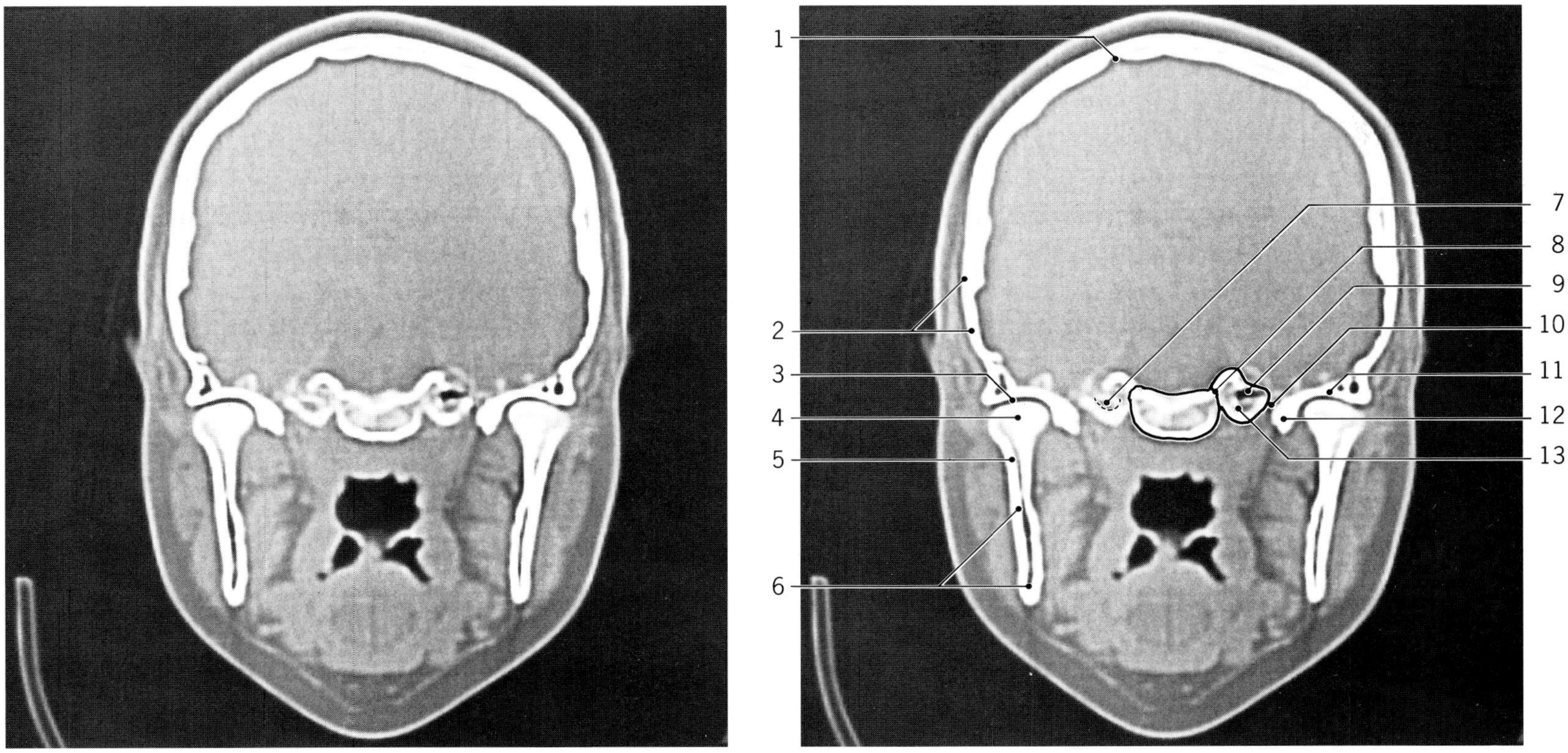

Temporomandibular joint, coronal CT (bone settings)

1: Granular foveola
2: Squamous part of temporal bone
3: Temporomandibular joint
4: Head of mandible
5: Neck of mandible
6: Ramus of mandible
7: Carotid canal, anterior bend
8: Petro-occipital fissure
9: Air cell in petrous bone
10: Sphenopetrous fissure
11: Mandibular fossa
12: Spine of sphenoid bone
13: Apex of petrous bone

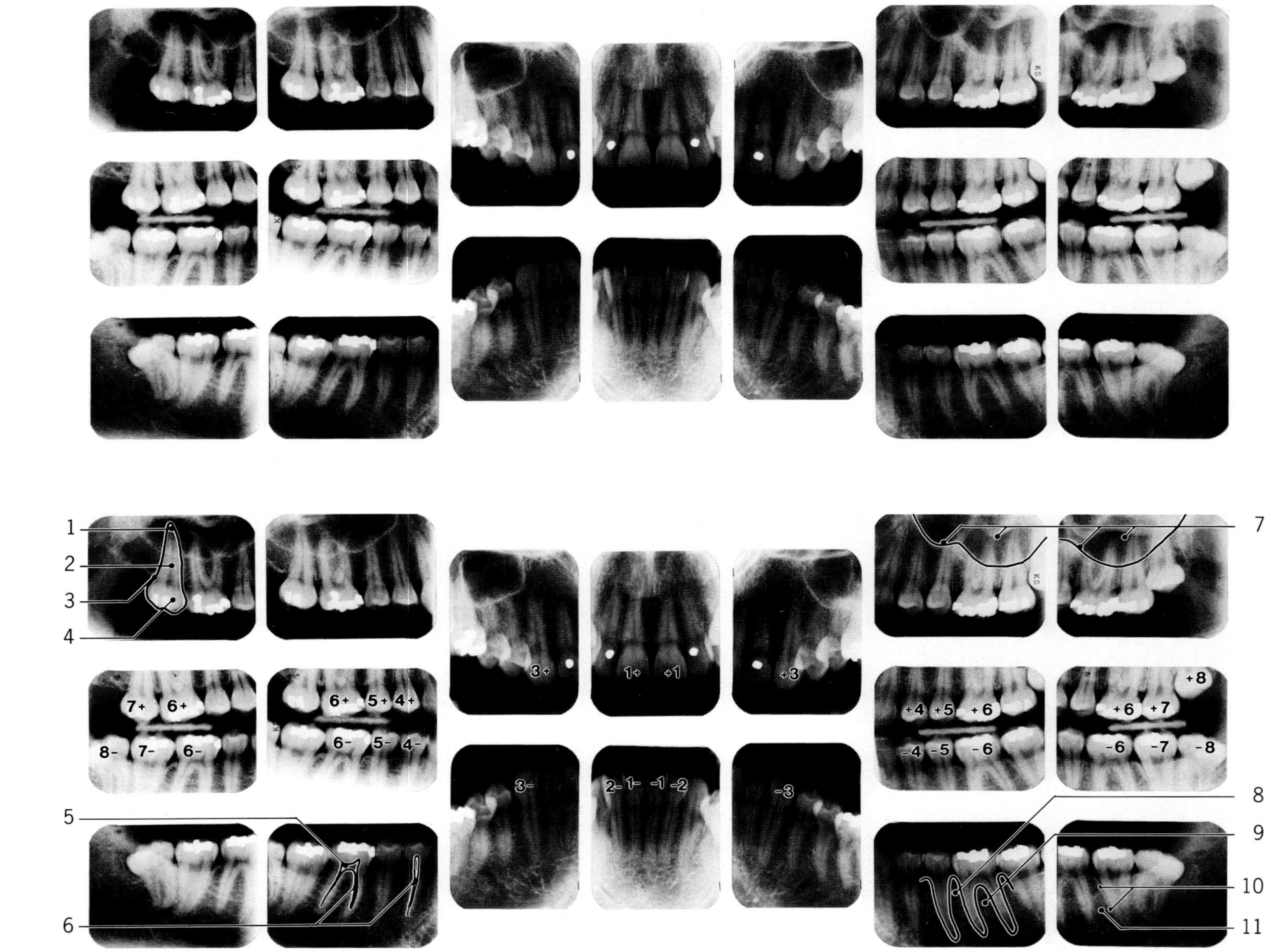

Teeth, "bite-wing" X-ray

Teeth are numbered according to the Haderup formula

1: Apex of root
2: Radix dentis (root)
3: Cervical margin
4: Crown
5: Pulp chamber
6: Pulp canal
7: Maxillary sinus
8: Interalveolar septum
9: Interradicular septum
10: Lamina dura of dental alveolus
11: Cancellous bone

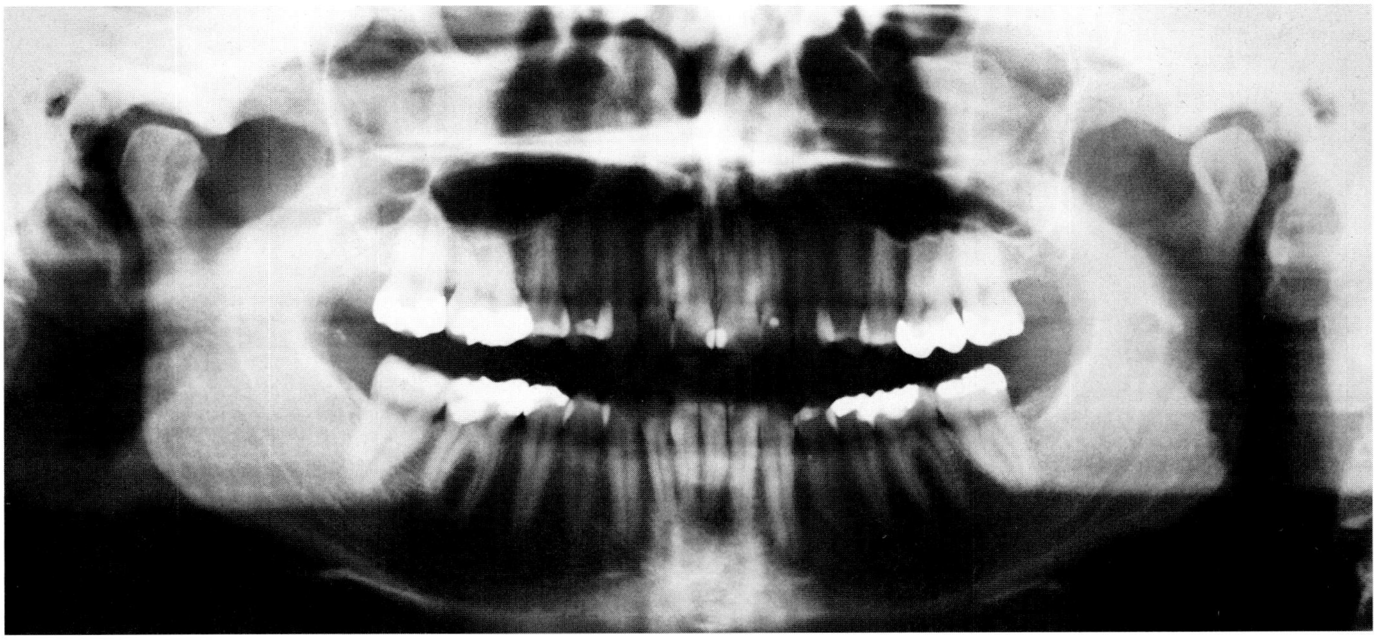

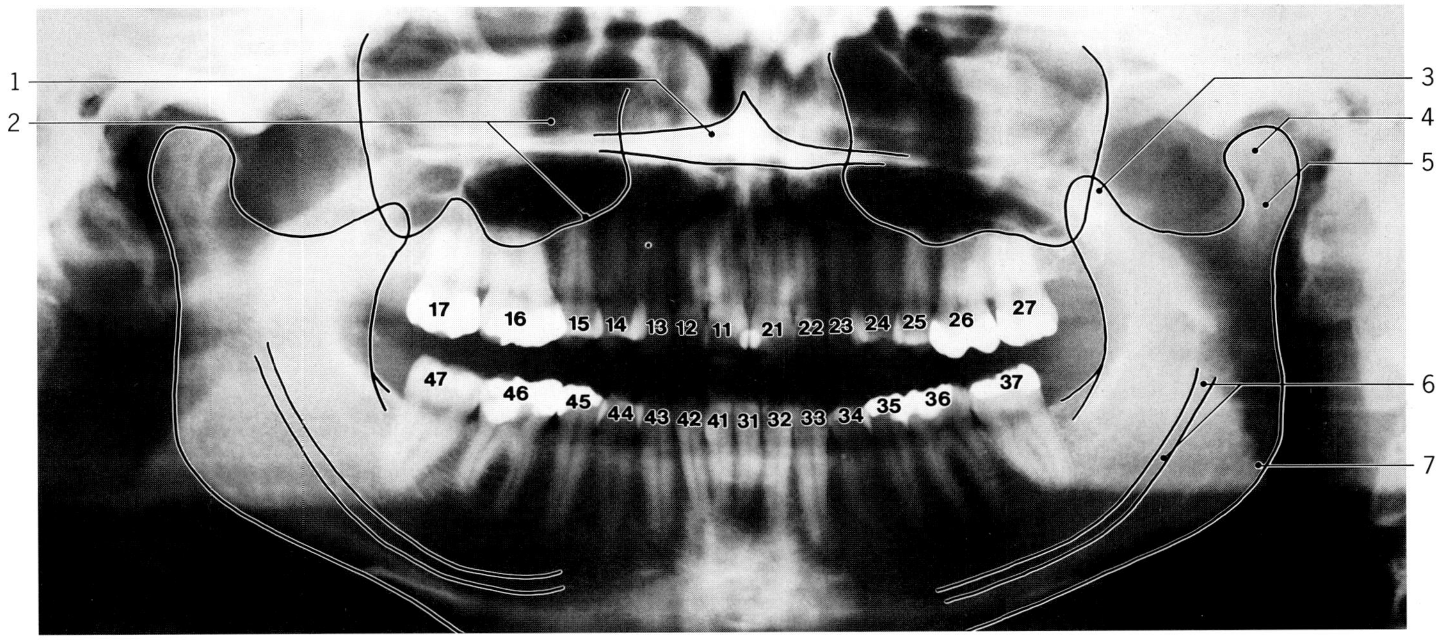

Teeth, panoramic X-ray, tomography

Teeth are numbered according to the international formula

1: Hard palate
2: Maxillary sinus
3: Coronoid process of mandible
4: Head of mandible
5: Neck of mandible
6: Mandibular canal
7: Angle of mandible

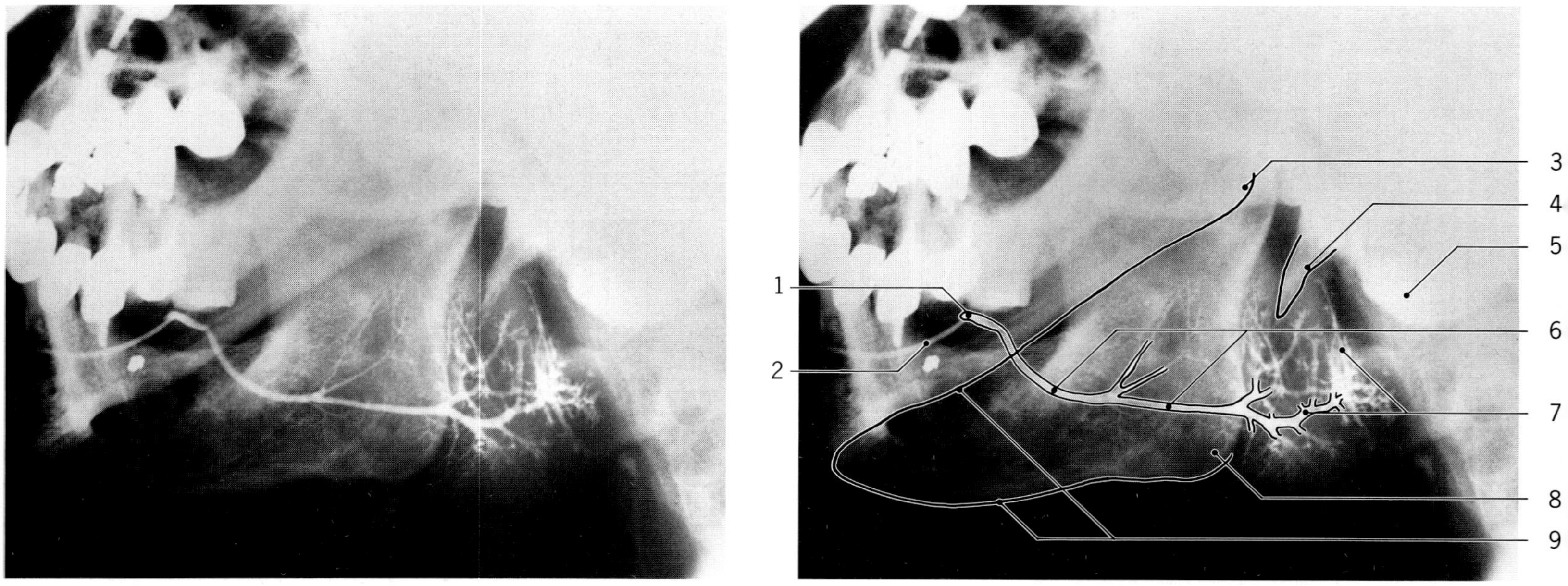

Parotid gland, oblique X-ray, sialography

1: Orifice of parotid duct
2: Cannula
3: Angle of mandible (contralateral)
4: Styloid process
5: Mastoid process
6: Parotid duct
7: Intraglandular ducts
8: Angle of mandible (ipsilateral)
9: Base of mandible

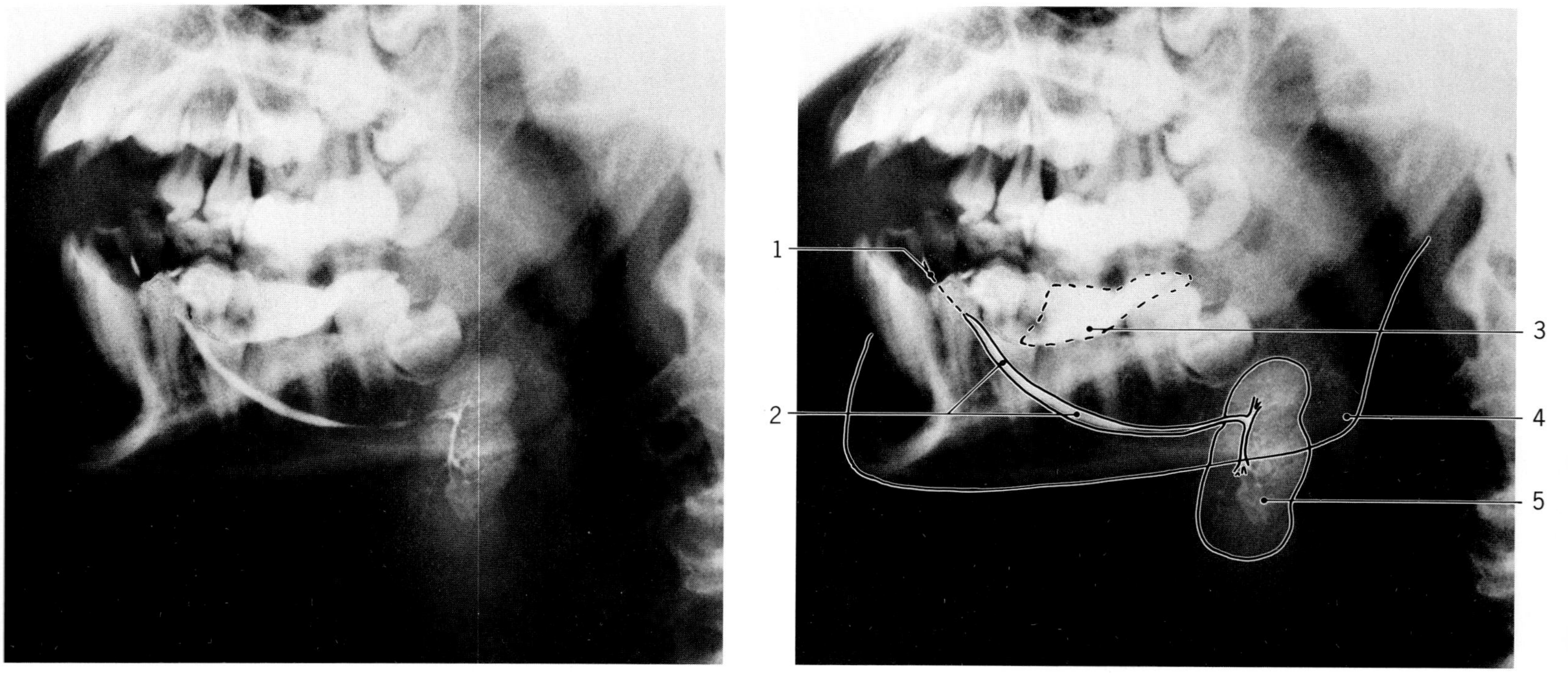

Submandibular gland, lateral X-ray, sialography

1: Cannula
2: Submandibular duct
3: Contrast medium in mouth
4: Angle of mandible
5: Submandibular gland

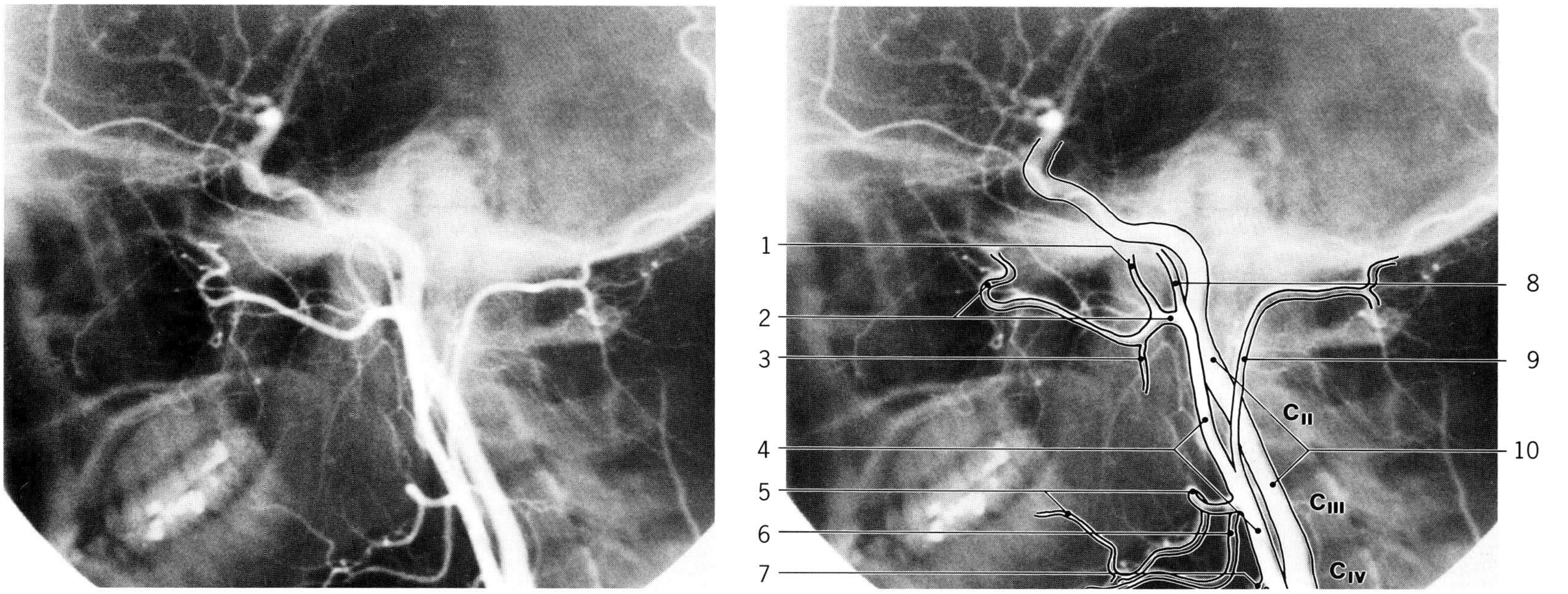

Carotid arteries, lateral X-ray, arteriography

1: Middle meningeal artery
2: Maxillary artery
3: Inferior alveolar artery
4: External carotid artery
5: Facial artery
6: Lingual artery
7: Superior thyroid artery
8: Superficial temporal artery
9: Occipital artery
10: Internal carotid artery

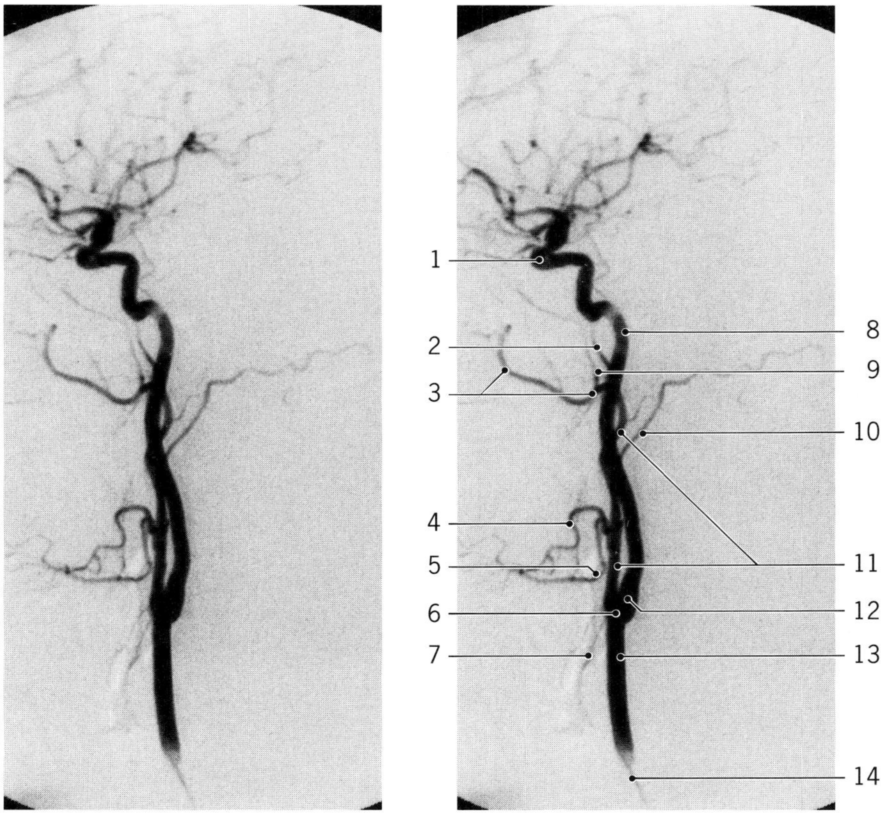

Carotid arteries, lateral X-ray, digital subtraction arteriography

1: Carotid "syphon"
2: Superficial temporal artery
3: Maxillary artery
4: Facial artery
5: Lingual artery
6: Carotid bifurcation
7: Superior thyroid artery
8: Internal carotid artery
9: Middle meningeal artery
10: Occipital artery
11: External carotid artery
12: Carotid sinus
13: Common carotid artery
14: Catheter

Brain

Axial CT-series

Median MR

Coronal MR-series

Arteries and veins

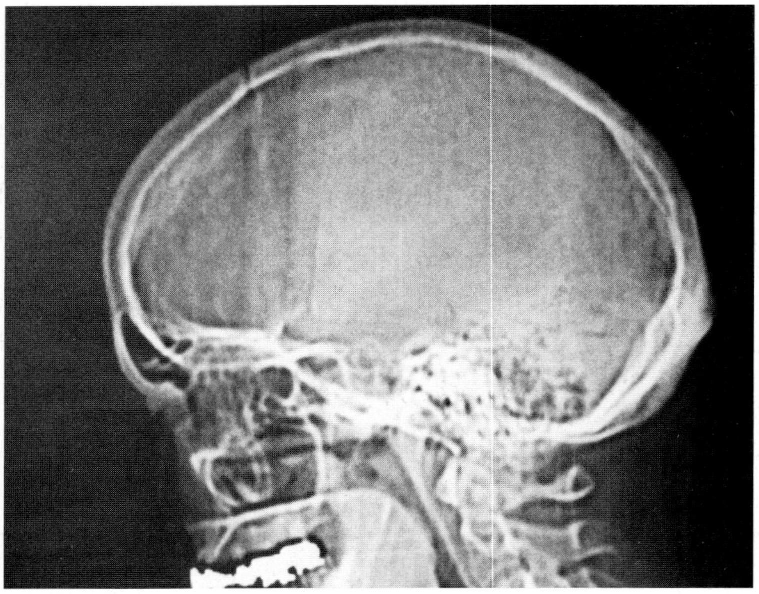

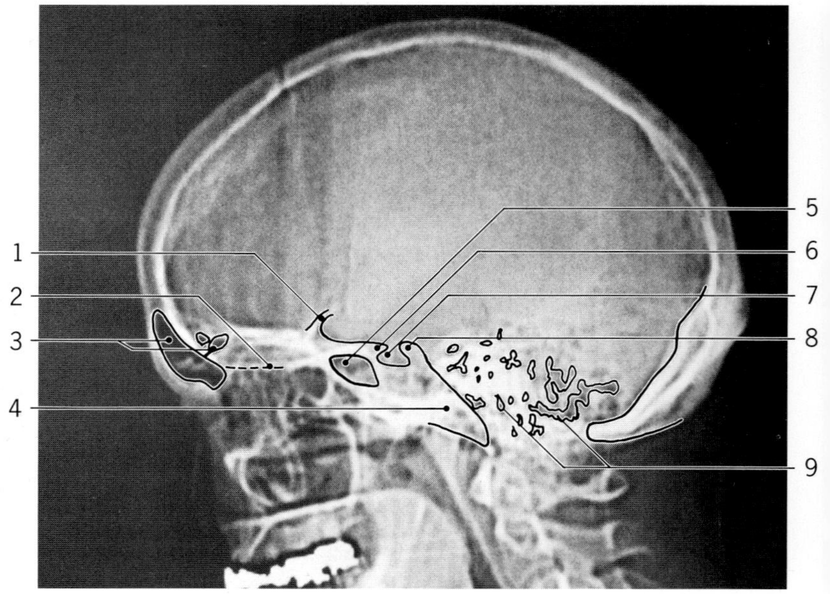

Scout view

1: Lesser wing of sphenoid bone
2: Cribriform plate
3: Frontal sinus
4: Clivus
5: Sphenoidal sinus
6: Anterior clinoid process
7: Hypophyseal fossa
8: Posterior clinoid process
9: Air cells in temporal bone

Scout view

Lines #1-15 indicate positions of axial sections in the following CT series.

Sections #1-6 are 3 mm thick, recorded at intervals of 5 mm, i.e. with 2 mm spacing.

Sections #7-15 are consecutive 10 mm sections.

Note change of angle between section #6 and #7

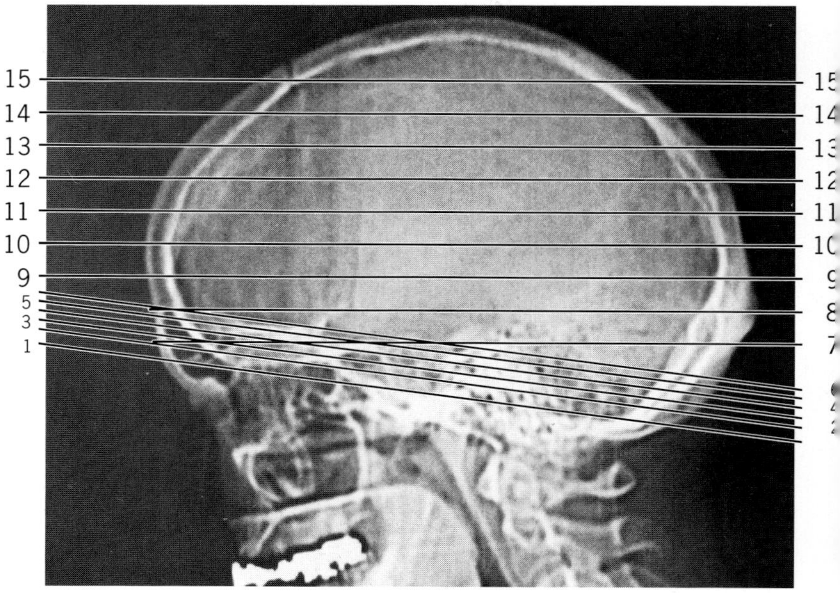

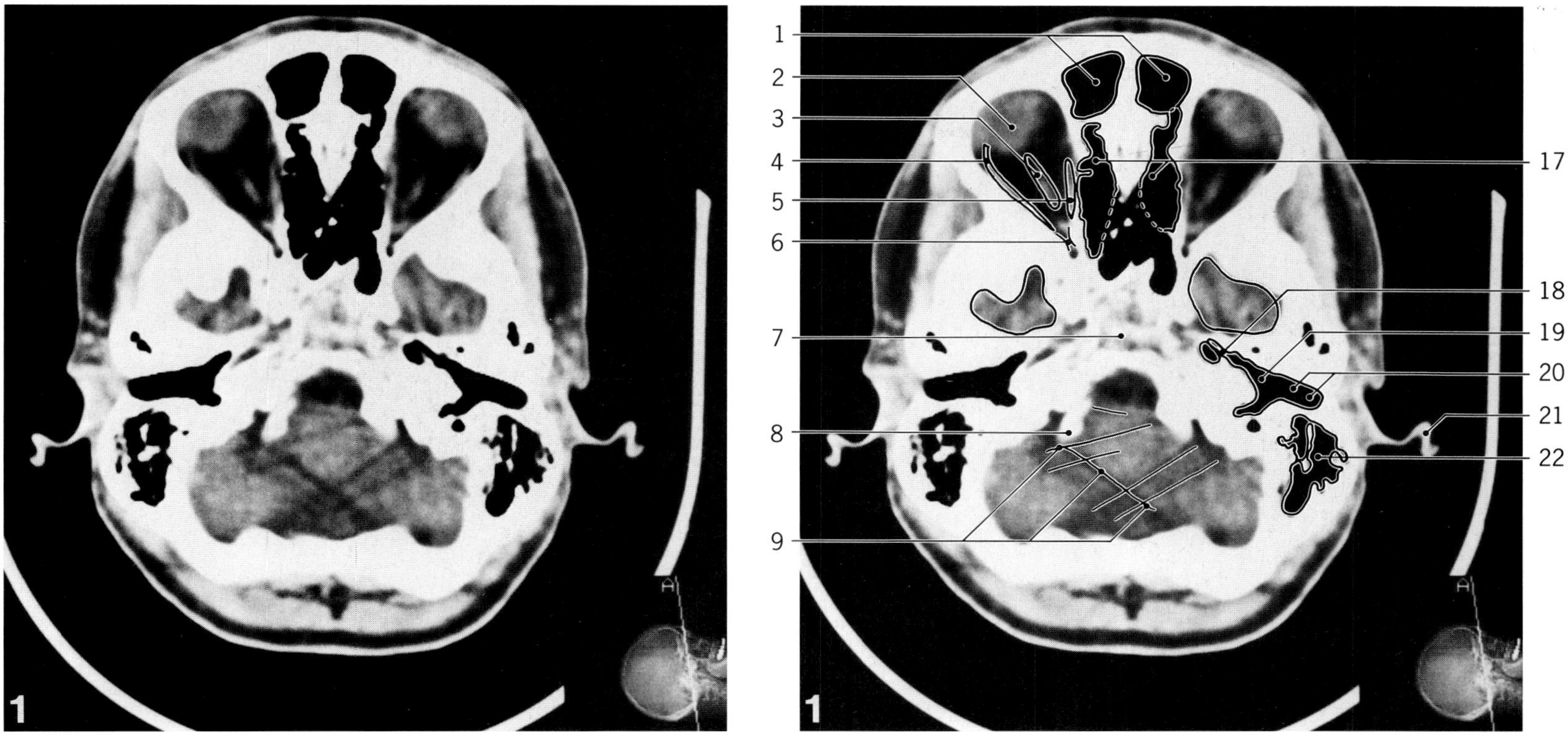

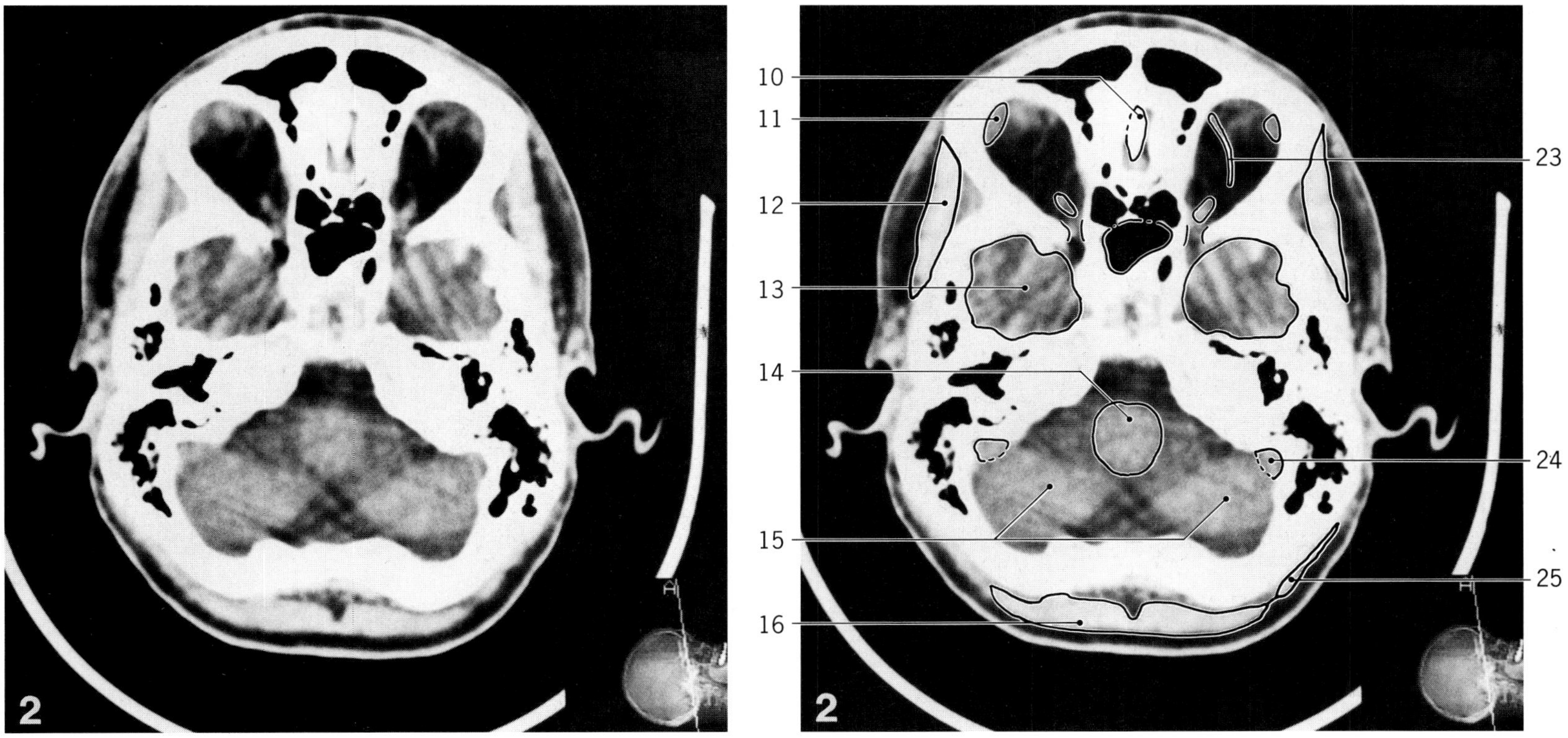

Brain, axial CT

Scout view on opposite page

1: Frontal sinus
2: Eye ball
3: Optic nerve
4: Rectus lateralis
5: Rectus medialis
6: Superior orbital fissure
7: Clivus
8: Jugular tubercle
9: Artefacts
10: Crista galli
11: Lacrimal gland
12: Temporalis
13: Temporal lobe
14: Medulla oblongata
15: Cerebellar hemispheres
16: Trapezius
17: Ethmoidal air cells
18: Auditory tube
19: Tympanic cavity
20: External auditory meatus
21: Auricle
22: Mastoid air cells
23: Ophthalmic artery
24: Sigmoid sinus
25: Splenius capitis

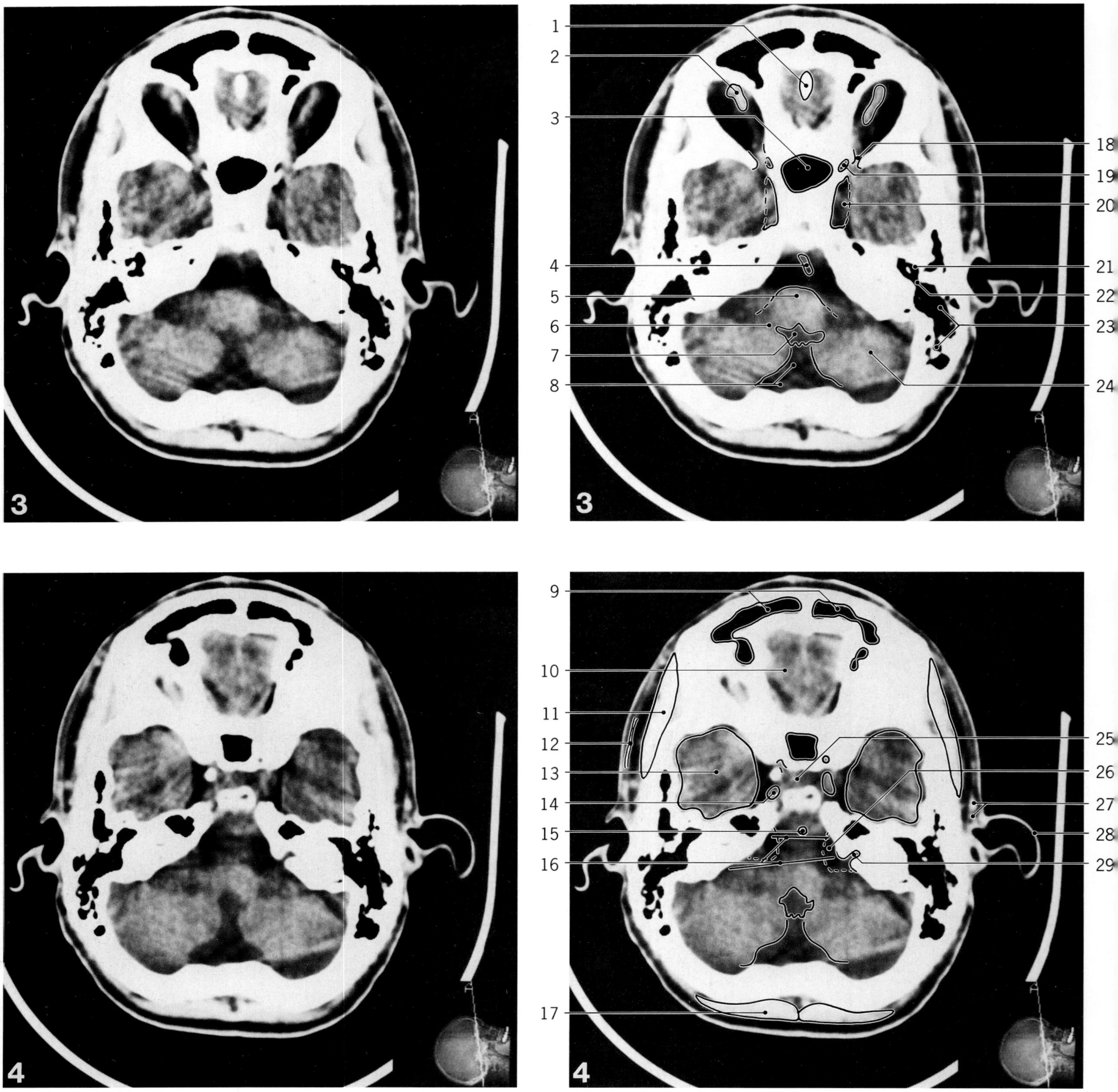

Brain, axial CT

Scout view on page 160

1: Crista galli
2: Rectus superior and levator palpebrae
3: Sphenoidal sinus
4: Basilar artery
5: Pons
6: Middle cerebellar peduncle
7: Fourth ventricle
8: Cerebello-medullary cistern
9: Frontal sinus
10: Frontal lobe
11: Temporalis muscle
12: Galea aponeurotica
13: Temporal lobe
14: Internal carotid artery
15: Basilary artery
16: Artefacts
17: Trapezius
18: Superior orbital fissure
19: Optic canal
20: Internal carotid artery in cavernous sinus
21: Tympanic cavity
22: Aditus ad antrum
23: Mastoid air cells
24: Cerebellar hemisphere
25: Hypophysis
26: Cerebellopontine cistern
27: Superficial temporal artery and vein
28: Auricle
29: Internal acoustic meatus

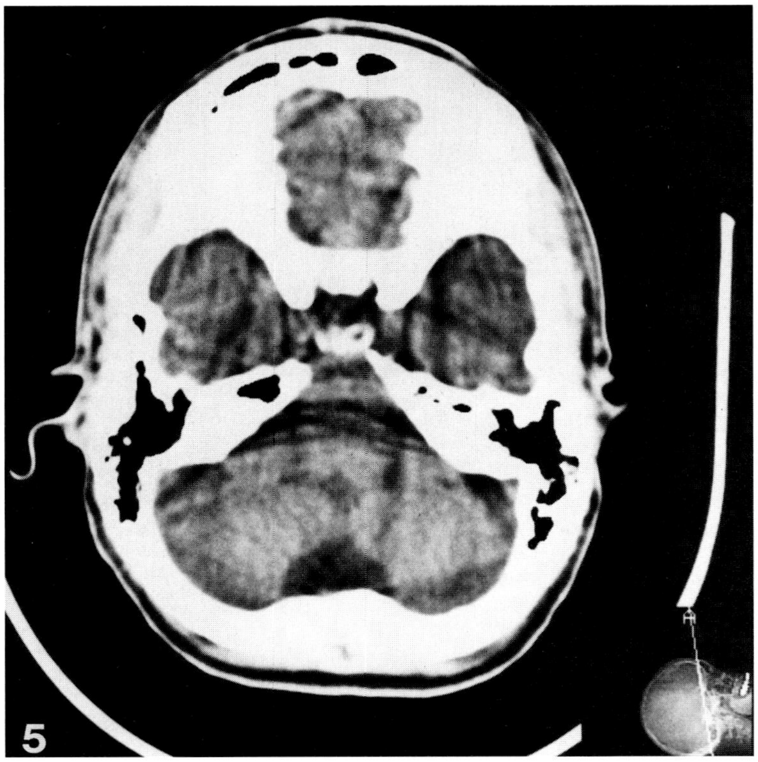

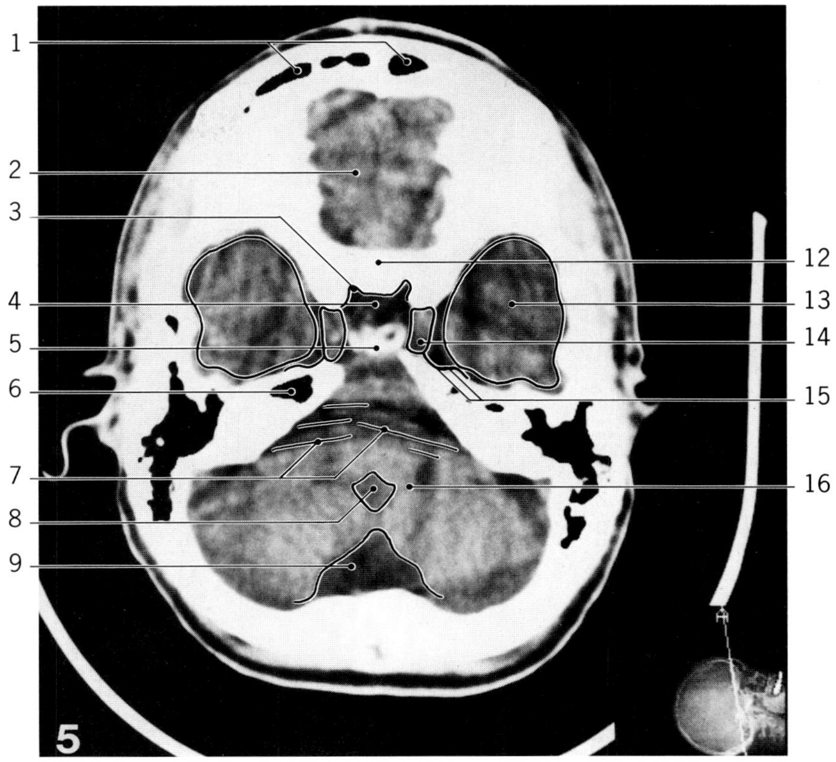

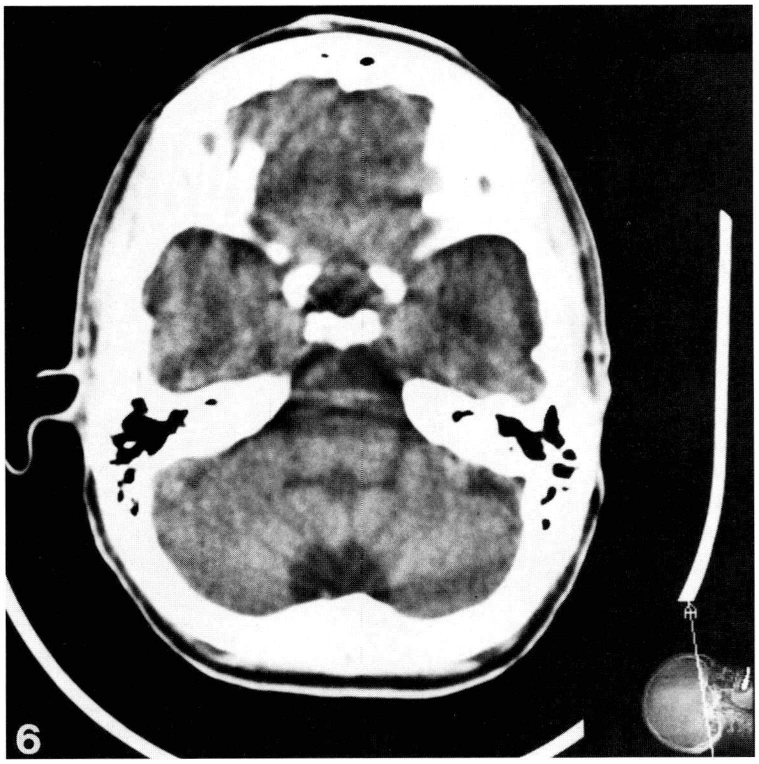

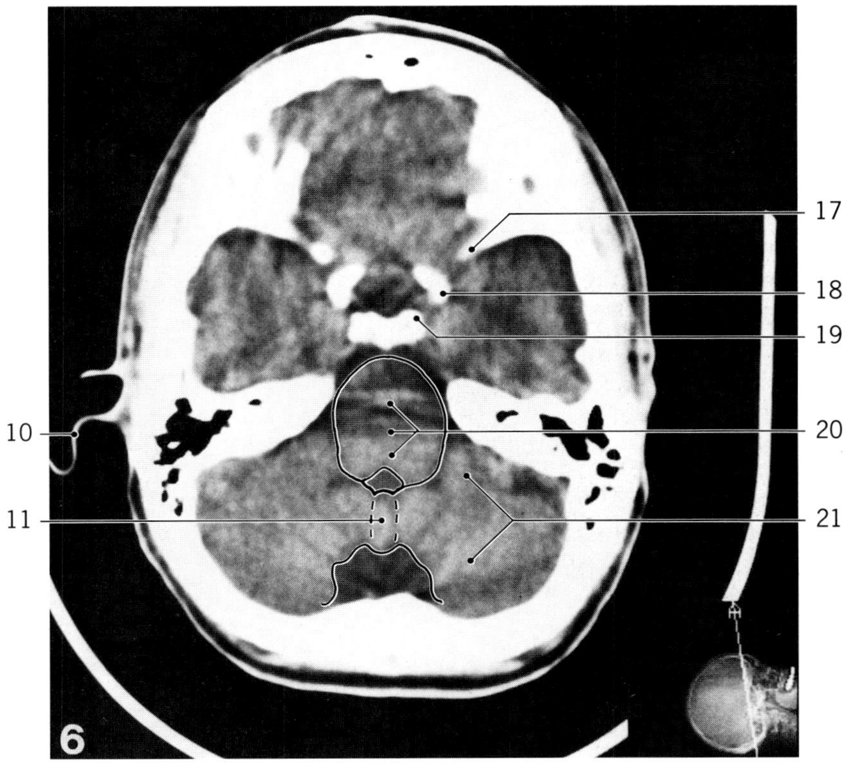

Brain, axial CT

Scout view on page 160

1: Frontal sinus
2: Frontal lobe
3: Optic canal
4: Optic chiasma
5: Dorsum sellae
6: Air cells anteriorly in petrous bone
7: Artefacts
8: Fourth ventricle
9: Cerebello-medullary cistern
10: Auricle
11: Vermis of cerebellum
12: Jugum sphenoidale
13: Temporal lobe
14: Internal carotid artery in cavernous sinus
15: Trigeminal impression
16: Superior cerebellar peduncle
17: Lesser wing of sphenoid bone
18: Anterior clinoid process
19: Posterior clinoid process
20: Pons
21: Cerebellar hemisphere

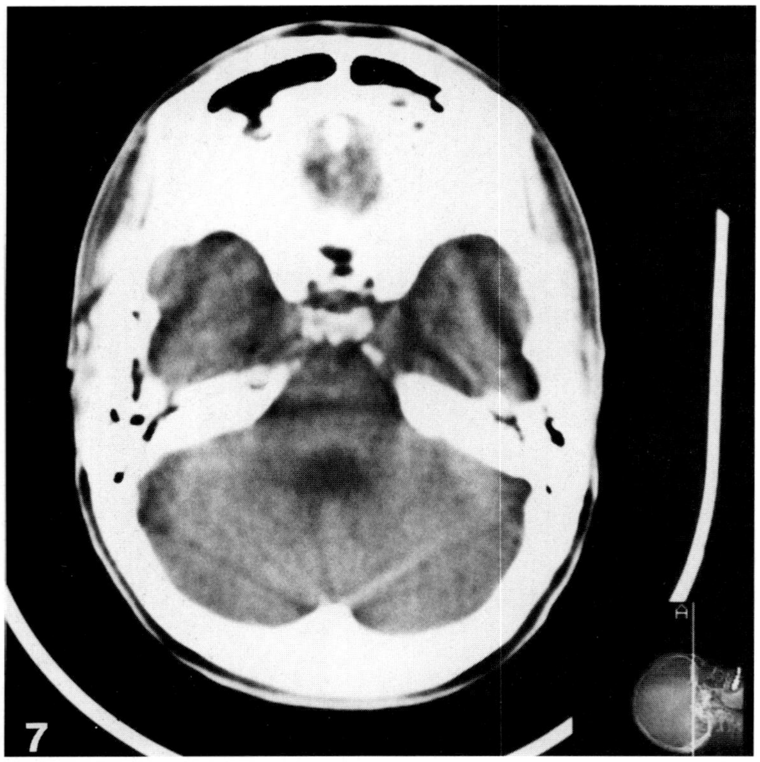

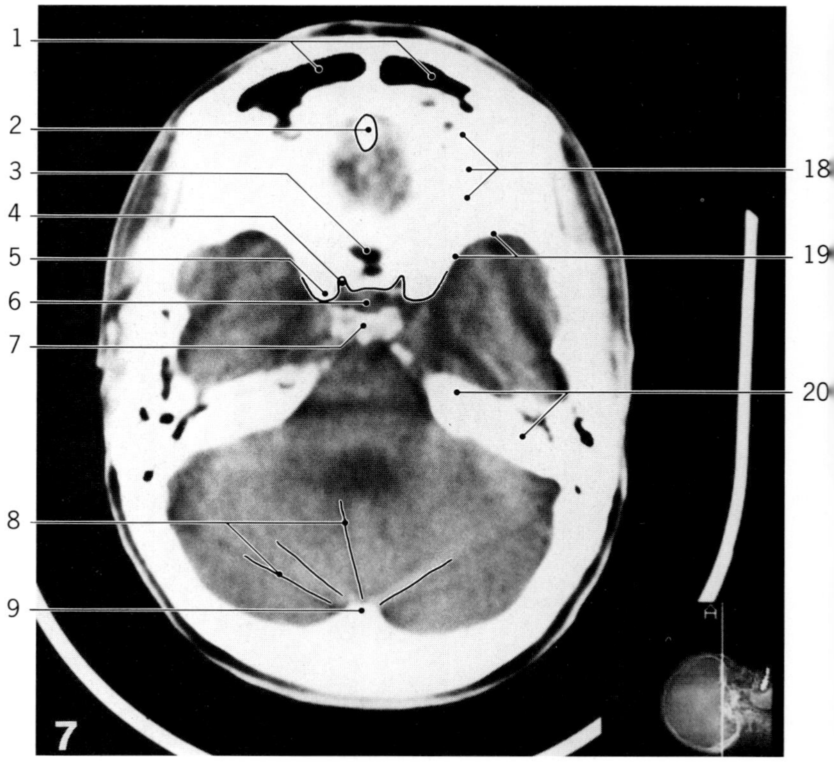

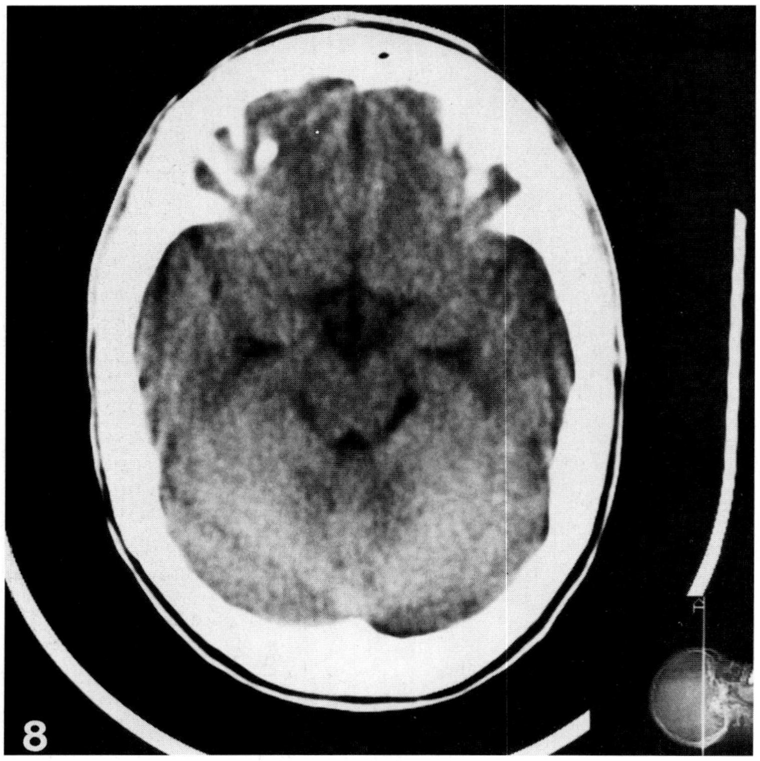

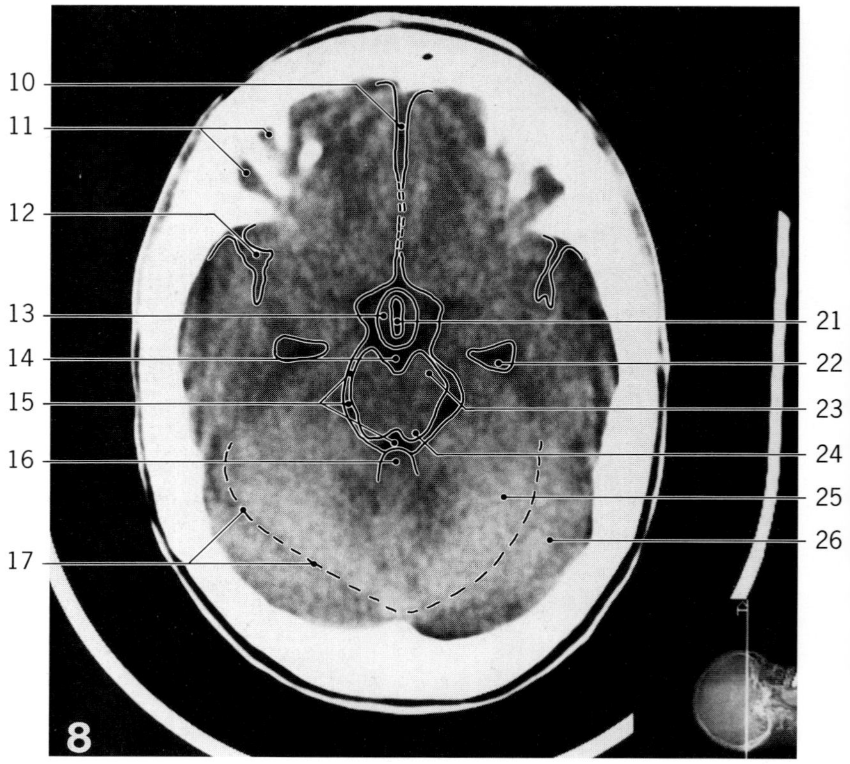

Brain, axial CT

Scout view on page 160

1: Frontal sinus
2: Crista galli
3: Sphenoidal sinus
4: Optic canal
5: Anterior clinoid process
6: Hypophysis
7: Dorsum sellae
8: Artefacts
9: Internal occipical protuberance
10: Longitudinal fissure of cerebrum
11: Impressions of cerebral gyri
12: Lateral sulcus (Sylvian)
13: Hypothalamus
14: Interpeduncular cistern
15: Cisterna ambiens
16: Vermis of cerebellum
17: Tentorium cerebelli
18: Orbital plate of frontal bone
19: Lesser wing of sphenoid bone
20: Petrous part of temporal bone
21: Third ventricle
22: Lateral ventricle, temporal horn
23: Cerebral peduncle
24: Inferior colliculus
25: Cerebellum
26: Occipital lobe

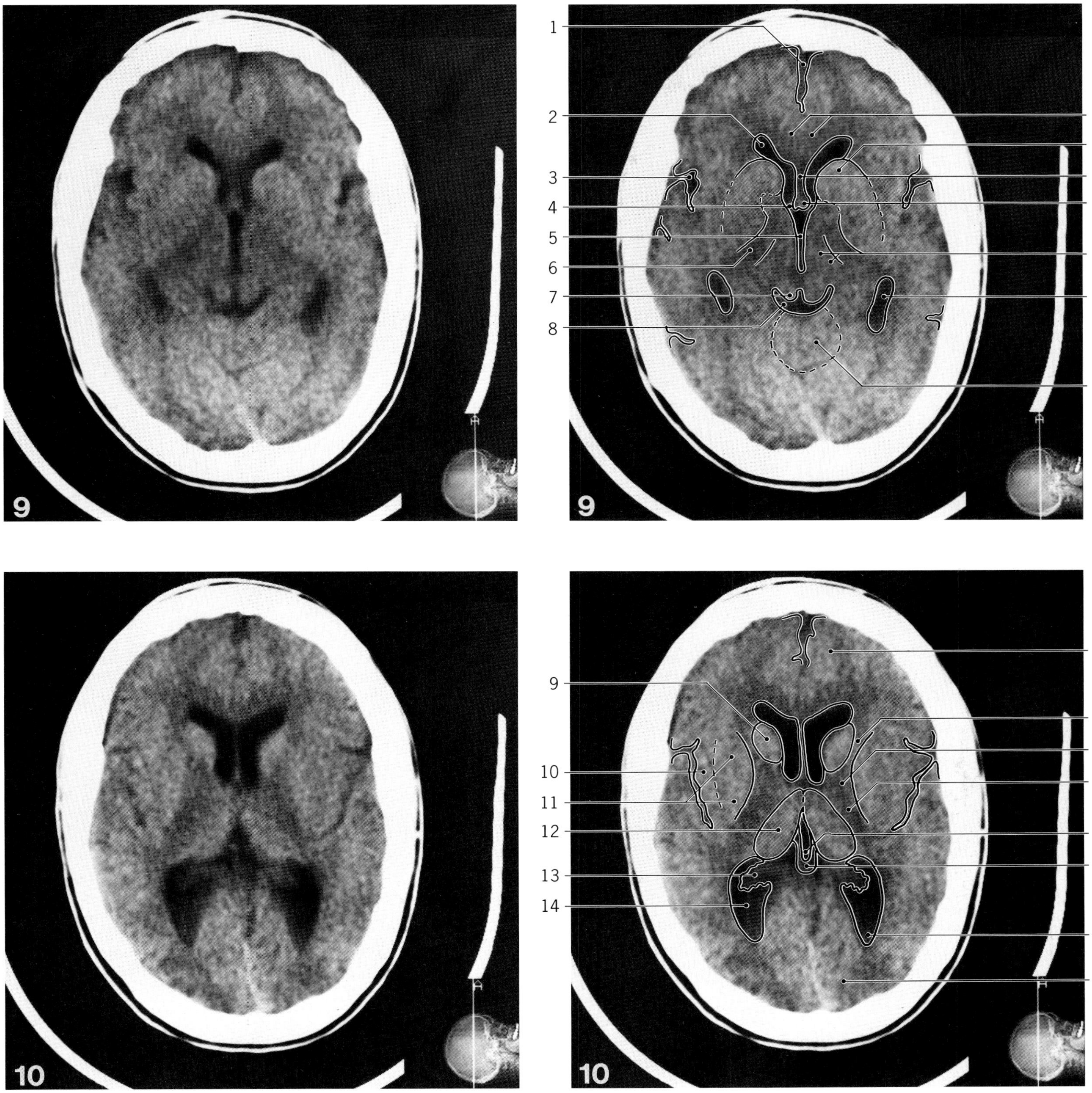

Brain, axial CT

Scout view on page 160

1: Longitudinal fissure
2: Lateral ventricle, frontal horn
3: Lateral sulcus (Sylvian)
4: Interventricular foramen (Monroi)
5: Third ventricle
6: Internal capsule, posterior limb
7: Superior colliculus
8: Cisterna ambiens
9: Head of caudate nucleus
10: Insula
11: Lentiform nucleus
12: Thalamus
13: Choroid plexus
14: Lateral ventricle
15: Genu of corpus callosum
16: Head of caudate nucleus, contiguous with lentiform nucleus
17: Septum pellucidum
18: Column of fornix
19: Subthalamus
20: Lateral ventricle, temporal horn
21: Cerebellum, quadrangular lobe
22: Frontal lobe
23: Internal capsule, anterior limb
24: Internal capsule, genu
25: Internal capsule, posterior limb
26: Pineal recess of third ventricle
27: Pineal gland
28: Lateral ventricle, occipital horn
29: Occipital lobe

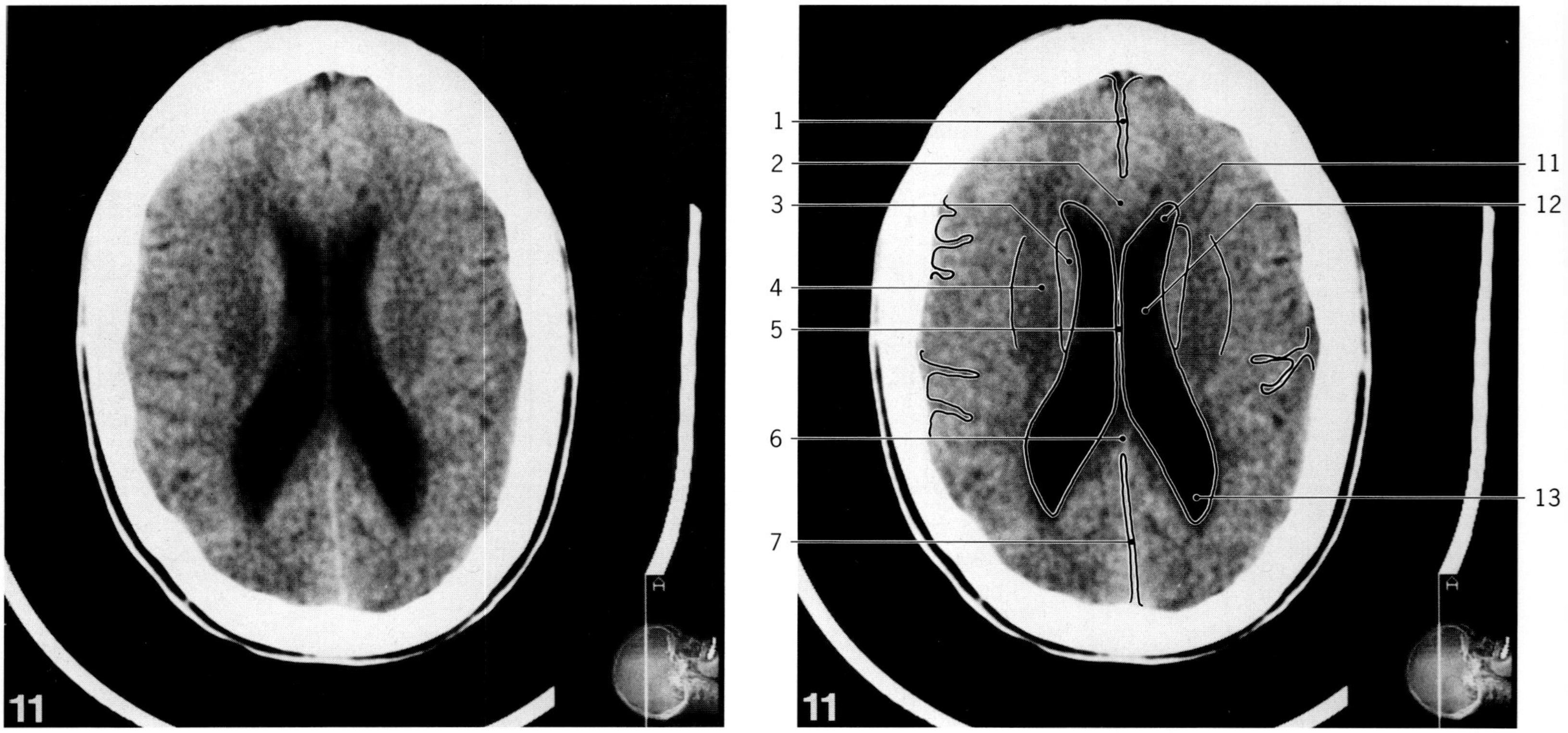

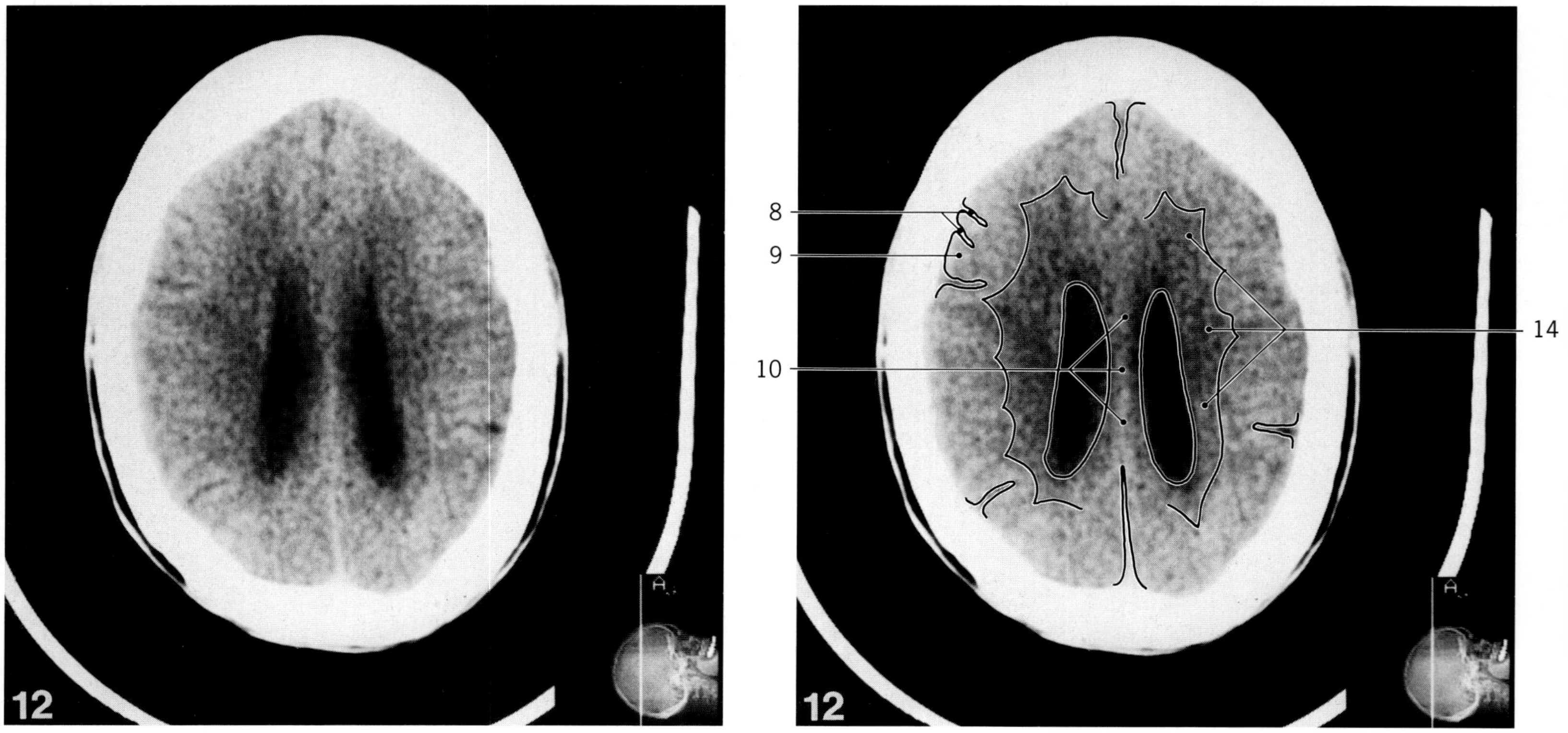

Brain, axial CT

Scout view on page 160

1: Longitudinal fissure of brain
2: Genu of corpus callosum
3: Body of caudate nucleus
4: Internal capsule
5: Septum pellucidum
6: Splenium of corpus callosum
7: Falx cerebri
8: Sulci of cerebral cortex
9: Gyrus of cerebral cortex
10: Corpus callosum
11: Lateral ventricle, frontal horn
12: Lateral ventricle, central part
13: Lateral ventricle, occipital horn
14: Corona radiata

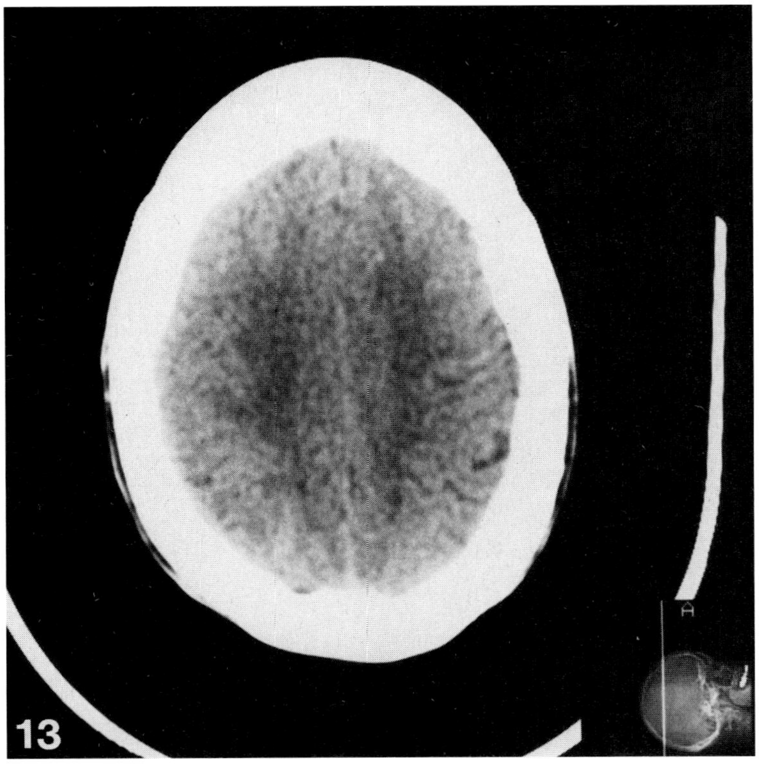

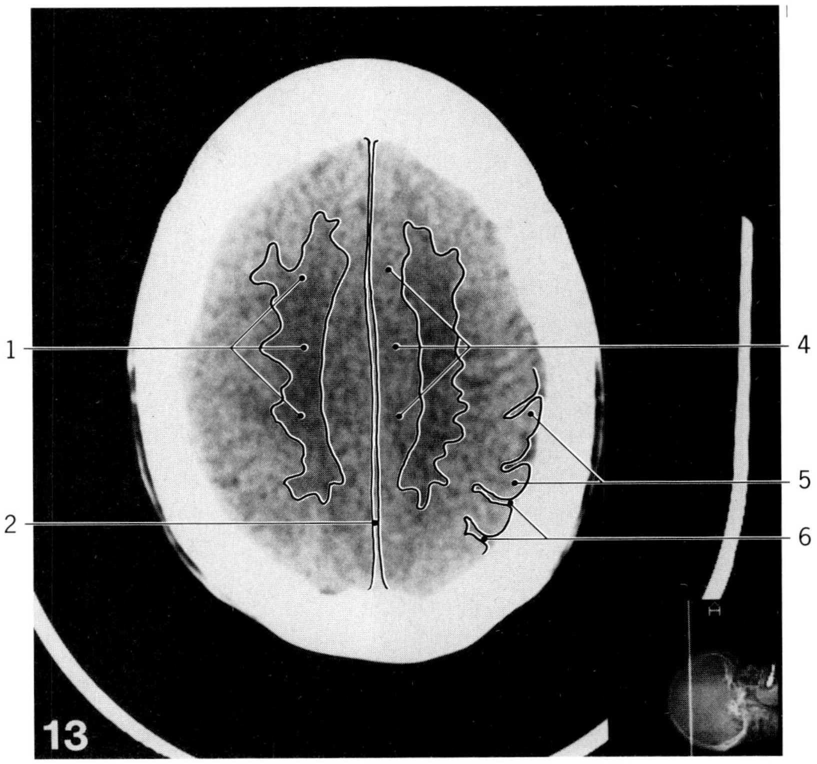

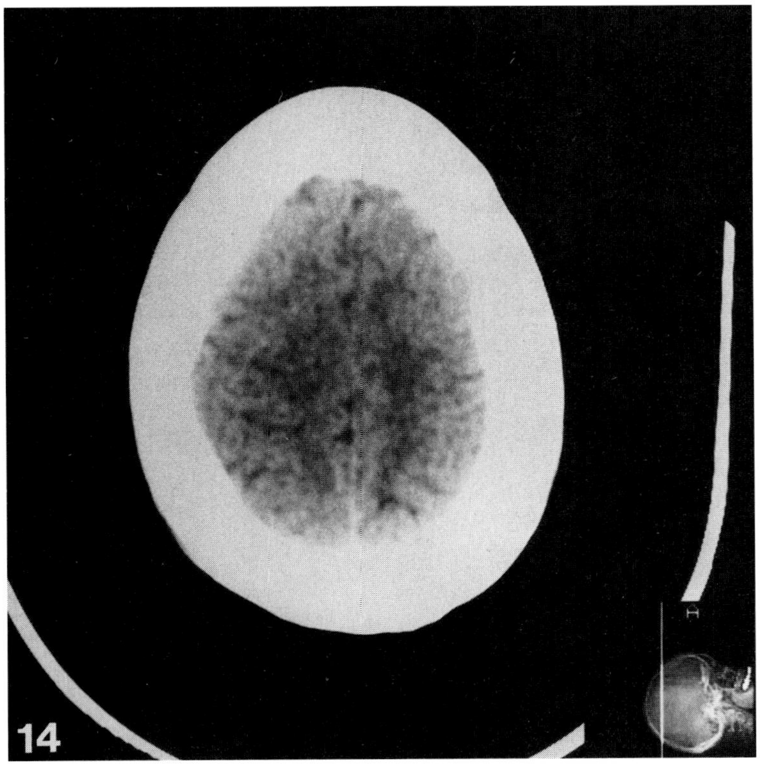

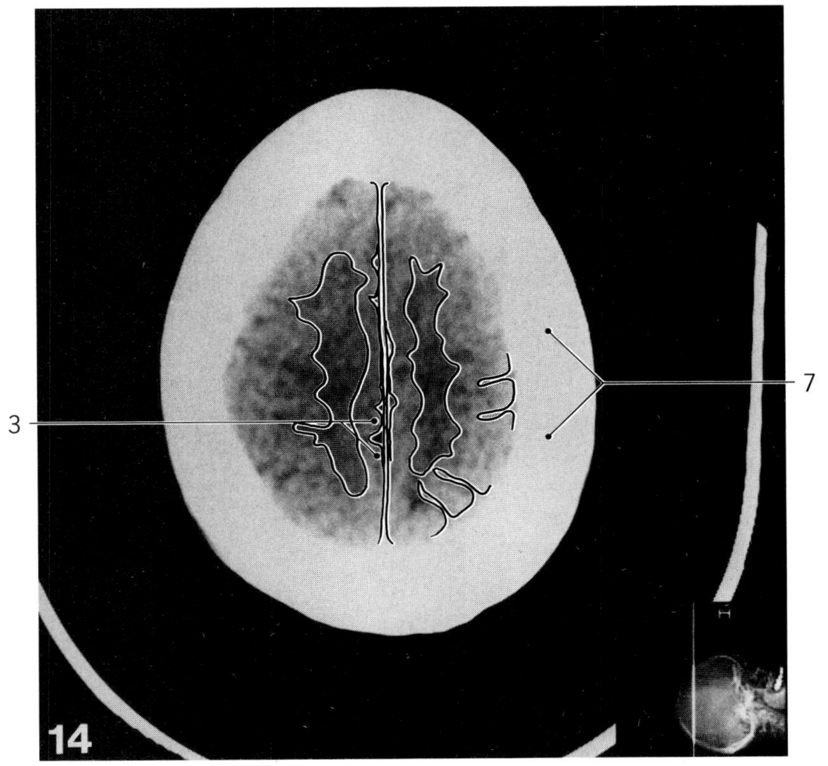

Brain, axial CT

Scout view on page 160

1: Corona radiata
2: Falx cerebri
3: Gyri on medial aspect of cerebral hemisphere
4: Cingulate gyrus
5: Gyri
6: Sulci
7: Calvaria

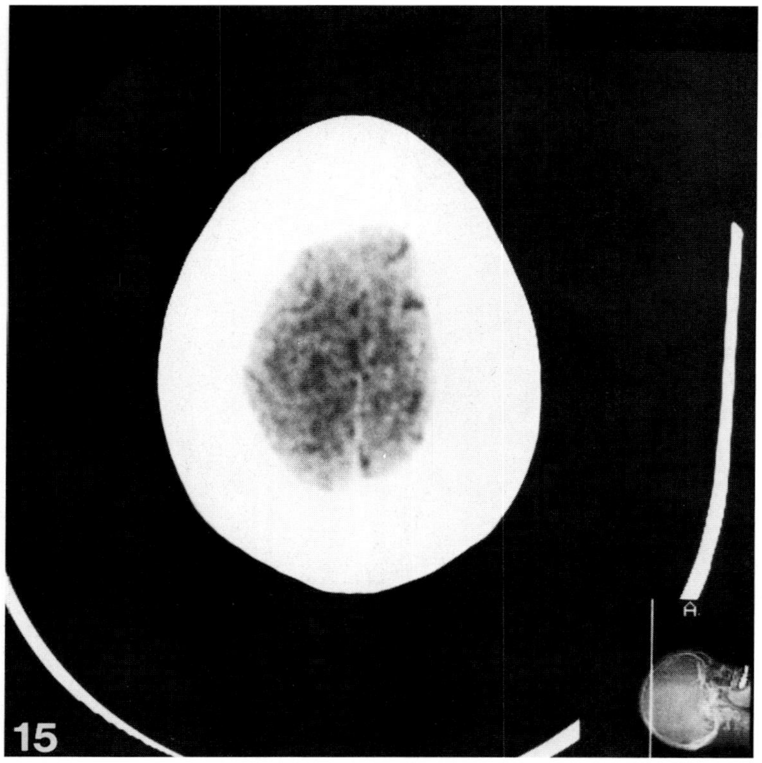

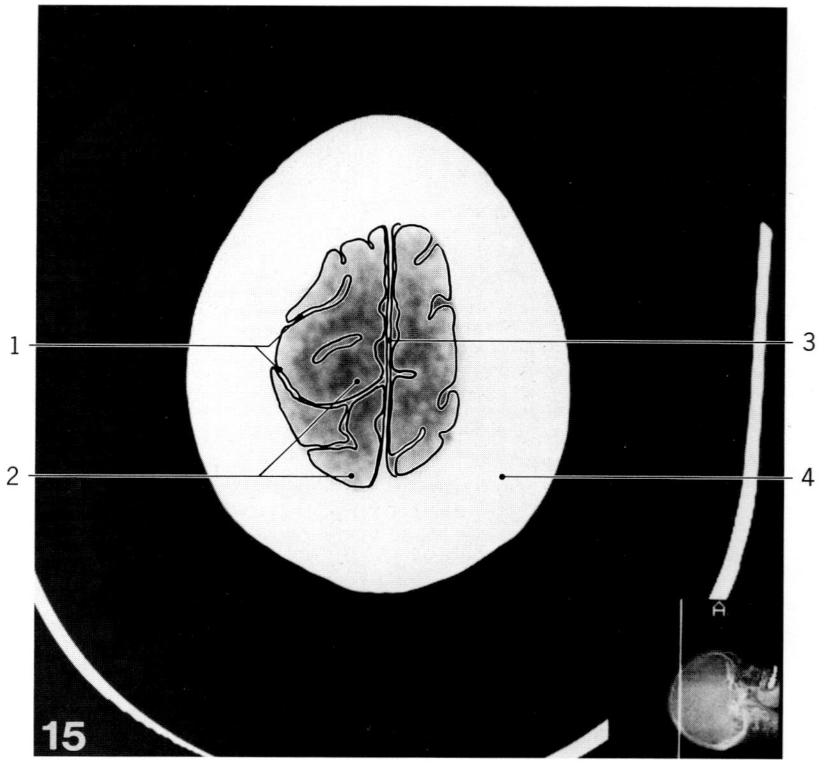

Brain, axial CT

Scout view on page 160

1: Sulci
2: Gyri
3: Falx cerebri
4: Calvaria

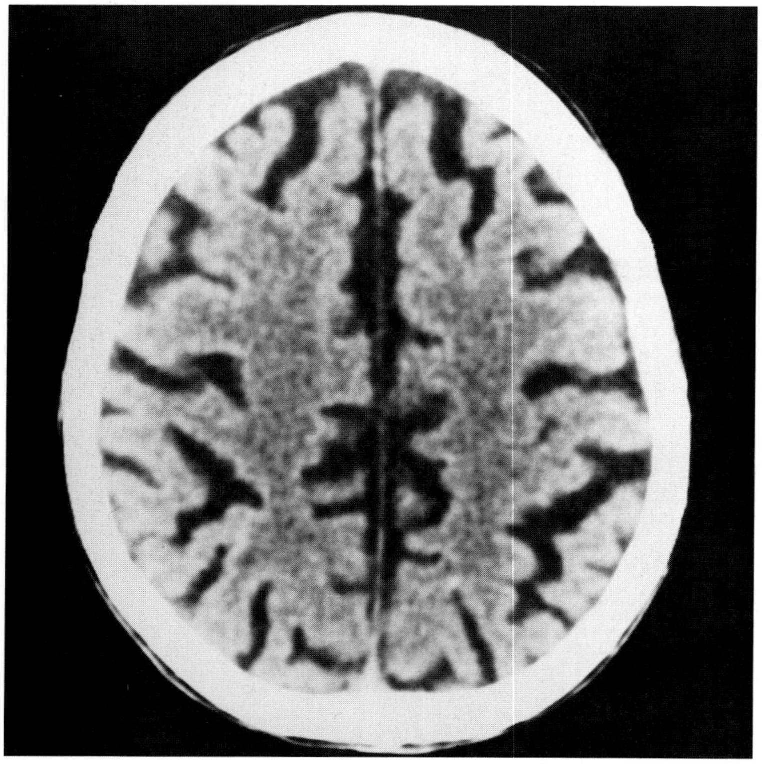

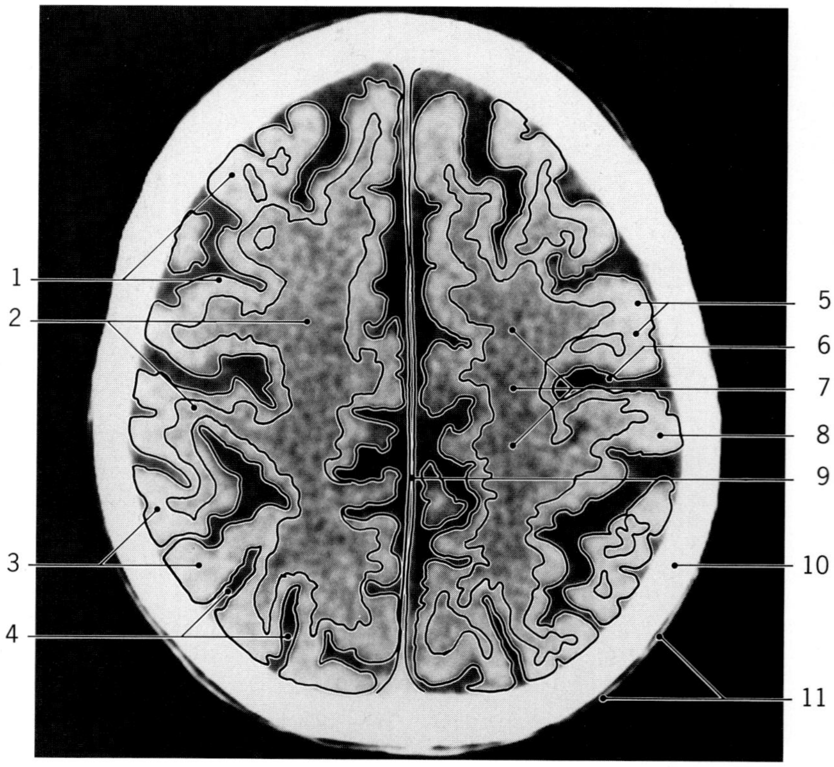

Brain, atrophic, axial CT

1: Grey matter
2: White matter
3: Gyri (atrophic)
4: Sulci (widened)
5: Precentral gyrus
6: Central sulcus
7: Corona radiata
8: Postcentral gyrus
9: Falx cerebri
10: Calvaria
11: Galea aponeurotica

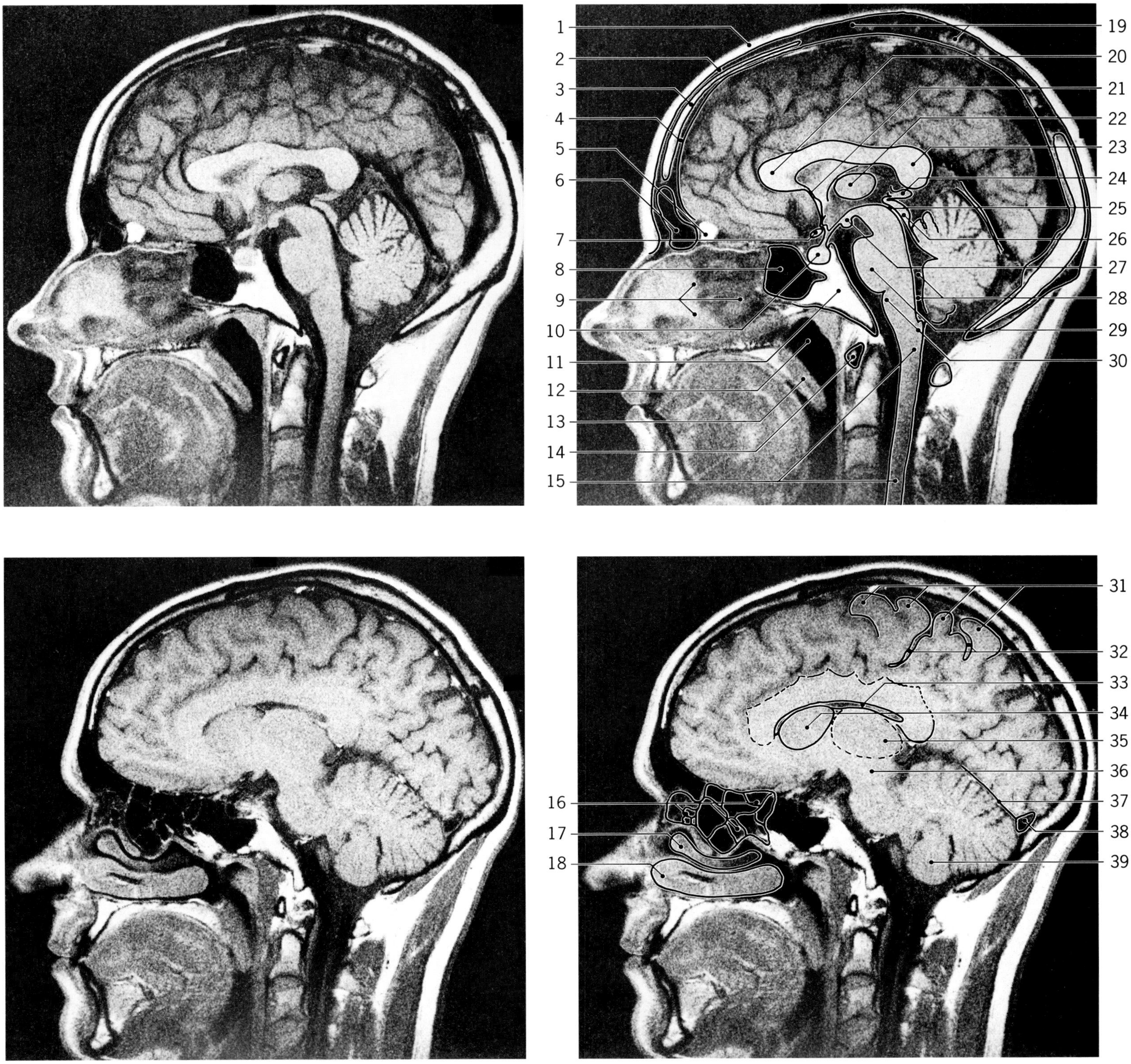

Brain, median (above) and paramedian section (below), MR

T1–weighted images

1: Subcutis of scalp
2: Outer table of calvaria
3: Diploë
4: Inner table of calvaria
5: Crista galli
6: Frontal sinus
7: Optic chiasm
8: Sphenoidal sinus
9: Nasal septum
10: Hypophysis
11: Clivus
12: Nasal part of pharynx
13: Uvula
14: Anterior arch of atlas
15: Spinal cord
16: Ethmoid air cells
17: Middle nasal concha
18: Inferior nasal concha
19: Sagittal suture
20: Genu of corpus callosum
21: Rostrum of corpus callosum
22: Thalamus
23: Splenium of corpus callosum
24: Pineal gland
25: Cerebral aqueduct
26: Tectum of mesencephalon
27: Mammillary body
28: Fourth ventricle
29: Pons
30: Medulla oblongata
31: Gyri of cerebral cortex
32: Sulci of cerebral cortex
33: Lateral ventricle
34: Head of caudate nucleus
35: Thalamus
36: Cerebral peduncle
37: Tentorium cerebelli
38: Transverse sinus
39: Cerebellar tonsil

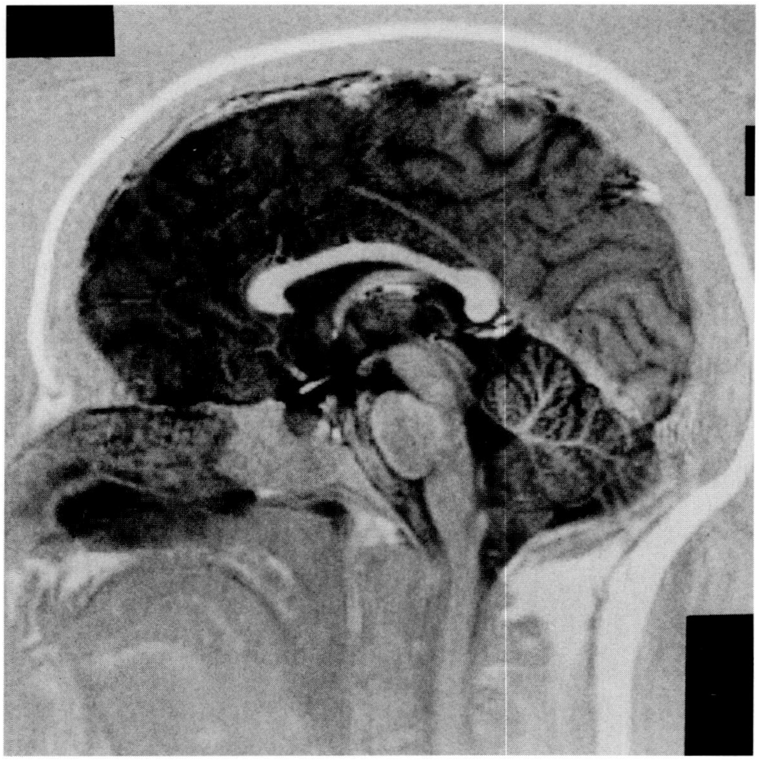

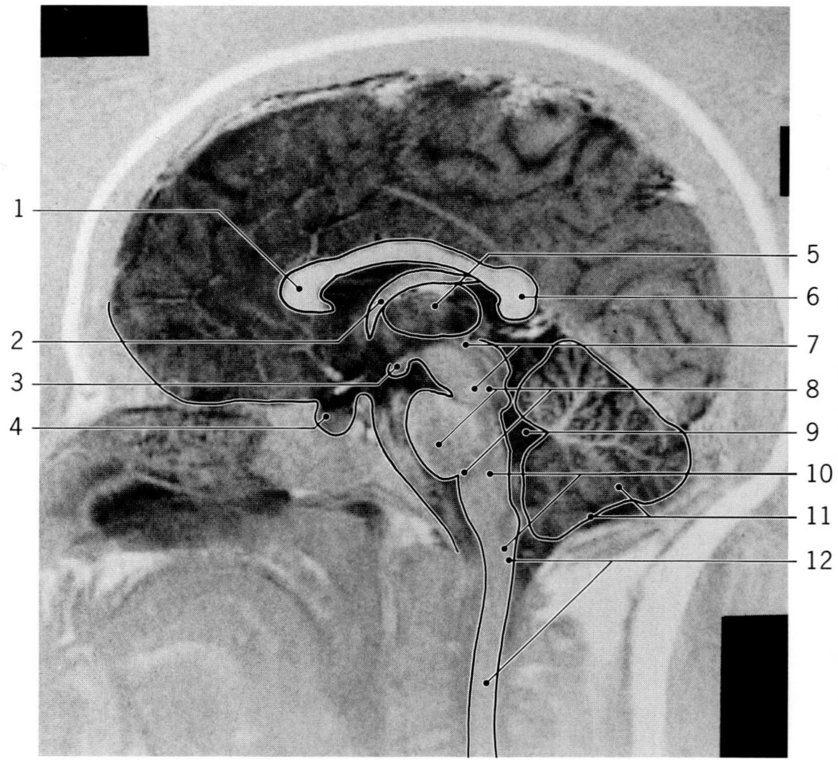

Scout view

1: Genu of corpus callosum
2: Fornix
3: Mammillary body
4: Hypophysis
5: Thalamus
6: Splenium of corpus callosum
7: Midbrain (mesencephalon)
8: Pons
9: Fourth ventricle
10: Medulla oblongata
11: Cerebellum
12: Spinal cord

Scout view

Lines #1-17 indicate positions of coronal sections in the following MR series.

Consecutive sections, 10 mm thick.

T_1–weighted recording

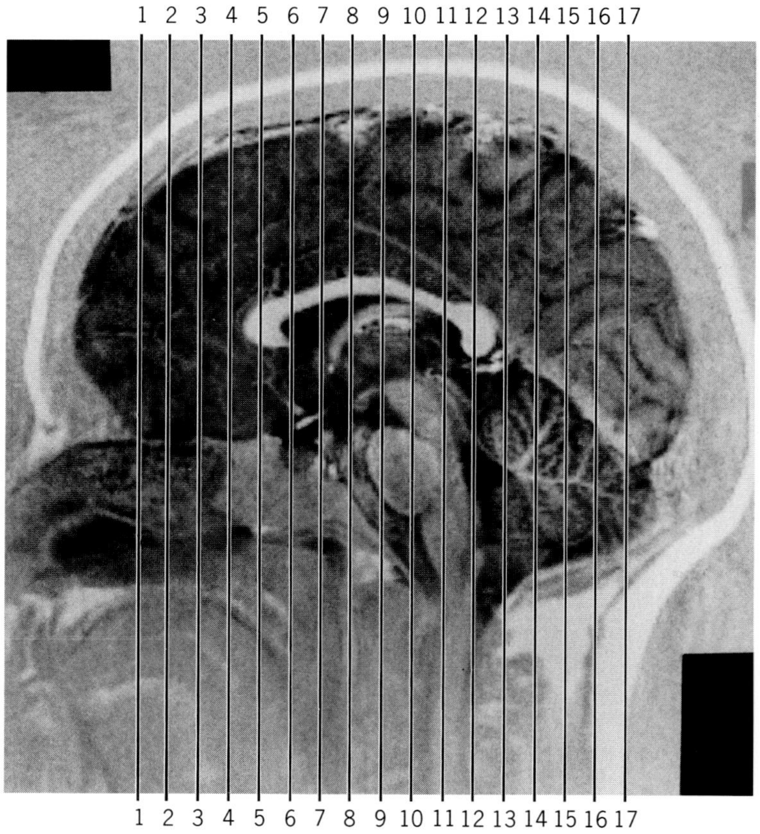

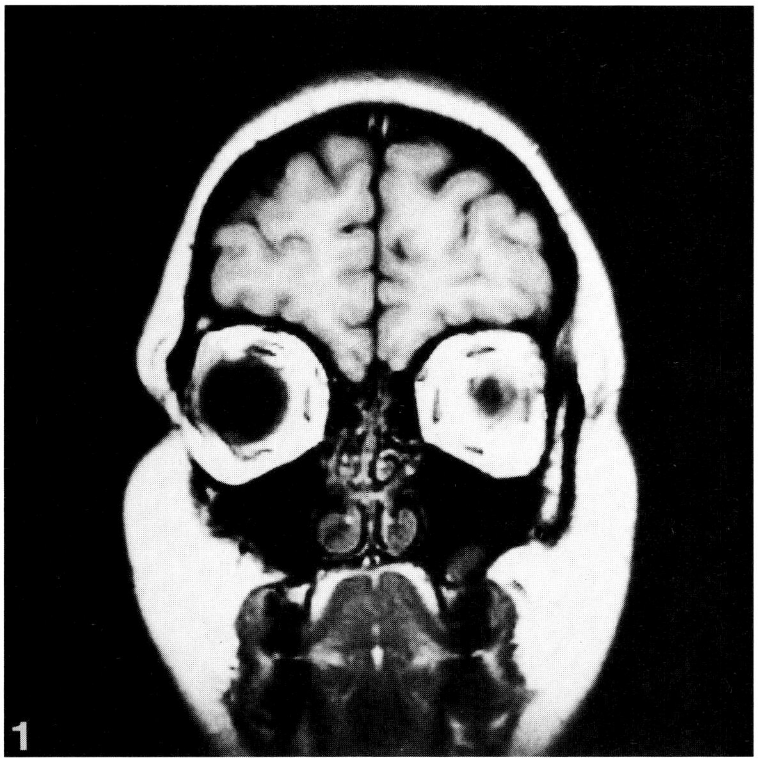

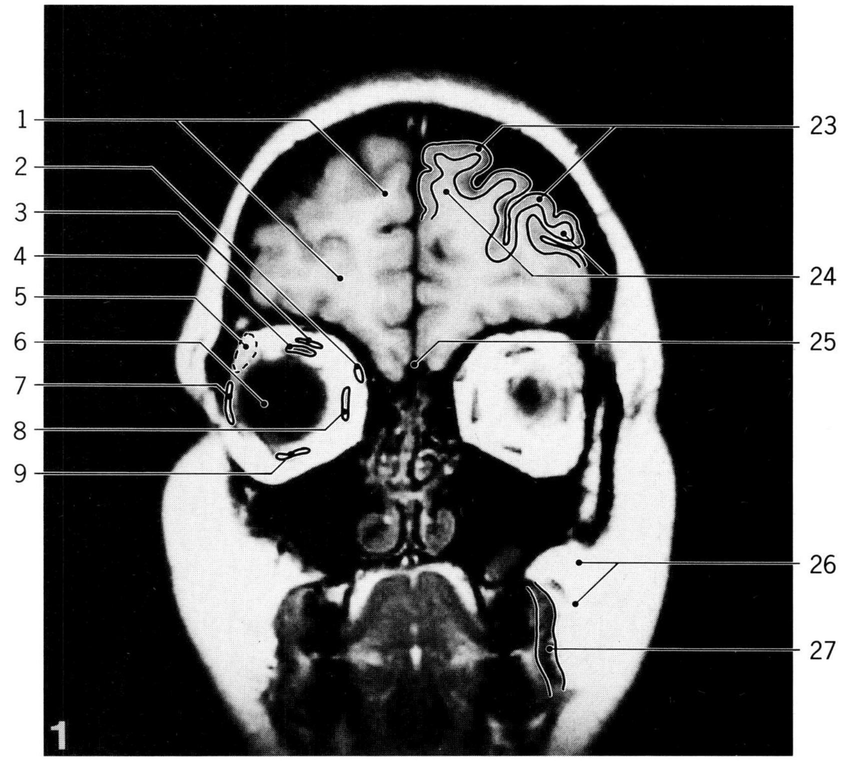

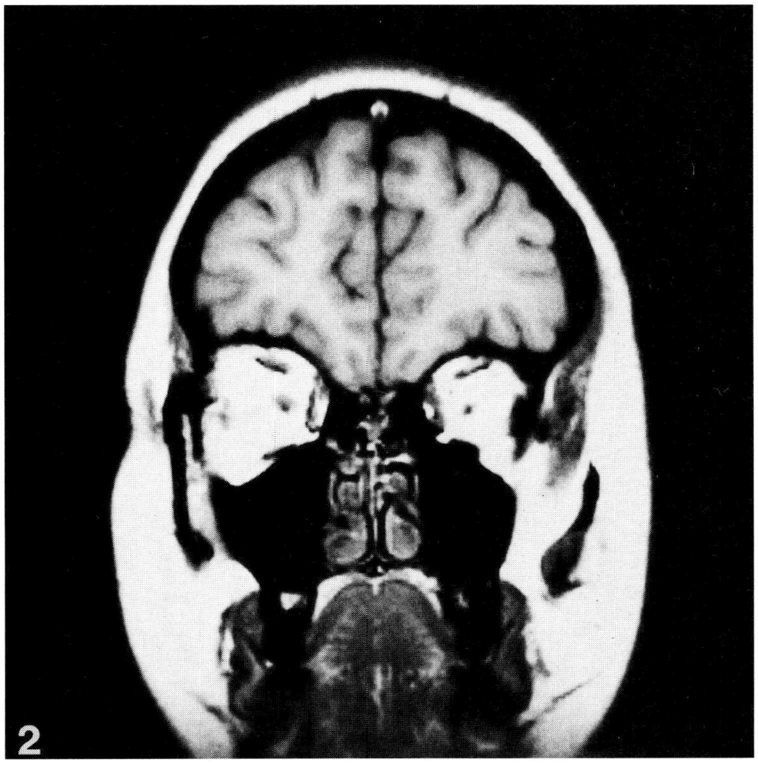

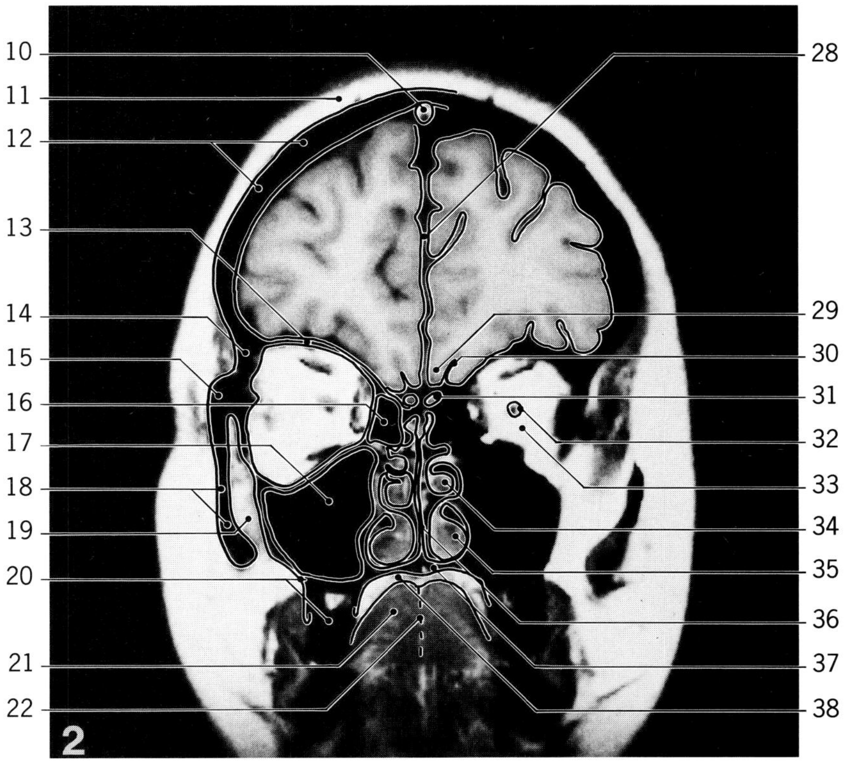

Brain, coronal MR

Scout view on previous page

1: Frontal lobe
2: Obliquus superior
3: Levator palpebrae
4: Rectus superior
5: Lacrimal gland
6: Eye ball
7: Rectus lateralis
8: Rectus medialis
9: Rectus inferior
10: Superior sagittal sinus
11: Scalp
12: Squamous part of frontal bone
13: Orbital plate of frontal bone
14: Zygomatic process of frontal bone
15: Frontal process of zygomatic bone
16: Ethmoidal air cells
17: Maxillary sinus
18: Body of zygomatic bone
19: Infratemporal fossa
20: Alveolar process with tooth
21: Tongue
22: Septum of tongue
23: Grey matter
24: White matter
25: Crista galli
26: Corpus adiposum buccae
27: Buccinator
28: Longitudinal fissure of cerebrum
29: Gyrus rectus
30: Sulcus rectus
31: Olfactory bulb
32: Optic nerve
33: Corpus adiposum orbitae
34: Middle nasal concha
35: Inferior nasal concha
36: Nasal septum
37: Hard palate
38: Palatal mucosa with glands and fat

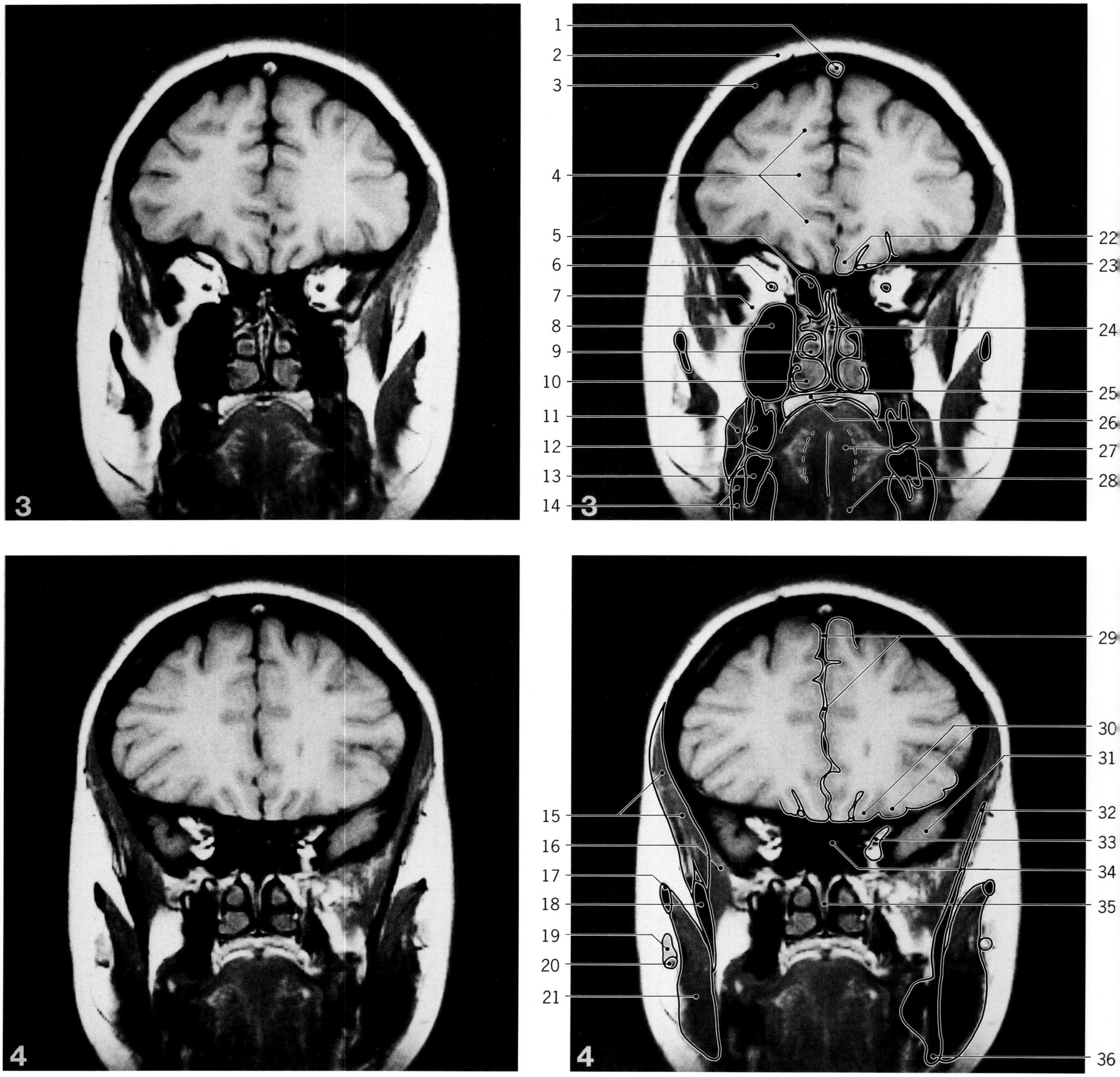

Brain, coronal MR

Scout view on page 170

1: Superior sagittal sinus
2: Scalp
3: Squamous part of frontal bone
4: Frontal lobe
5: Ethmoidal air cells
6: Optic nerve
7: Inferior orbital fissure
8: Maxillary sinus
9: Middle nasal concha
10: Inferior nasal concha
11: Buccinator
12: Third upper molar
13: Third lower molar
14: Alveolar part of mandible
15: Temporalis muscle
16: Lateral pterygoid muscle
17: Zygomatic arch
18: Coronoid process
19: Accessory parotid gland
20: Parotid duct
21: Masseter
22: Gyrus rectus
23: Olfactory tract
24: Nasal septum
25: Hard palate
26: Palatal glands and fat
27: Genioglossus
28: Geniohyoideus
29: Longitudinal fissure of cerebrum
30: Orbital gyri
31: Temporal lobe (pole)
32: Temporalis (tendon)
33: Superior orbital fissure
34: Sphenoidal sinus
35: Vomer
36: Ramus of mandible

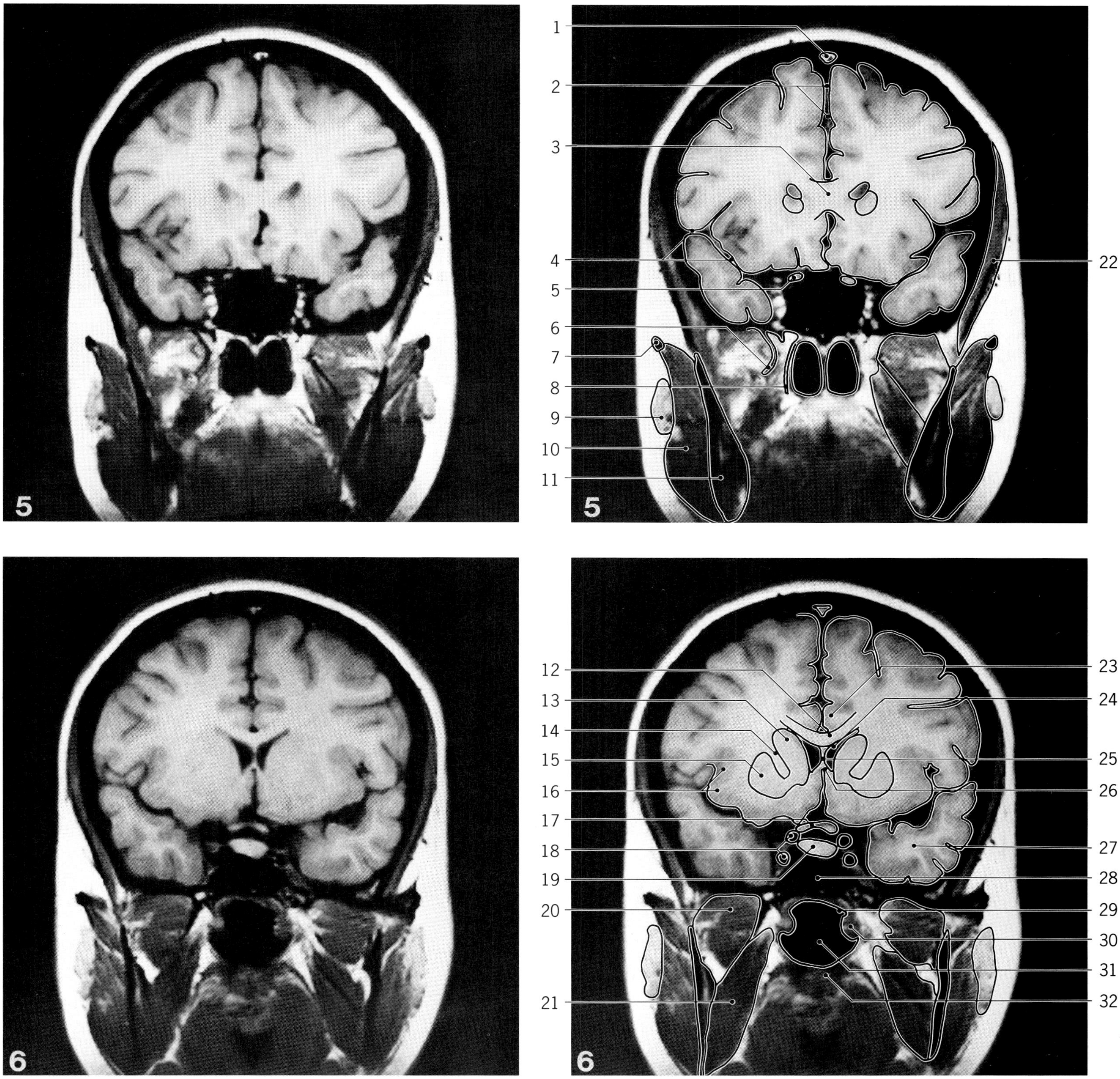

Brain, coronal MR

Scout view on page 170

1: Superior sagittal sinus
2: Longitudinal fissure of cerebrum
3: Genu of corpus callosum
4: Lateral sulcus (Sylvian)
5: Optic nerve
6: Lateral plate of pterygoid process
7: Zygomatic arch
8: Medial plate of pterygoid process
9: Parotid gland
10: Masseter
11: Ramus of mandible
12: Trunk of corpus callosum
13: Head of caudate nucleus
14: Internal capsule
15: Lentiform nucleus
16: Insula
17: Optic chiasm
18: Internal carotid artery ("Syphon")
19: Hypophysis
20: Lateral pterygoid muscle
21: Medial pterygoid muscle
22: Temporalis muscle
23: Cingulate gyrus
24: Lateral ventricle, frontal horn
25: Septum pellucidum
26: Rostrum of corpus callosum
27: Temporal lobe
28: Sphenoidal sinus
29: Lateral recess of pharynx
30: Torus levatorius
31: Nasal part of pharynx
32: Soft palate

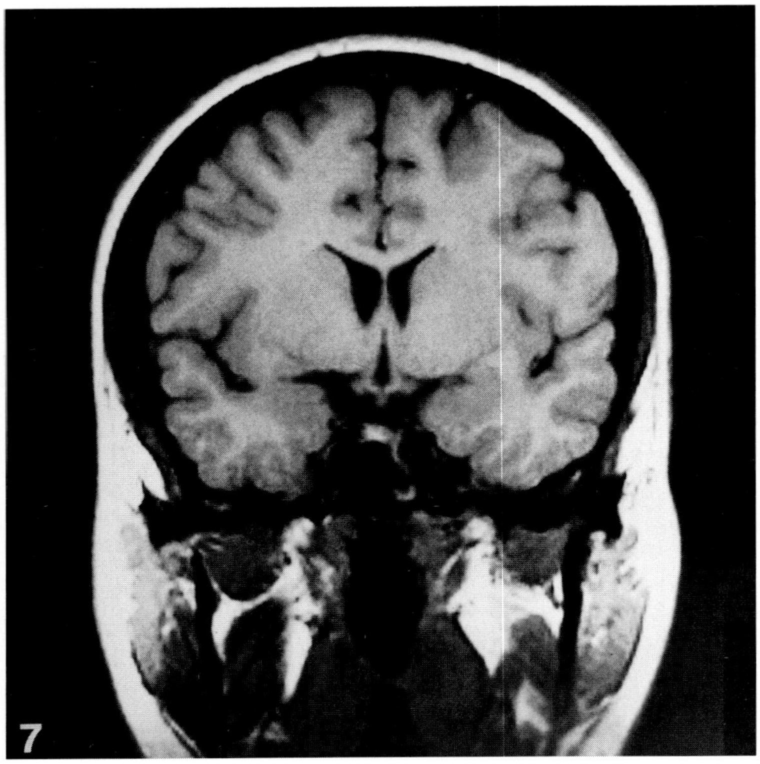

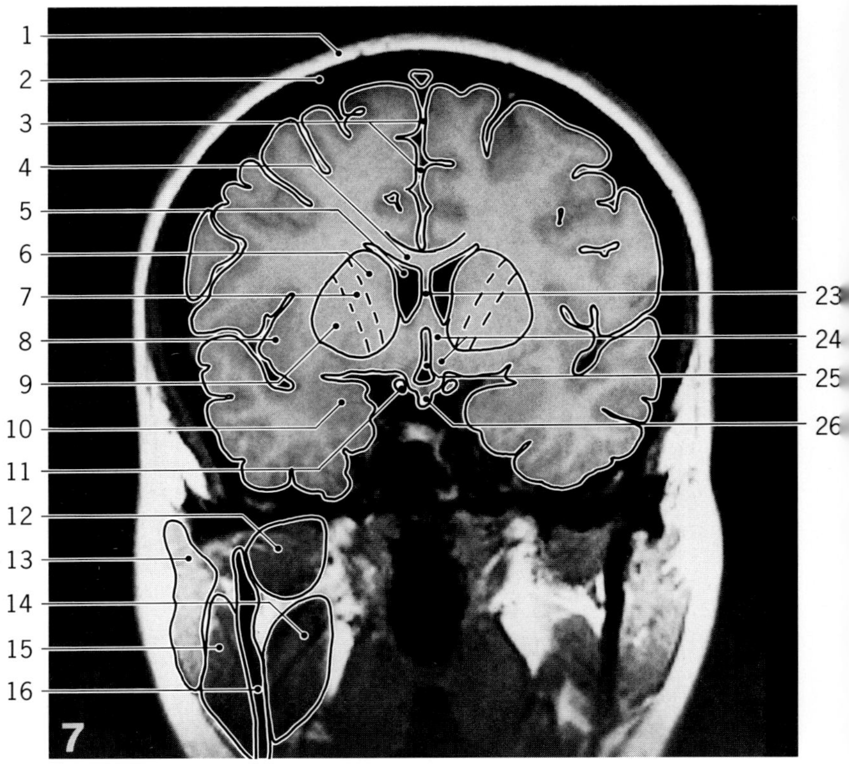

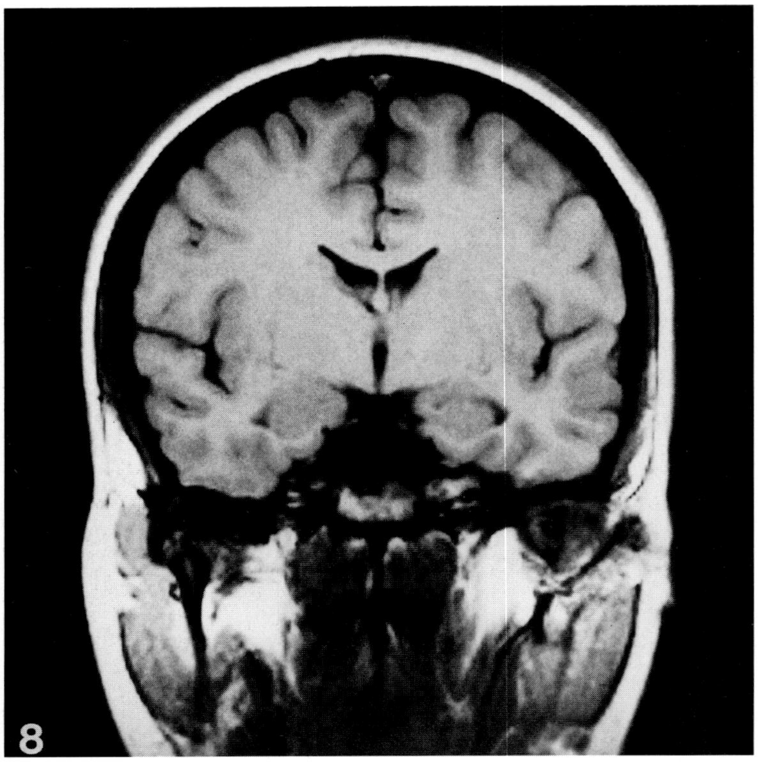

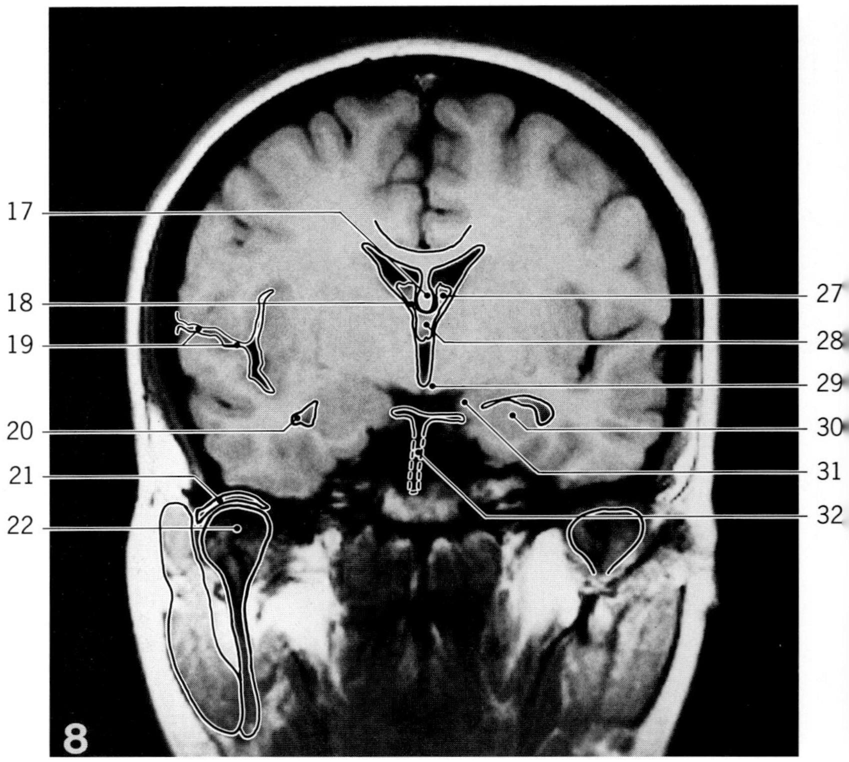

Brain, coronal MR

Scout view on page 170

1: Scalp
2: Calvaria
3: Longitudinal fissure of cerebrum
4: Trunk of corpus callosum
5: Lateral ventricle, central part
6: Body of caudate nucleus
7: Internal capsule
8: Insula
9: Lentiform nucleus
10: Amygdaloid nucleus
11: Optic tract
12: Lateral pterygoid muscle
13: Parotid gland
14: Medial pterygoid muscle
15: Masseter
16: Ramus of mandible
17: Body of fornix
18: Interventricular foramen with choroid plexus
19: Lateral sulcus (Sylvian)
20: Lateral ventricle, temporal horn
21: Articular disc in temporomandibular joint
22: Head of mandible
23: Septum pellucidum
24: Hypothalamus
25: Third ventricle
26: Infundibulum
27: Choroid plexus in lateral ventricle
28: Choroid plexus in third ventricle
29: Mammillary body
30: Hippocampus
31: Uncus of temporal lobe
32: Basilar artery

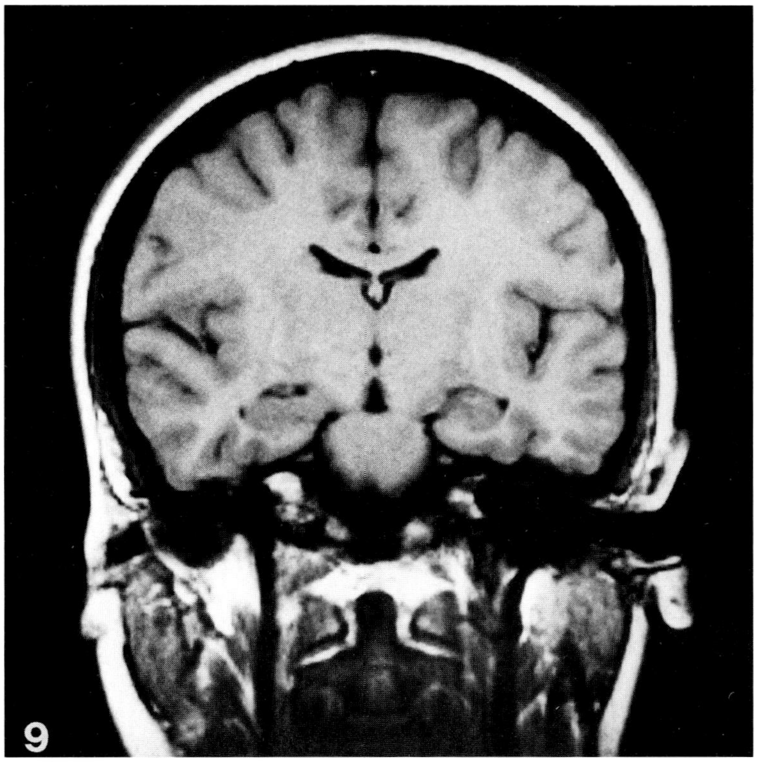

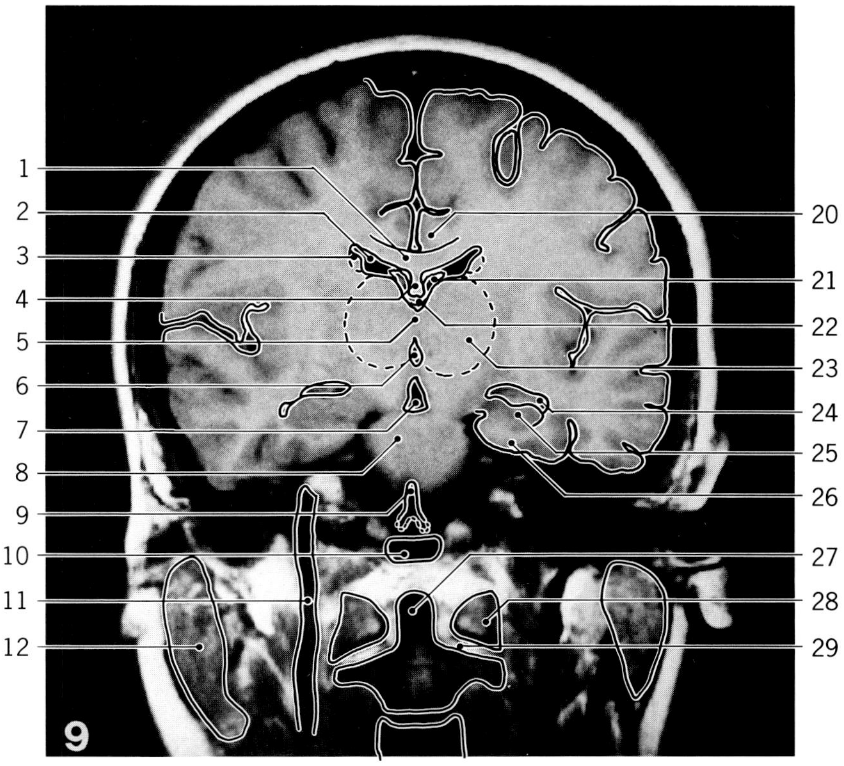

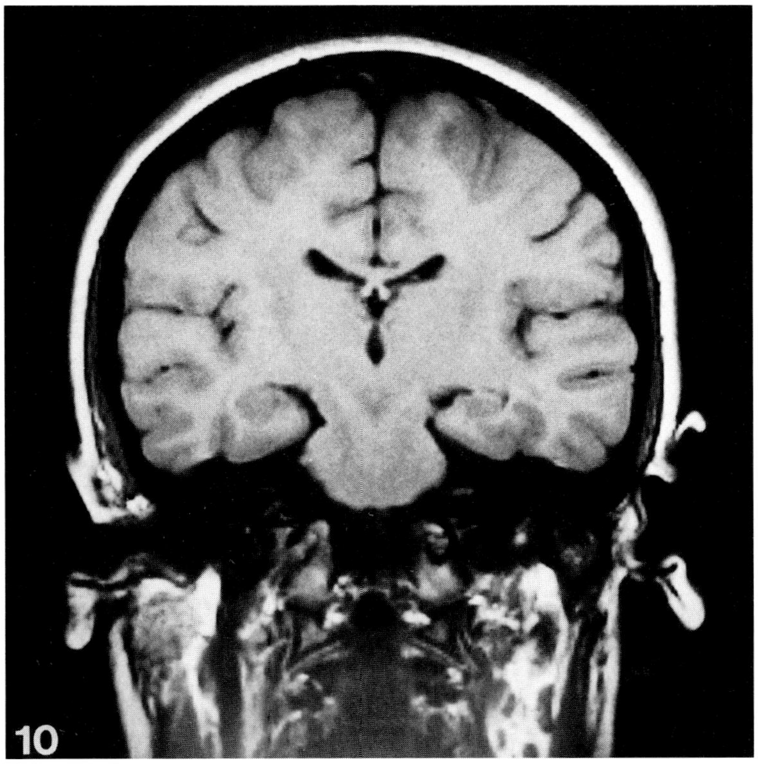

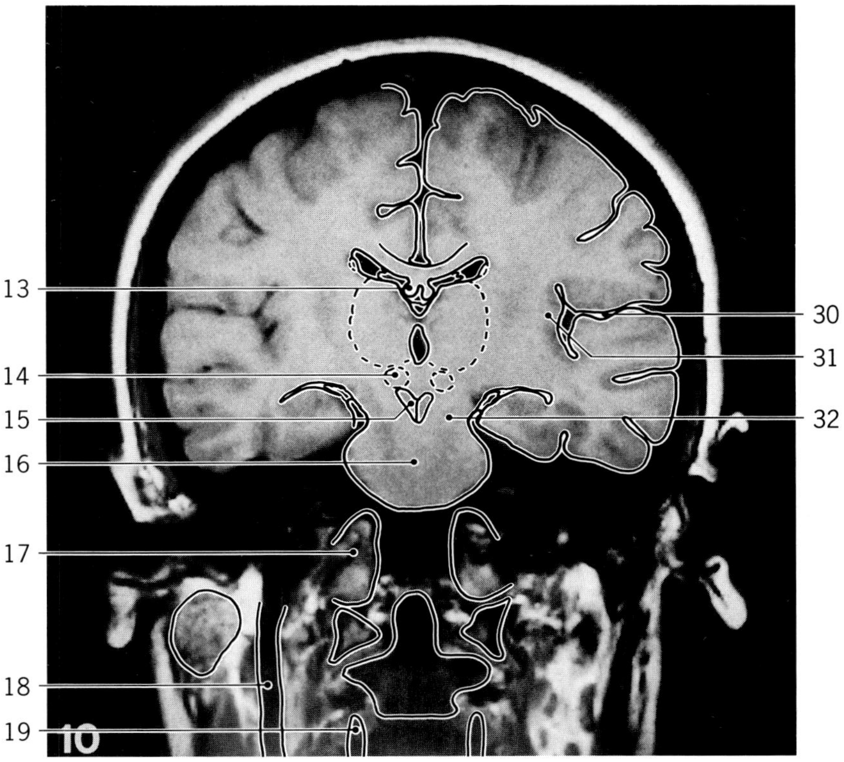

Brain, coronal MR

Scout view on page 170

1: Trunk of corpus callosum
2: Lateral ventricle, central part
3: Caudate nucleus
4: Body of fornix
5: Interthalamic adhesion
6: Third ventricle
7: Interpeduncular cistern
8: Pons
9: Basilar artery
10: Clivus (edge)
11: Internal carotid artery
12: Parotid gland
13: Crus of fornix
14: Nucleus ruber
15: Substantia nigra
16: Pons
17: Occipital condyle
18: Internal jugular vein
19: Vertebral artery
20: Cingulate gyrus
21: Choroid plexus in lateral ventricle
22: Choroid plexus in third ventricle
23: Thalamus
24: Lateral ventricle, temporal horn
25: Hippocampus
26: Parahippocampal gyrus
27: Dens axis
28: Lateral mass of atlas
29: Lateral atlanto-axial joint
30: Lateral sulcus (Sylvian)
31: Insula
32: Cerebral peduncle

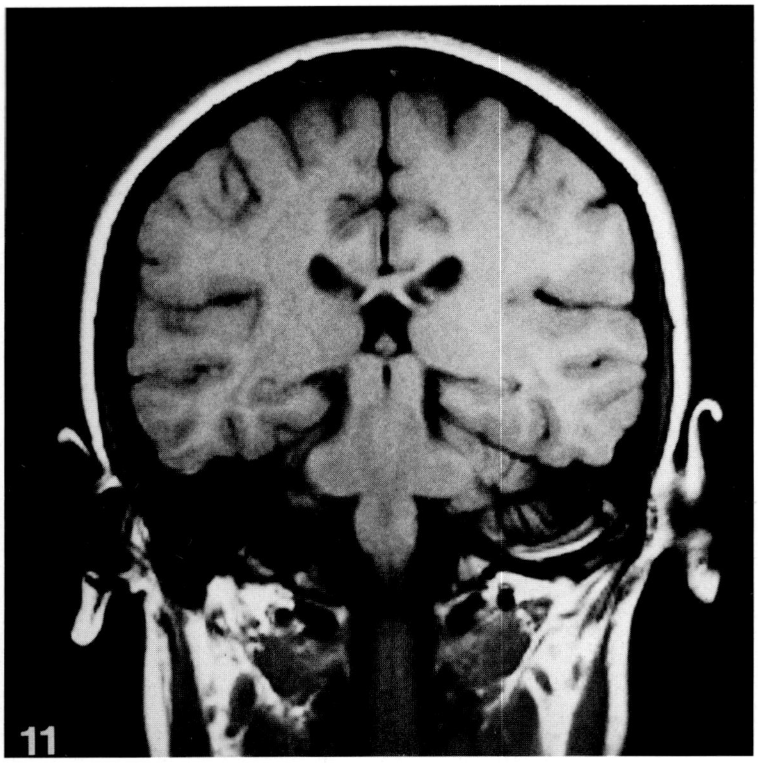

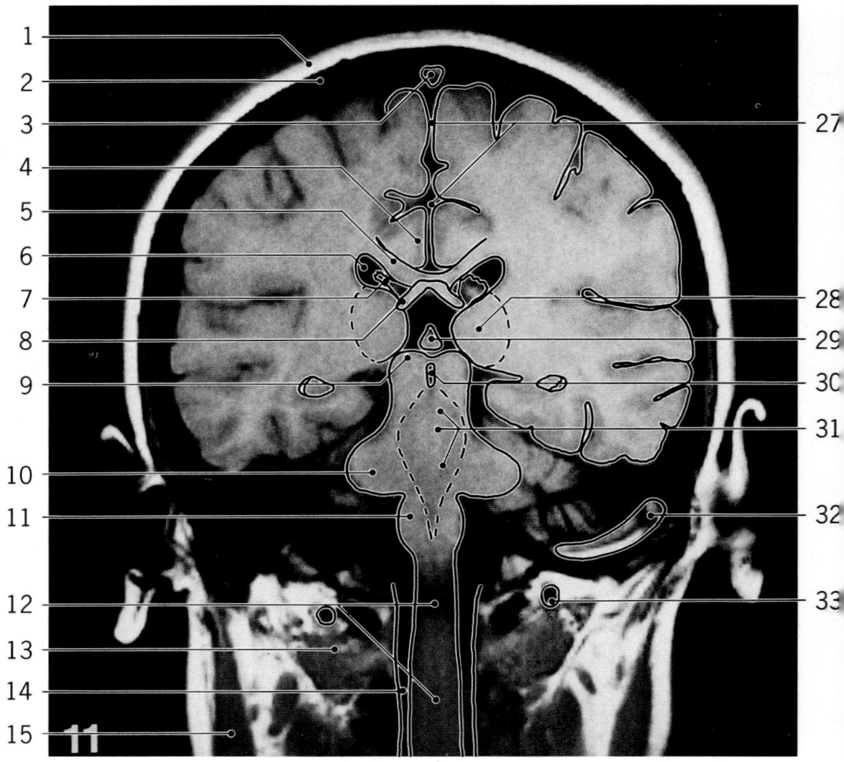

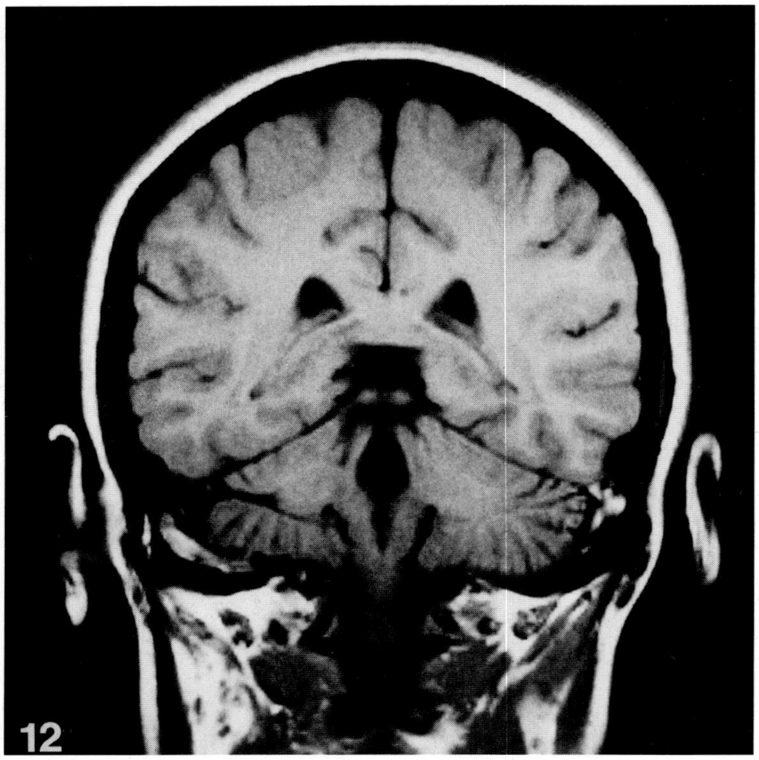

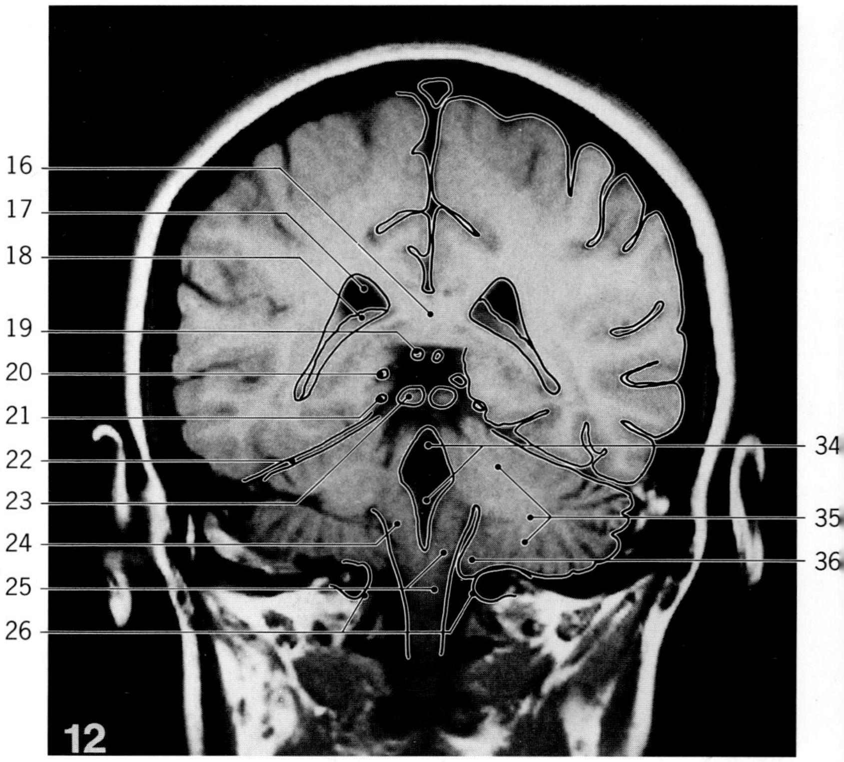

Brain, coronal MR

Scout view on page 170

1: Scalp
2: Calvaria
3: Superior sagittal sinus
4: Cingulate gyrus
5: Trunk of corpus callosum
6: Lateral ventricle
7: Choroid plexus
8: Crus of fornix
9: Superior colliculus
10: Middle cerebellar peduncle
11: Olive
12: Spinal cord
13: Obliquus capitis inferior
14: Subarachnoid space
15: Sternocleidomastoid
16: Splenium of corpus callosum
17: Lateral ventricle
18: Choroid plexus
19: Internal cerebral vein
20: Posterior cerebral artery
21: Superior cerebellar artery
22: Tentorium cerebelli
23: Inferior colliculus
24: Inferior cerebellar peduncle
25: Medulla oblongata
26: Foramen magnum
27: Longitudinal fissure
28: Thalamus
29: Pineal gland
30: Cerebral aqueduct
31: Cranial nerve nuclei
32: Sigmoid sinus
33: Vertebral artery
34: Rhomboid fossa
35: Cerebellum
36: Cerebellar tonsil

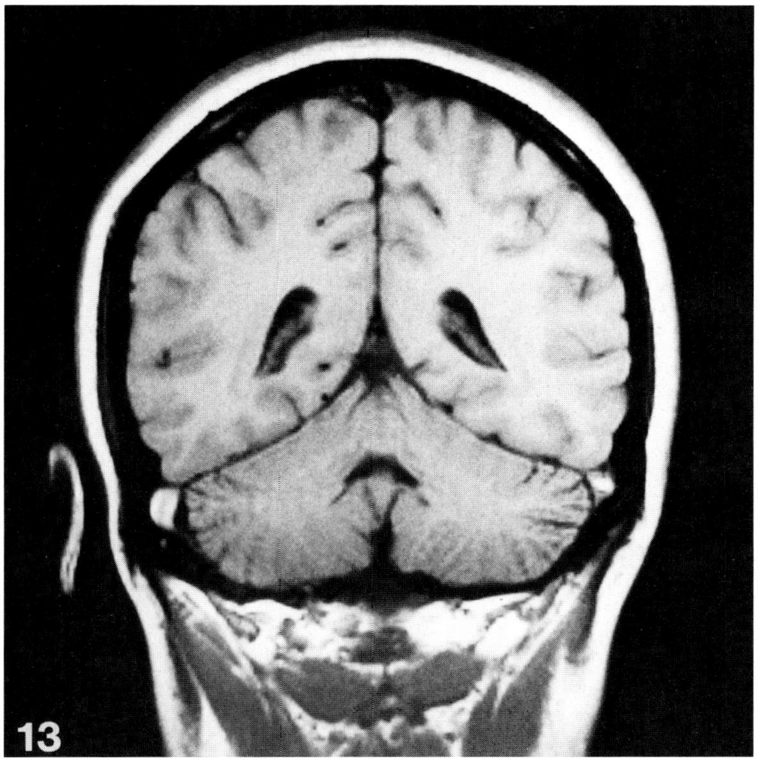

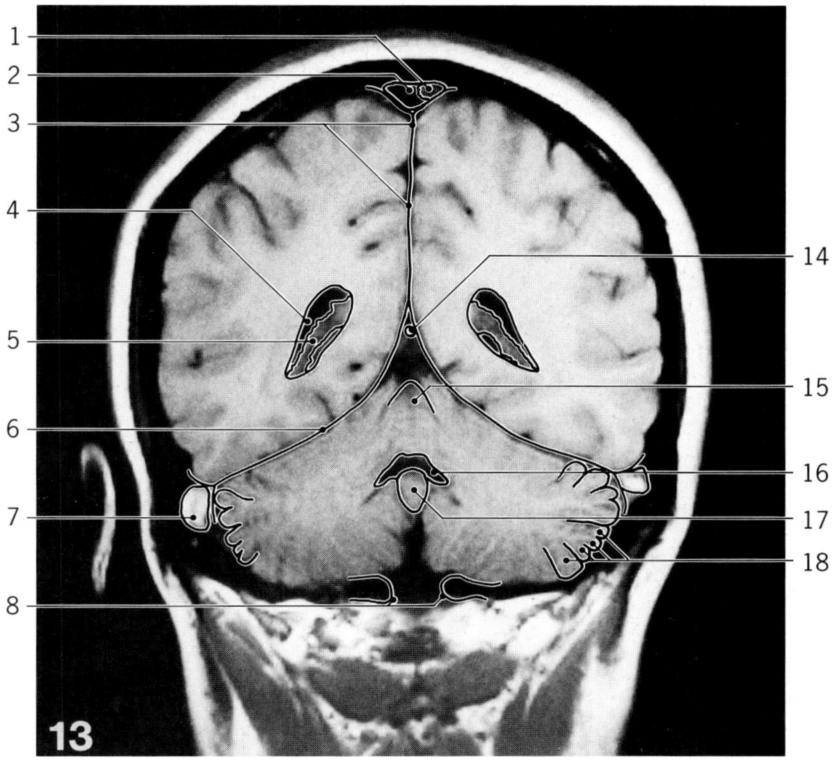

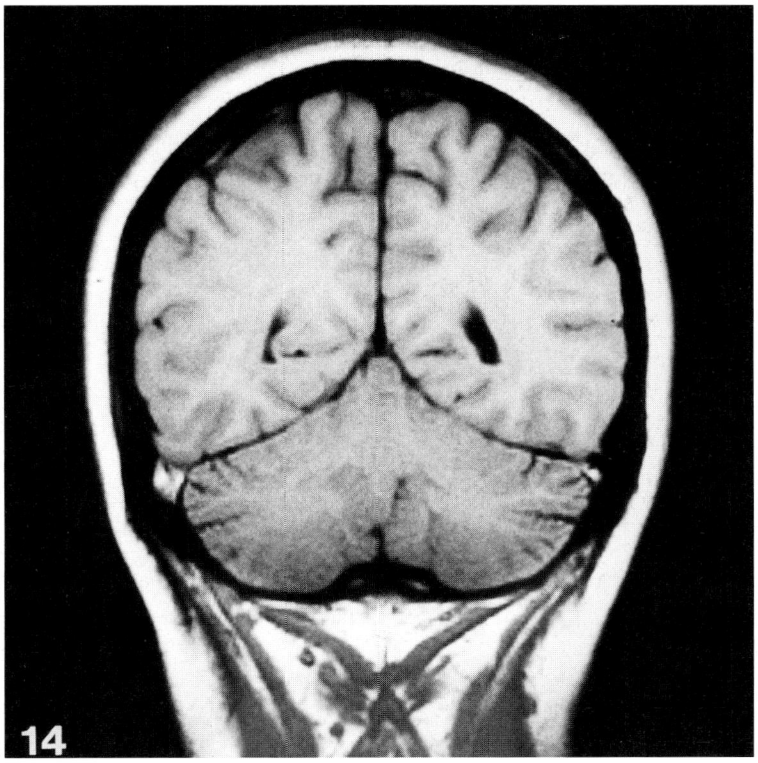

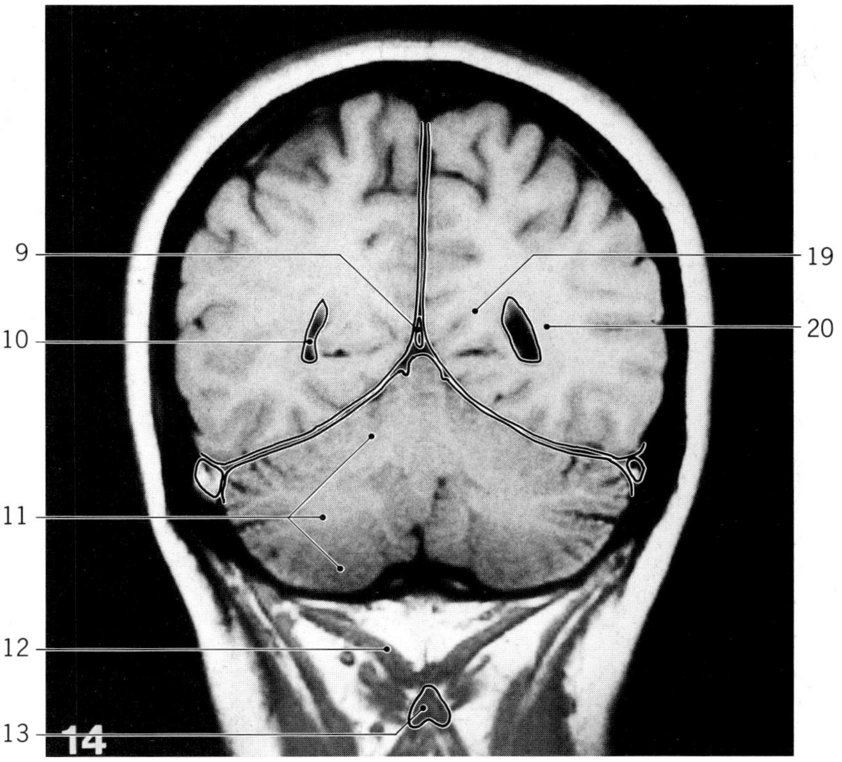

Brain, coronal MR

Scout view on page 170

1: Arachnoid villi
2: Superior sagittal sinus
3: Falx cerebri
4: Lateral ventricle
5: Choroid plexus
6: Tentorium cerebelli
7: Sigmoid sinus
8: Foramen magnum
9: Straight sinus
10: Lateral ventricle, occipital horn
11: Cerebellum (hemisphere)
12: Rectus capitis posterior major
13: Spinous process of axis
14: Great cerebral vein (Galen)
15: Vermis of cerebellum
16: Fourth ventricle
17: Nodule of vermis
18: Foliae of cerebellum
19: Posterior radiation of corpus callosum (forceps occipitalis major)
20: Optic radiation

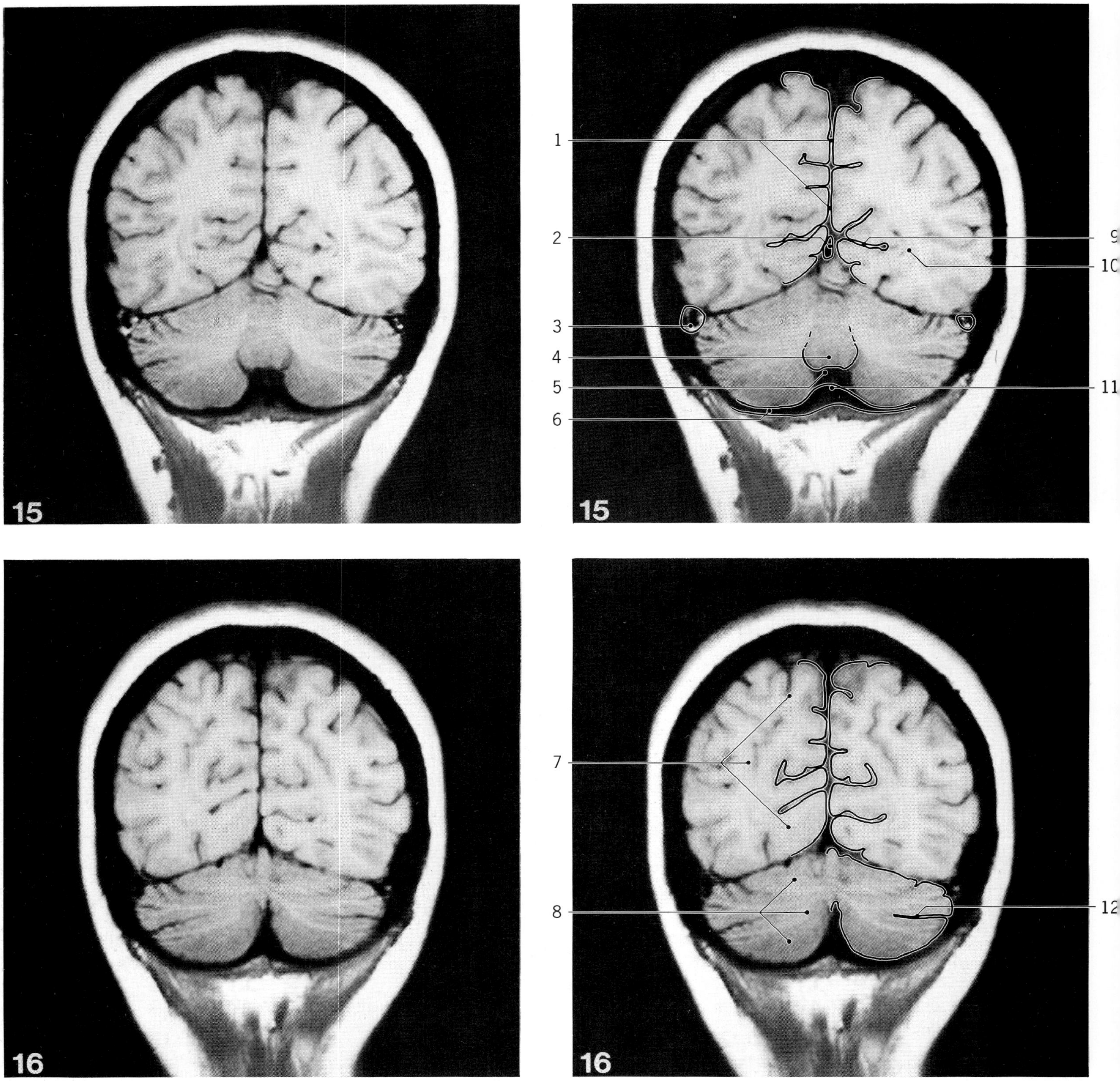

Brain, coronal MR

Scout view on page 170

1: Longitudinal fissure
2: Straight sinus
3: Sigmoid sinus
4: Pyramis vermis
5: Cerebello-medullary cistern
6: Squamous part of occipital bone
7: Occipital lobe
8: Cerebellum (hemisphere)
9: Calcarine sulcus
10: Optic radiation
11: Internal occipital crest
12: Horizontal fissure of cerebellum

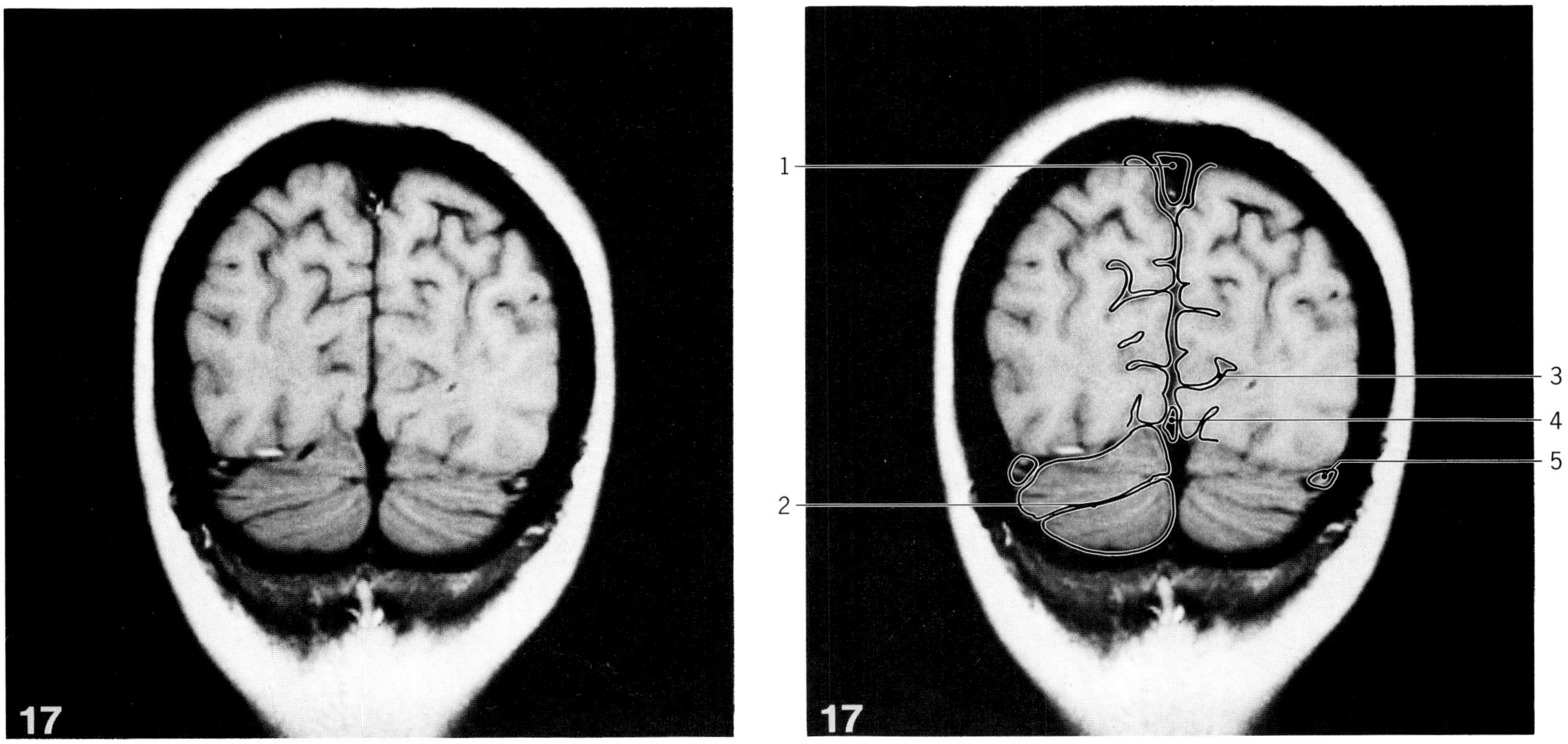

Brain, coronal MR

Scout view on page 170

1: Superior sagittal sinus
2: Horizontal fissure of cerebellum
3: Calcarine sulcus
4: Straight sinus
5: Transverse sinus

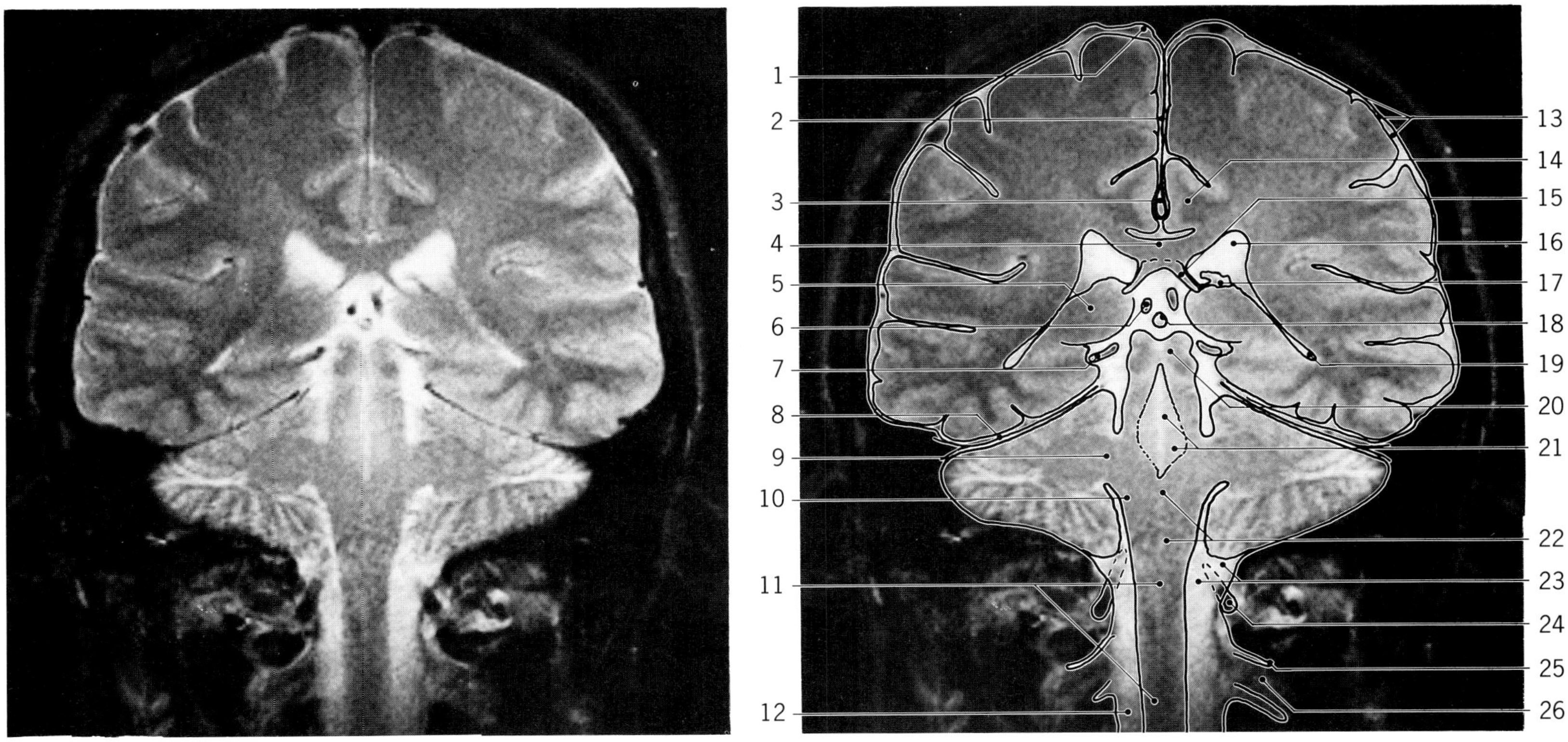

Brain, coronal MR. T_2–weighted image (compare section #12, page 176)

1: Arachnoid granulations in superior sagittal sinus
2: Falx cerebri
3: Inferior sagittal sinus
4: Splenium of corpus callosum
5: Thalamus (pulvinar)
6: Internal cerebral vein
7: Posterior cerebral artery
8: Tentorium cerebelli
9: Middle cerebellar peduncle
10: Inferior cerebellar peduncle
11: Spinal cord
12: Subarachnoid space
13: Subarachnoid space
14: Cingulate gyrus
15: Crus of the fornix
16: Lateral ventricle, central part
17: Choroid plexus
18: Pineal gland
19: Lateral ventricle, temporal horn
20: Tectum mesencephali (quadrigeminal plate)
21: Fourth ventricle
22: Medulla oblongata
23: Cerebello-medullary cistern
24: Vertebral artery
25: Root pouch of second cervical spinal nerve
26: Second cervical spinal nerve

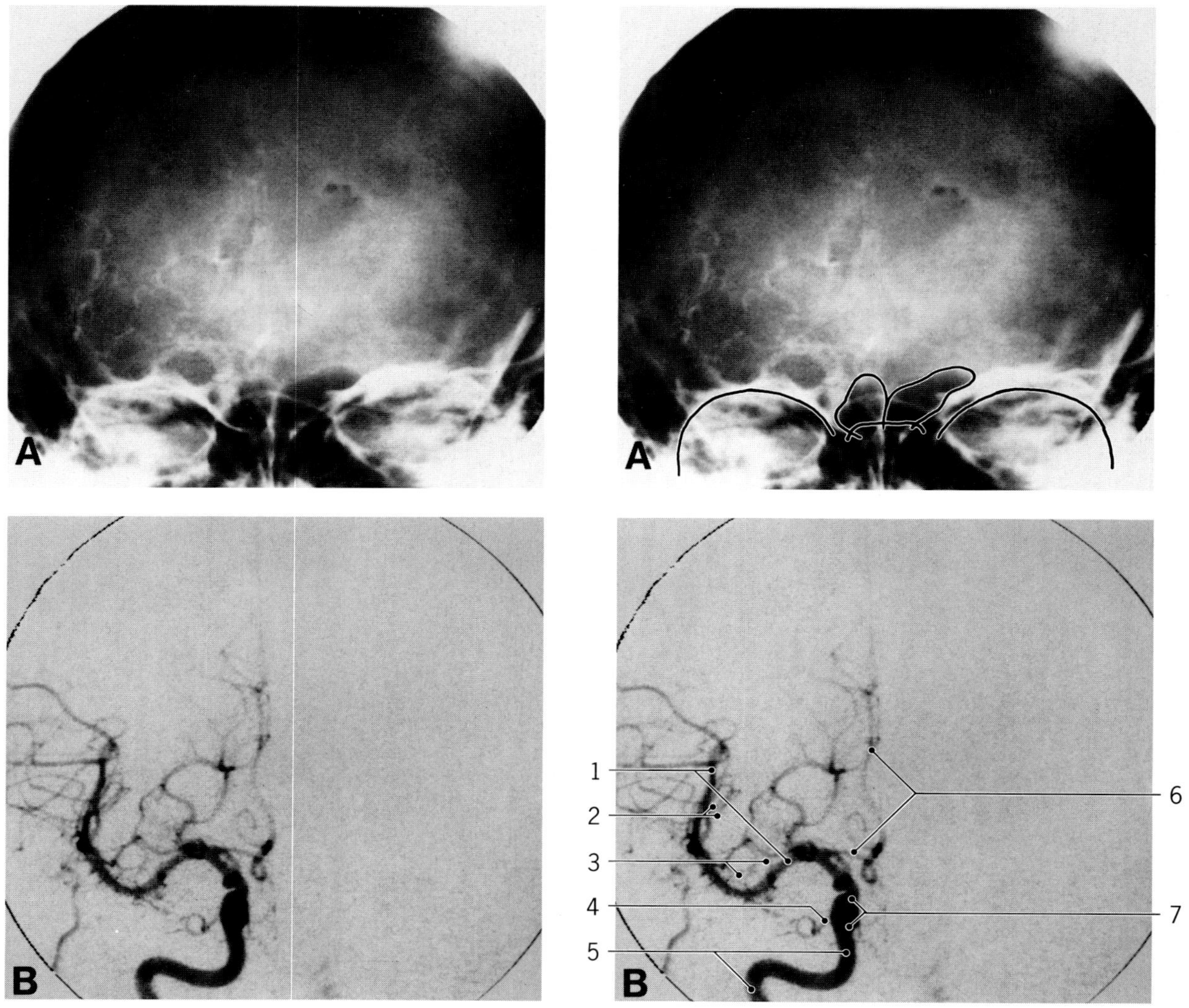

Internal carotid artery, a-p X-ray, arteriography

A: Unprocessed X-ray, B: After digital subtraction

1: Middle cerebral artery
2: Insular arteries
3: Lateral thalamostriate arteries
4: Ophthalmic artery
5: Internal carotid artery in carotid canal
6: Anterior cerebral artery
7: Carotid "syphon"

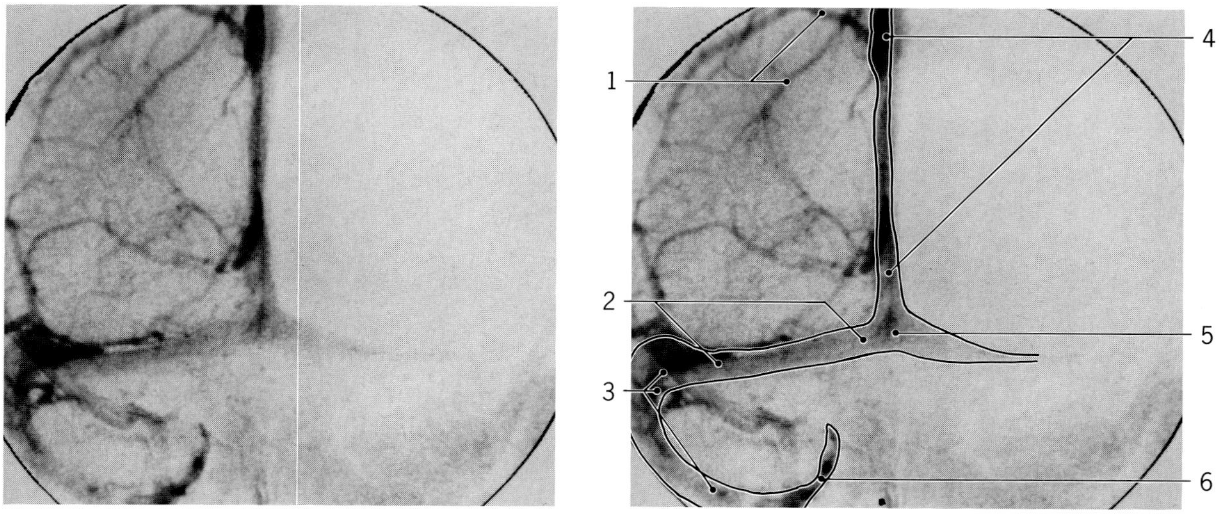

Cerebral veins, a-p X-ray, venous phase of arteriography (Digital subtraction)

1: Superior cerebral veins
2: Transverse sinus
3: Sigmoid sinus
4: Superior sagittal sinus
5: Confluens of sinuses
6: Inferior petrous sinus

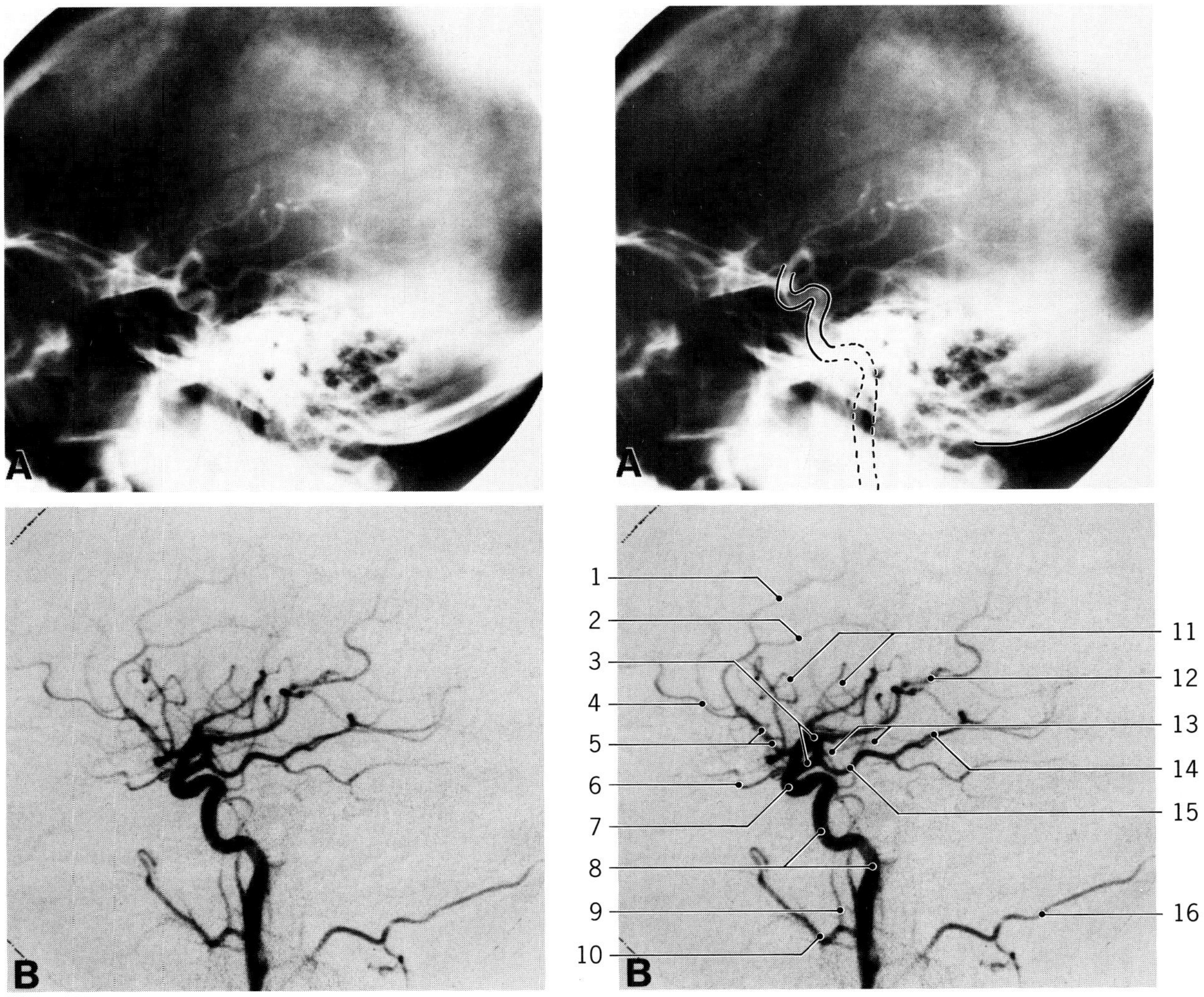

Internal carotid artery, lateral X-ray, arteriography A: Unprocessed X-ray, B: After digital subtraction

1: Callosomarginal artery
2: Pericallosal artery
3: Middle cerebral artery
4: Frontopolar artery
5: Anterior cerebral artery
6: Ophthalmic artery
7: Carotid "syphon"
8: Internal carotid artery in carotid canal
9: Middle meningeal artery
10: Maxillary artery
11: Insular arteries
12: Middle cerebral artery, parietal branches
13: Anterior choroid artery
14: Posterior cerebral artery
15: Posterior communicating artery
16: Occipital artery

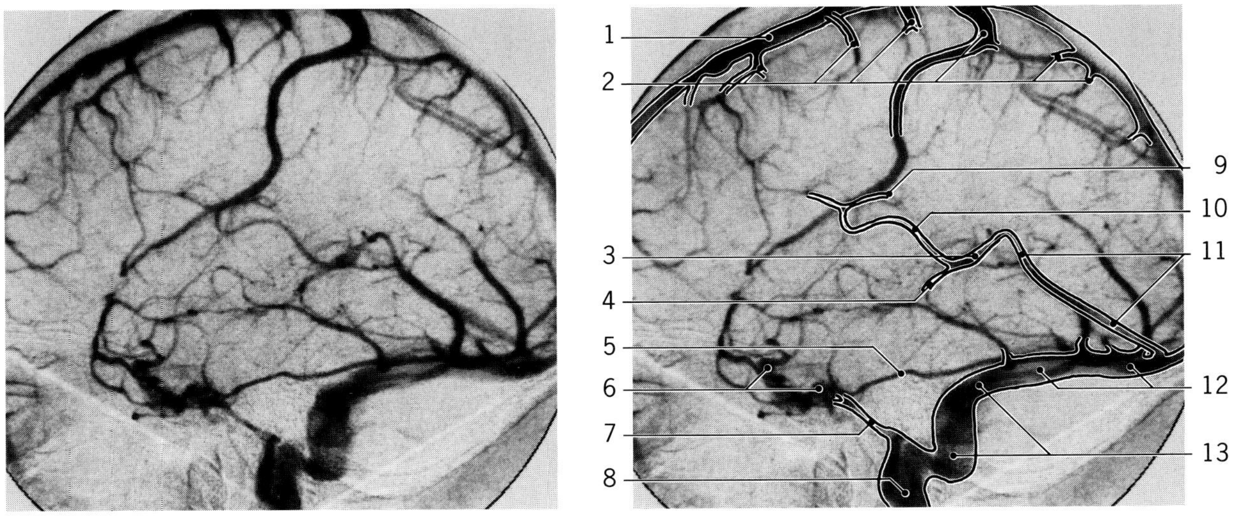

Cerebral veins, lateral X-ray, venous phase of arteriography (Digital subtraction)

1: Superior sagittal sinus
2: Superior cerebral veins
3: Great cerebral vein (Galen)
4: Basal vein (Rosenthal)
5: Superior petrous sinus
6: Cavernous sinus
7: Inferior petrous sinus
8: Bulb of internal jugular vein
9: Thalamostriate vein
10: Internal cerebral vein
11: Straight sinus
12: Transverse sinus
13: Sigmoid sinus

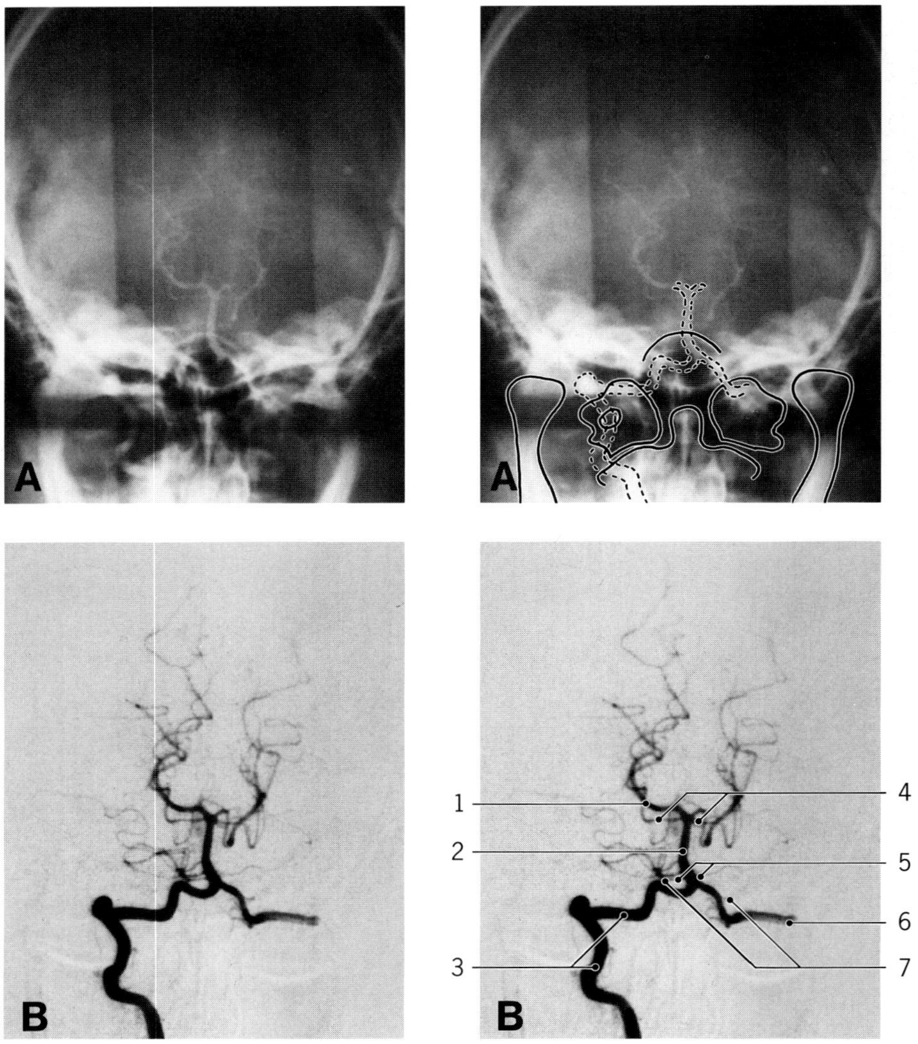

Vertebral artery, a-p X-ray, arteriography

A: Unprocessed X-ray, B: After digital subtraction

1: Posterior cerebral artery
2: Basilar artery
3: Vertebral artery
4: Superior cerebellar arteries
5: Anterior inferior cerebellar arteries ("AICA")
6: Overflow in contralateral vertebral artery
7: Posterior inferior cerebellar arteries ("PICA")

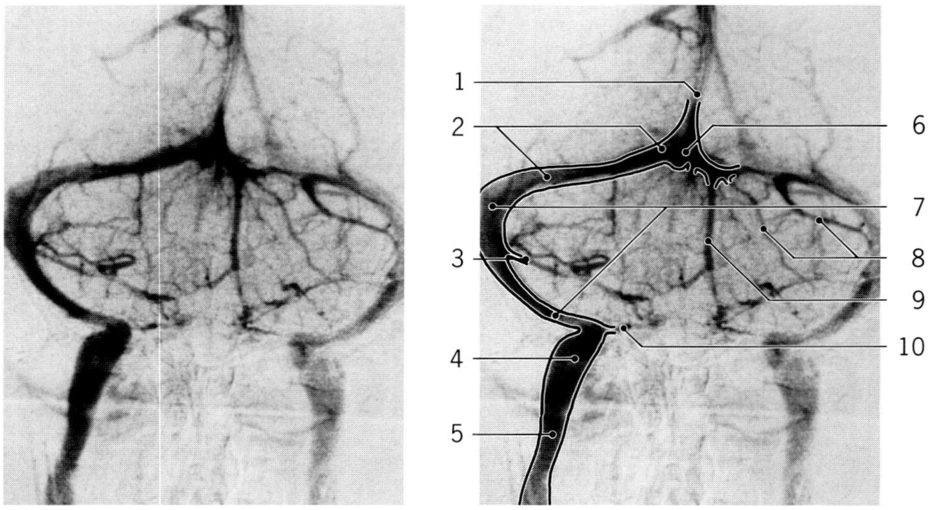

Cerebral veins, a-p X-ray, venous phase of arteriography (Digital subtraction)

1: Superior sagittal sinus
2: Transverse sinus
3: Superior petrous sinus
4: Bulb of internal jugular vein
5: Internal jugular vein
6: Confluence of sinuses
7: Sigmoid sinus
8: Inferior veins of cerebellar hemisphere
9: Inferior vermis vein
10: Inferior petrous sinus

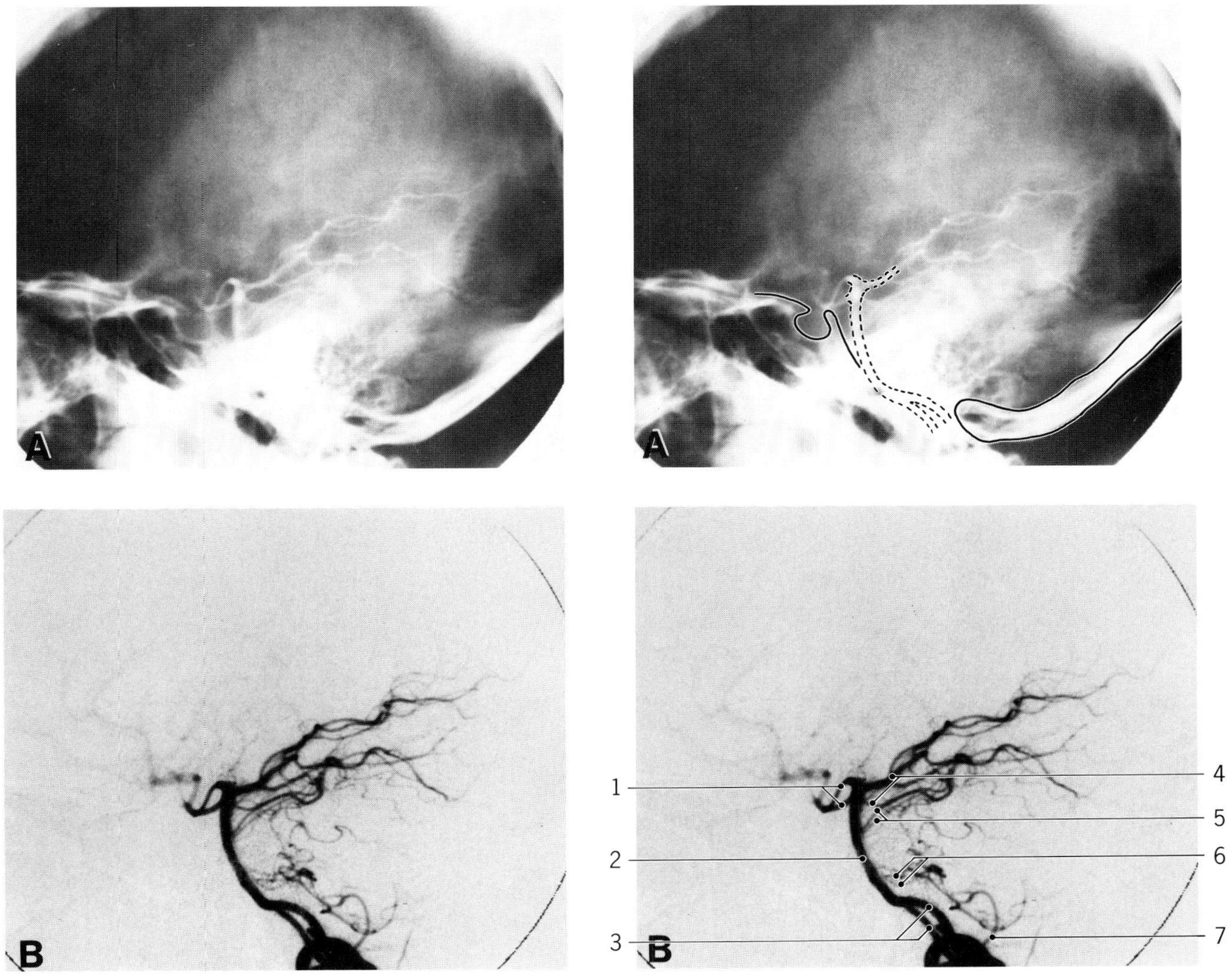

Vertebral artery, lateral X-ray, arteriography

A: Unprocessed X-ray, B: After digital subtraction

1: Posterior communicating arteries
2: Basilar artery
3: Vertebral arteries
4: Posterior cerebral arteries
5: Superior cerebellar arteries
6: Anterior inferior cerebellar arteries ("AICA")
7: Posterior inferior cerebellar artery ("PICA")

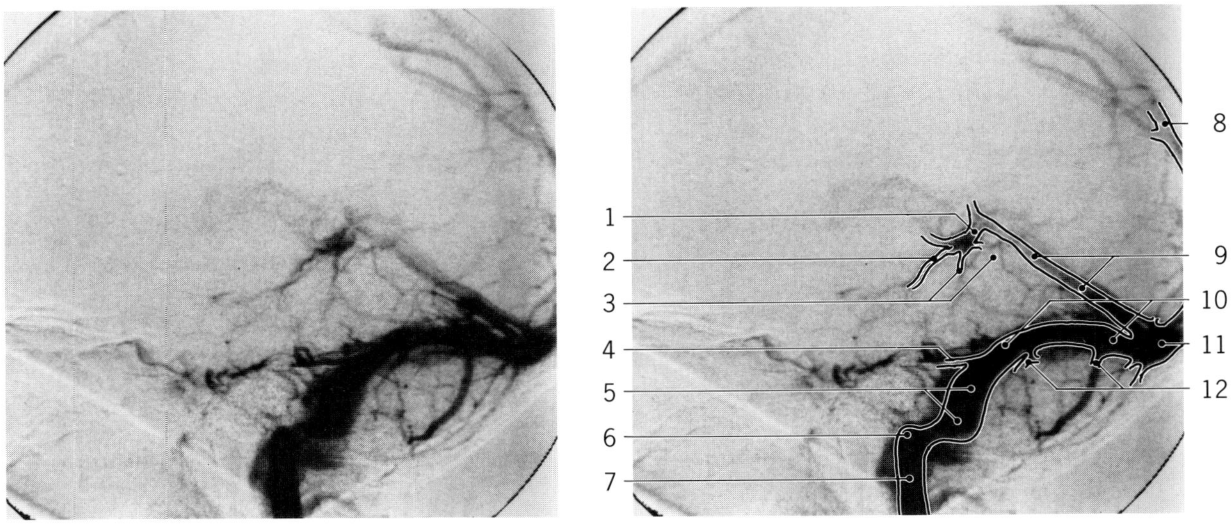

Cerebral veins, lateral X-ray, venous phase of arteriography (Digital subtraction)

1: Great cerebral vein
2: Basal vein (Rosenthal)
3: Superior cerebellar veins
4: Superior petrous sinus
5: Sigmoid sinus
6: Bulb of the internal jugular vein
7: Internal jugular vein
8: Superior sagittal sinus
9: Straight sinus
10: Transverse sinus
11: Confluence of sinuses
12: Inferior cerebellar veins

NECK

Larynx

Pharynx

Neck, axial CT-series

Thyroid gland

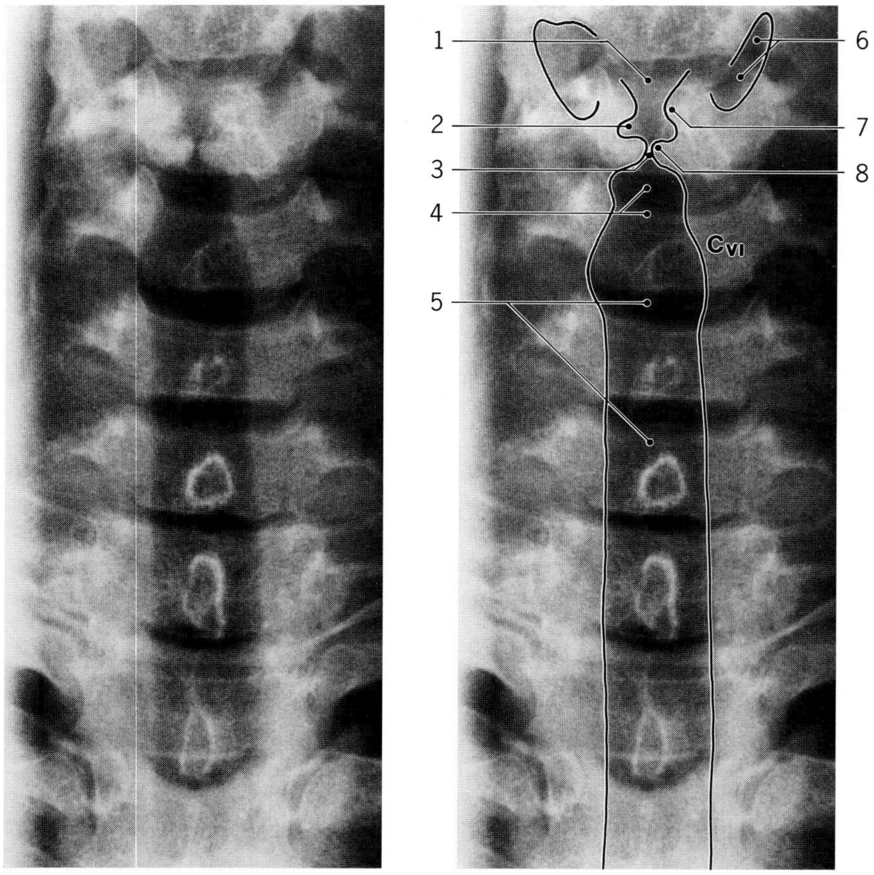

Larynx, a-p X-ray

1: Vestibule of larynx
2: Sinus (ventricle) of the larynx
3: Rima glottidis
4: Infraglottic cavity
5: Trachea
6: Piriform fossa
7: Vestibular fold
8: Vocal fold

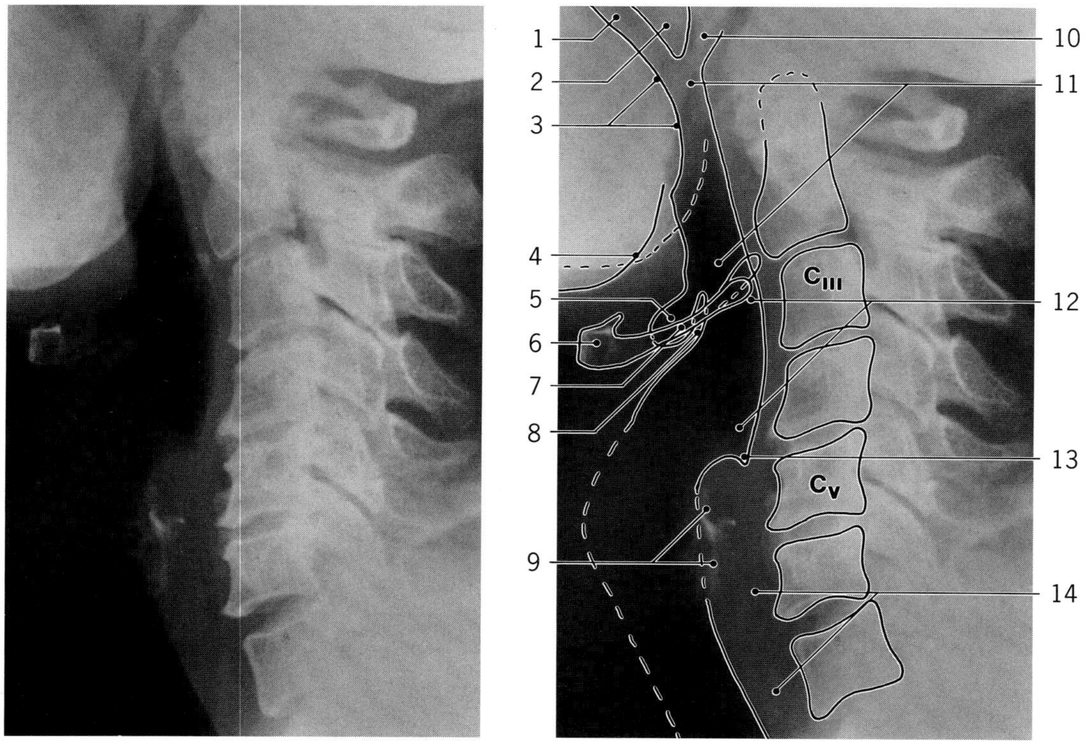

Larynx, lateral X-ray

1: Oral cavity
2: Uvula
3: Root of tongue
4: Angle of mandible
5: Vallecula
6: Body of hyoid bone
7: Greater cornu of hyoid bone
8: Epiglottis
9: Lamina of cricoid cartilage (calcified)
10: Nasal part of pharynx
11: Oral part of pharynx
12: Laryngeal part of pharynx
13: Entrance to oesophagus
14: Oesophagus

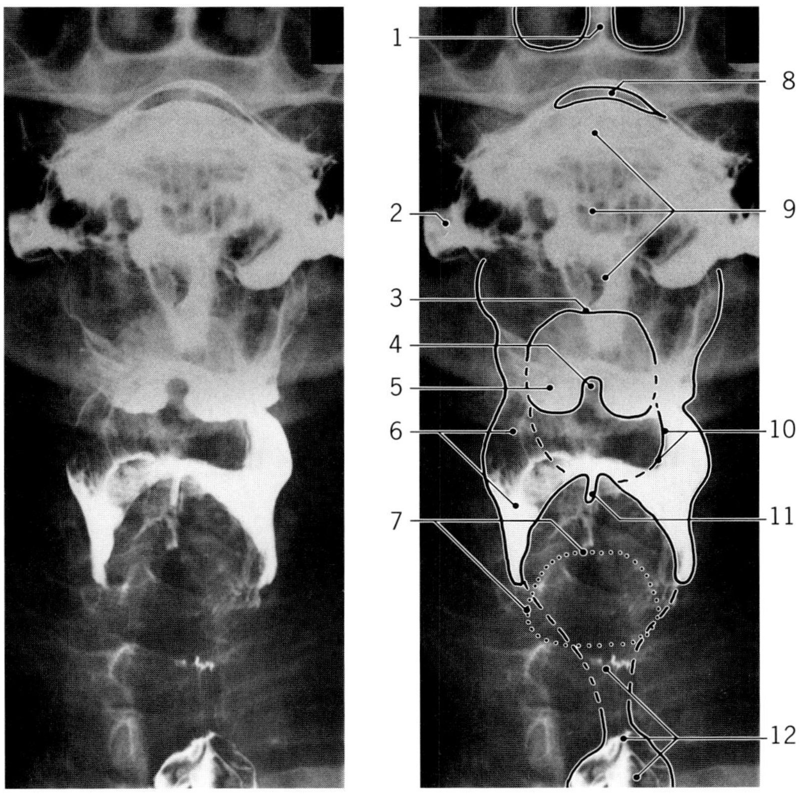

Pharynx, a-p X-ray, barium swallow

1: Nasal septum
2: Vestibule of the mouth
3: Epiglottis
4: Median glosso-epiglottic fold
5: Vallecula
6: Piriform fossa
7: Contour of lamina of cricoid cartilage
8: Air between tongue and palate
9: Barium in mouth and pharynx
10: Ary-epiglottic fold
11: Interarytenoid notch
12: Oesophagus

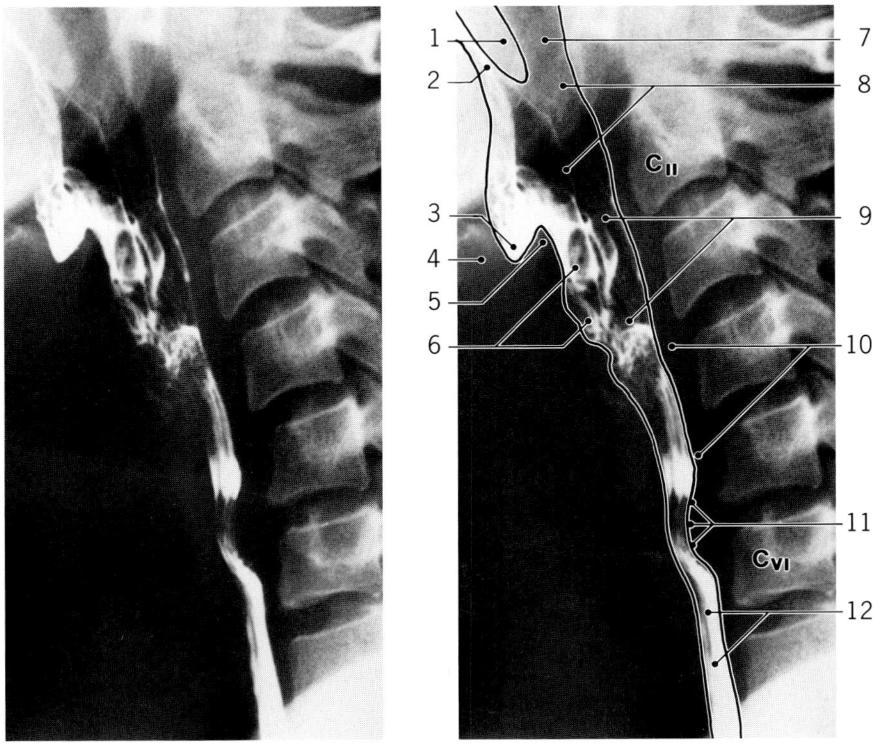

Pharynx, lateral X-ray, barium swallow

1: Uvula
2: Oral cavity
3: Vallecula
4: Hyoid bone
5: Epiglottis
6: Piriform fossa
7: Nasal part of pharynx (nasopharynx)
8: Oral part of pharynx (oropharynx)
9: Laryngeal part of pharynx (laryngopharynx)
10: Retropharyngeal space
11: Impression of cricopharyngeus muscle
12: Oesophagus

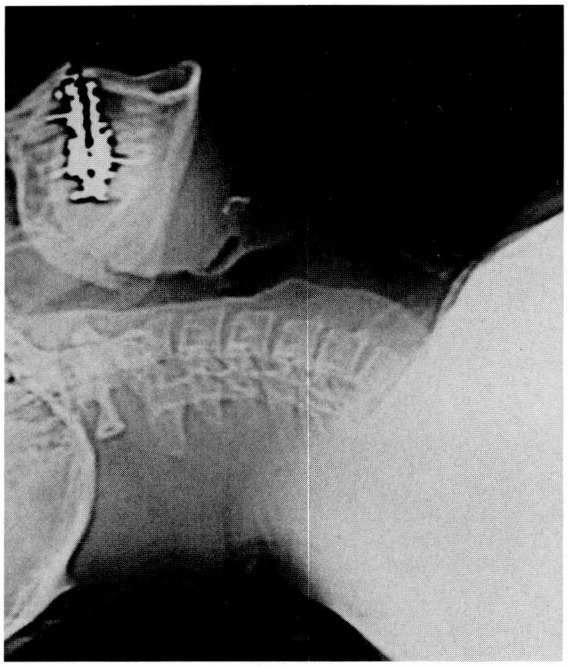

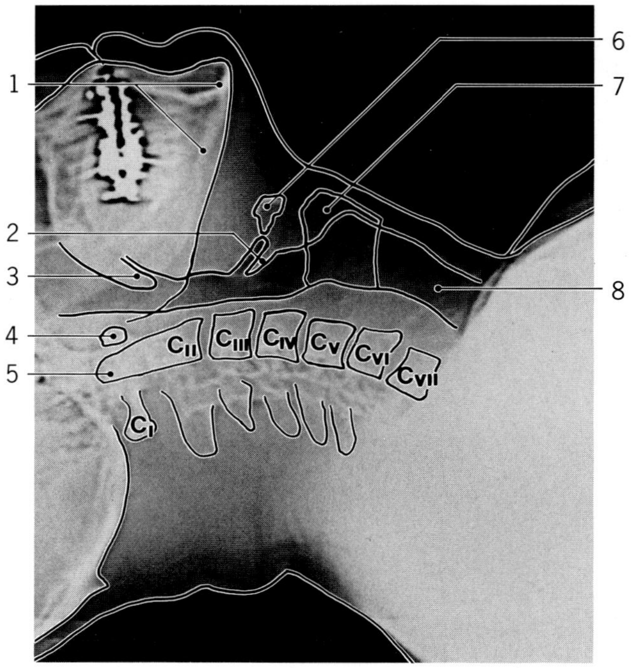

Scout view

1: Mandible
2: Epiglottis
3: Uvula
4: Anterior arch of atlas
5: Dens axis
6: Hyoid bone
7: Thyroid cartilage
8: Trachea

Scout view

Lines #1-15 indicate positions of sections in the following CT-series.

Consecutive sections, 10 mm thick

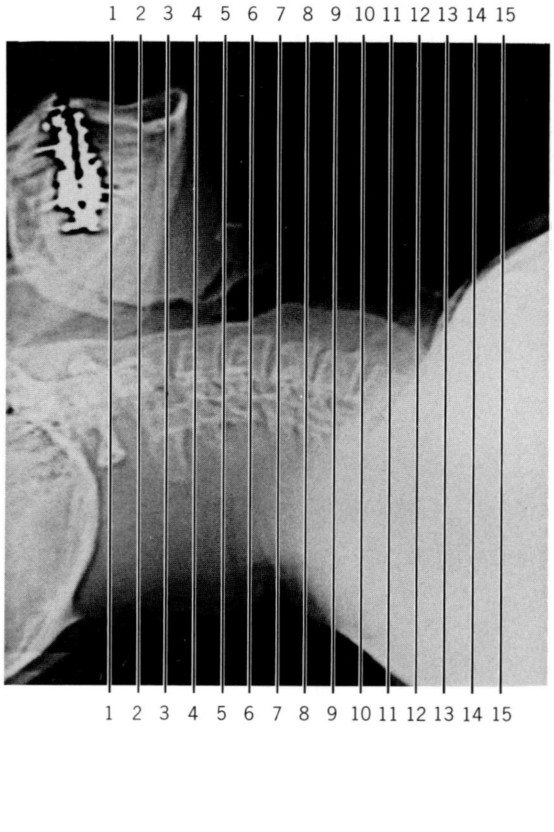

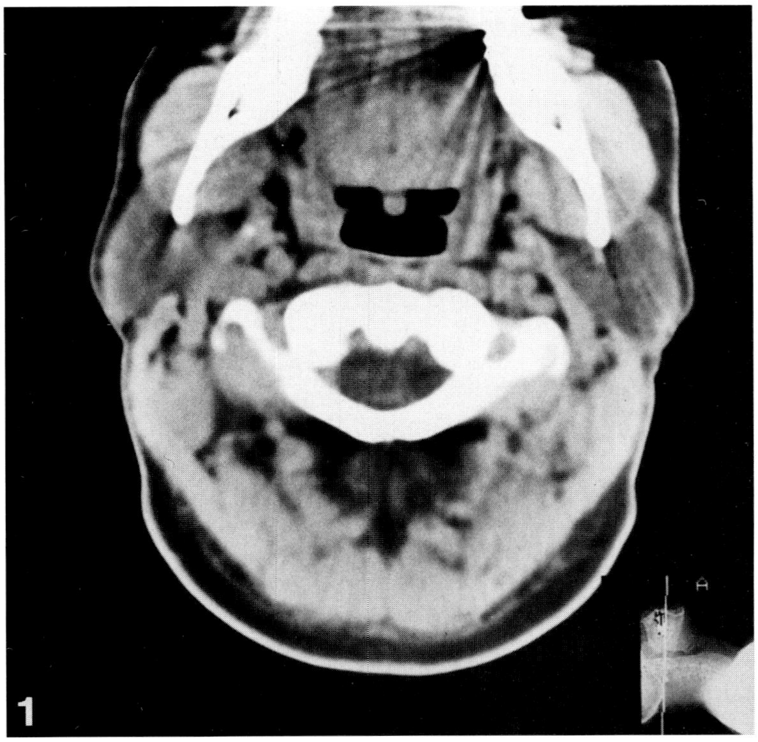

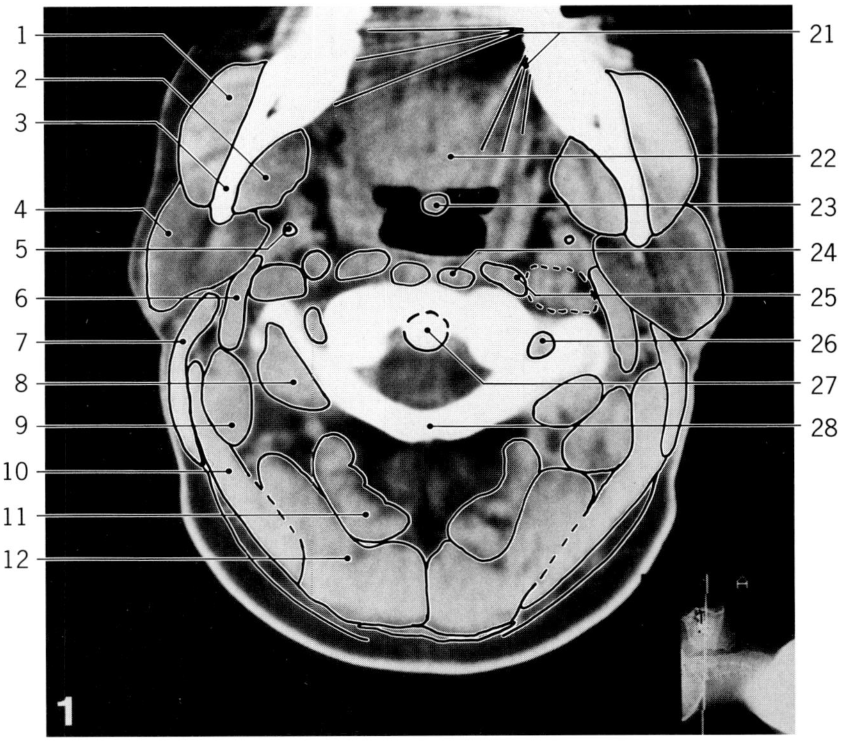

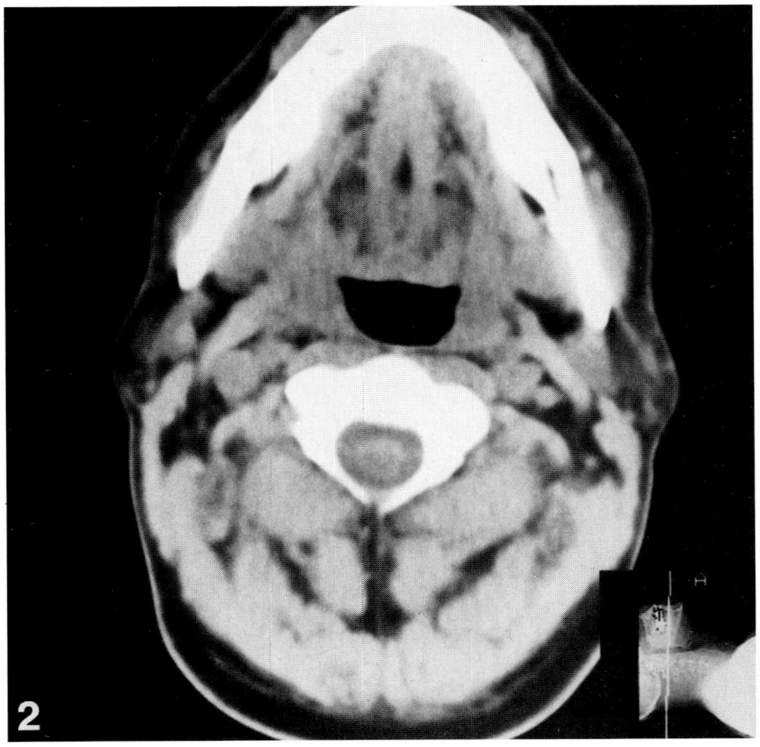

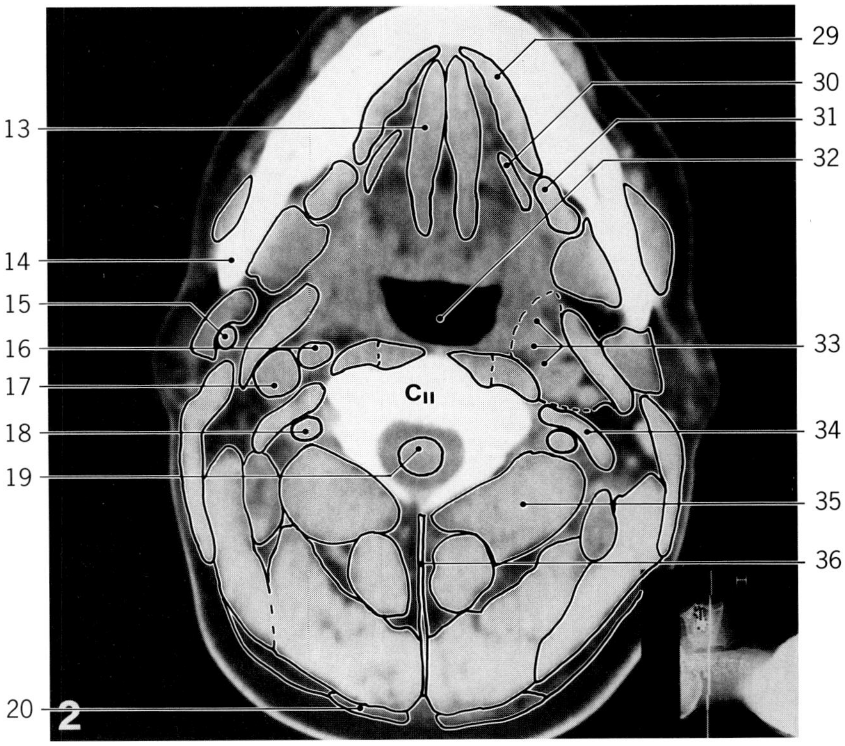

Neck, axial CT

Scout view on opposite page

1: Masseter
2: Medial pterygoid muscle
3: Ramus of mandible
4: Parotid gland
5: Styloid process
6: Posterior belly of digastricus
7: Sternocleidomastoid
8: Obliquus capitis inferior
9: Longissimus capitis
10: Splenius capitis
11: Rectus capitis posterior major
12: Semispinalis capitis
13: Genioglossus
14: Angle of mandible
15: Retromandibular vein
16: Internal carotid artery
17: Internal jugular vein
18: Vertebral artery
19: Spinal cord
20: Trapezius
21: Artefacts from dental filling
22: Tongue
23: Uvula
24: Longus colli
25: Longus capitis
26: Foramen transversarium of atlas
27: Dens axis
28: Posterior arch of atlas
29: Mylohyoideus
30: Hyoglossus
31: Submandibular gland
32: Oral part of pharynx
33: Lateropharyngeal space
34: Levator scapulae, and splenius cervicis
35: Obliquus capitis inferior
36: Lig. nuchae

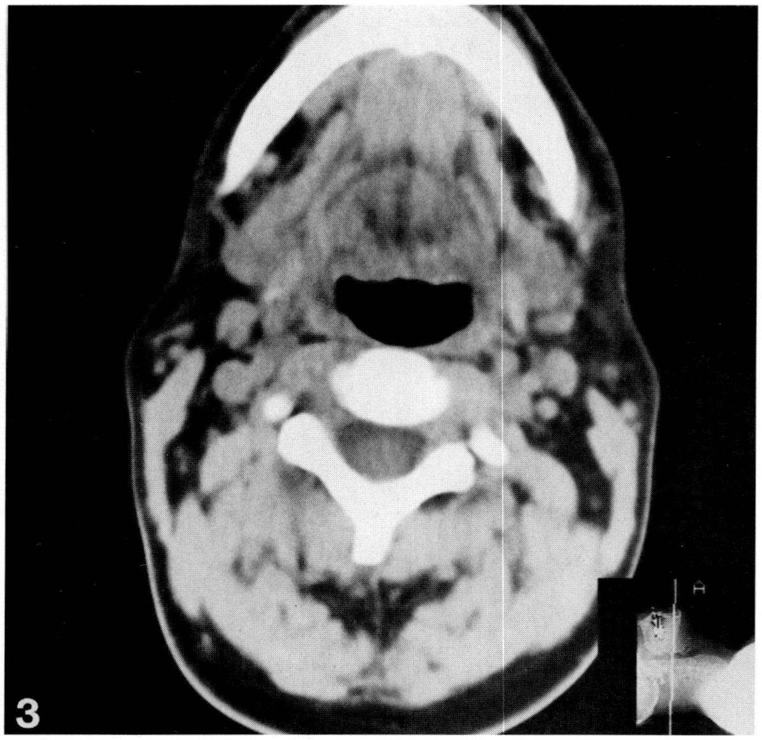

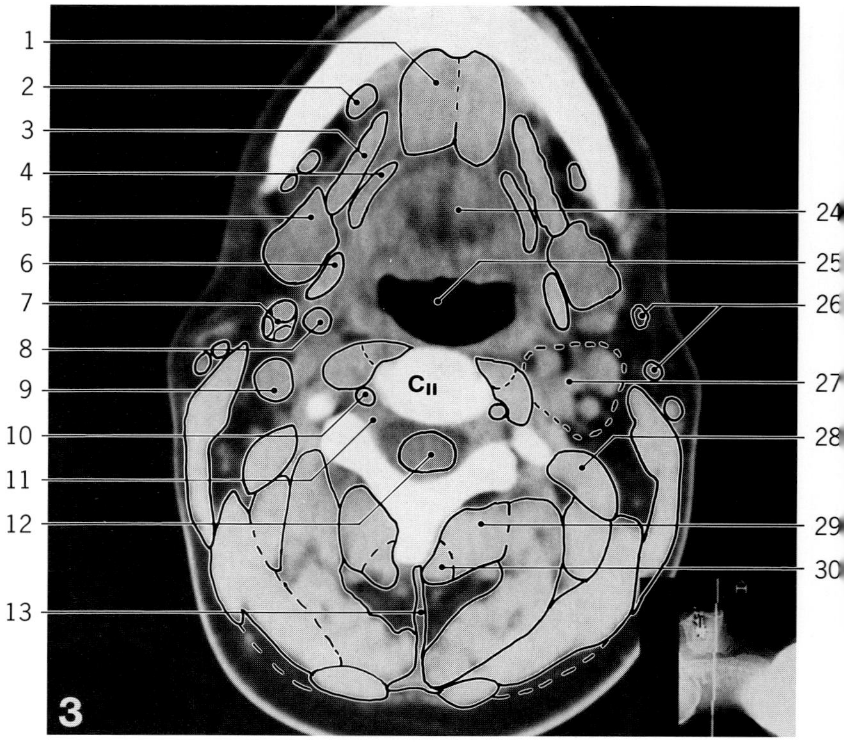

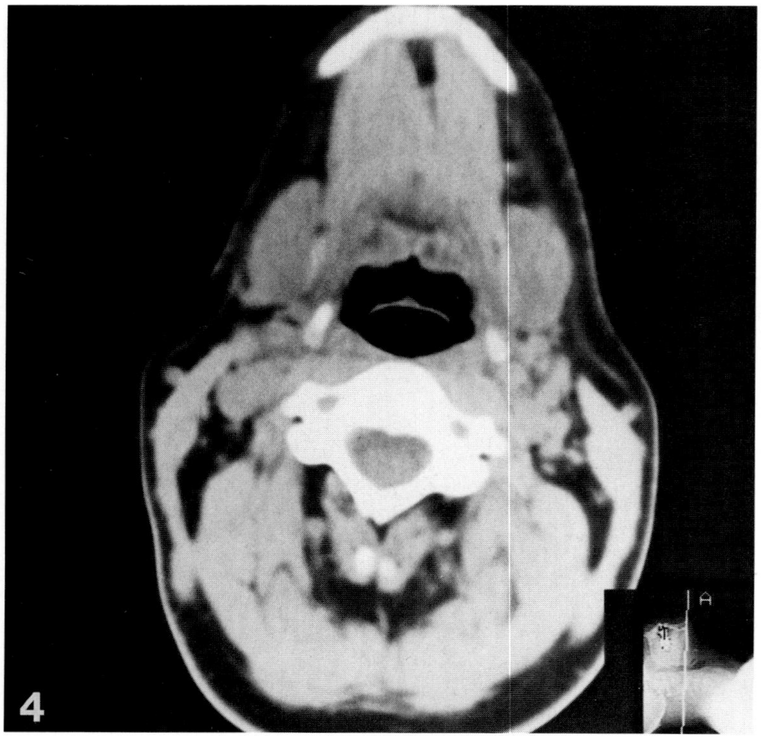

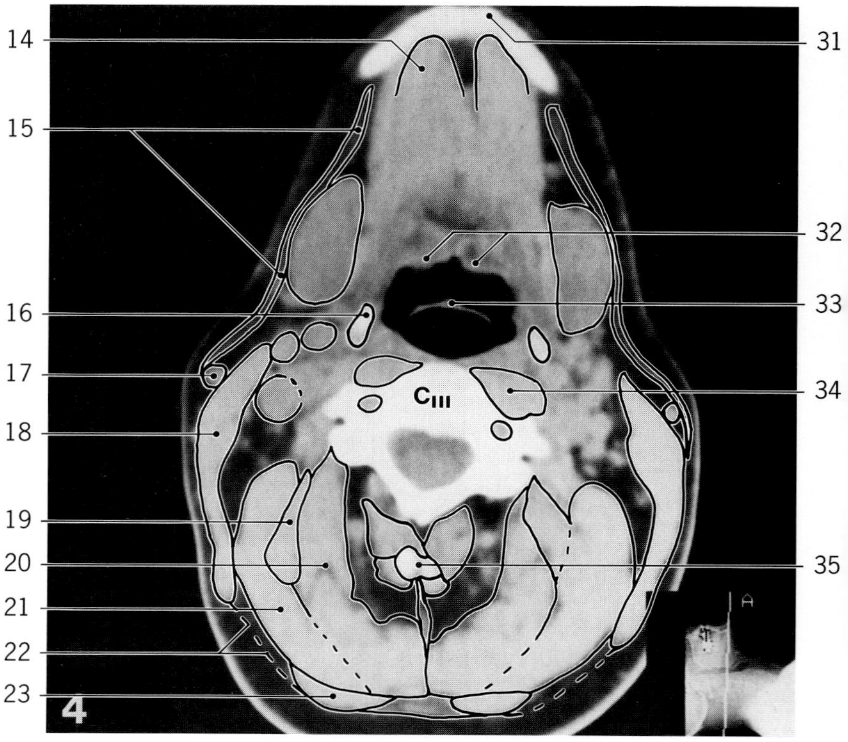

Neck, axial CT

Scout view on page 188

1: Geniohyoideus
2: Submandibular lymph node
3: Mylohyoideus
4: Hyoglossus
5: Submandibular gland
6: Digastricus and stylohyoideus
7: External carotid artery (branching)
8: Internal carotid artery
9: Internal jugular vein
10: Vertebral artery
11: Intervertebral foramen with spinal nerve
12: Spinal cord
13: Lig. nuchae
14: Digastricus, anterior belly
15: Platysma
16: Greater cornu of hyoid bone
17: External jugular vein
18: Sternocleidomastoid
19: Longissimus capitis
20: Semispinalis capitis
21: Splenius capitis
22: Superficial lamina of deep cervical fascia
23: Trapezius
24: Root of tongue
25: Oral part of pharynx
26: External jugular lymph nodes
27: Lateropharyngeal space with vessels, nerves and internal jugular lymph nodes
28: Splenius cervicis, and levator scapulae
29: Obliquus capitis inferior
30: Rectus capitis posterior major
31: Mental tuberosity
32: Lingual tonsil
33: Epiglottis
34: Longus colli, and longus capitis
35: Spinous process of C II

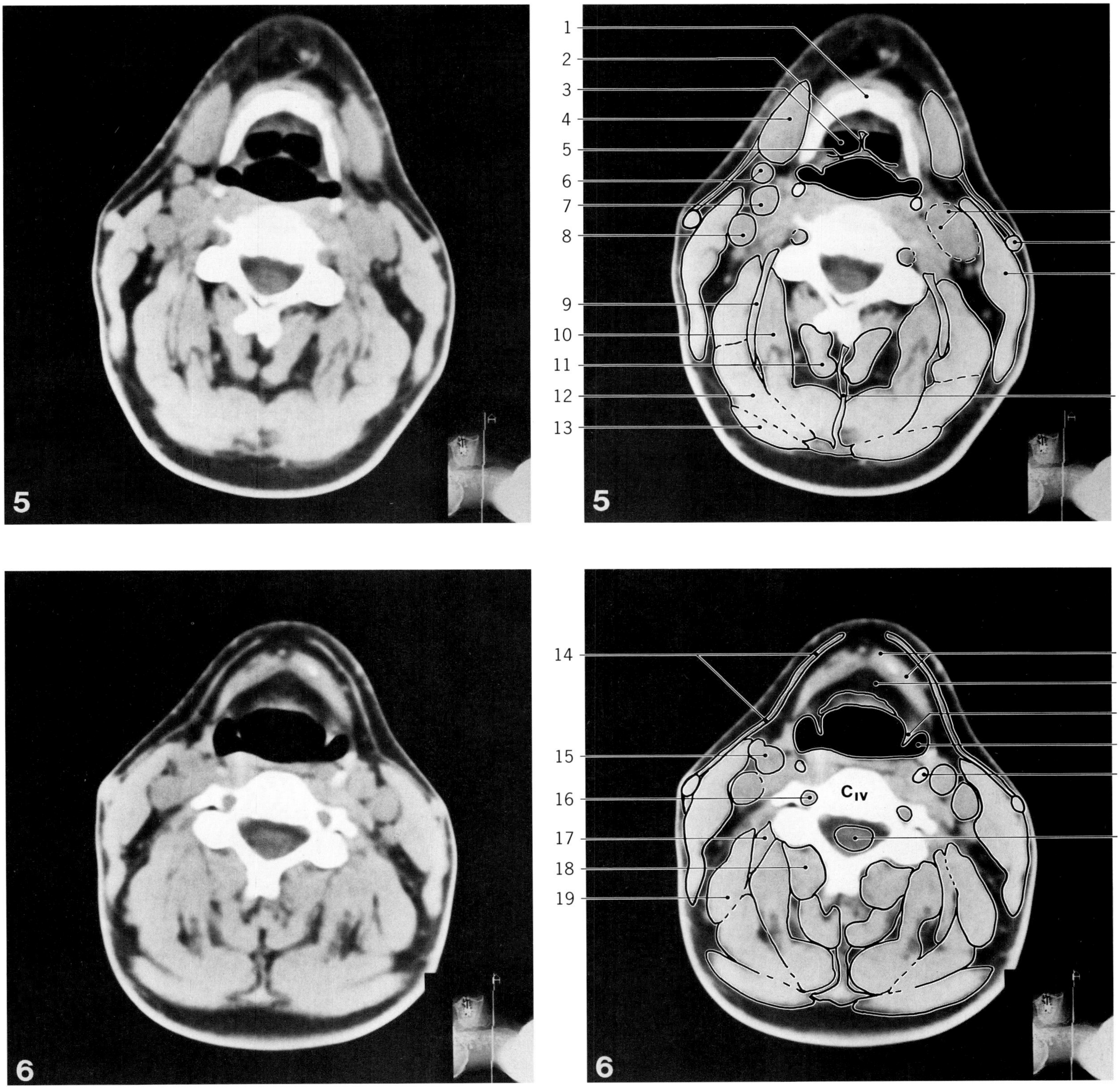

Neck, axial CT

Scout view on page 188

1: Body of hyoid bone
2: Median glosso-epiglottic fold
3: Vallecula
4: Submandibular gland
5: Epiglottis
6: External carotid artery
7: Carotid sinus
8: Internal jugular vein
9: Longissimus capitis
10: Semispinalis capitis
11: Semispinalis cervicis
12: Splenius capitis
13: Trapezius
14: Platysma
15: Carotid bifurcation
16: Vertebral artery
17: Longissimus cervicis
18: Rotator and multifidus muscles
19: Levator scapulae
20: Lateropharyngeal space
21: External jugular vein
22: Sternocleidomastoid
23: Lig. nuchae
24: Infrahyoid muscles
25: Laryngeal fat pad
26: Ary-epiglottic fold
27: Piriform fossa
28: Superior cornu of thyroid cartilage
29: Spinal cord

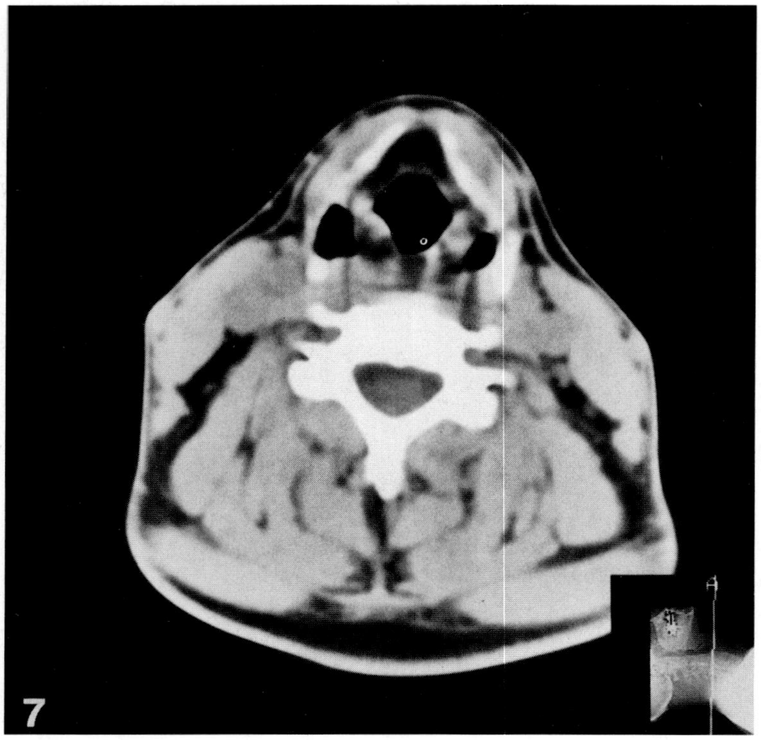

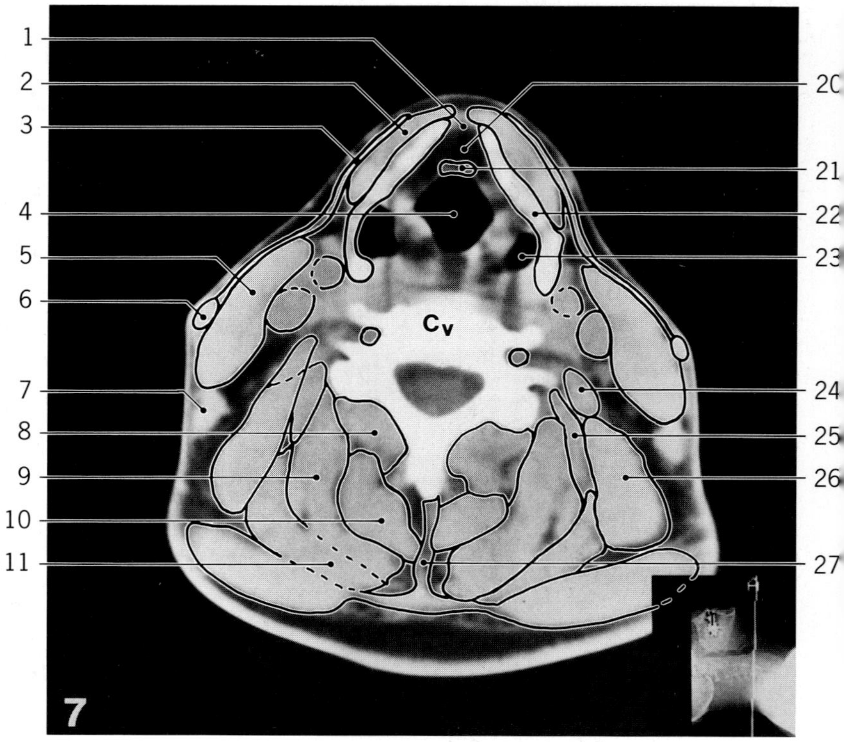

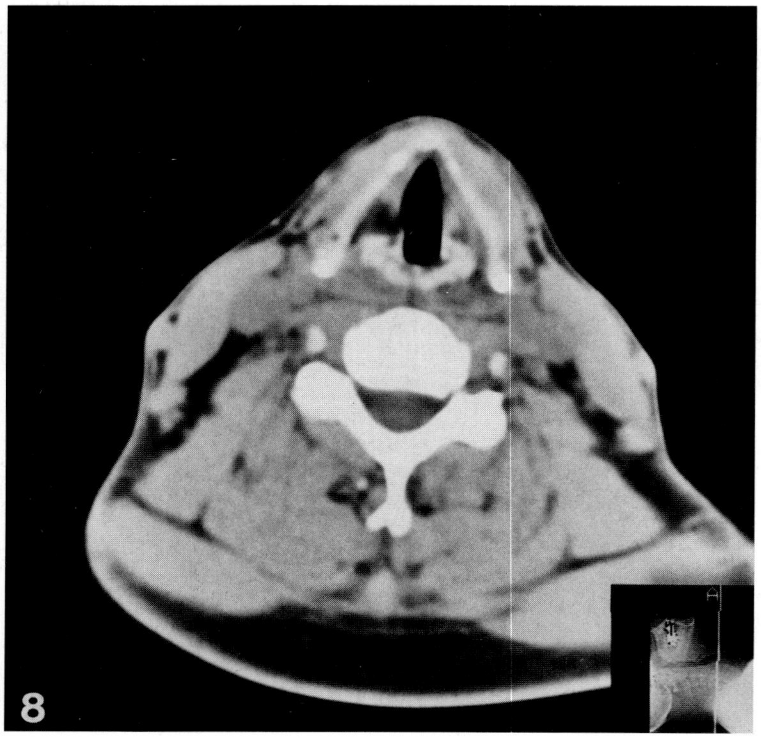

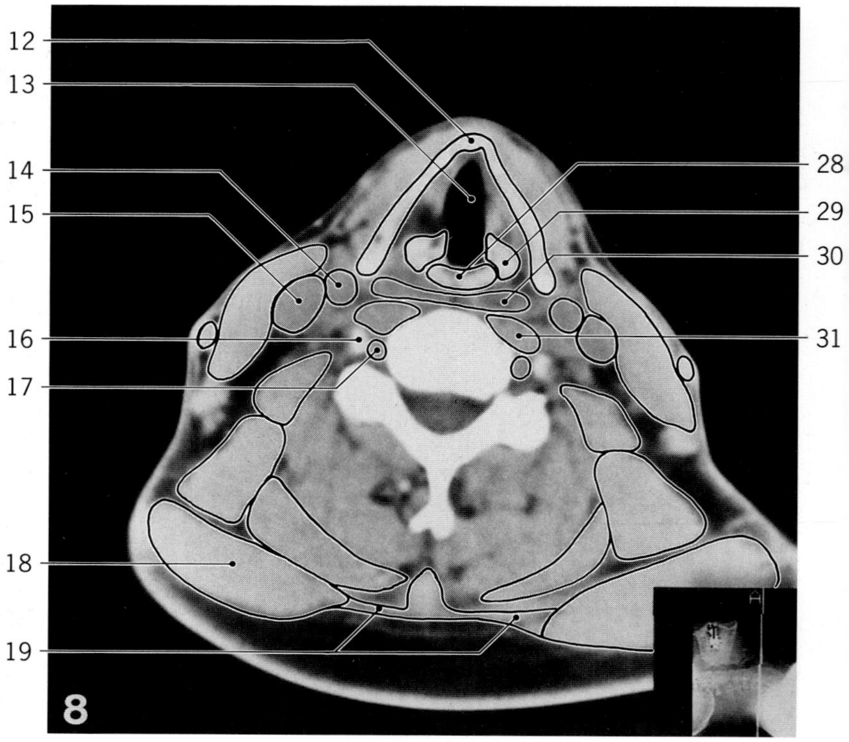

Neck, axial CT

Scout view on page 188

1: Thyroid notch
2: Infrahyoid muscles
3: Platysma
4: Vestibule of larynx
5: Sternocleidomastoid
6: External jugular vein
7: Lymph node
8: Rotatores and multifidi muscles
9: Semispinalis capitis
10: Semispinalis cervicis
11: Splenius capitis
12: Laryngeal prominence
13: Rima glottidis
14: Common carotid artery
15: Internal jugular vein
16: Anterior tubercle of transverse process
17: Vertebral artery
18: Trapezius
19: Speculum rhomboideum
20: Laryngeal fat pad
21: Epiglottis
22: Lamina of thyroid cartilage
23: Piriform fossa
24: Scalenus medius
25: Longissimus cervicis
26: Levator scapulae
27: Lig. nuchae
28: Lamina of cricoid cartilage
29: Arythenoid cartilage
30: Laryngeal part of pharynx
31: Longus colli and longus capitis

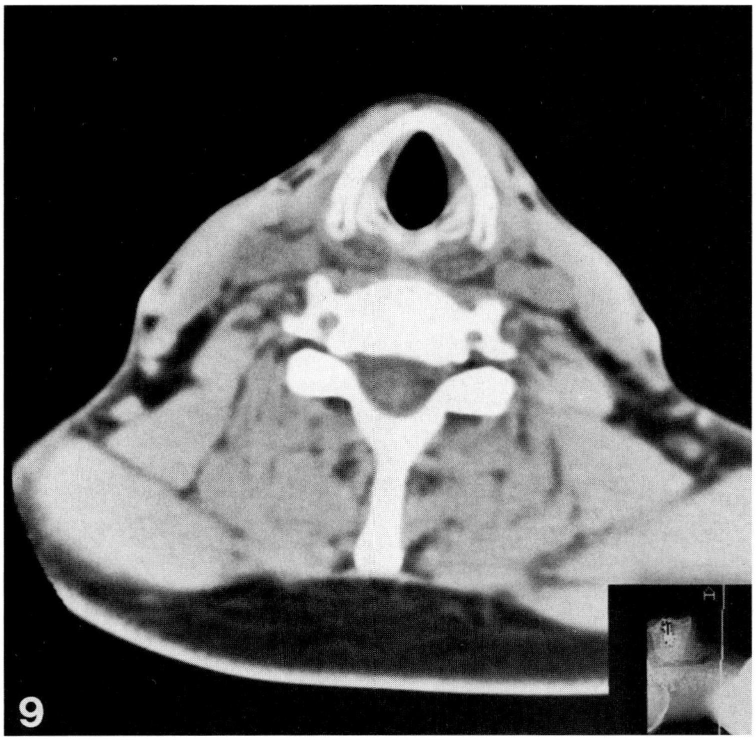

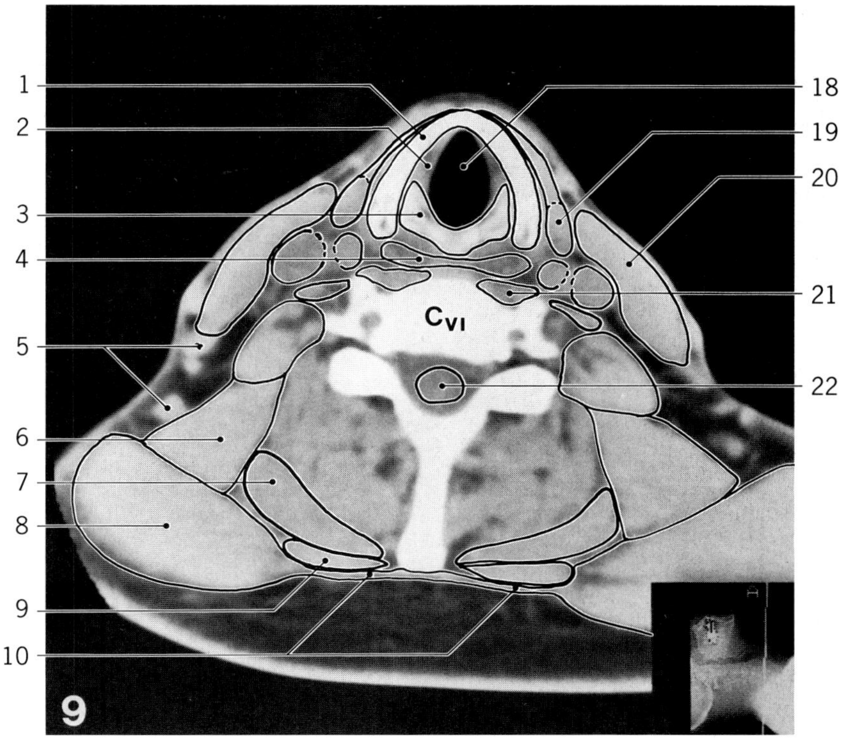

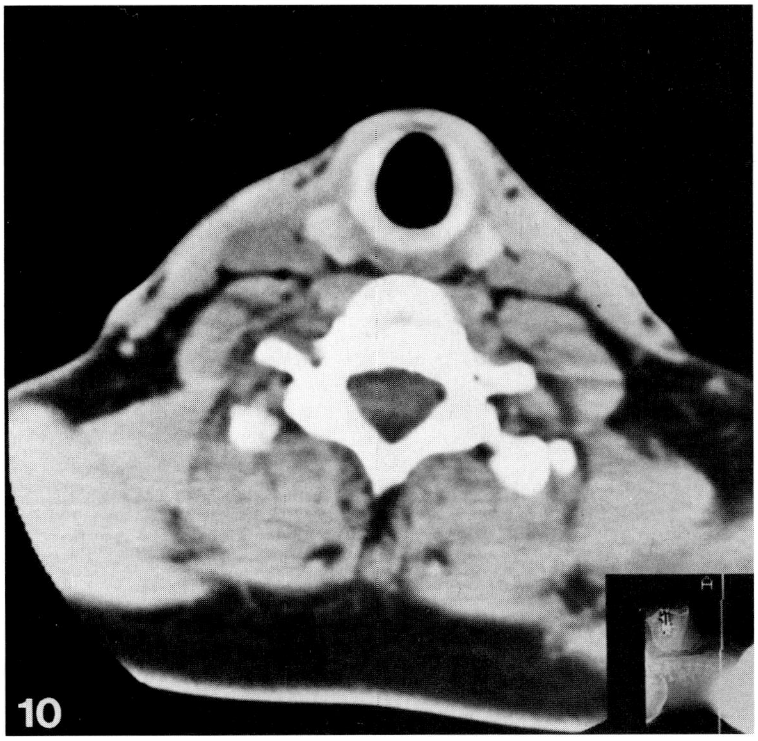

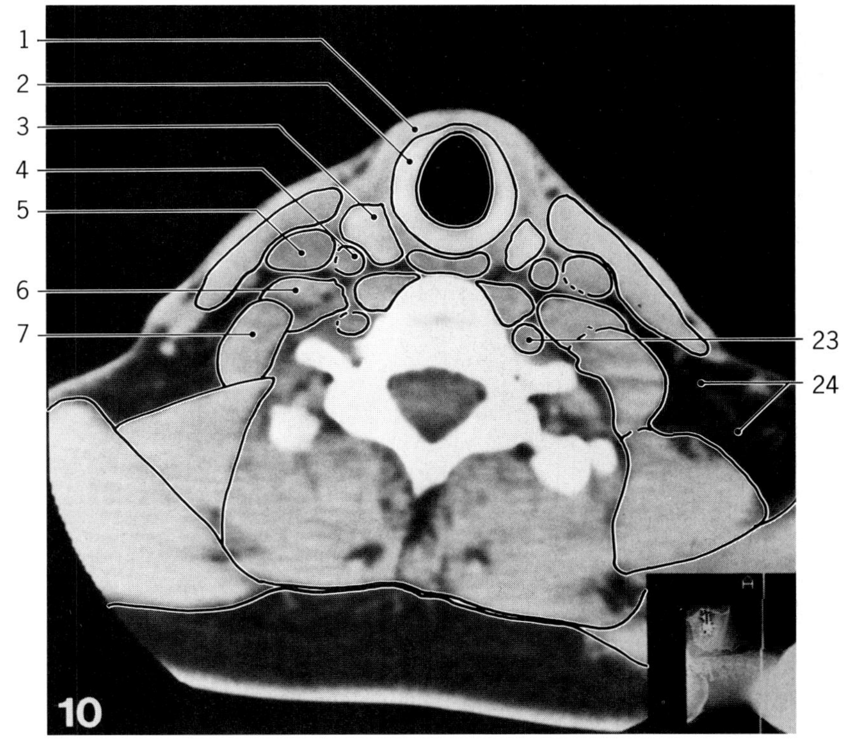

Neck, axial CT

Scout view on page 188

1: Lamina of thyroid cartilage
2: Conus elasticus
3: Lamina of cricoid cartilage
4: Laryngeal part of pharynx
5: Superficial cervical lymph nodes
6: Levator scapulae
7: Splenius
8: Trapezius
9: Rhomboideus
10: Speculum rhomboideum
11: Infrahyoid muscles
12: Arch of cricoid cartilage
13: Thyroid gland
14: Common carotid artery
15: Internal jugular vein
16: Scalenus anterior
17: Scalenus medius
18: Cavitas infraglottica
19: Omohyoideus, superior belly
20: Sternocleidomastoid
21: Longus colli and longus capitis
22: Spinal cord
23: Vertebral artery and vein
24: Lateral cervical region

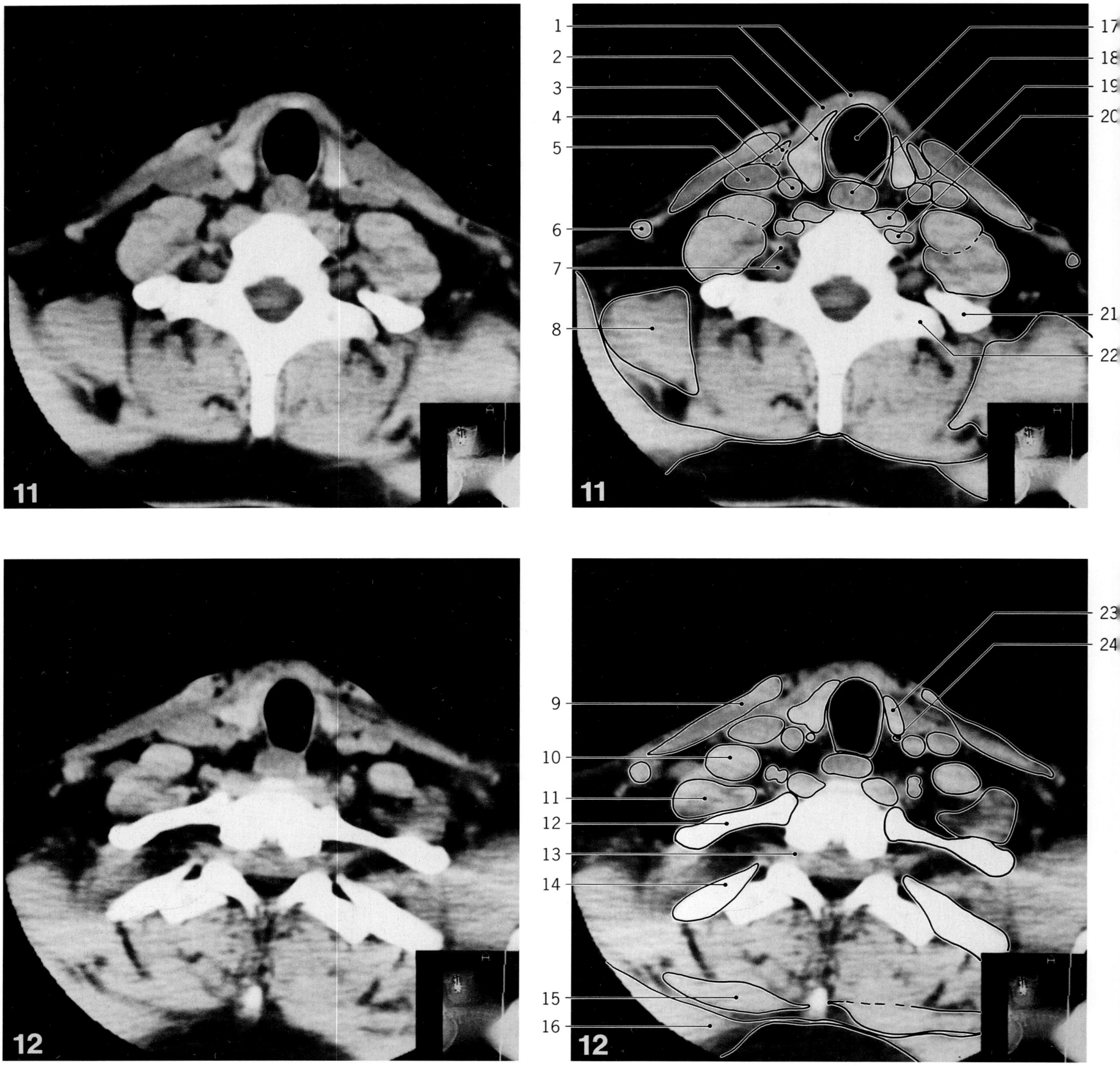

Neck, axial CT

Scout view on page 188

1: Sternohyoid, and sternothyroid muscles
2: Right lobe of thyroid gland
3: Omohyoideus, superior belly
4: Common carotid artery
5: Internal jugular vein
6: External jugular vein
7: Roots of brachial plexus
8: Levator scapulae
9: Sternocleidomastoid
10: Scalenus anterior
11: Scalenus medius
12: Neck of first rib
13: First thoracic spinal nerve
14: Second rib
15: Rhomboideus
16: Trapezius
17: Trachea
18: Oesophagus
19: Longus colli
20: Vertebral artery and vein
21: Tubercle of first rib
22: Transverse process of thoracic vertebra I
23: Left lobe of thyroid gland
24: Inferior thyroid artery

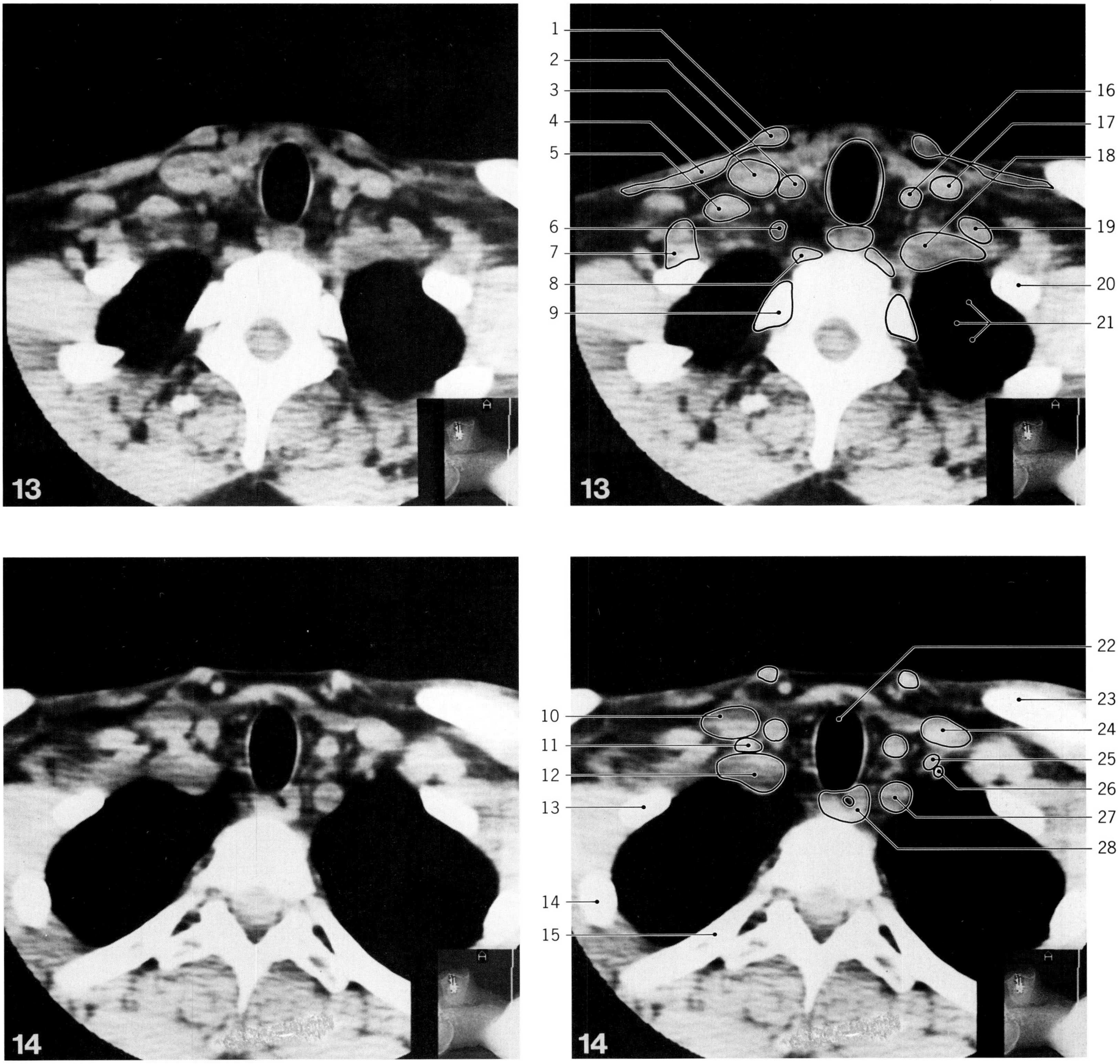

Neck, axial CT

Scout view on page 188

1: Sternal head of sternocleidomastoid
2: Right common carotid artery
3: Right internal jugular vein joining with right subclavian vein
4: Clavicular head of sternocleidomastoid
5: Right scalenus anterior
6: Right vertebral artery
7: Scalenus medius
8: Longus colli
9: Head of costa II
10: Right subclavian vein
11: Right vertebral vein
12: Right subclavian artery
13: First rib
14: Second rib
15: Third rib
16: Left common carotid artery
17: Left internal jugular vein
18: Left subclavian artery
19: Left scalenus anterior
20: First rib
21: Apex of lung
22: Trachea
23: Clavicle
24: Left subclavian vein
25: Left vertebral vein
26: Internal thoracic artery
27: Left subclavian artery
28: Oesophagus

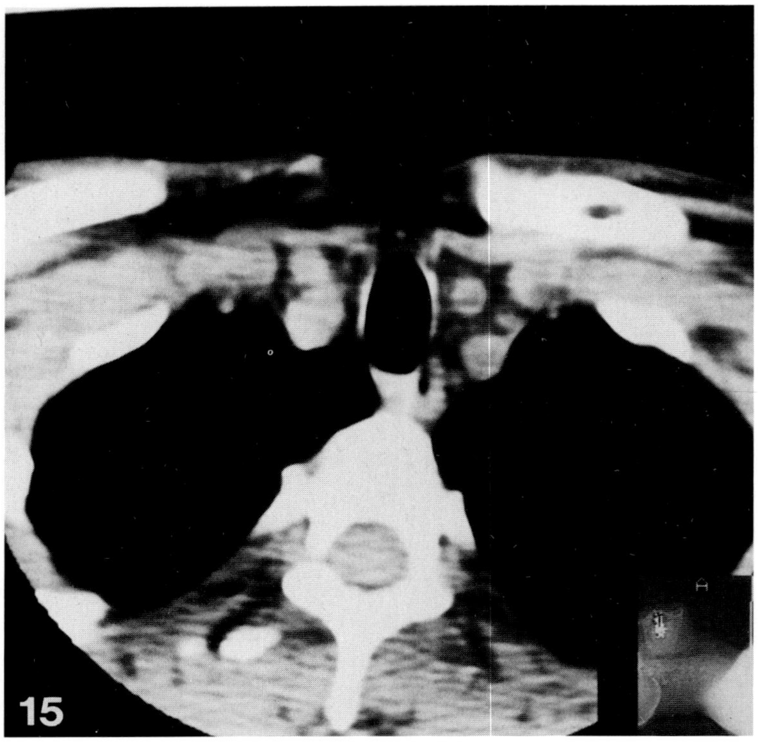

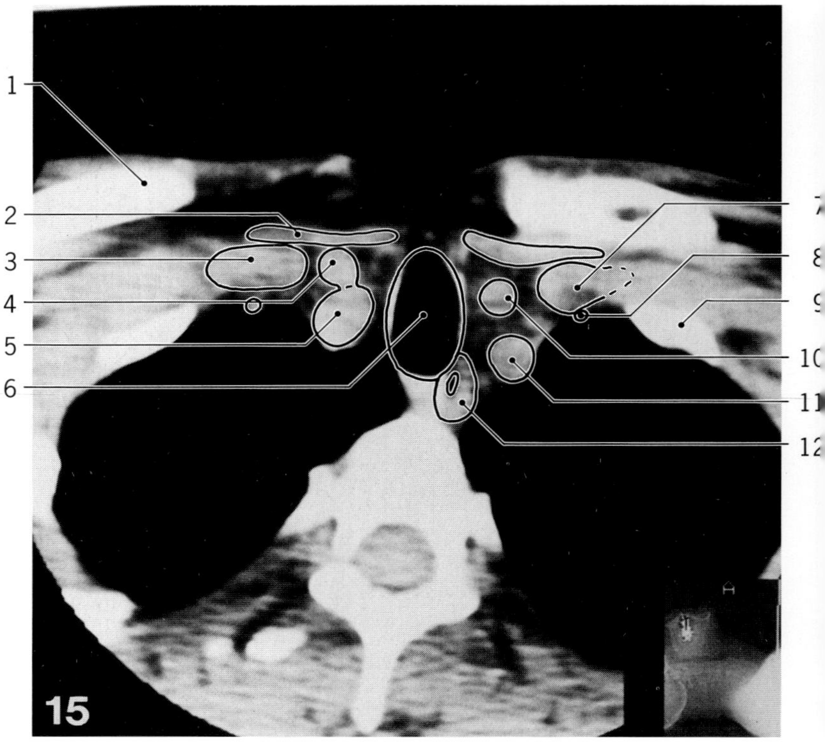

Neck, axial CT

Scout view on page 188

1: Clavicle
2: Infrahyoid muscles
3: Right subclavian vein
4: Right common carotid artery
5: Brachiocephalic trunk
6: Trachea
7: Left subclavian vein
8: Internal thoracic artery
9: First rib
10: Left common carotid artery
11: Left subclavian artery
12: Oesophagus

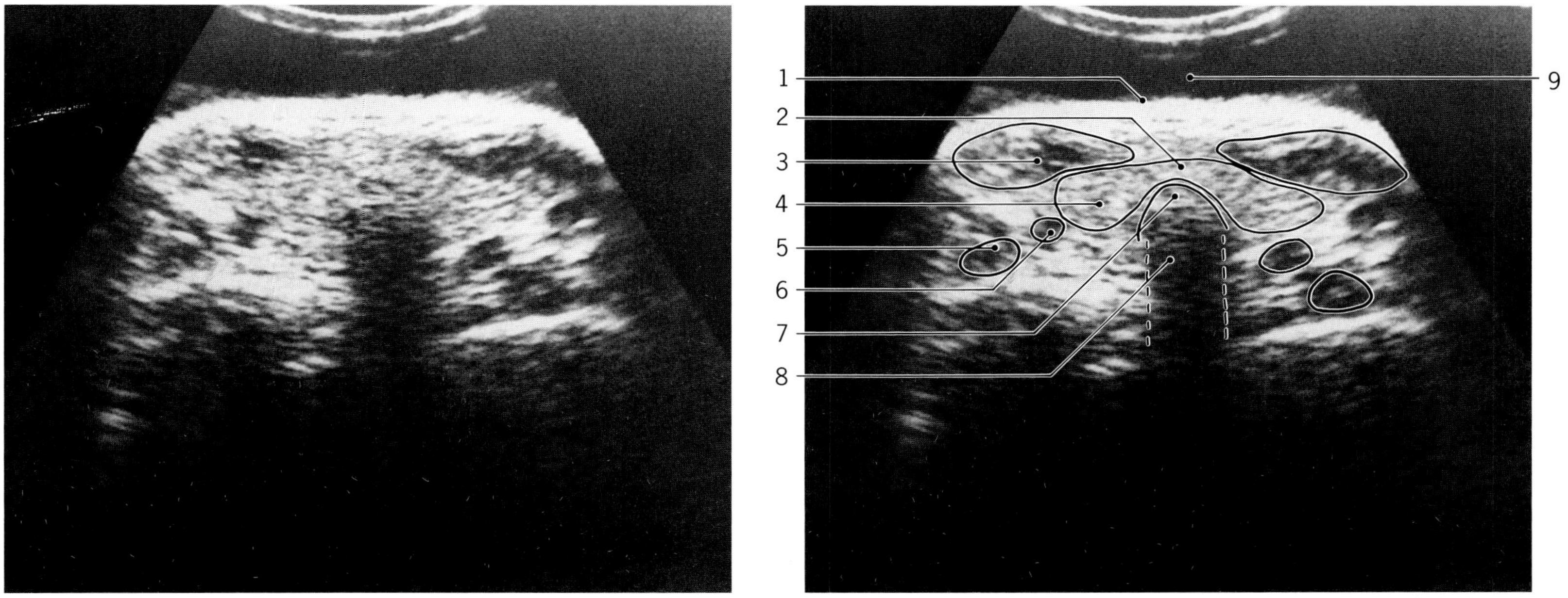

Thyroid gland, transverse section, US

1: Skin
2: Isthmus of thyroid gland
3: Sternocleidomastoid
4: Right lobe of thyroid gland
5: Internal jugular vein
6: Common carotid artery
7: Trachea
8: Acoustic "shadow"
9: Gel spacer between skin and ultrasound probe

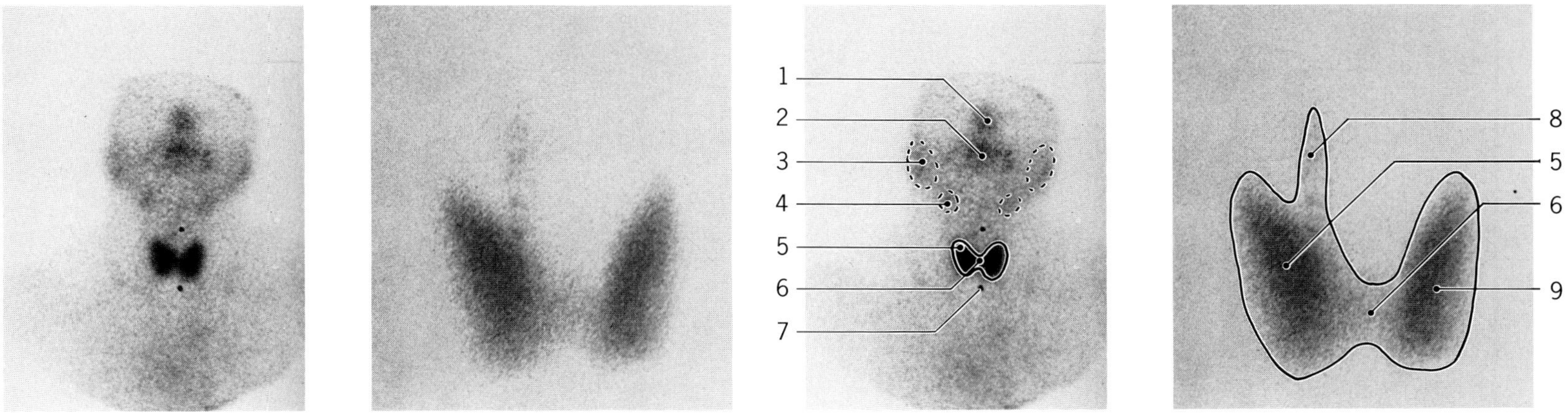

Thyroid gland, anterior view, ^{131}J-scintigraphy

(Note: salivary glands and mucous glands of the nose excrete iodine)

1: Nose
2: Mouth
3: Parotid gland
4: Submandibular gland
5: Right lobe of thyroid gland
6: Isthmus of thyroid gland
7: Marker at jugular incisure
8: Pyramidal lobe of thyroid gland
9: Left lobe of thyroid gland

THORAX

Thoracic cage

Lungs

Axial CT-series

Heart and great vessels

Oesophagus

Breast

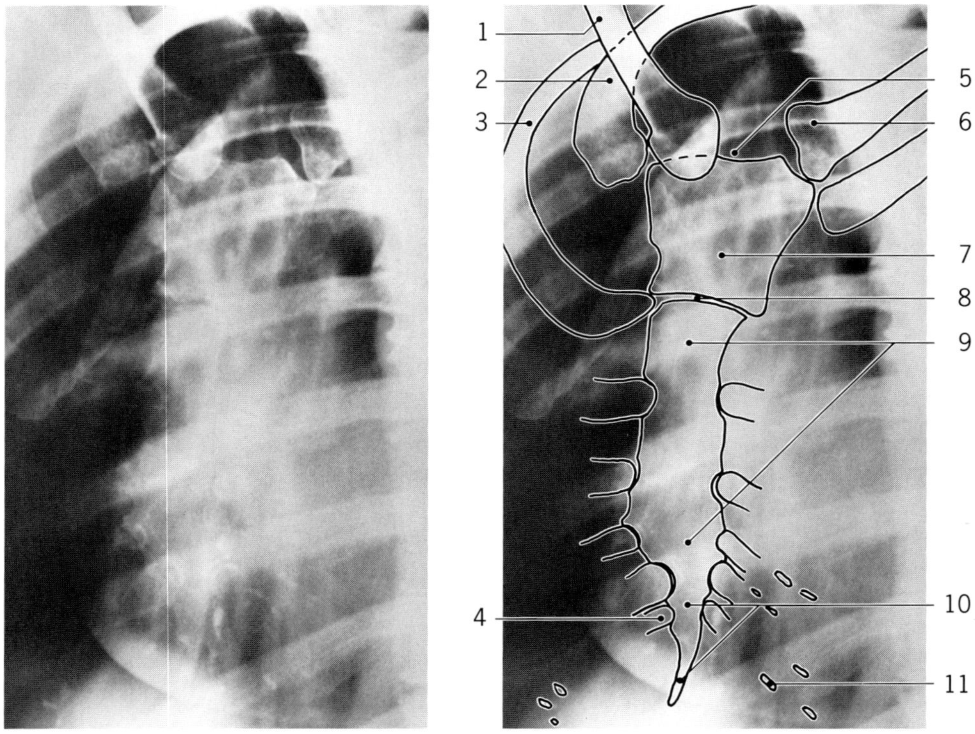

Sternum, oblique X-ray

1: Body of clavicle
2: First rib
3: Second rib
4: Seventh rib
5: Jugular incisure
6: Sternal end of clavicle
7: Manubrium of sternum
8: Sternal angle
9: Body of sternum
10: Xiphoid process
11: Calcified costal cartilage

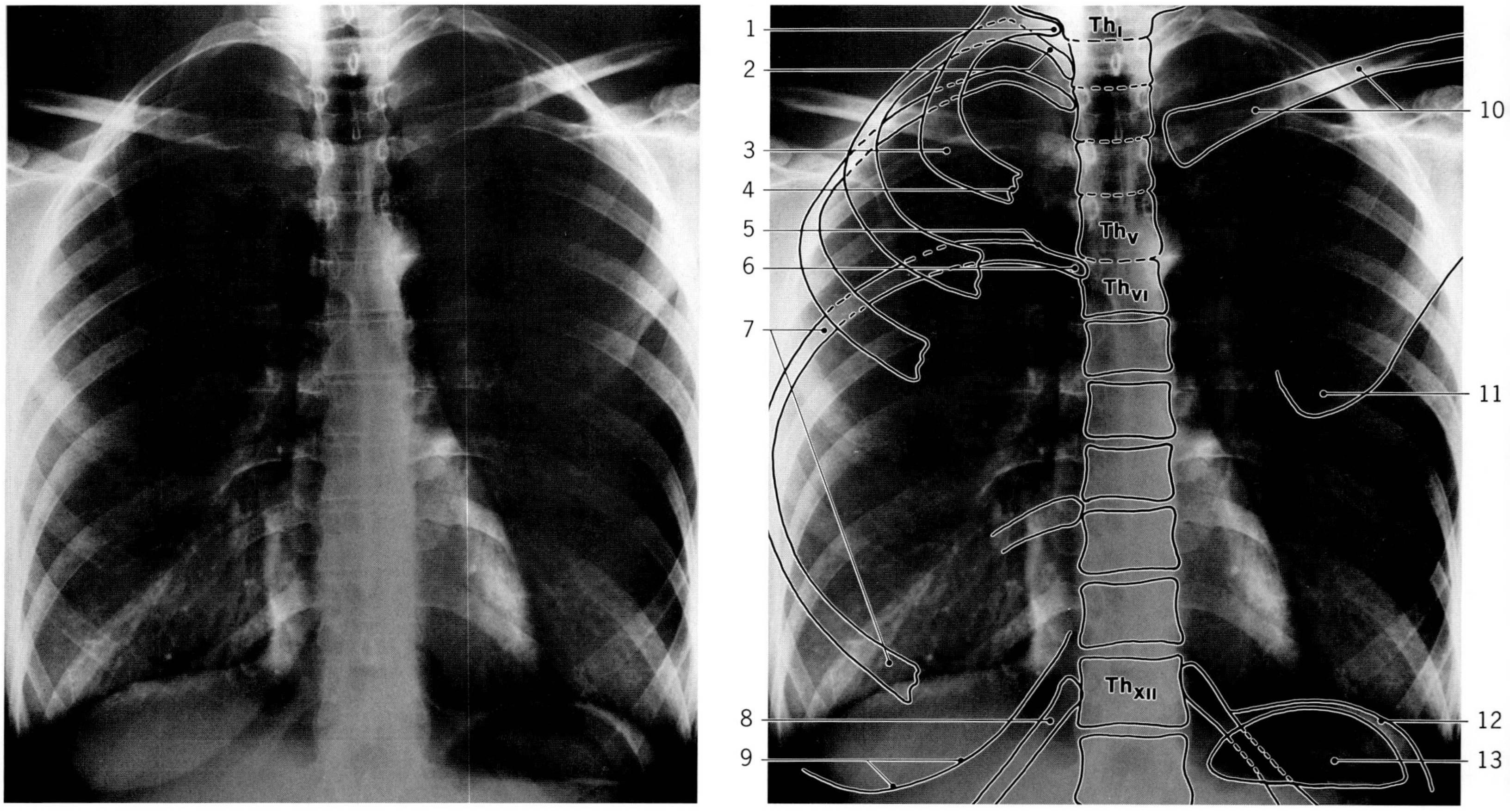

Thoracic cage, a-p X-ray

1: Head of first rib
2: Neck of second rib
3: Shaft of first rib
4: Osteochondral junction
5: Tuberculum of costa VI
6: Head of sixth rib
7: Shaft of sixth rib
8: 12th rib
9: Mamma
10: Clavicle
11: Inferior angle of scapula
12: Diaphragm
13: Gastric air

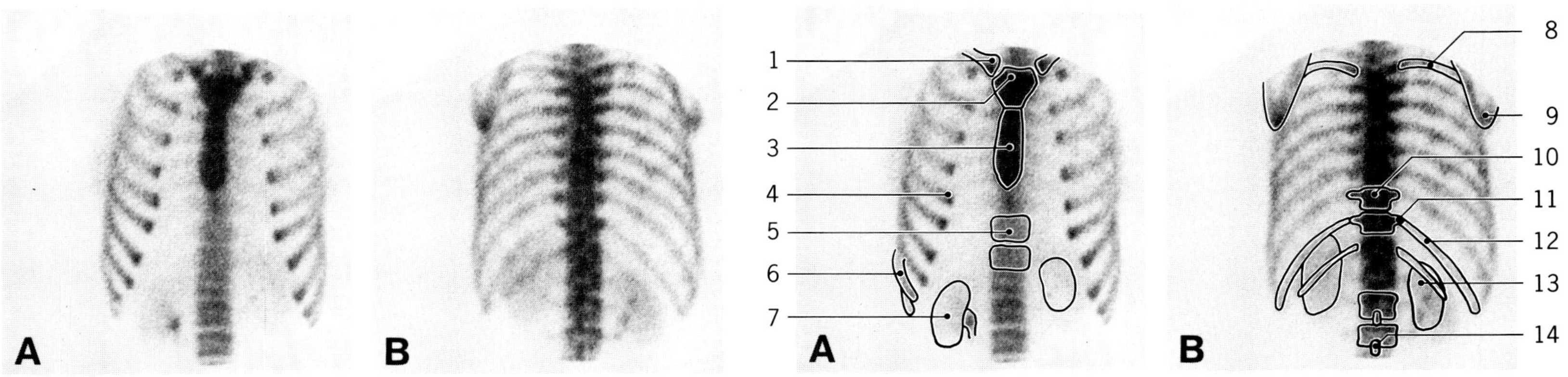

Thorax, ^{99m}Tc-MDP, scintigraphy

A: Anterior view, B: Posterior view

1: Sternal end of clavicle
2: Manubrium of sternum
3: Body of sternum
4: Osteochondral junction (5th rib)
5: Body of thoracic vertebra (Th X)
6: Ninth rib
7: Right kidney
8: Fourth rib
9: Inferior angle of scapula
10: Body of thoracic vertebra (Th X)
11: Transverse process of vertebra, and neck of rib
12: 11th rib
13: Right kidney
14: Spinous process of lumbar vertebra

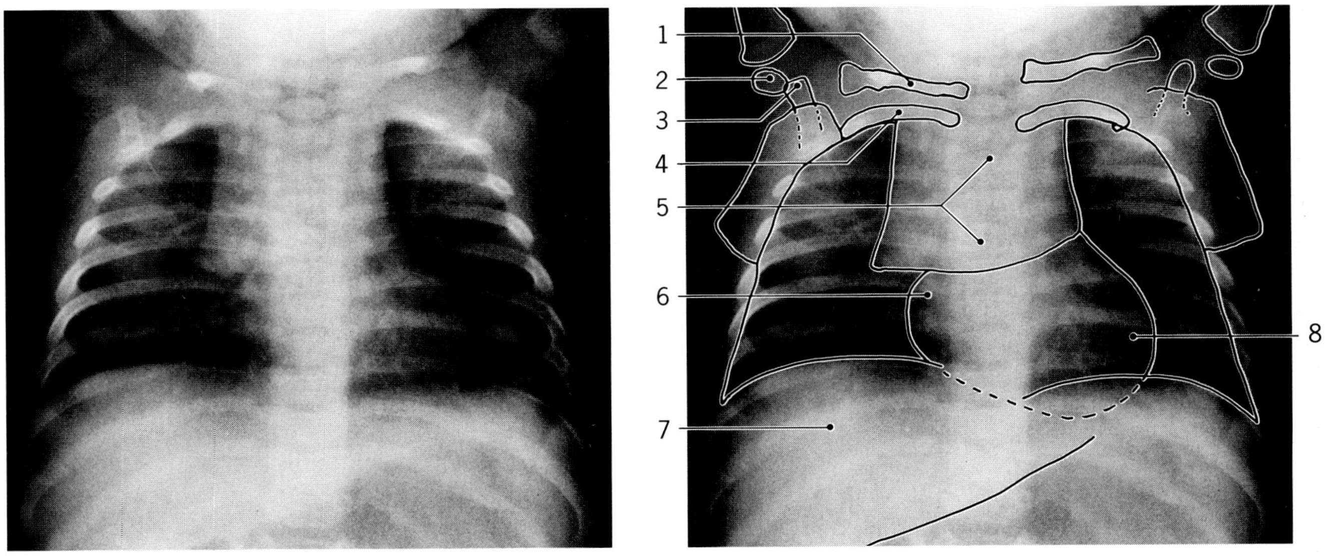

Thorax, a-p X-ray, child 1 month

1: Clavicle
2: Humeral head (ossification center)
3: Acromion
4: First rib
5: Thymus
6: Right atrium
7: Liver
8: Left ventricle

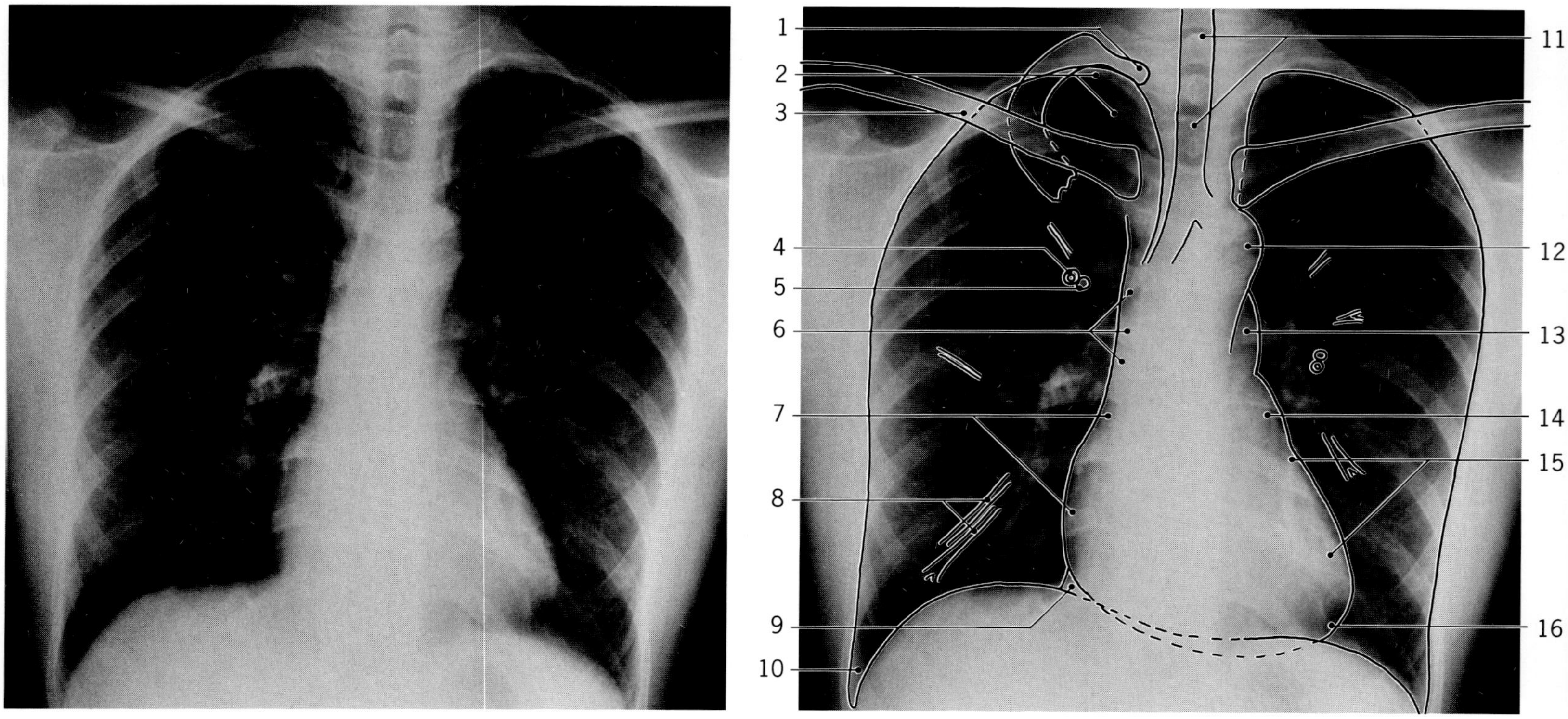

Thorax, p-a X-ray, deep inspiration

1: Head of first rib
2: Apex of lung
3: Clavicle
4: Bronchus (longitudinal view)
5: Lung vessel (longitudinal view)
6: Superior caval vein
7: Right atrium
8: Lung vessels
9: Inferior caval vein
10: Costodiaphragmatic sulcus
11: Trachea
12: Aortic arch
13: Pulmonary trunk
14: Left auricle
15: Left ventricle
16: Apex of heart

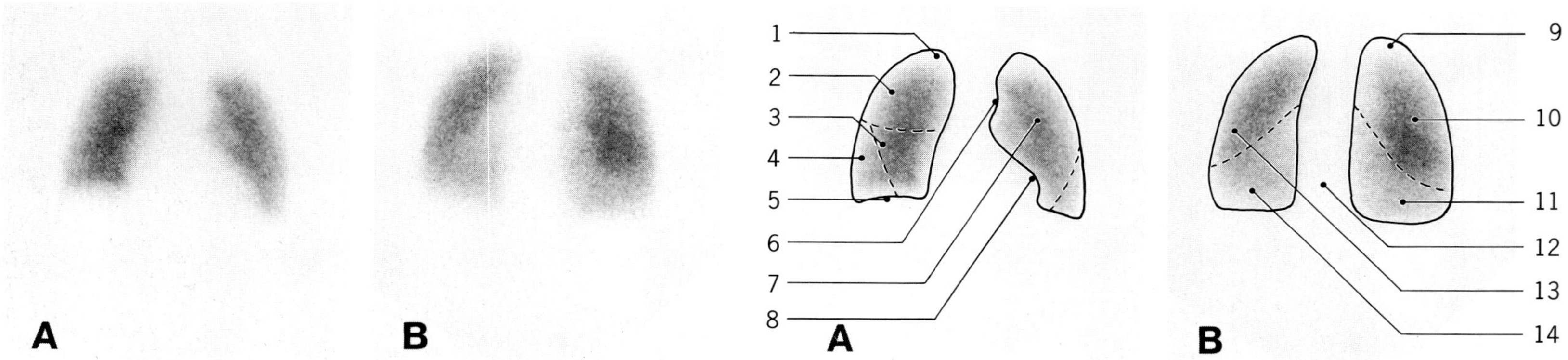

Lungs, ^{133}Xe inhalation, scintigraphy

A: Anterior view, B: Posterior view

1: Apex of right lung
2: Superior lobe of right lung
3: Middle lobe of right lung
4: Inferior lobe of right lung
5: Base of right lung
6: Impression from aorta
7: Superior lobe of left lung
8: Cardiac incisure
9: Apex of right lung
10: Superior lobe of right lung
11: Inferior lobe of right lung
12: Mediastinum
13: Superior lobe of left lung
14: Inferior lobe of left lung

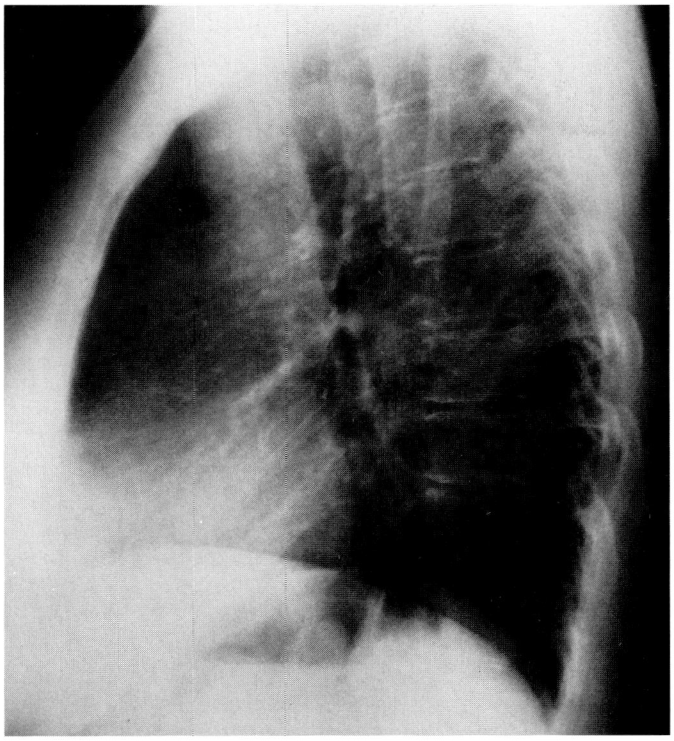

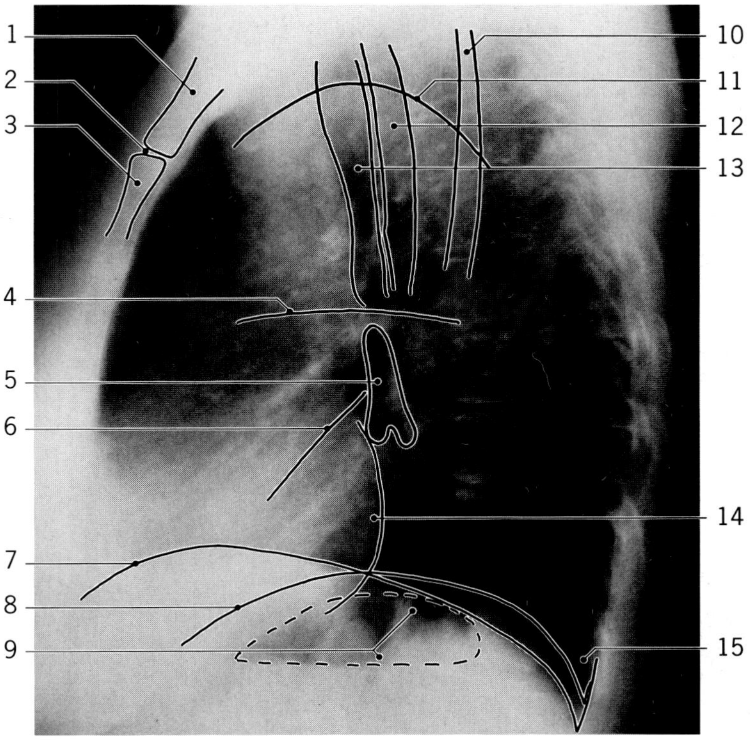

Thorax, lateral X-ray

1: Manubrium of sternum
2: Angle of sternum
3: Body of sternum
4: Horizontal fissure of right lung
5: Bronchus
6: Oblique fissure of lung
7: Diaphragm, right dome
8: Diaphragm, left dome
9: Air in fundus of stomach
10: Scapula
11: Aortic arch
12: Oesophagus (with air)
13: Trachea
14: Left atrium
15: Costodiaphragmatic sulcus

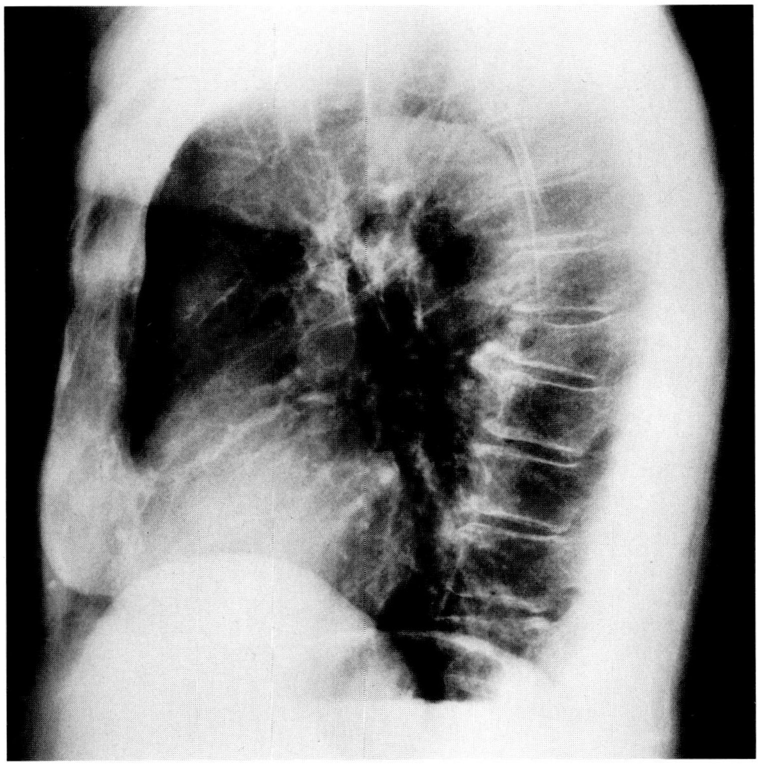

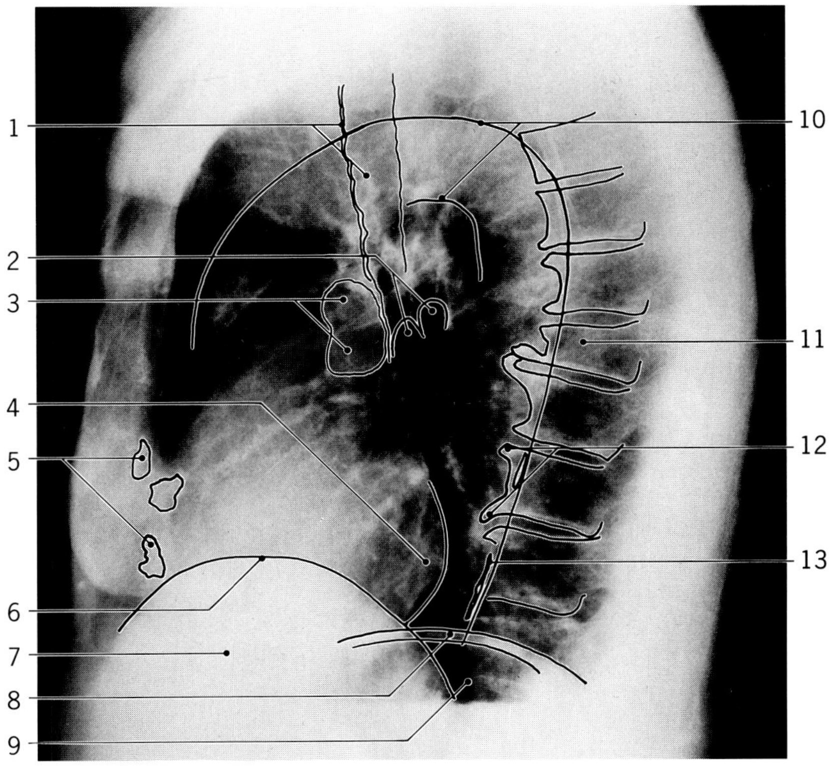

Thorax of old age, lateral X-ray

1: Trachea with calcified cartilage
2: Principal bronchi
3: Pulmonary arteries
4: Left ventricle (enlarged)
5: Calcified costal cartilage
6: Right dome of diaphragm (relaxed)
7: Liver
8: Left dome of diaphragm
9: Gastric air
10: Aortic arch (dilated)
11: Body of vertebra (collapsed)
12: Osteophytes
13: Calcification of aortic wall

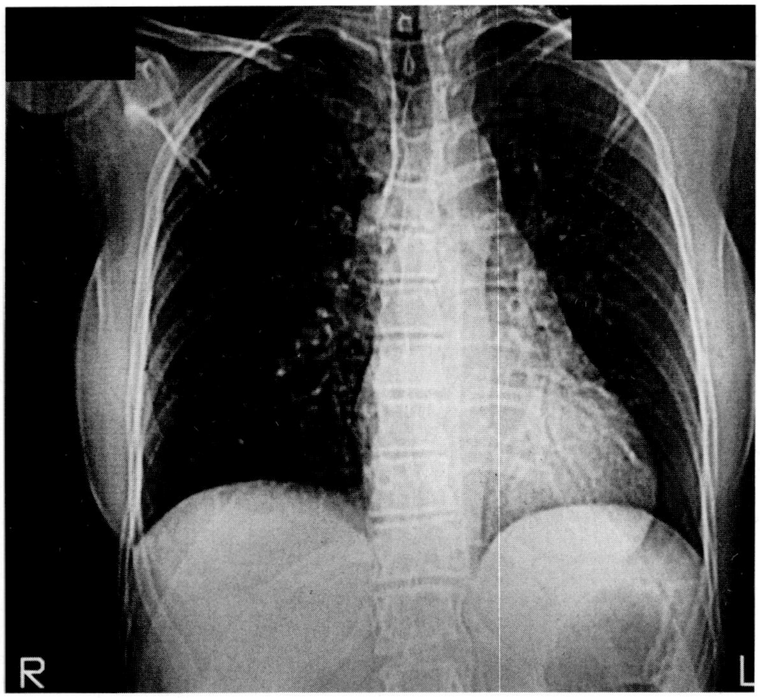

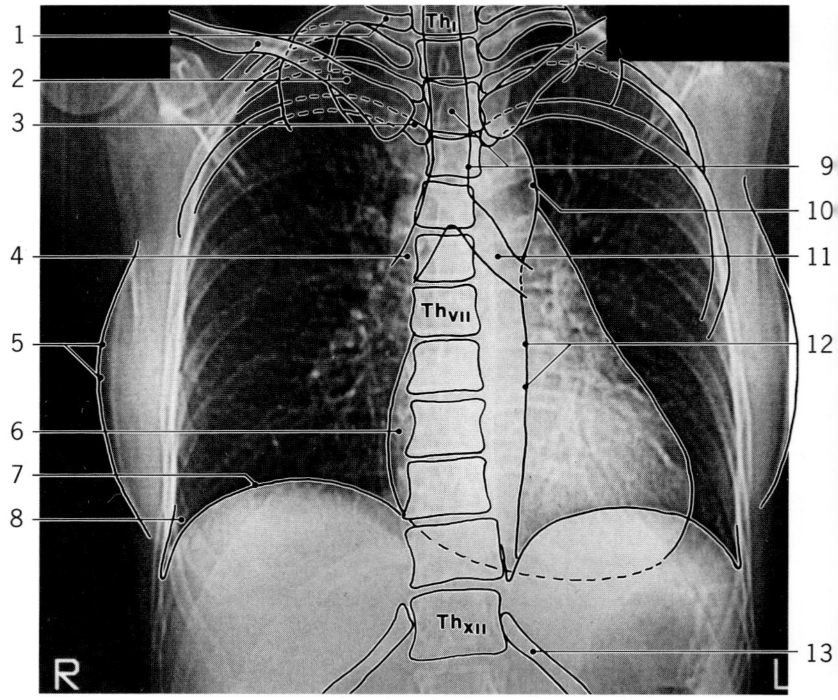

Scout view

1: Neck of first rib
2: Clavicle
3: Head of fourth rib
4: Right principal bronchus
5: Breast
6: Right atrium
7: Diaphragm
8: Costodiaphragmatic sulcus
9: Trachea
10: Aortic arch
11: Left principal bronchus
12: Thoracic aorta
13: 12th rib

Scout view

Lines #1-20 indicate positions of sections in the following CT series.

Sections are 10 mm thick, recorded at intervals of 15 mm, i.e. with 5 mm spacing.

Each section is displayed with soft tissue settings (above) and with lung settings (below)

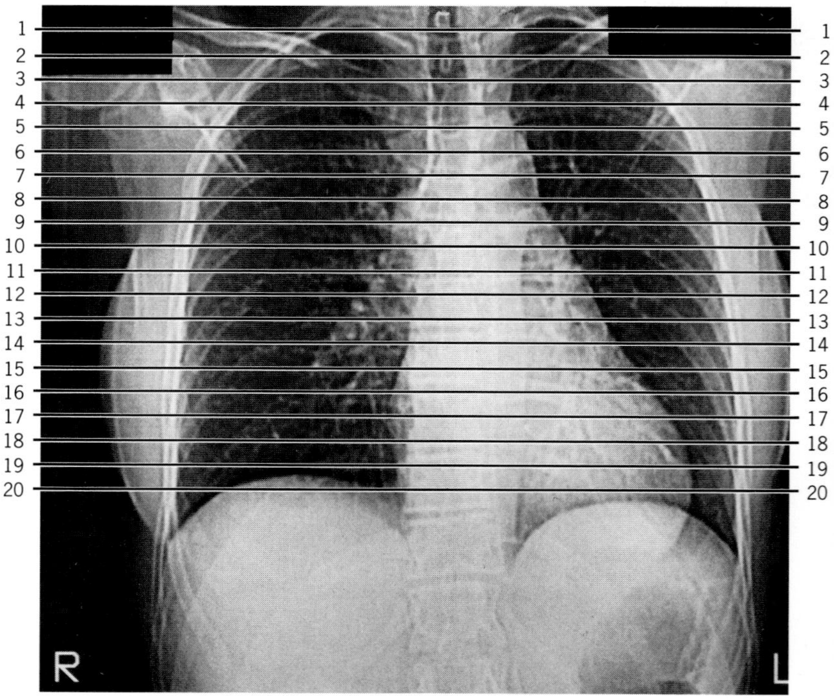

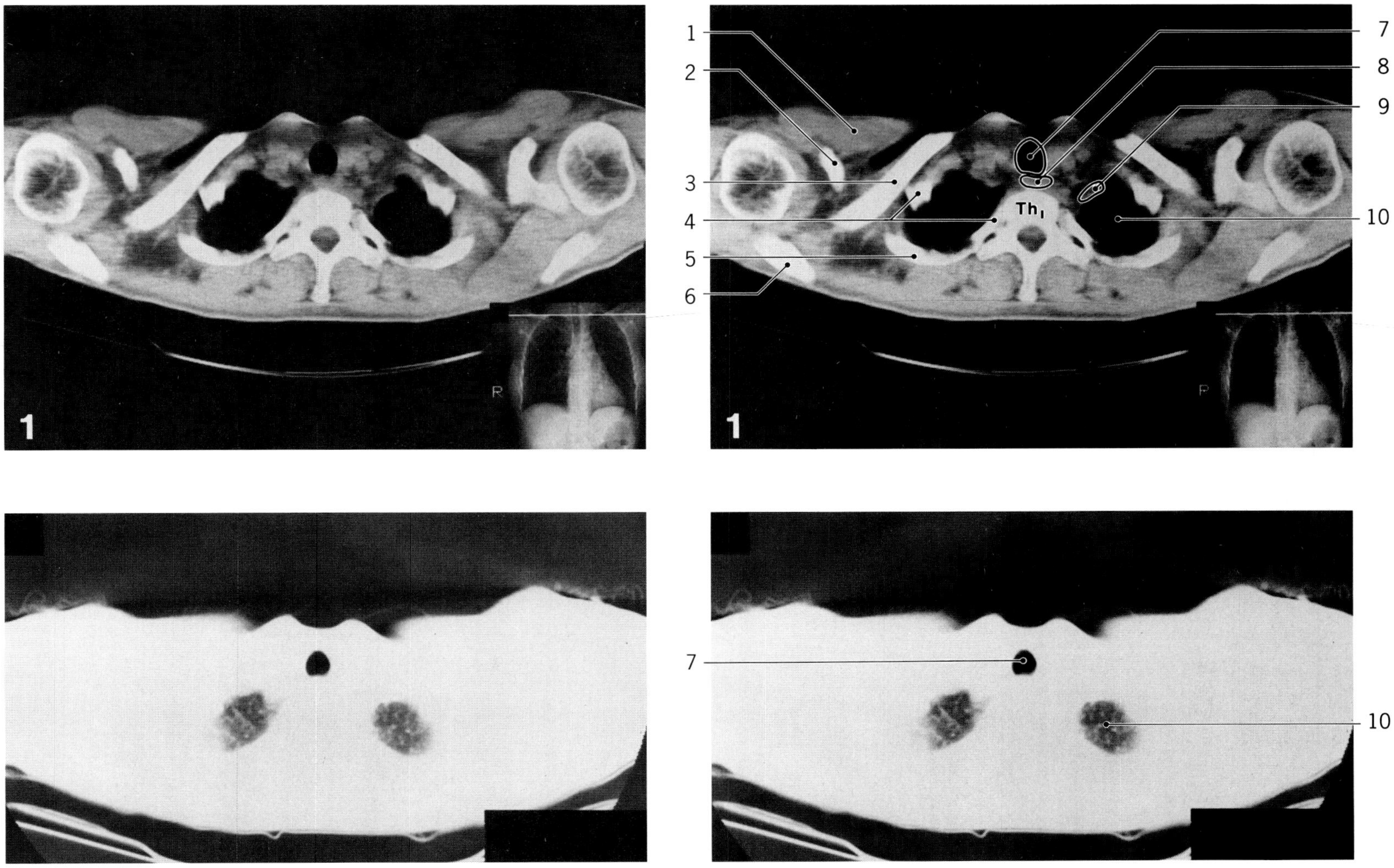

Thorax, axial CT

Scout view on opposite page

1: Pectoralis major (arm elevated)
2: Coracoid process
3: Clavicle
4: First rib
5: Second rib
6: Acromion
7: Trachea
8: Oesophagus
9: Left subclavian artery
10: Apex of lung

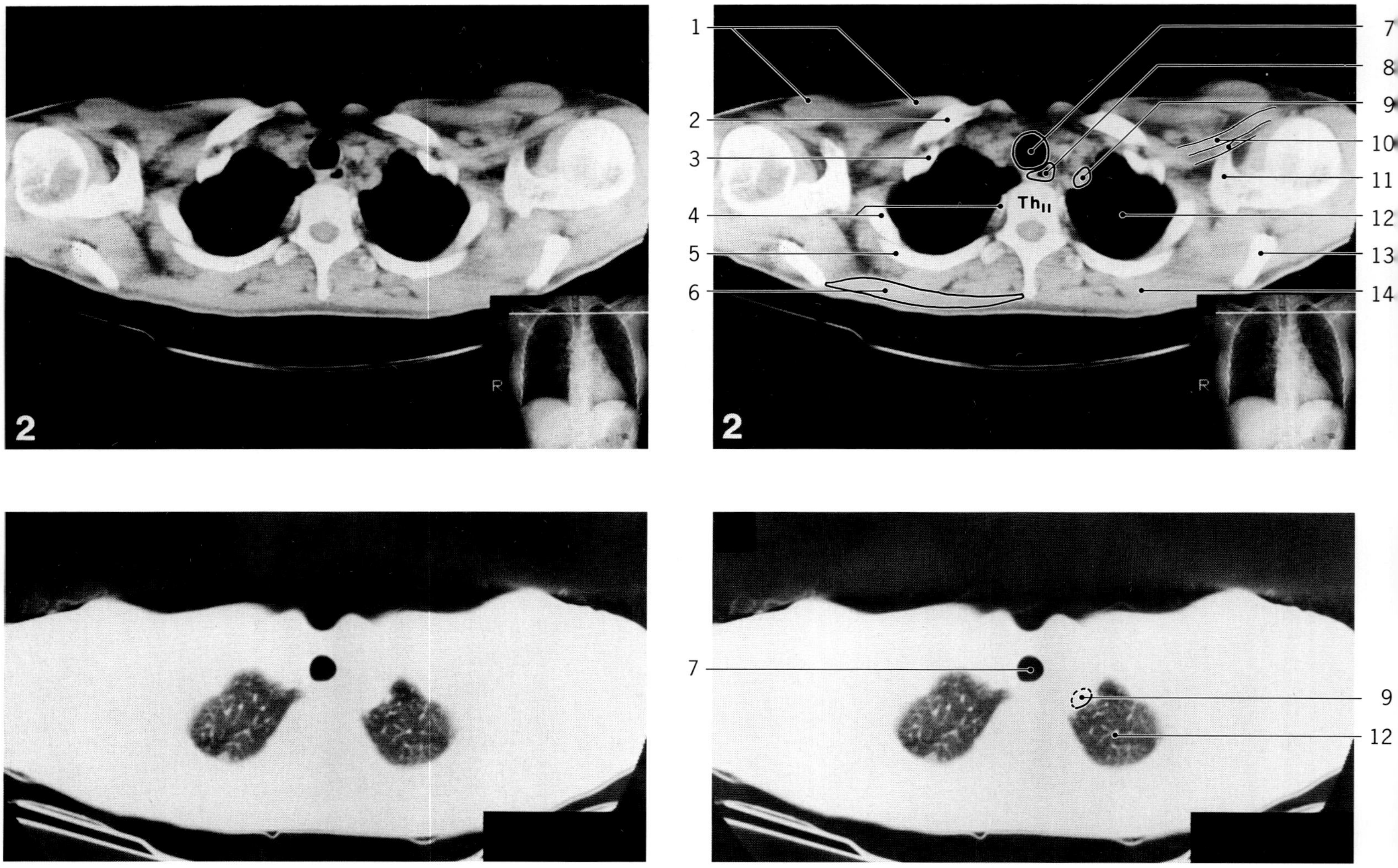

Thorax, axial CT

Scout view on page 204

1: Pectoralis major (arm elevated)
2: Clavicle
3: First rib
4: Second rib
5: Third rib
6: Trapezius
7: Trachea
8: Oesophagus
9: Left subclavian artery
10: Axillary vessels, and brachial plexus
11: Coracoid process
12: Apex of lung
13: Acromion
14: Levator scapulae

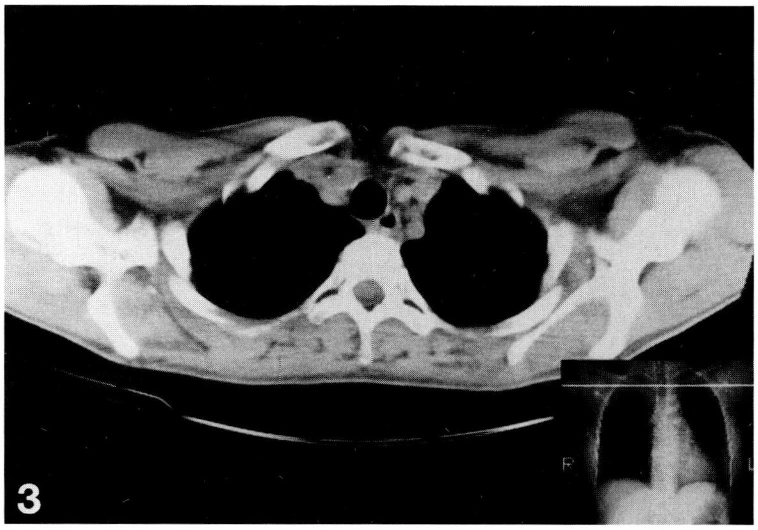

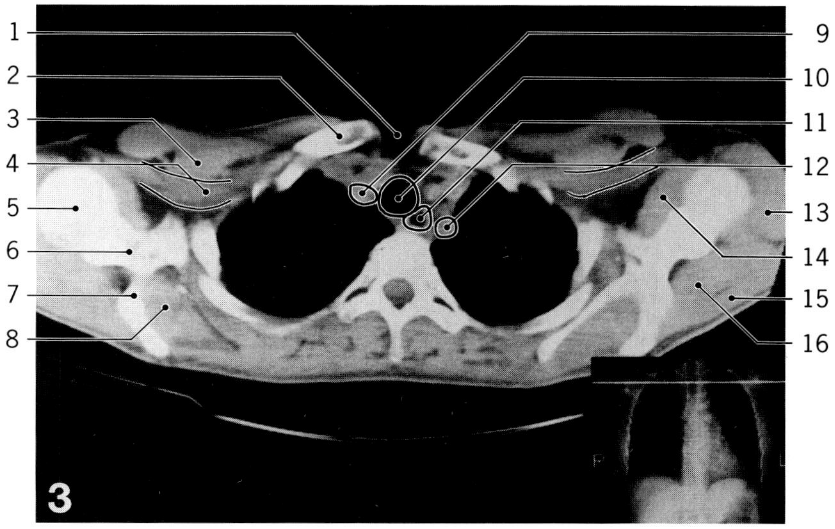

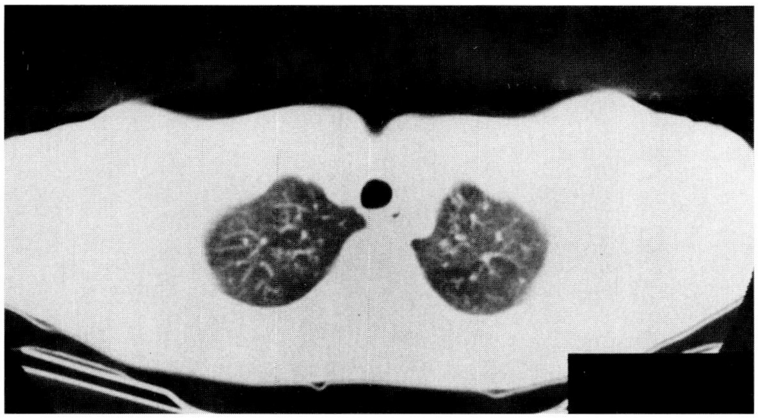

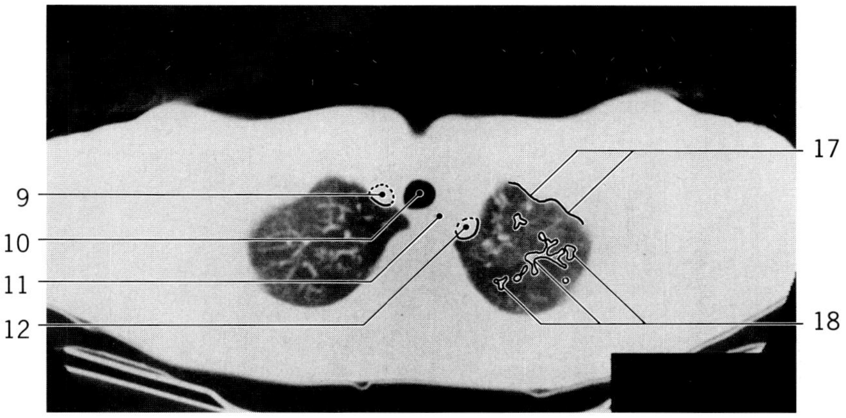

Thorax, axial CT

Scout view on page 204

1: Jugular notch
2: Clavicle
3: Pectoralis minor
4: Axillary vessels, and brachial plexus
5: Head of humerus
6: Neck of scapula
7: Spine of scapula
8: Supraspinatus
9: Right internal jugular vein
10: Trachea
11: Oesophagus (with air)
12: Left subclavian artery
13: Latissimus dorsi, and teres major (arms elevated)
14: Subscapularis
15: Deltoid
16: Infraspinatus, and teres minor
17: Impressions in lung from ribs
18: Lung vessels

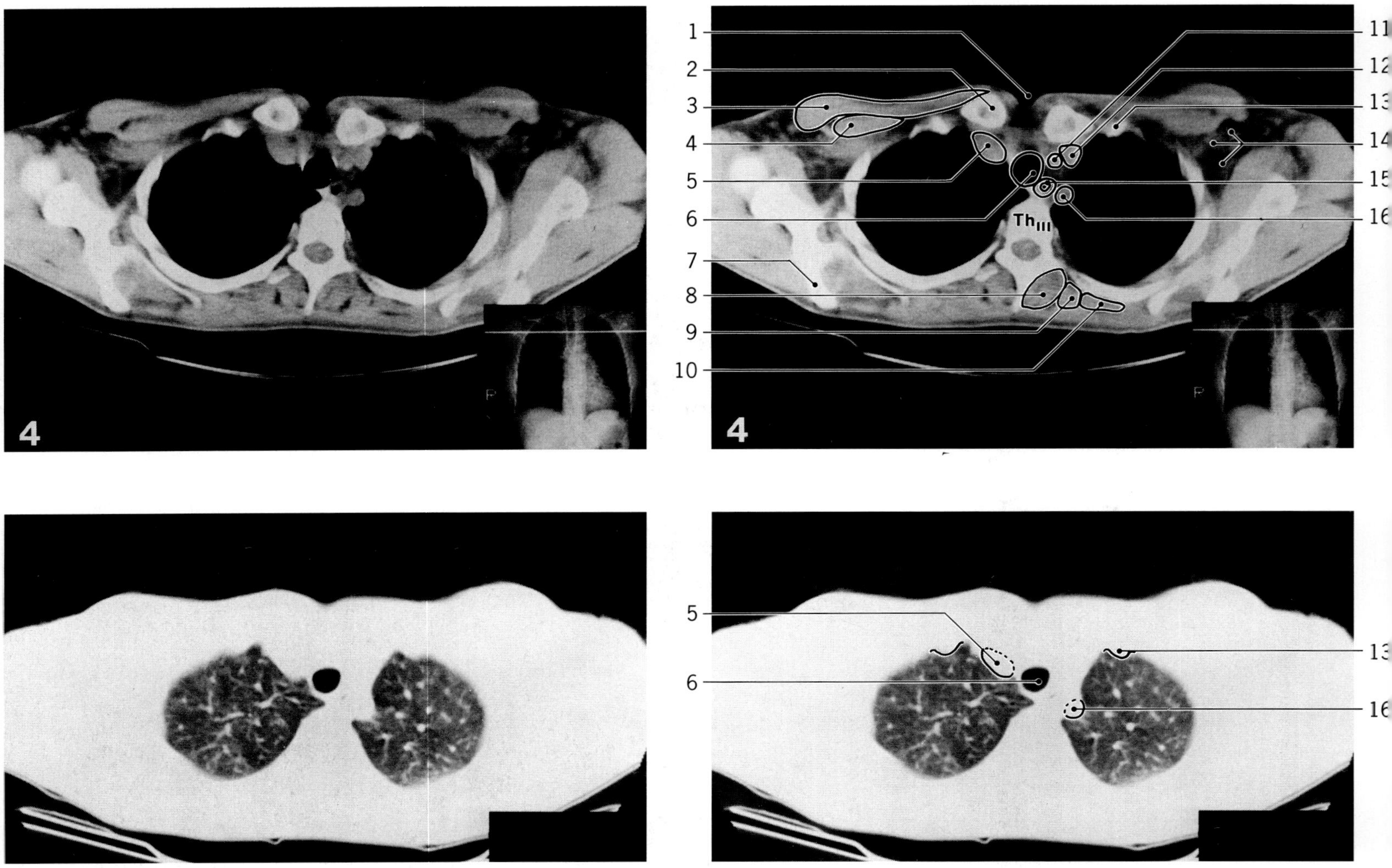

Thorax, axial CT

Scout view on page 204

1: Jugular notch
2: Sternal end of clavicle
3: Pectoralis major
4: Pectoralis minor
5: Right brachiocephalic vein
6: Trachea
7: Spine of scapula
8: Transversospinal muscles
9: Longissimus thoracis
10: Iliocostalis thoracis
11: Left common carotid artery
12: Left internal jugular vein
13: First rib
14: Axillary fat with lymph nodes and vessels
15: Oesophagus (with air)
16: Left subclavian artery

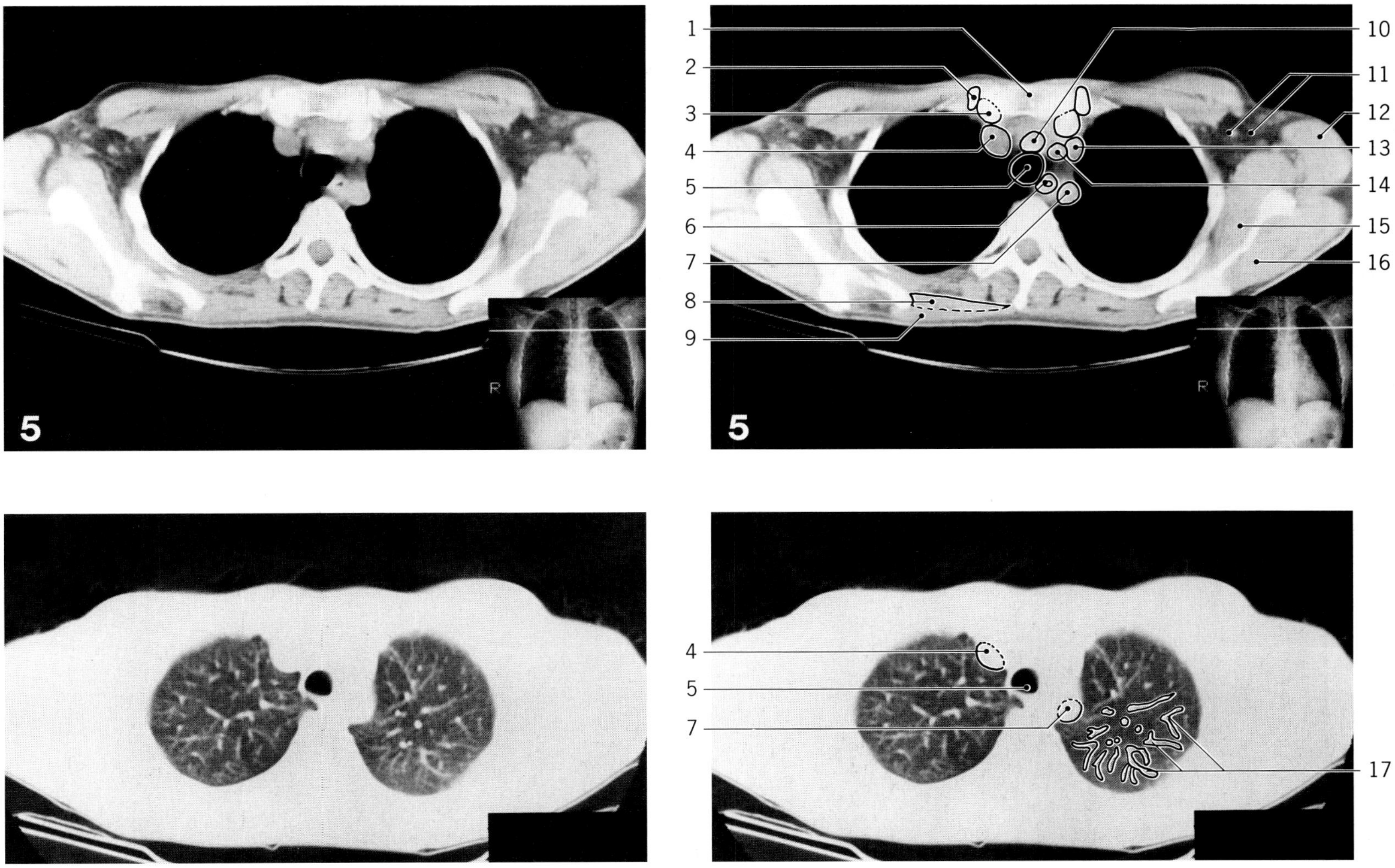

Thorax, axial CT

Scout view on page 204

1: Manubrium of sternum
2: First rib
3: Sternal end of clavicle
4: Right brachiocephalic vein
5: Trachea
6: Oesophagus
7: Left subclavian artery
8: Rhomboideus
9: Trapezius
10: Brachiocephalic trunk
11: Axillary fat with lymph nodes and vessels
12: Latissimus dorsi, and teres major (arms elevated)
13: Left internal jugular vein
14: Left common carotid artery
15: Subscapularis
16: Infraspinatus
17: Lung vessels

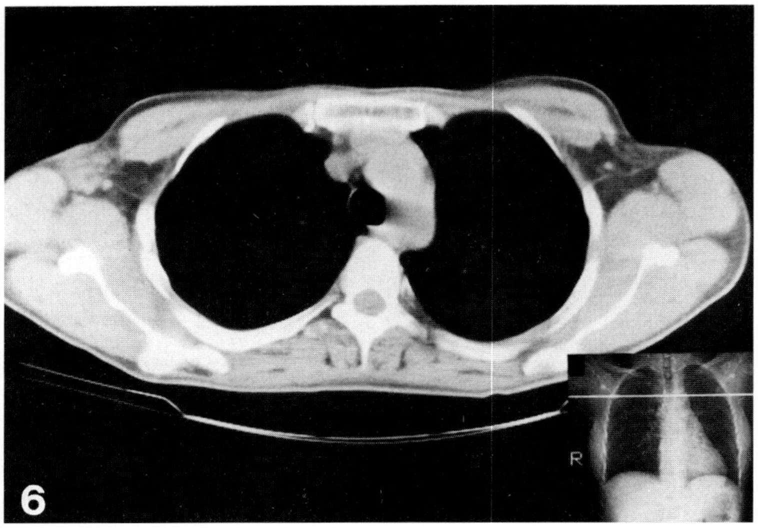

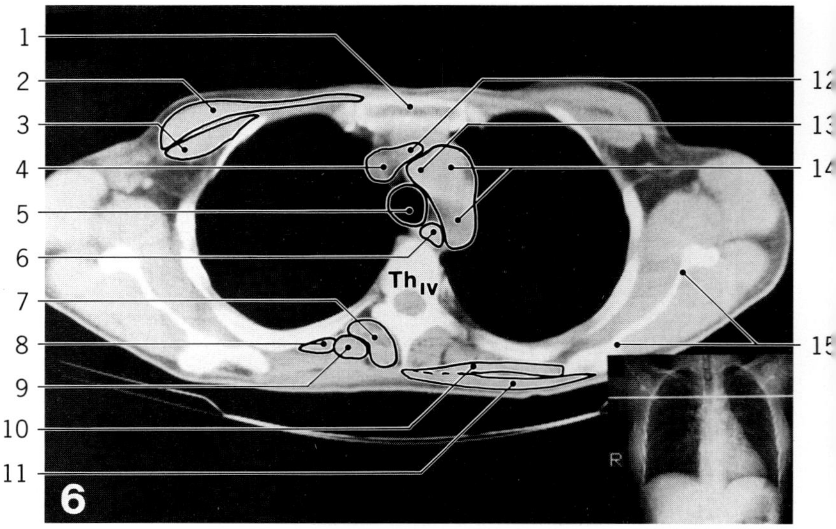

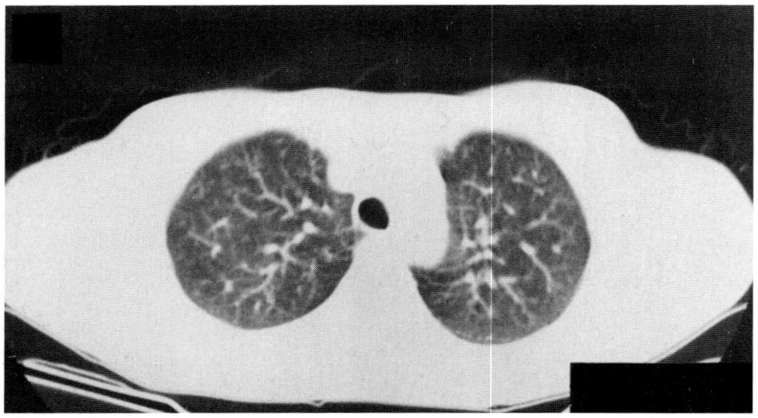

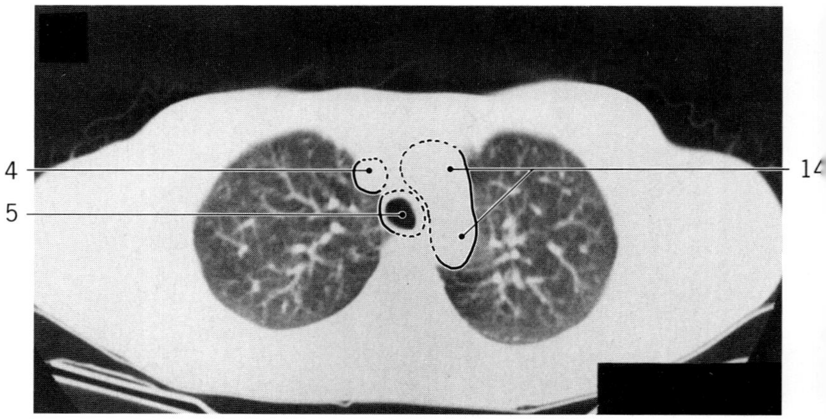

Thorax, axial CT

Scout view on page 204

1: Manubrium of sternum
2: Pectoralis major
3: Pectoralis minor
4: Right brachiocephalic vein
5: Trachea
6: Oesophagus
7: Transversospinal muscles
8: Iliocostalis thoracis
9: Longissimus thoracis
10: Rhomboideus
11: Trapezius
12: Left brachiocephalic vein
13: Brachiocephalic trunk (origin)
14: Aortic arch
15: Scapula

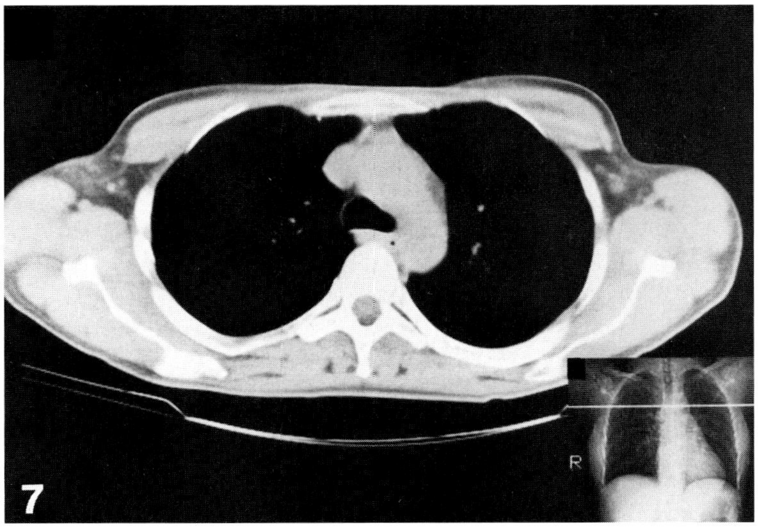

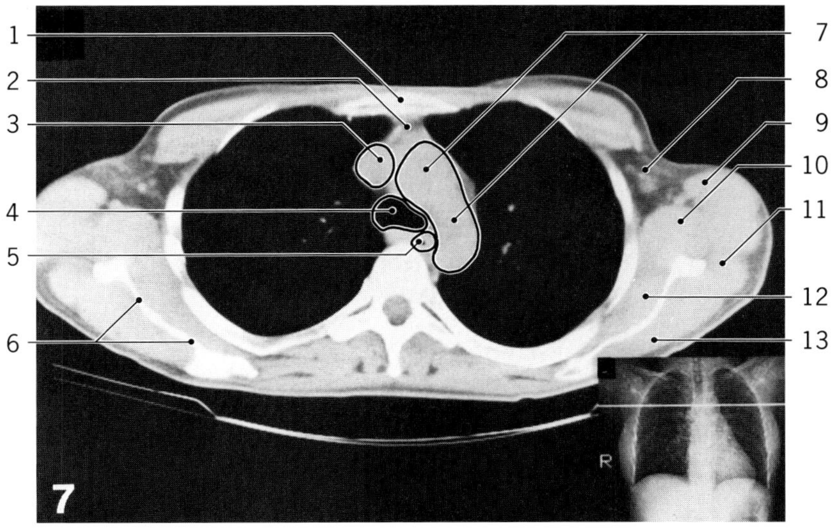

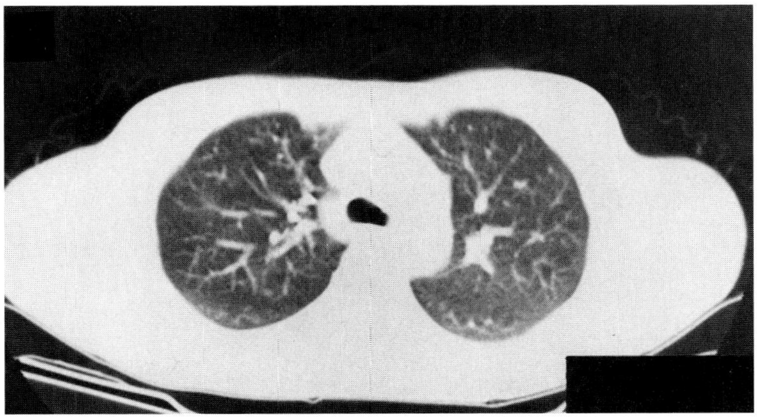

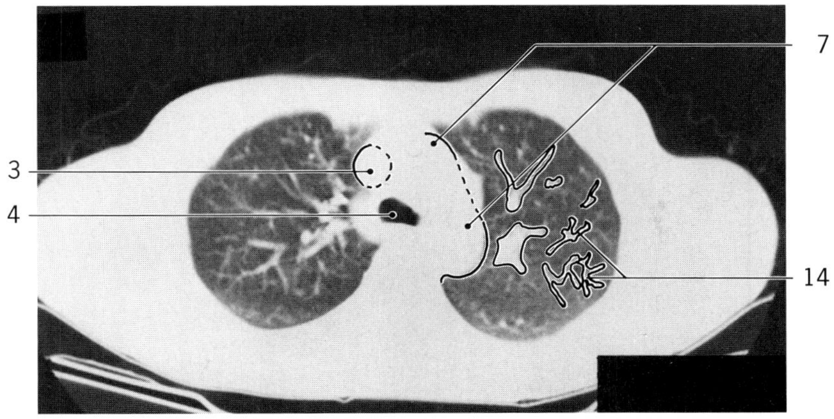

Thorax, axial CT

Scout view on page 204

1: Sternum
2: Superior mediastinum with thymic residues
3: Superior caval vein
4: Trachea
5: Oesophagus
6: Scapula
7: Aortic arch
8: Axillary fat with lymph nodes and vessels
9: Latissimus dorsi (arm elevated)
10: Teres major
11: Teres minor
12: Subscapularis
13: Infraspinatus
14: Lung vessels

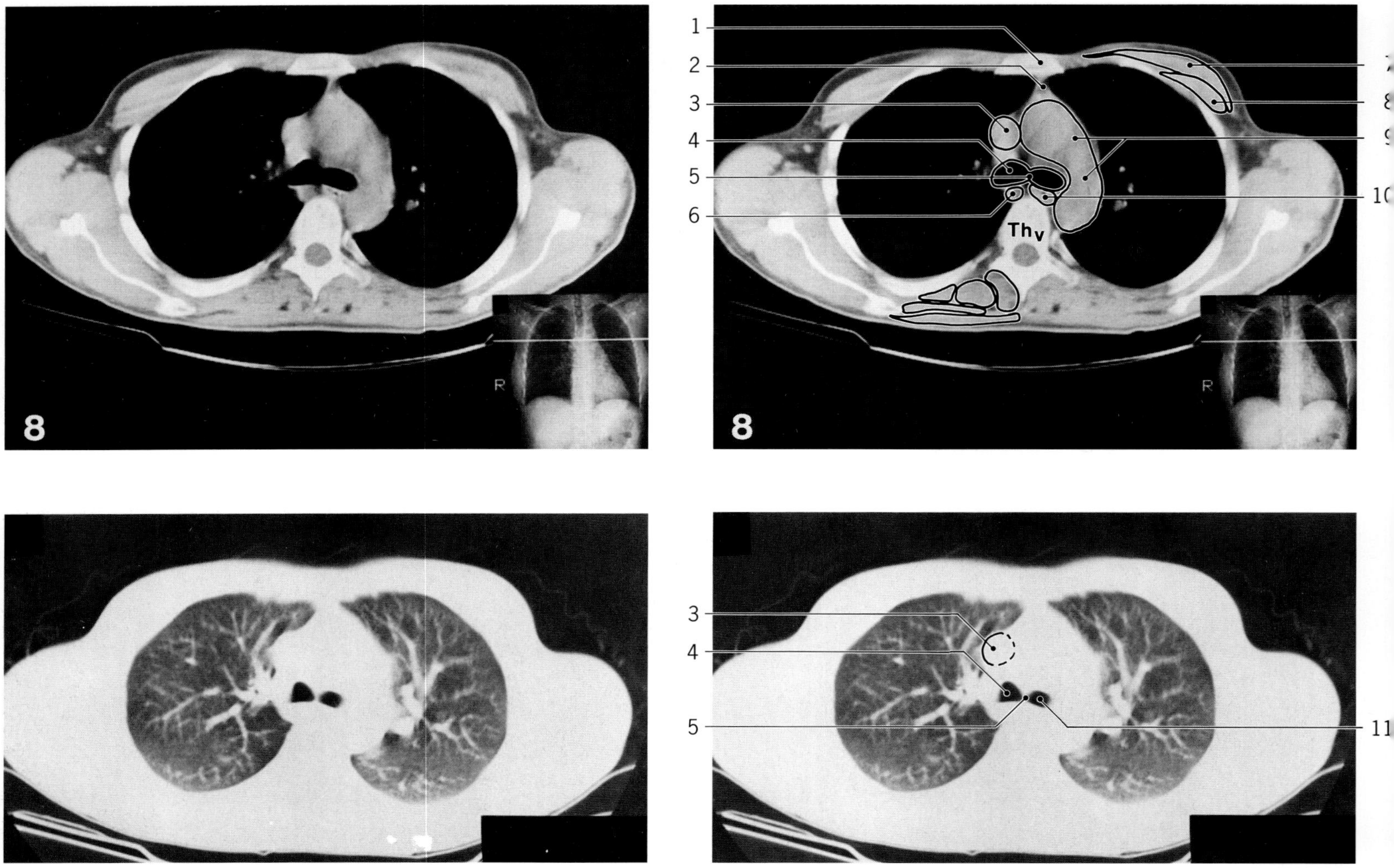

Thorax, axial CT

Scout view on page 204

1: Sternum
2: Anterior mediastinum
3: Superior caval vein
4: Right principal bronchus
5: Carina
6: Azygos vein
7: Pectoralis major
8: Pectoralis minor
9: Aortic arch
10: Oesophagus
11: Left principal bronchus

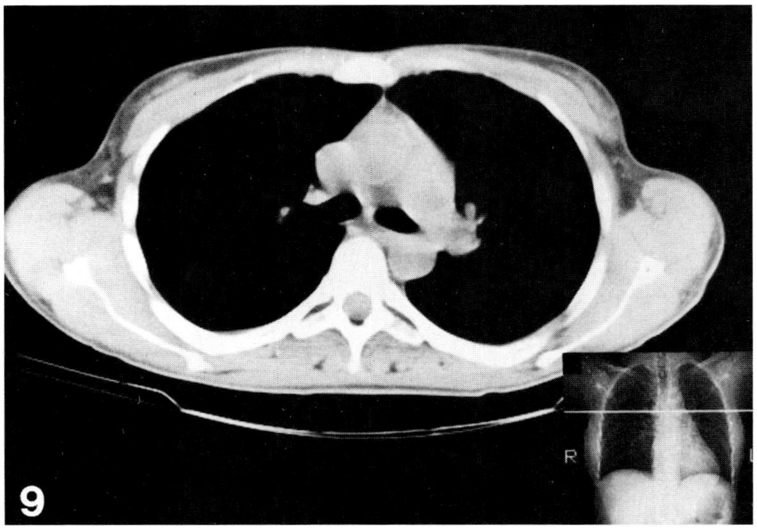

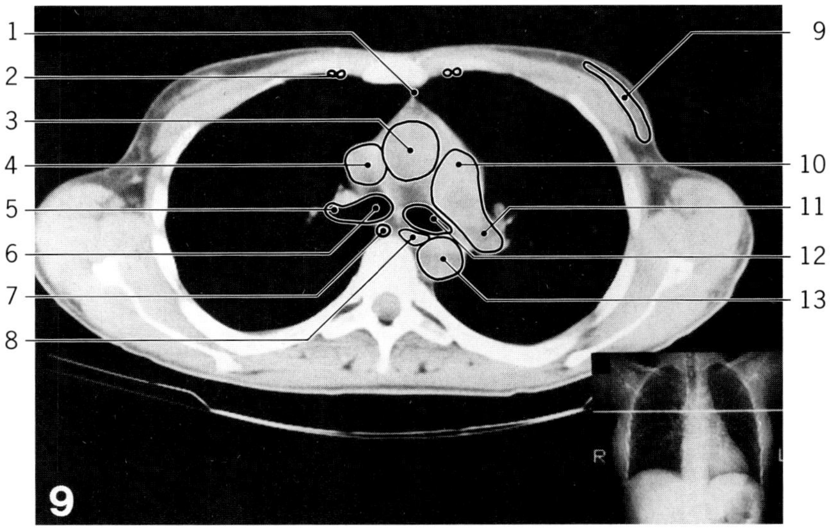

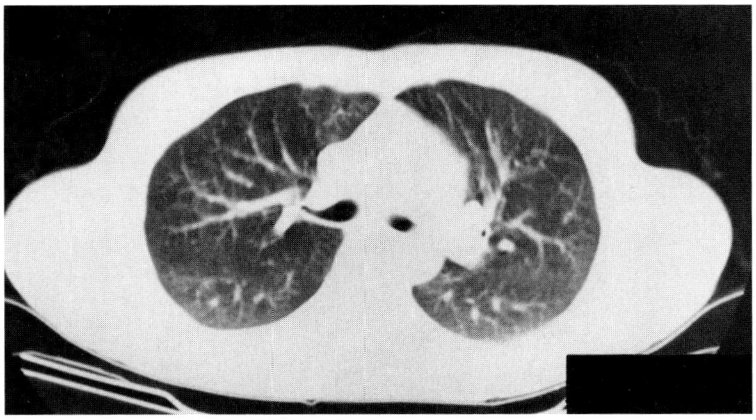

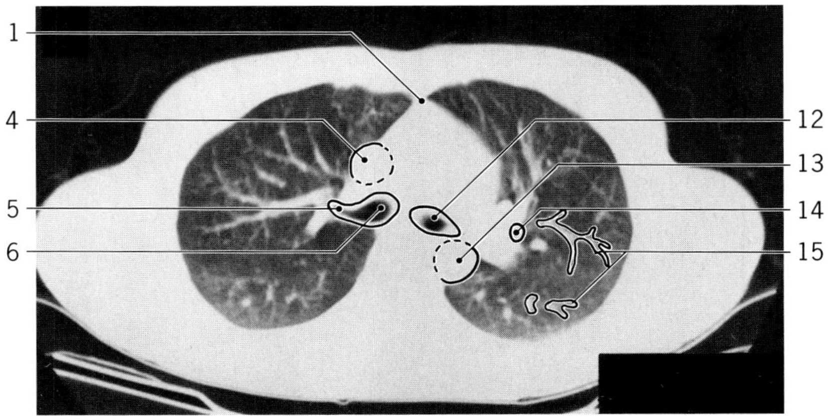

Thorax, axial CT

Scout view on page 204

1: Anterior mediastinum
2: Internal thoracic vein and artery
3: Ascending aorta
4: Superior caval vein
5: Right superior lobar bronchus
6: Right principal bronchus
7: Azygos vein
8: Oesophagus
9: Axillary process of mammary gland
10: Pulmonary trunk
11: Left pulmonary artery
12: Left principal bronchus
13: Thoracic (descending) aorta
14: Left superior lobar bronchus
15: Lung vessels

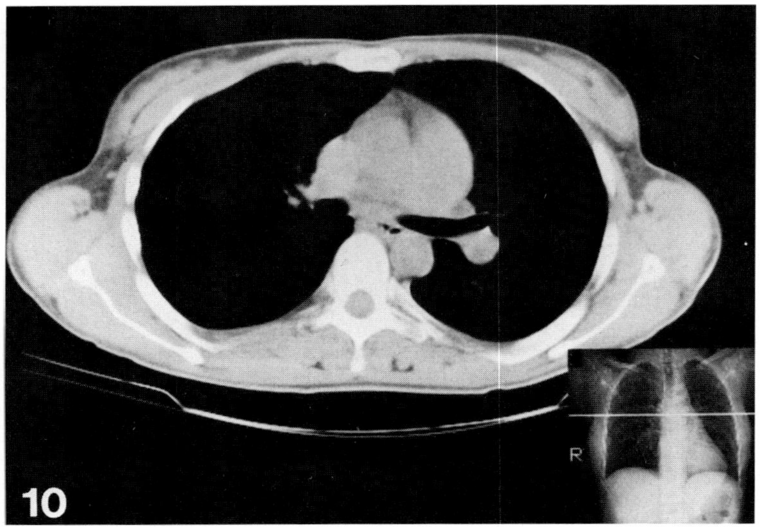

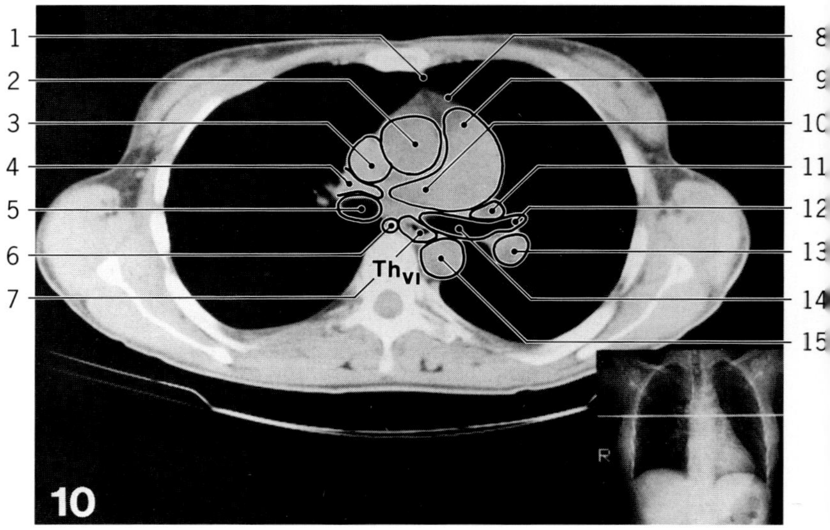

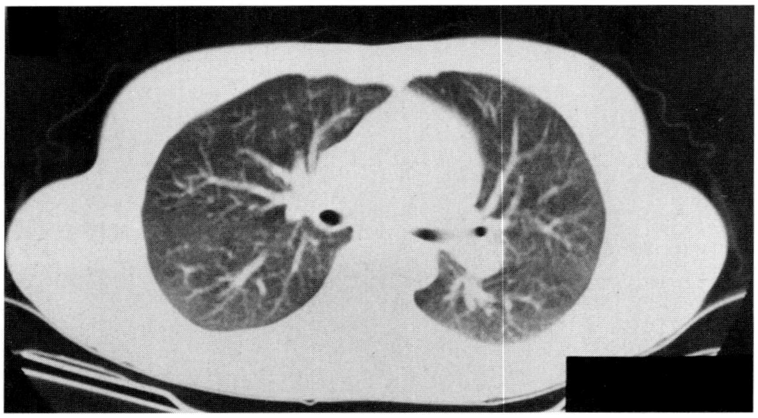

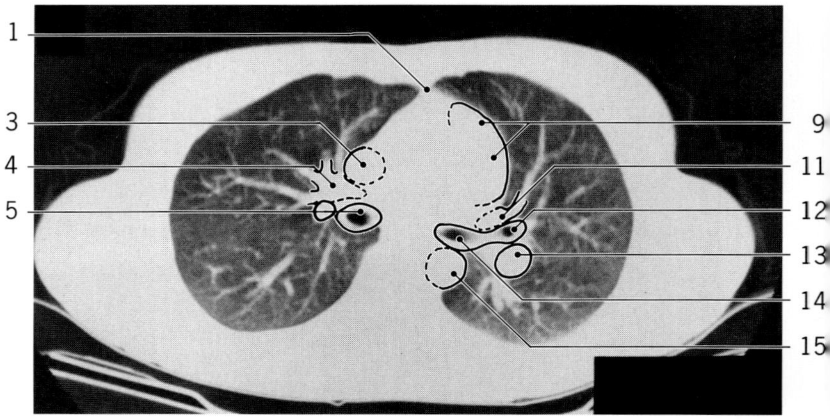

Thorax, axial CT

Scout view on page 204

1: Anterior mediastinum
2: Ascending aorta
3: Superior caval vein
4: Right superior pulmonary vein, and apical branches of right pulmonary artery
5: Right intermediate bronchus
6: Azygos vein
7: Oesophagus
8: Pericardium
9: Pulmonary trunk
10: Right pulmonary artery
11: Left superior pulmonary vein
12: Left superior lobar bronchus
13: Left pulmonary artery
14: Left principal bronchus
15: Thoracic aorta

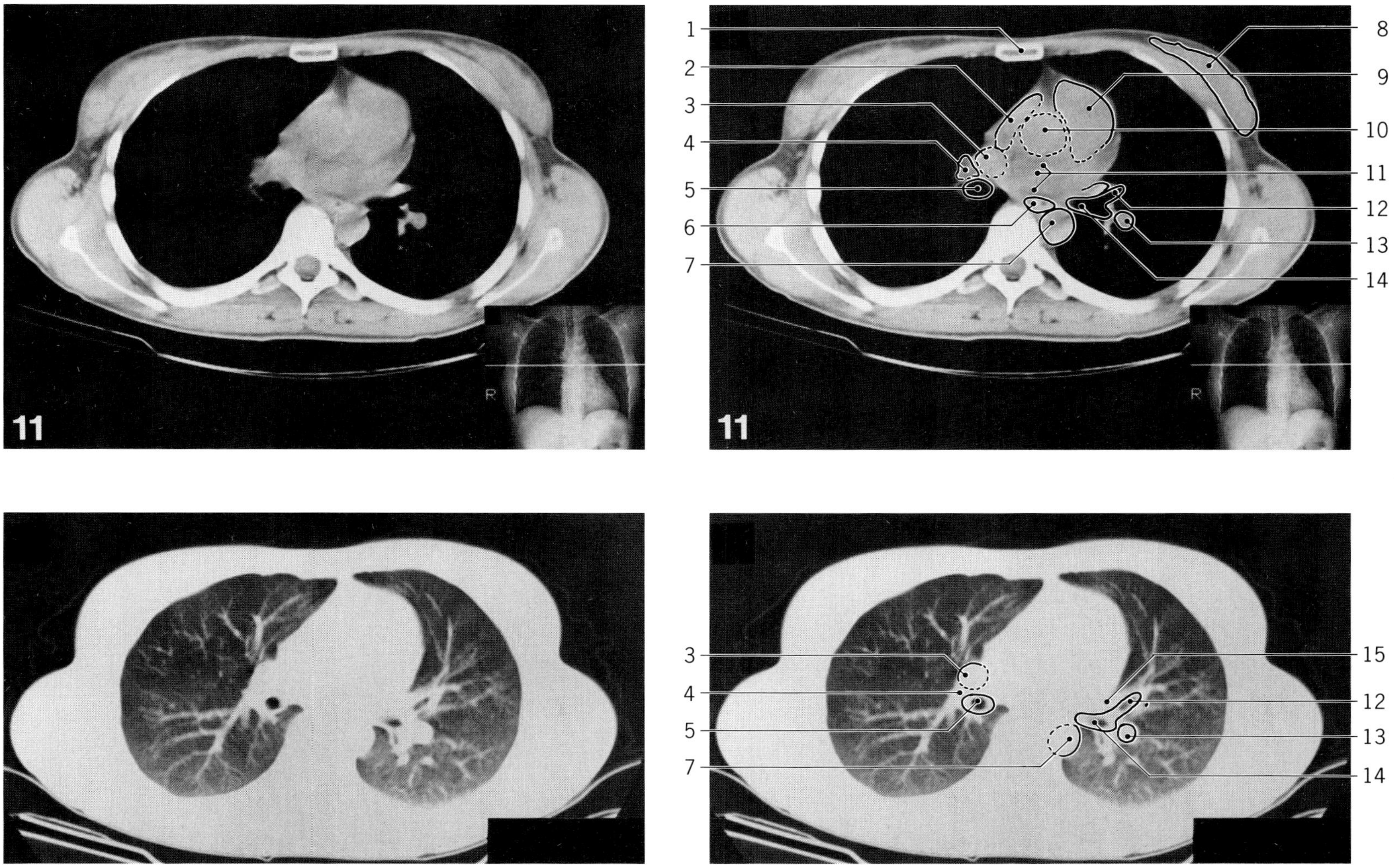

Thorax, axial CT

Scout view on page 204

1: Body of sternum
2: Right auricle
3: Superior caval vein
4: Branches of right pulmonary artery, and superior pulmonary vein
5: Right intermediate bronchus
6: Oesophagus
7: Thoracic aorta
8: Body of mammary gland
9: Pulmonary trunk
10: Ascending aorta
11: Left atrium
12: Left superior lobar bronchus
13: Branch of left pulmonary artery
14: Left intermediate bronchus
15: Left superior pulmonary vein

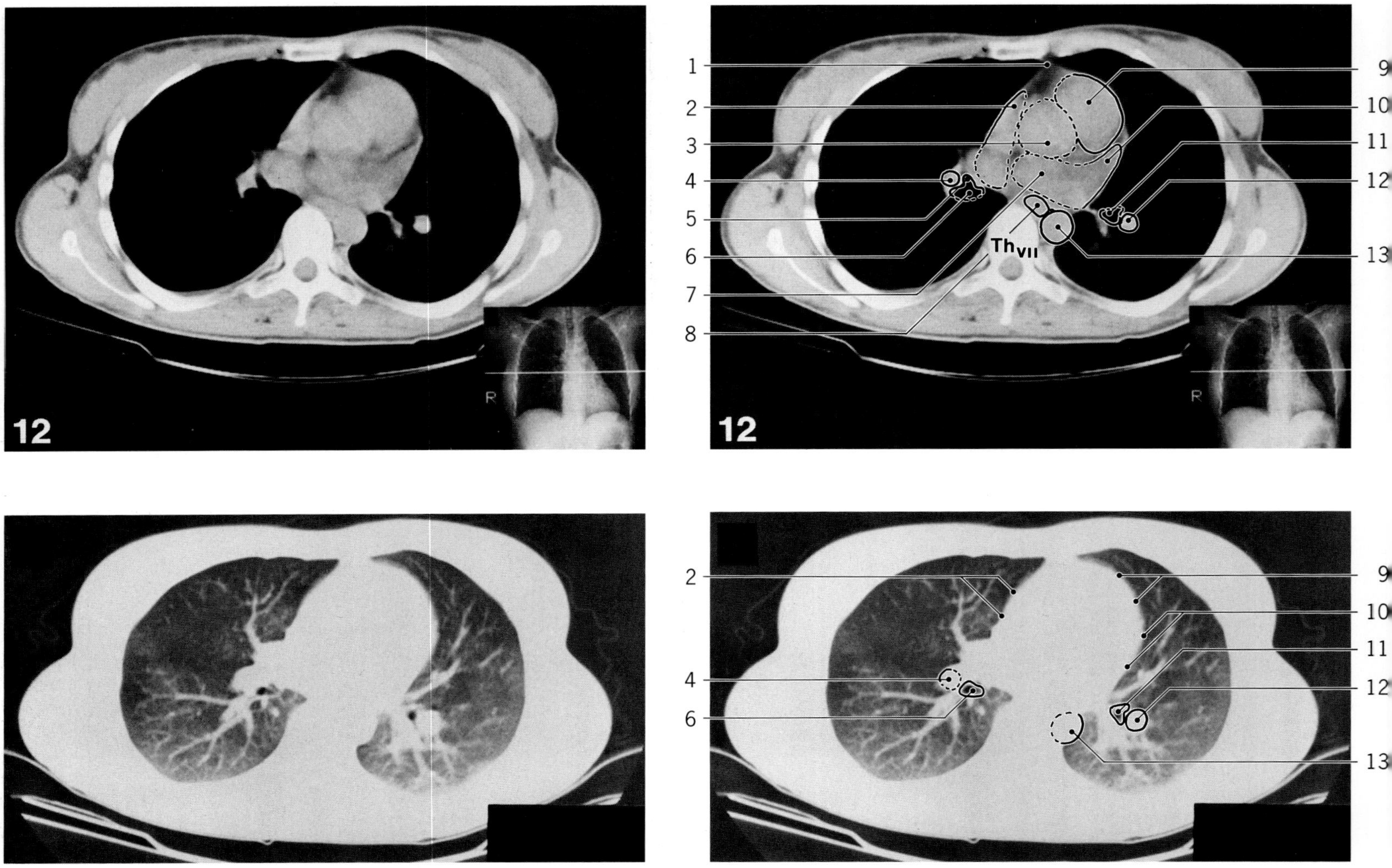

Thorax, axial CT

Scout view on page 204

1: Anterior mediastinum
2: Right auricle
3: Aortic bulb
4: Right pulmonary artery, branch to middle and lower lobes
5: Middle lobar bronchus
6: Right inferior lobar bronchus
7: Left atrium
8: Oesophagus
9: Truncus arteriosus
10: Left auricle
11: Left inferior lobar bronchus
12: Left pulmonary artery, branch to lower lobe
13: Thoracic aorta

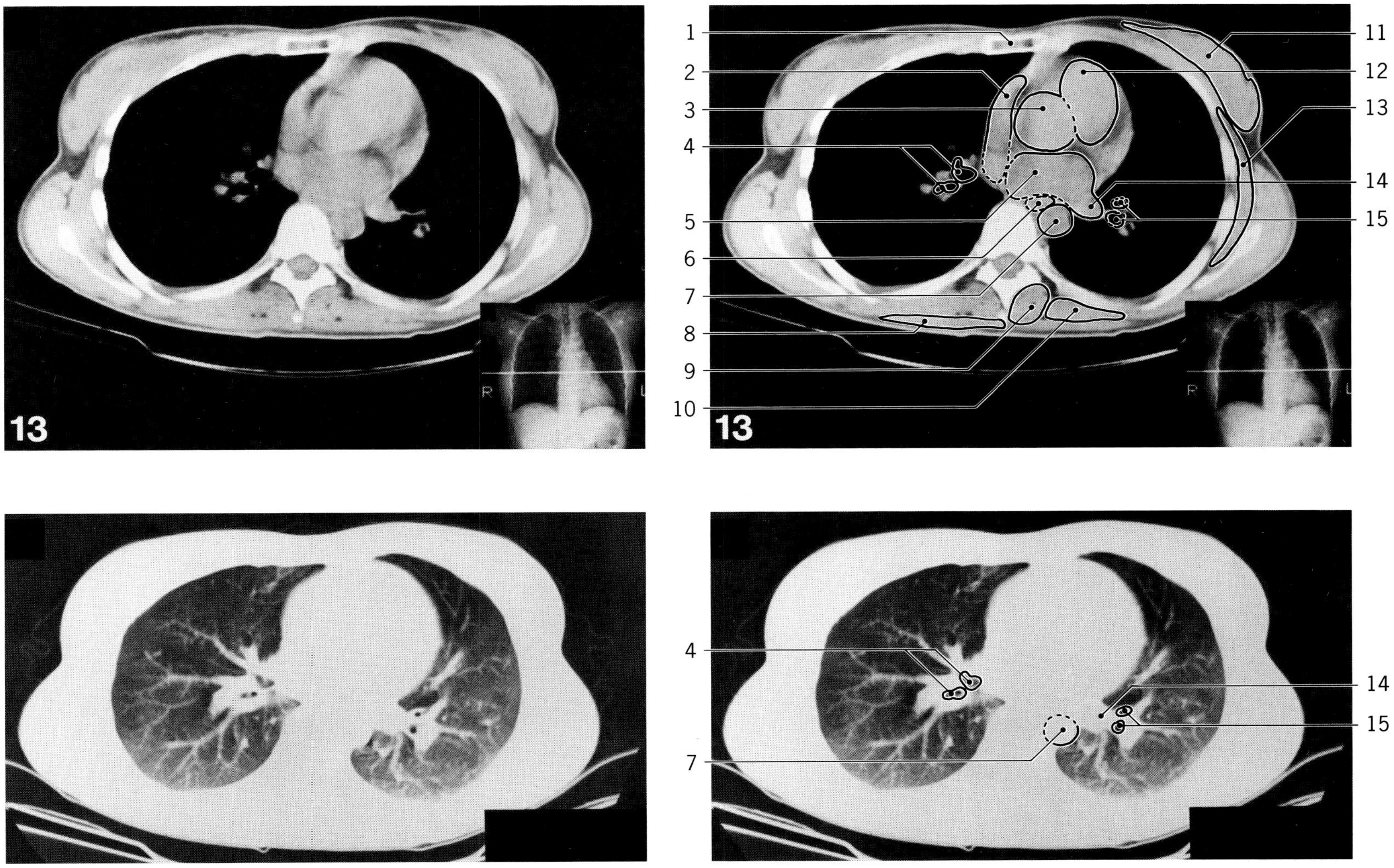

Thorax, axial CT

Scout view on page 204

1: Body of sternum
2: Right auricle
3: Aortic bulb
4: Bronchi to middle and lower lobes
5: Left atrium
6: Oesophagus
7: Thoracic aorta
8: Trapezius
9: Transversospinal muscles
10: Longissimus thoracis, and iliocostalis thoracis
11: Body of mammary gland
12: Truncus arteriosus
13: Serratus anterior
14: Left inferior pulmonary vein
15: Bronchi to left lower lobe

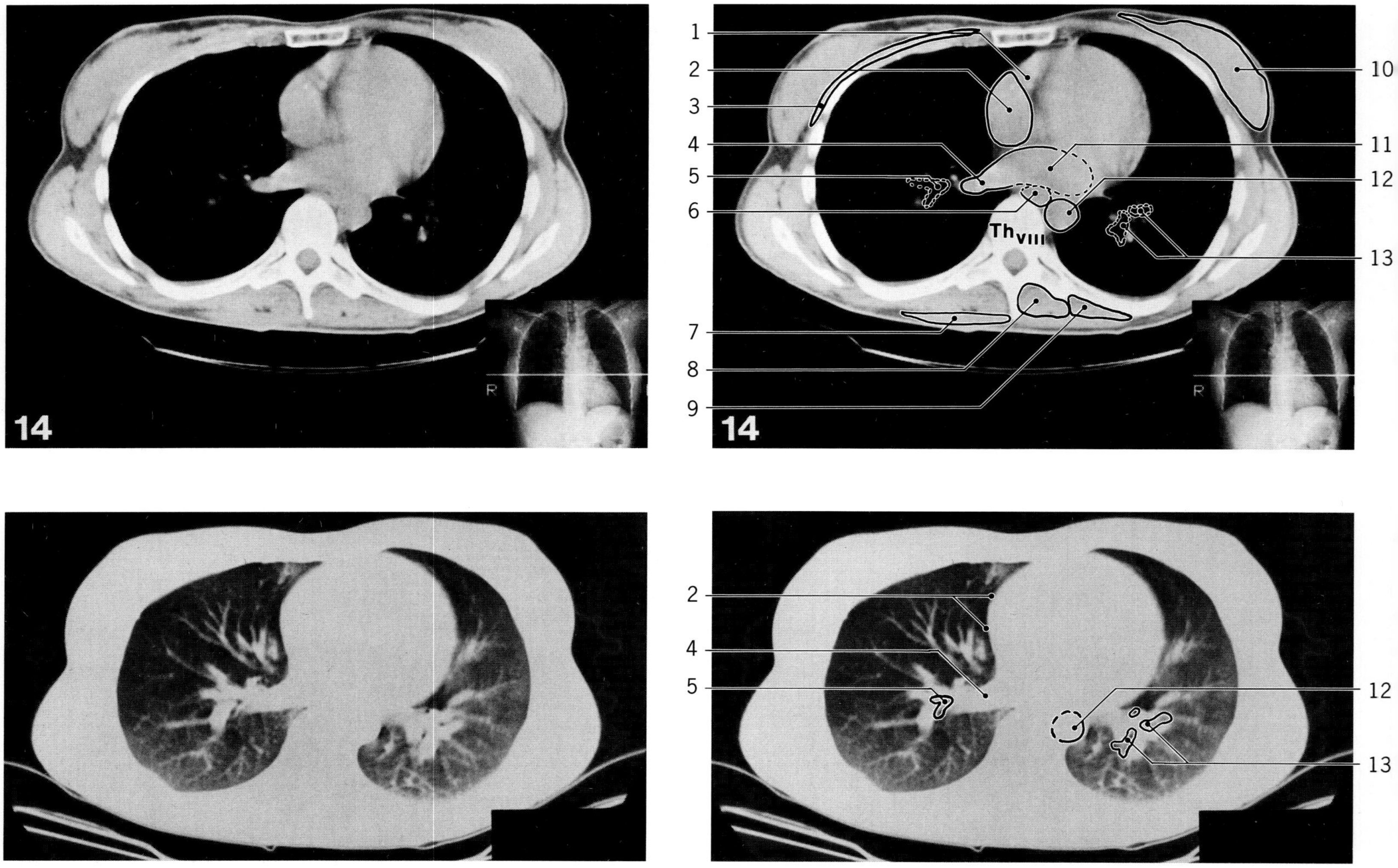

Thorax, axial CT

Scout view on page 204

1: Coronary sulcus with right coronary artery
2: Right atrium
3: Pectoralis major
4: Right inferior pulmonary vein
5: Segmental bronchi to right lower lobe
6: Oesophagus
7: Trapezius
8: Transversospinal muscles
9: Longissimus thoracis, and iliocostalis thoracis
10: Body of mammary gland
11: Left atrium
12: Thoracic aorta
13: Segmental bronchi to left lower lobe

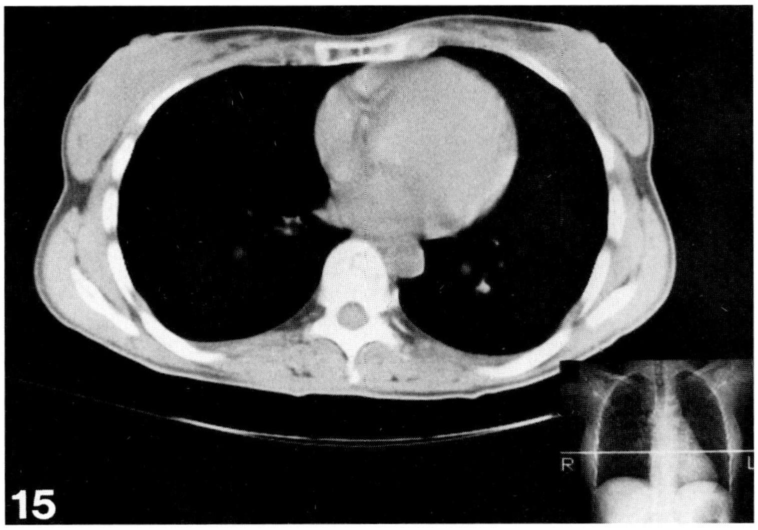

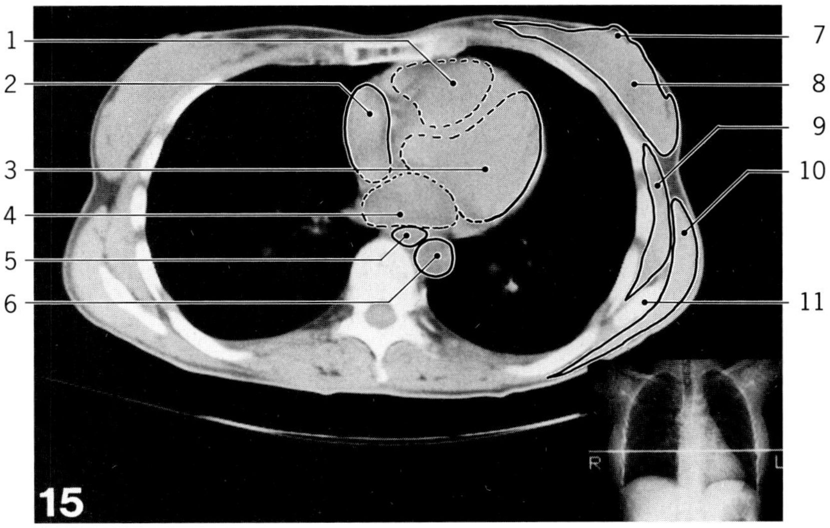

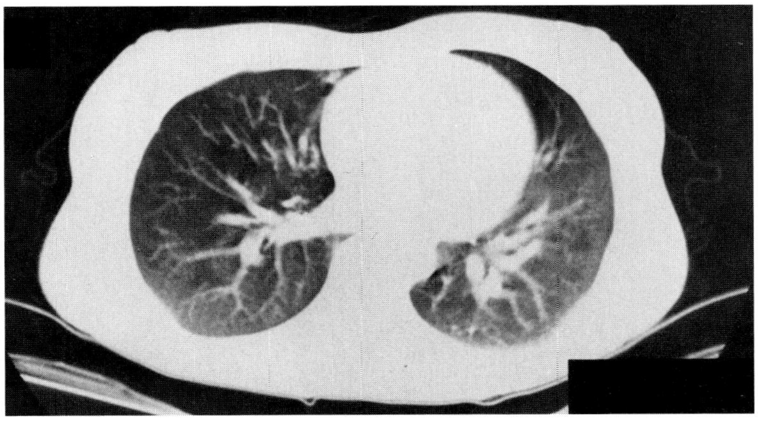

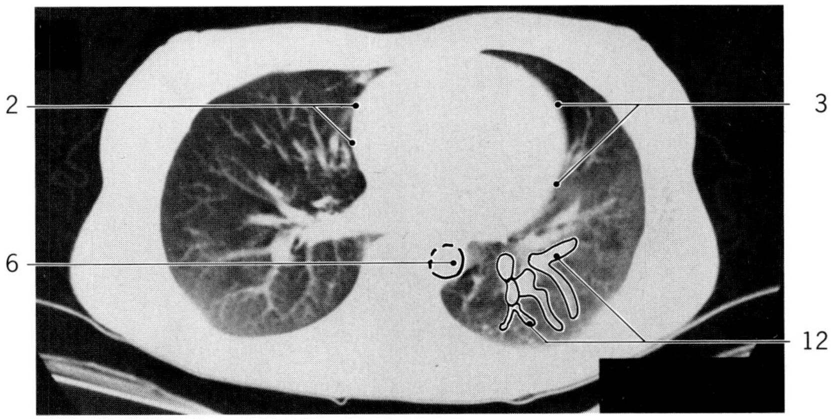

Thorax, axial CT

Scout view on page 204

1: Right ventricle
2: Right atrium
3: Left ventricle
4: Left atrium
5: Oesophagus
6: Thoracic aorta
7: Nipple
8: Body of mammary gland
9: Serratus anterior
10: Latissimus dorsi
11: Inferior angle of scapula
12: Lung vessels

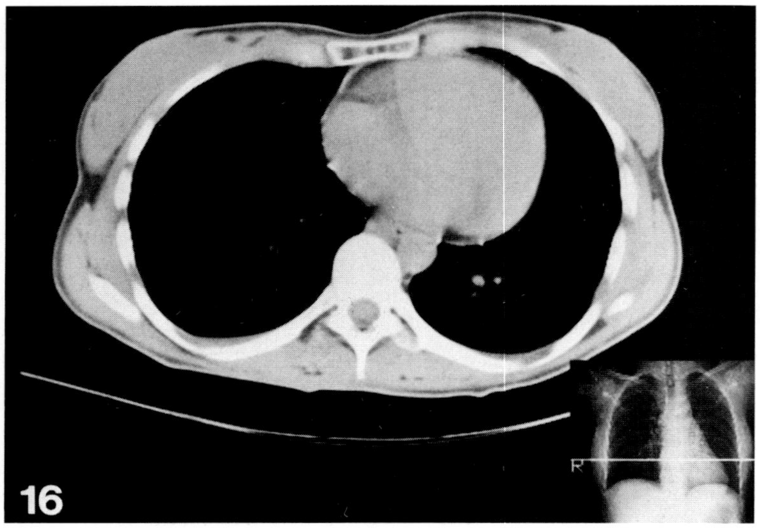

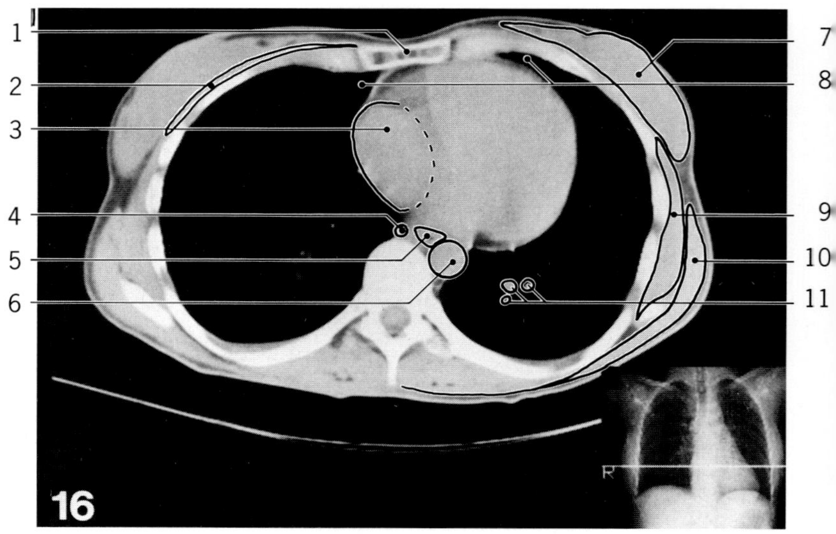

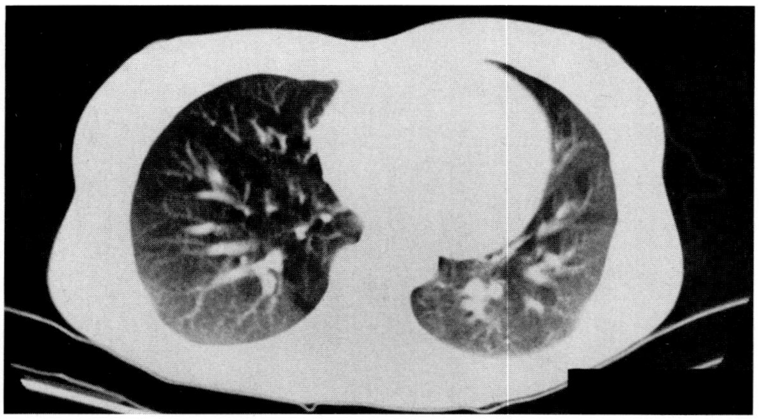

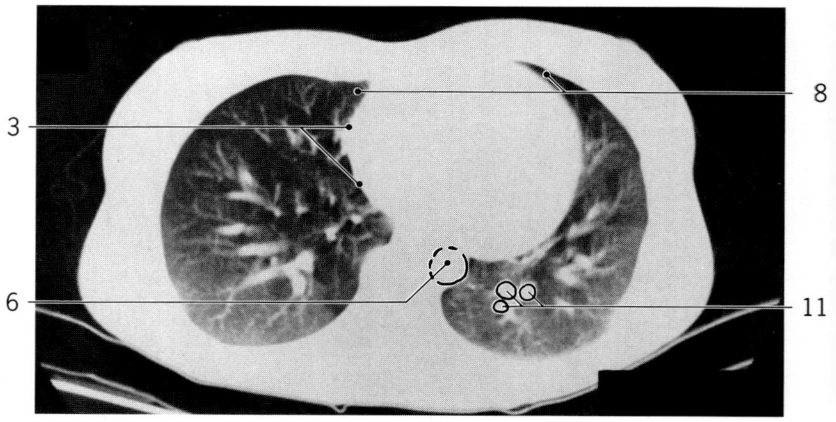

Thorax, axial CT

Scout view on page 204

1: Body of sternum
2: Pectoralis major
3: Right atrium
4: Azygos vein
5: Oesophagus
6: Thoracic aorta
7: Body of mammary gland
8: Costomediastinal sulcus
9: Serratus anterior
10: Latissimus dorsi
11: Lung vessels

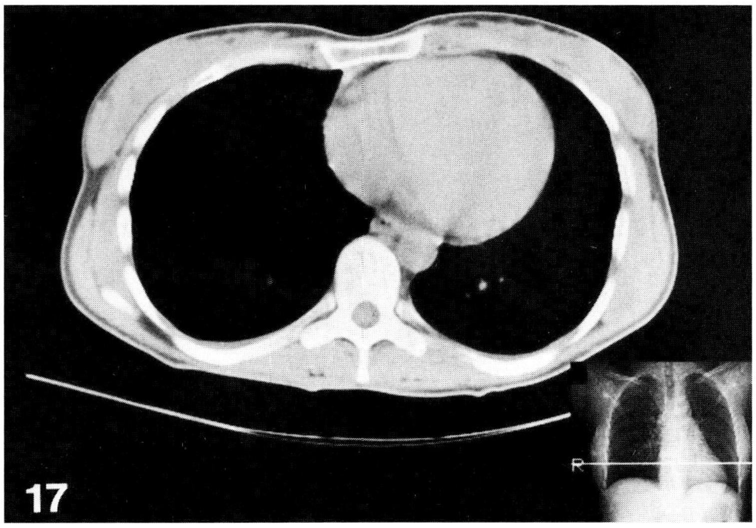

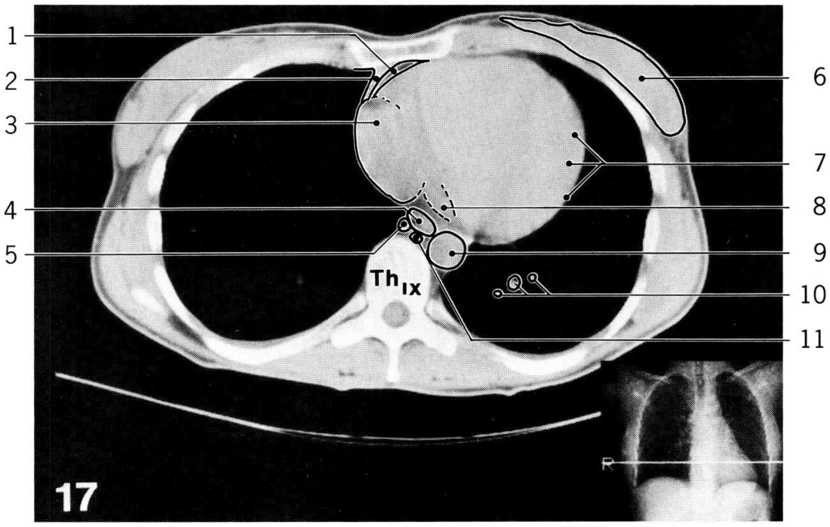

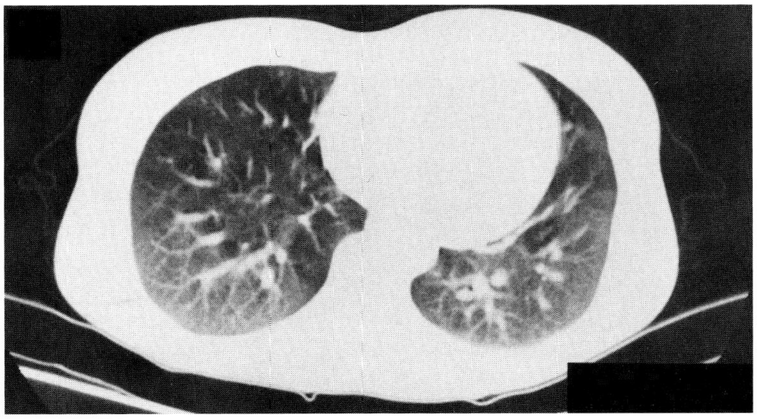

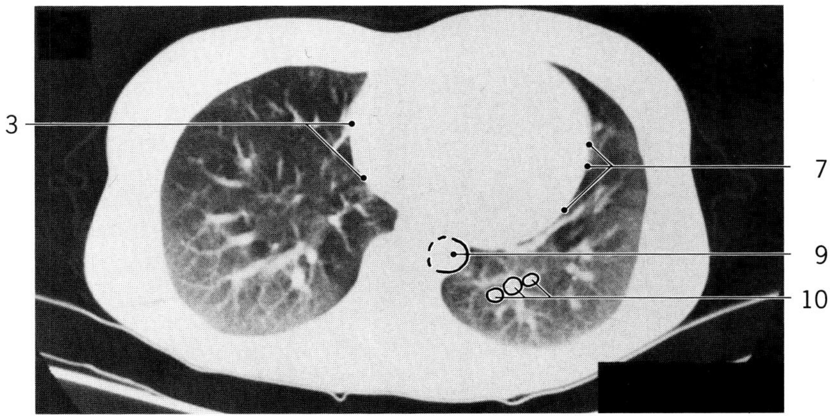

Thorax, axial CT

Scout view on page 204

1: Pericardial cavity with small volume of fluid
2: Pleura and pericardial sac
3: Right atrium
4: Oesophagus
5: Azygos vein
6: Body of mammary gland
7: Left ventricle
8: Coronary sinus
9: Thoracic aorta
10: Lung vessels
11: Thoracic duct

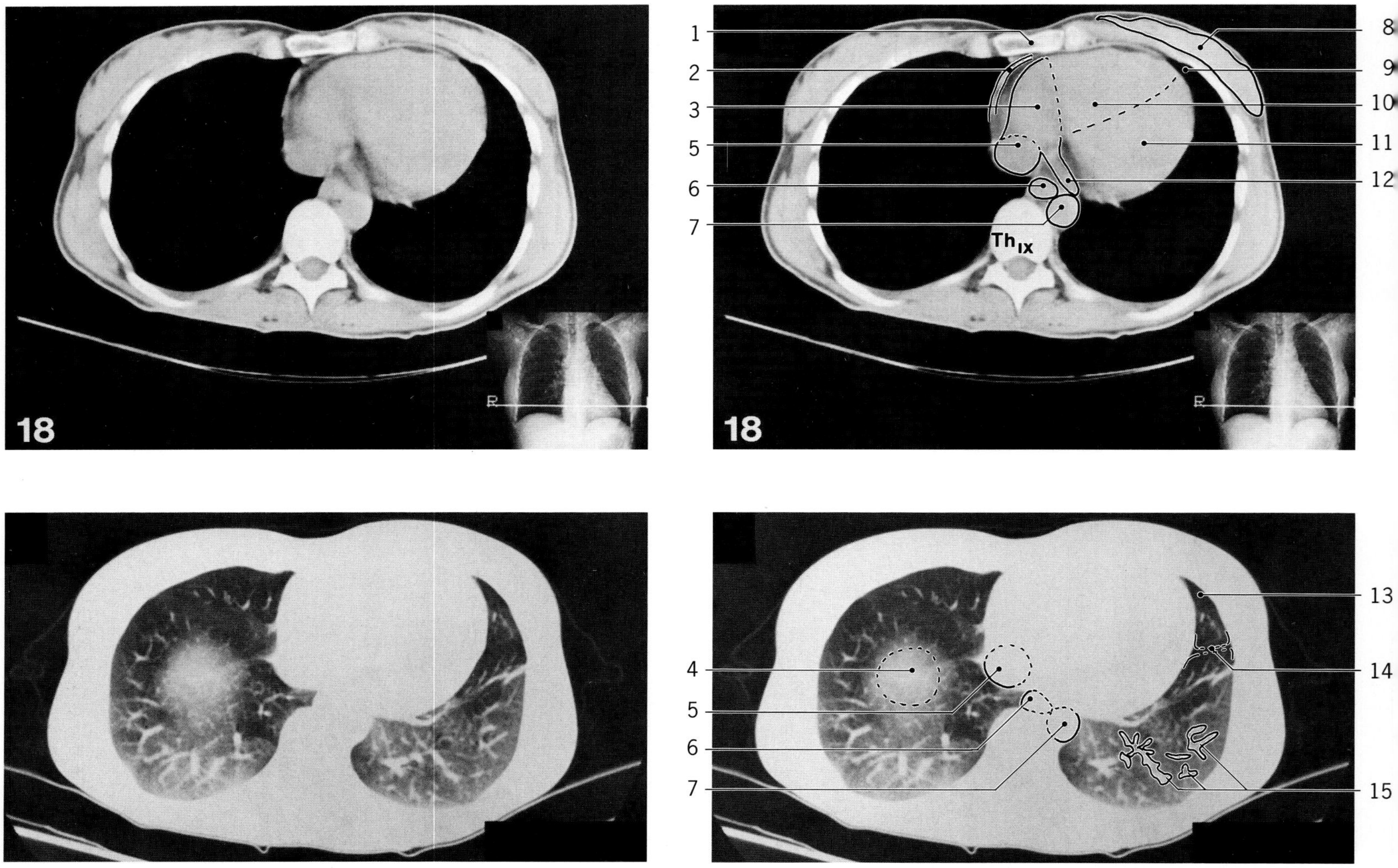

Thorax, axial CT

Scout view on page 204

1: Body of sternum
2: Pleura and pericardial sac
3: Right atrium
4: Diaphragm
5: Inferior caval vein
6: Oesophagus
7: Thoracic aorta
8: Mammary gland
9: Costomediastinal sulcus
10: Right ventricle
11: Left ventricle
12: Coronary sinus
13: Lingula of left lung
14: Oblique fissure of left lung
15: Lung vessels

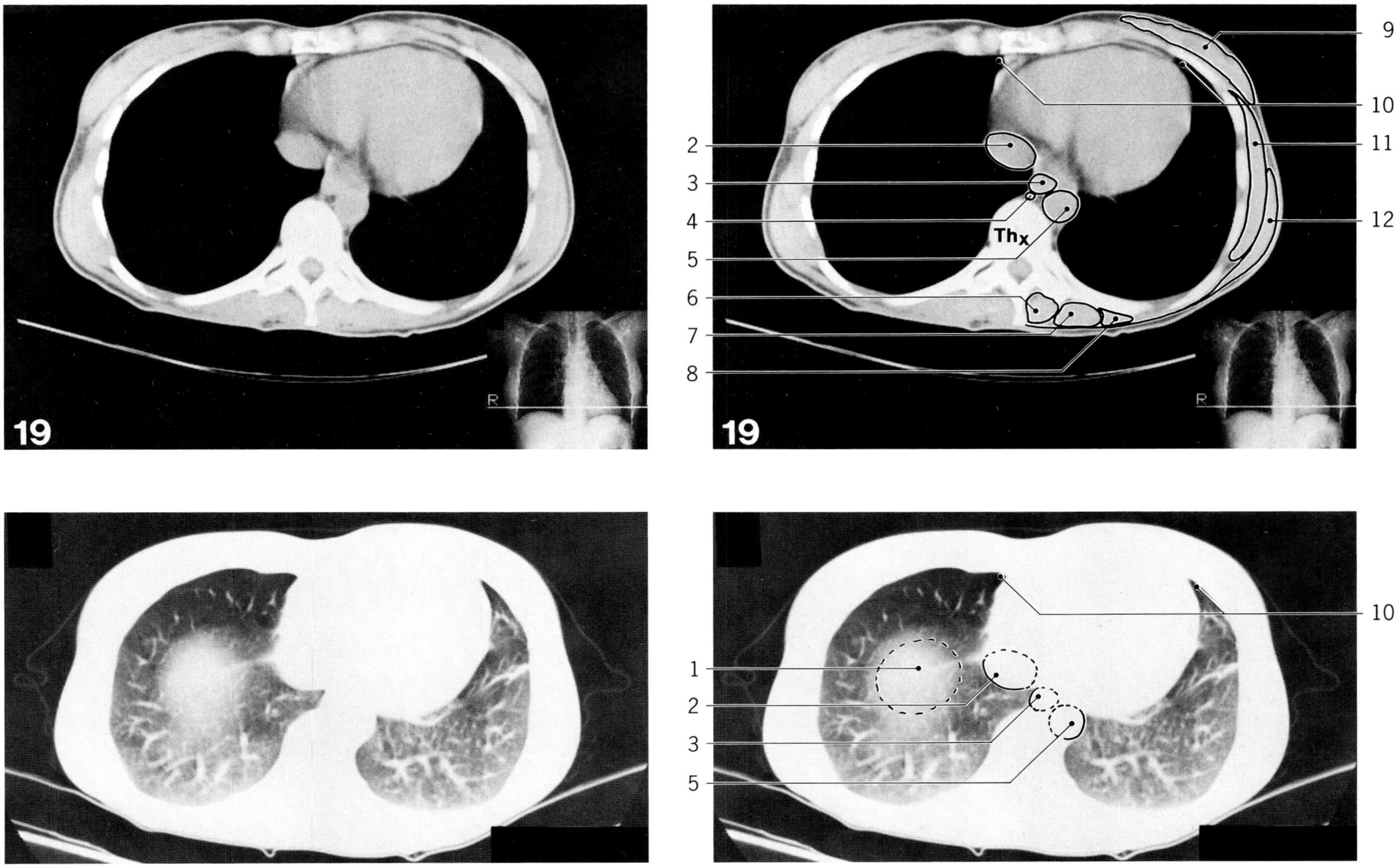

Thorax, axial CT

Scout view on page 204

1: Diaphragm
2: Inferior caval vein
3: Oesophagus
4: Azygos vein
5: Thoracic aorta
6: Transversospinal muscles
7: Longissimus
8: Iliocostalis
9: Mammary gland
10: Costomediastinal sulcus
11: Serratus anterior
12: Latissimus dorsi

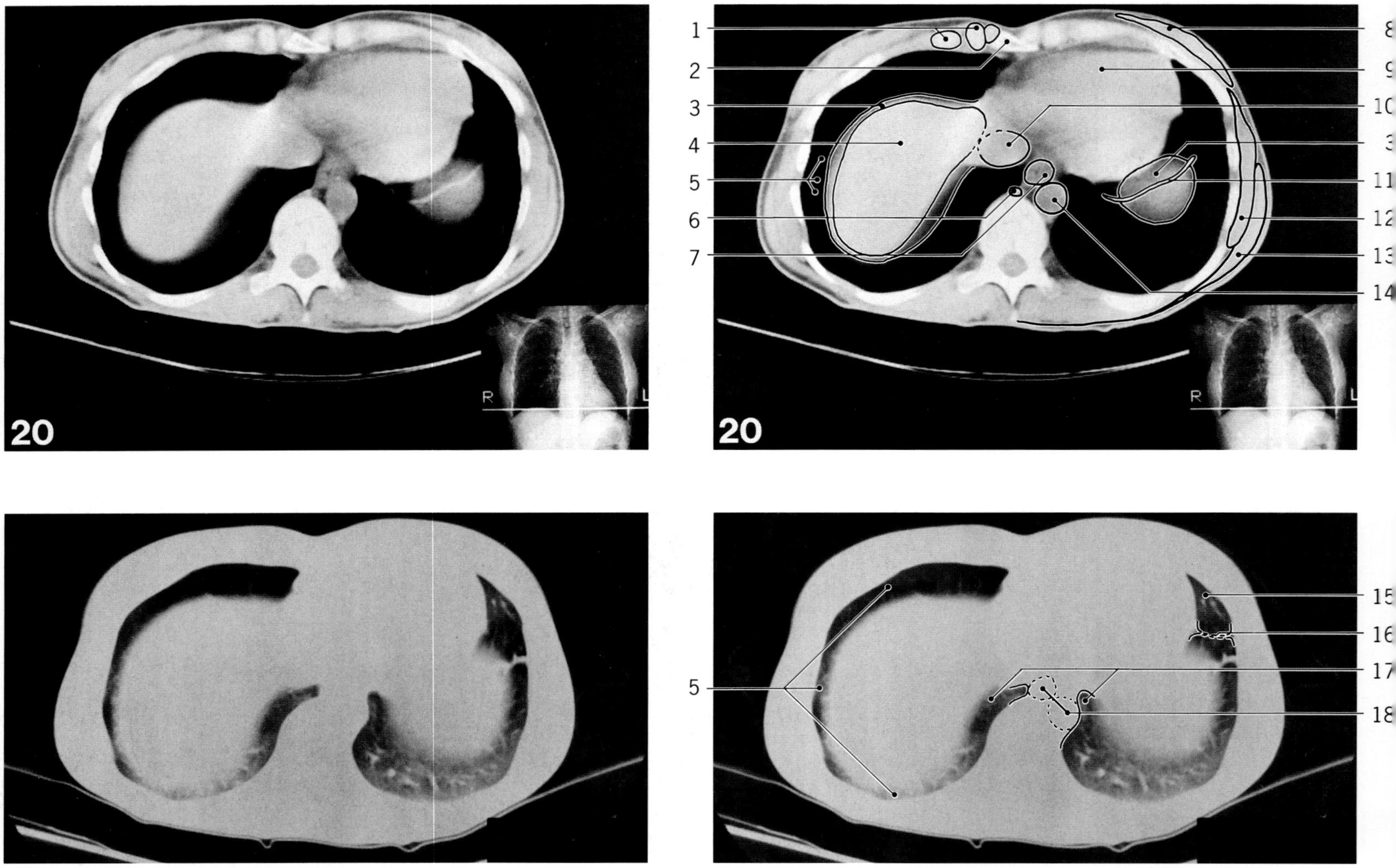

Thorax, axial CT

Scout view on page 204

1: Cartilage of ribs
2: Xiphoid process
3: Diaphragm
4: Liver
5: Costodiaphragmatic sulcus
6: Azygos vein
7: Oesophagus
8: Mammary gland
9: Heart
10: Inferior caval vein
11: Inferior phrenic artery
12: Serratus anterior
13: Latissimus dorsi
14: Thoracic aorta
15: Lingula of left lung
16: Oblique fissure
17: Phrenicomediastinal sulcus
18: Oesophagus and aorta in posterior mediastinum

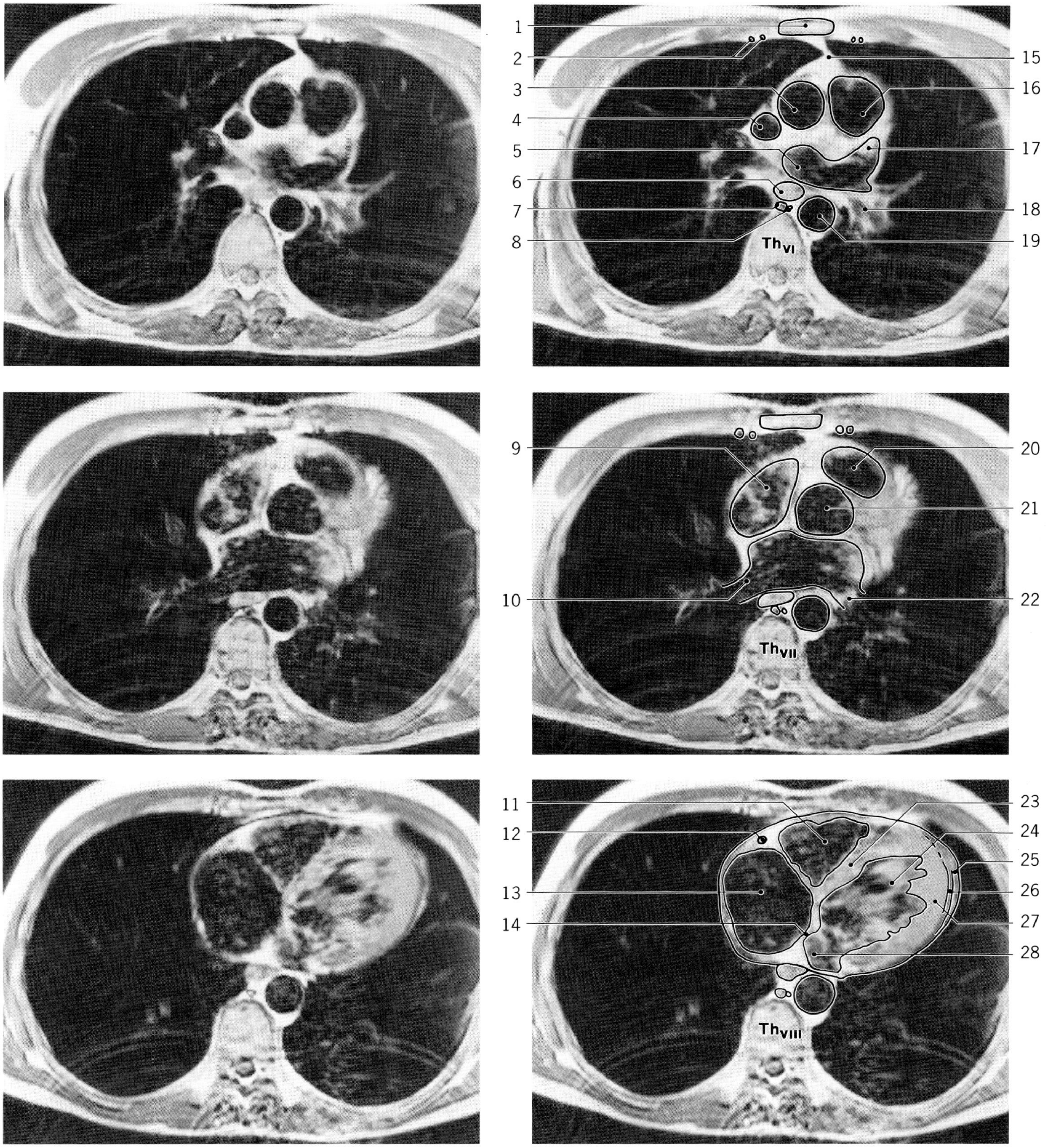

Heart, axial MR, level Th VI, Th VII and Th VIII

T_1-weighted recording

1: Body of sternum
2: Internal thoracic artery and vein
3: Ascending aorta
4: Superior caval vein
5: Left atrium
6: Oesophagus
7: Azygos vein
8: Thoracic duct
9: Right atrium
10: Right inferior pulmonary vein
11: Right ventricle
12: Right coronary artery
13: Right atrium
14: Interatrial septum
15: Anterior mediastinum (sternopericardial ligament)
16: Pulmonary trunk
17: Left auricle
18: Root of left lung
19: Thoracic aorta
20: Conus arteriosus
21: Bulb of aorta
22: Left inferior pulmonary vein
23: Interventricular septum
24: Left ventricle
25: Pericardial sac
26: Pericardial cavity
27: Myocardium of left ventricle
28: Left atrium

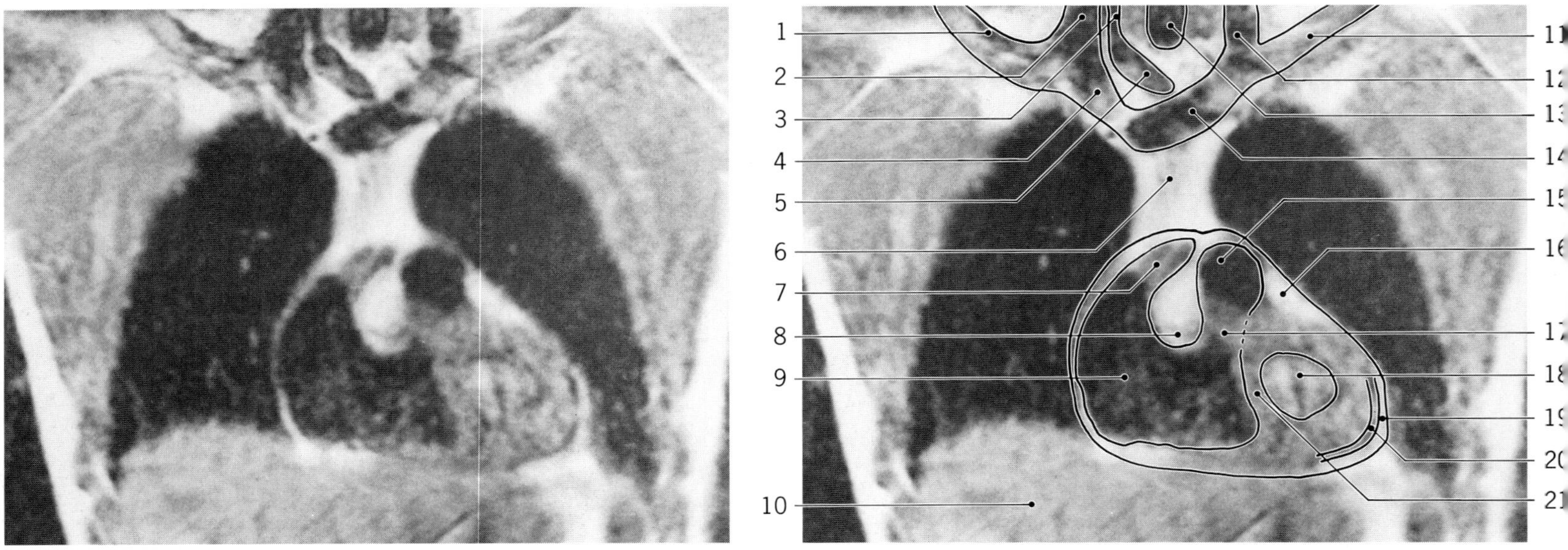

Heart, coronal MR

T1-weighted recording

1: Right subclavian vein
2: Right internal jugular vein
3: Right common carotid artery
4: Right brachiocephalic vein
5: Brachiocephalic trunk
6: Superior mediastinum
7: Right atrium
8: Supraventricular crest
9: Right ventricle
10: Liver
11: Left subclavian vein
12: Left internal jugular vein
13: Trachea
14: Left brachiocephalic vein
15: Pulmonary trunk
16: Epicardial fat
17: Conus arteriosus
18: Left ventricular cavity
19: Pericardial sac
20: Pericardial cavity
21: Interventricular septum

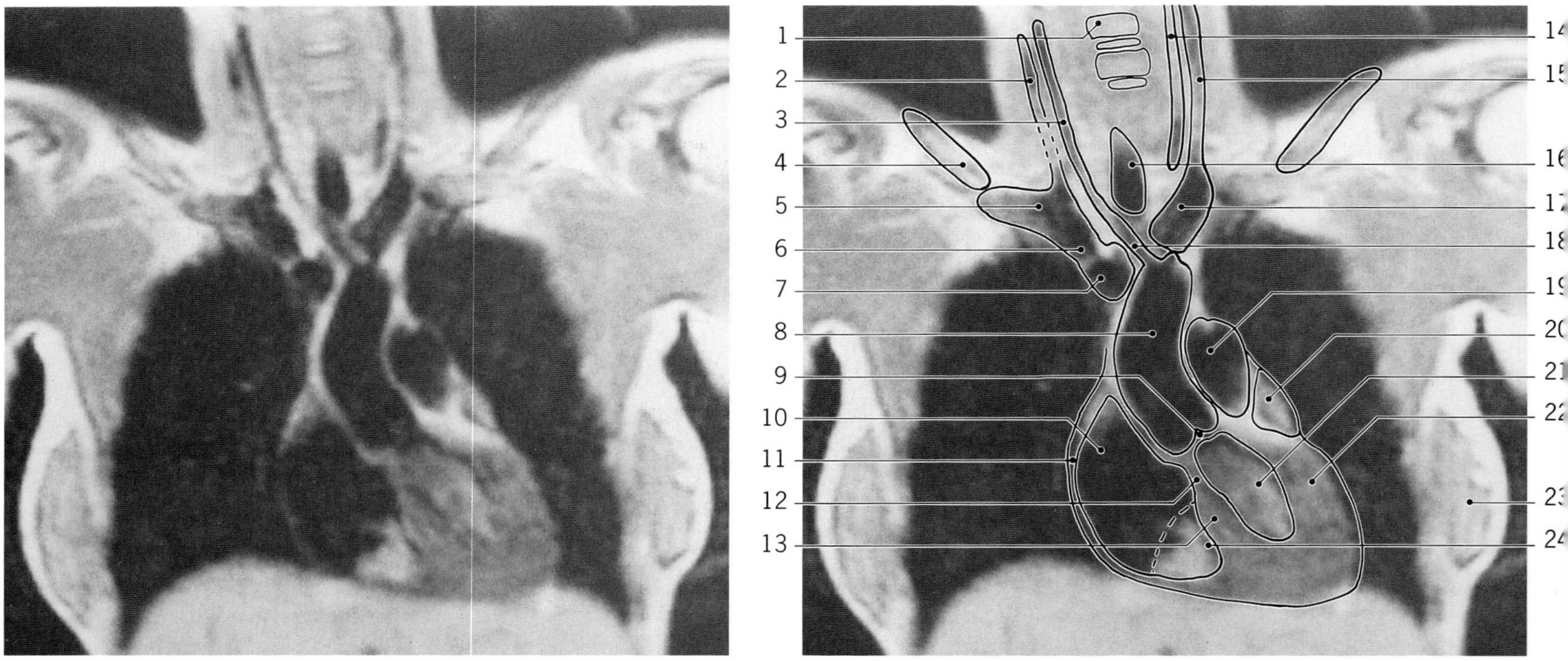

Heart, coronal MR

T1-weighted recording

1: Body of cervical vertebra
2: Right internal jugular vein
3: Right common carotid artery
4: Clavicle
5: Right subclavian vein
6: Right brachiocephalic vein
7: Superior caval vein
8: Ascending aorta
9: Aortic valve
10: Right atrium
11: Right atrial wall, pericardium and pleura
12: Interventricular septum, membranous part
13: Interventricular septum, muscular part
14: Left common carotid artery
15: Left internal jugular vein
16: Trachea
17: Left brachiocephalic vein
18: Brachiocephalic trunk
19: Pulmonary trunk
20: Left auricle
21: Left ventricle
22: Myocardium of left ventricle
23: Mamma
24: Right ventricle

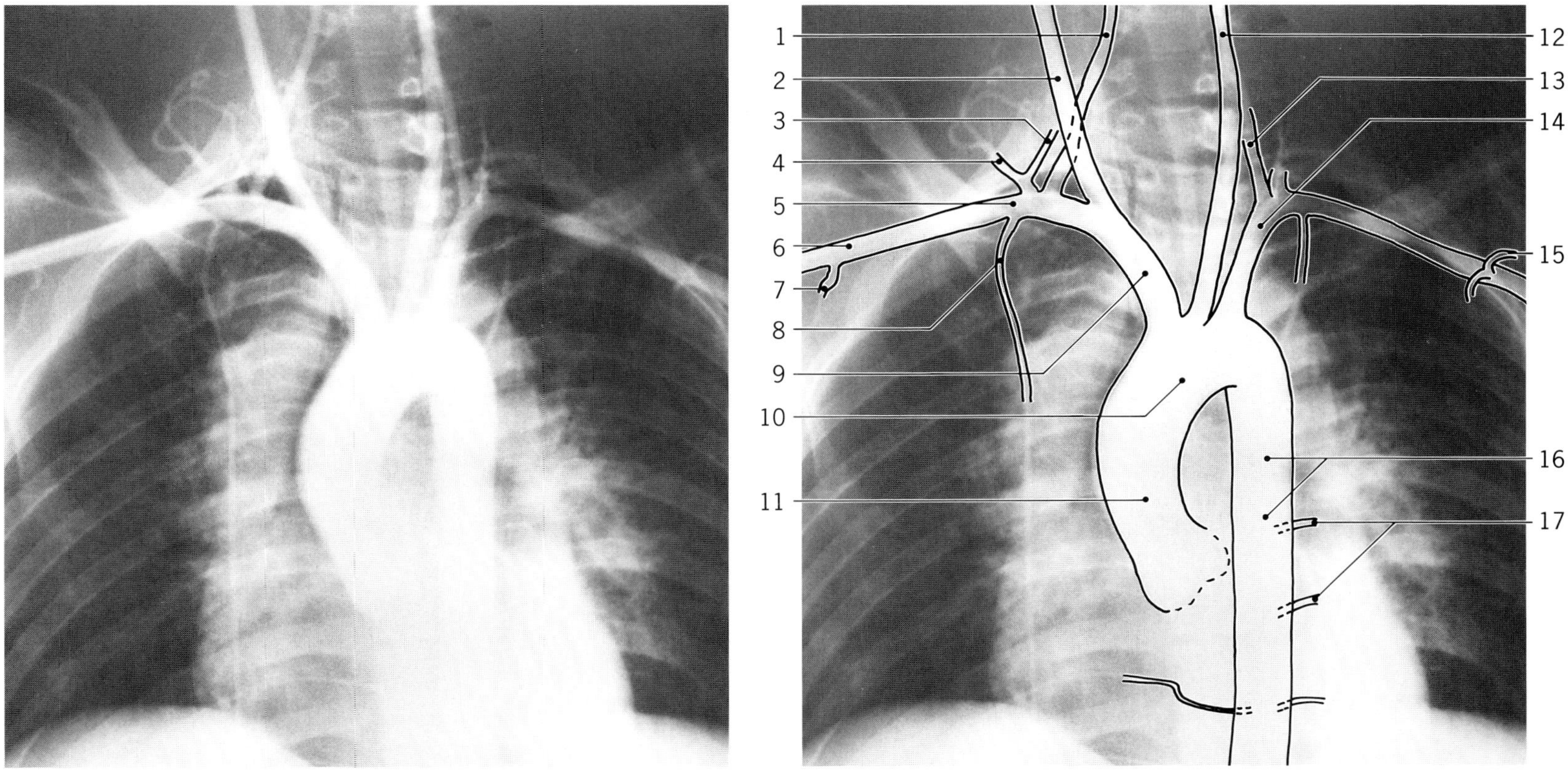

Aortic arch and great arteries, a-p X-ray, aortography

1: Right vertebral artery
2: Right common carotid artery
3: Inferior thyroid artery
4: Transverse cervical artery
5: Right subclavian artery
6: Axillary artery
7: Subscapular artery
8: Internal thoracic artery
9: Brachiocephalic trunk
10: Aortic arch
11: Ascending aorta
12: Left common carotid artery
13: Left vertebral artery
14: Left subclavian artery
15: Thoraco-acromial artery
16: Thoracic aorta
17: Intercostal arteries

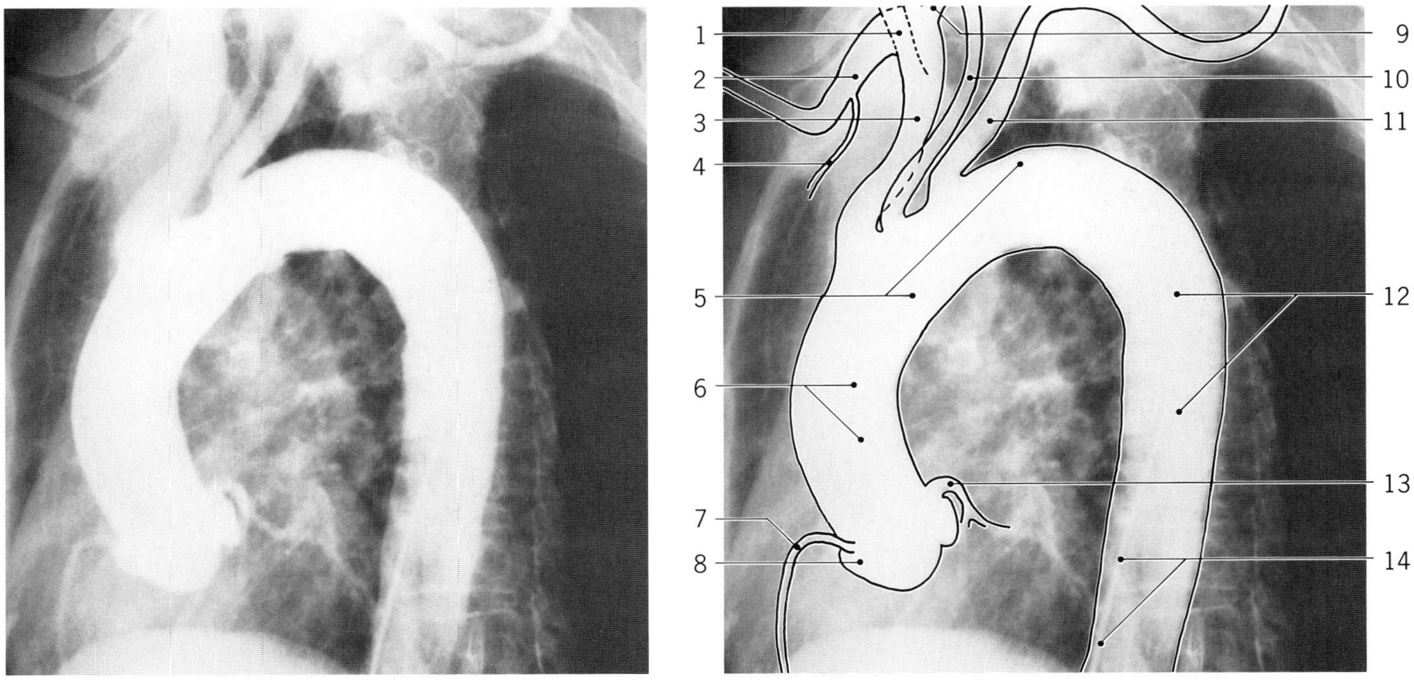

Aortic arch and great arteries, oblique X-ray, aortography

1: Right common carotid artery
2: Right subclavian artery
3: Brachiocephalic trunk
4: Internal thoracic artery
5: Aortic arch
6: Ascending aorta
7: Right coronary artery
8: Aortic sinus
9: Right vertebral artery
10: Left common carotid artery
11: Left subclavian artery
12: Thoracic aorta
13: Left coronary artery
14: Catheter

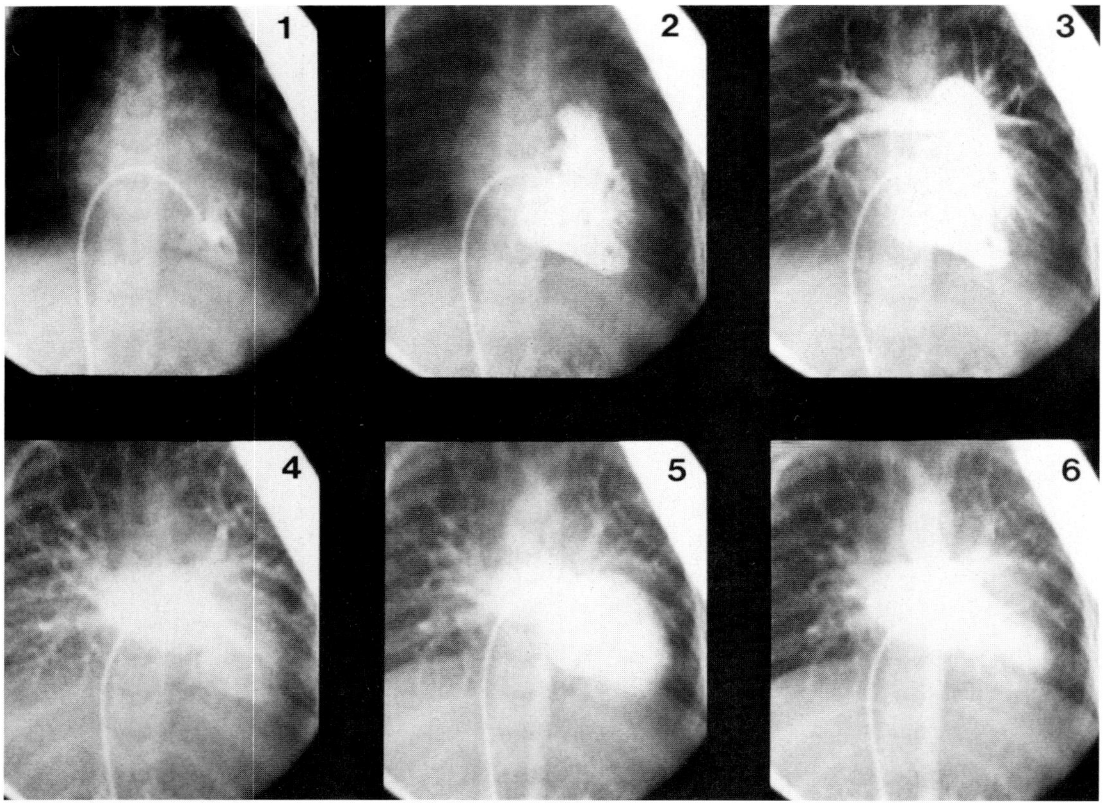

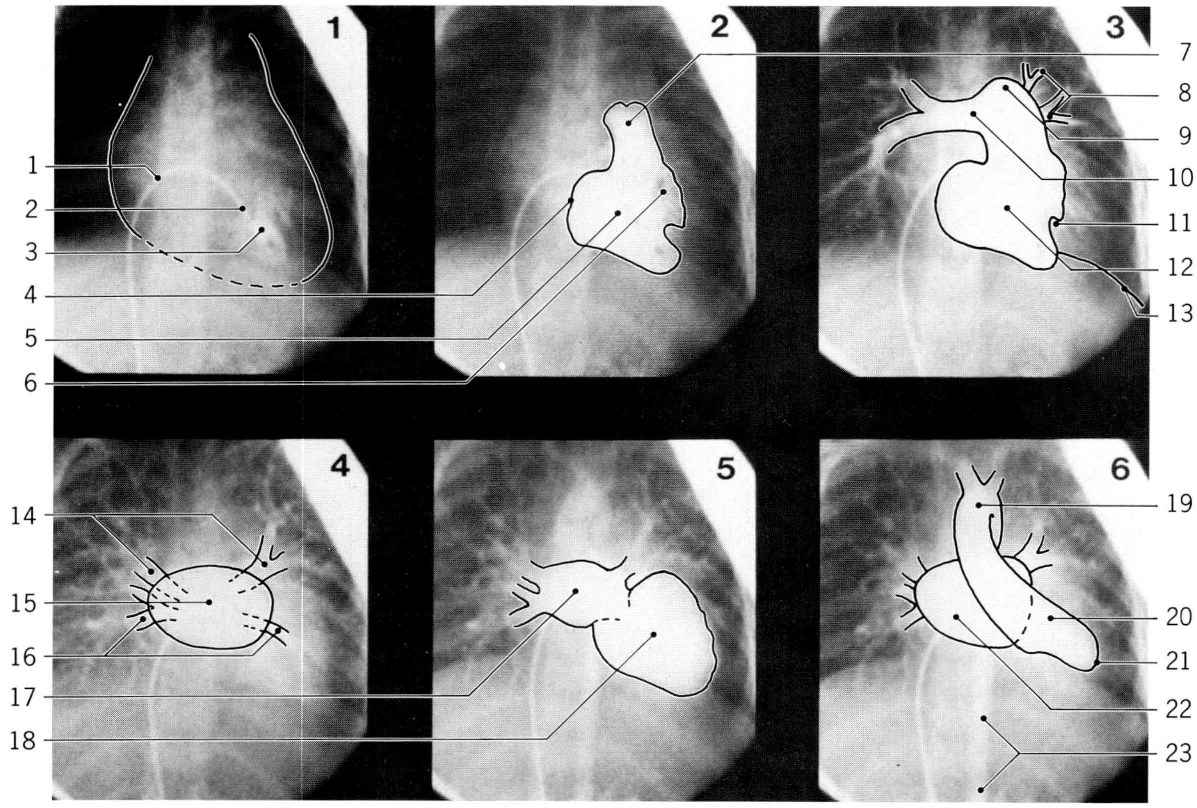

Heart, a-p, cardiac cineangiography, child

Six frames of a cardiac angiography sequence

1: Catheter in right atrium
2: Tip of catheter in right ventricle
3: Initial outflow of contrast medium
4: Tricuspid valve (closed)
5: Right ventricle (early systole)
6: Trabeculae carneae
7: Pulmonary trunk
8: Branches of left pulmonary artery
9: Left pulmonary artery
10: Right pulmonary artery
11: Anterior papillary muscle of right ventricle
12: Right ventricle (systole)
13: Diaphragm
14: Superior pulmonary veins
15: Left atrium (diastole)
16: Inferior pulmonary veins
17: Left atrium (systole)
18: Left ventricle (diastole)
19: Aortic arch
20: Left ventricle (systole)
21: Apex of left ventricle
22: Left atrium (diastole)
23: Abdominal aorta

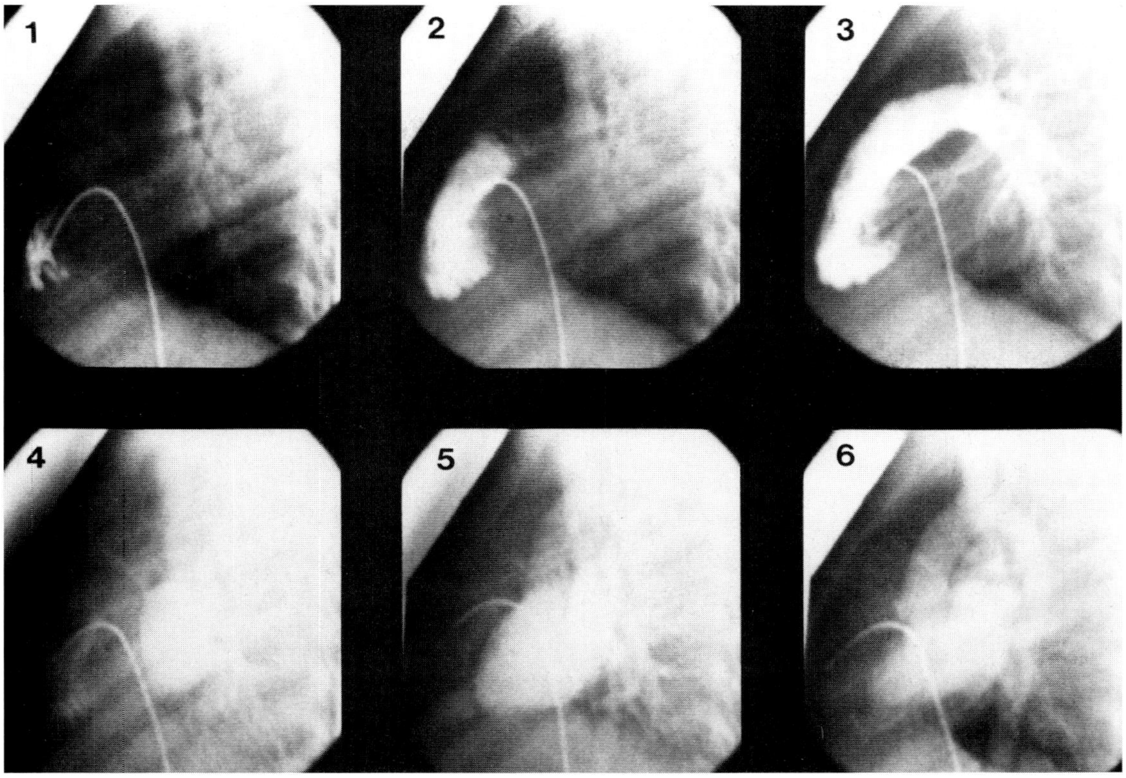

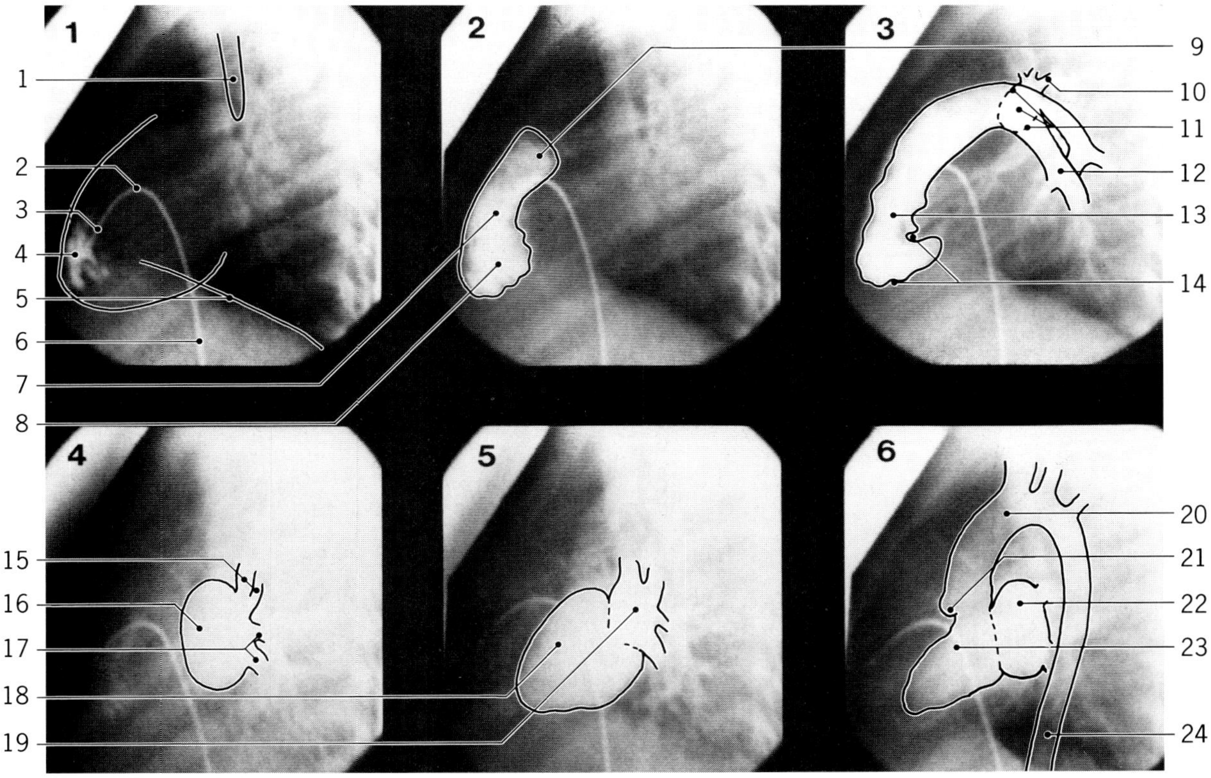

Heart, lateral, cardiac cineangiography, child

Six frames of a cardiac angiography sequence

1: Trachea
2: Catheter in right atrium
3: Tip of catheter in right ventricle
4: Initial outflow of contrast medium
5: Diaphragm
6: Catheter in inferior caval vein
7: Conus arteriosus (infundibulum)
8: Right ventricle (early systole)
9: Pulmonary trunk
10: Pulmonary artery branches to upper lobes
11: Right pulmonary artery (longitudinal view)
12: Branches of left pulmonary artery
13: Right ventricle (systole)
14: Trabeculae carneae
15: Superior pulmonary veins
16: Left atrium (diastole)
17: Inferior pulmonary veins
18: Left ventricle (diastole)
19: Left atrium (systole)
20: Aortic arch
21: Aortic sinus
22: Left atrium (diastole)
23: Left ventricle (systole)
24: Descending aorta

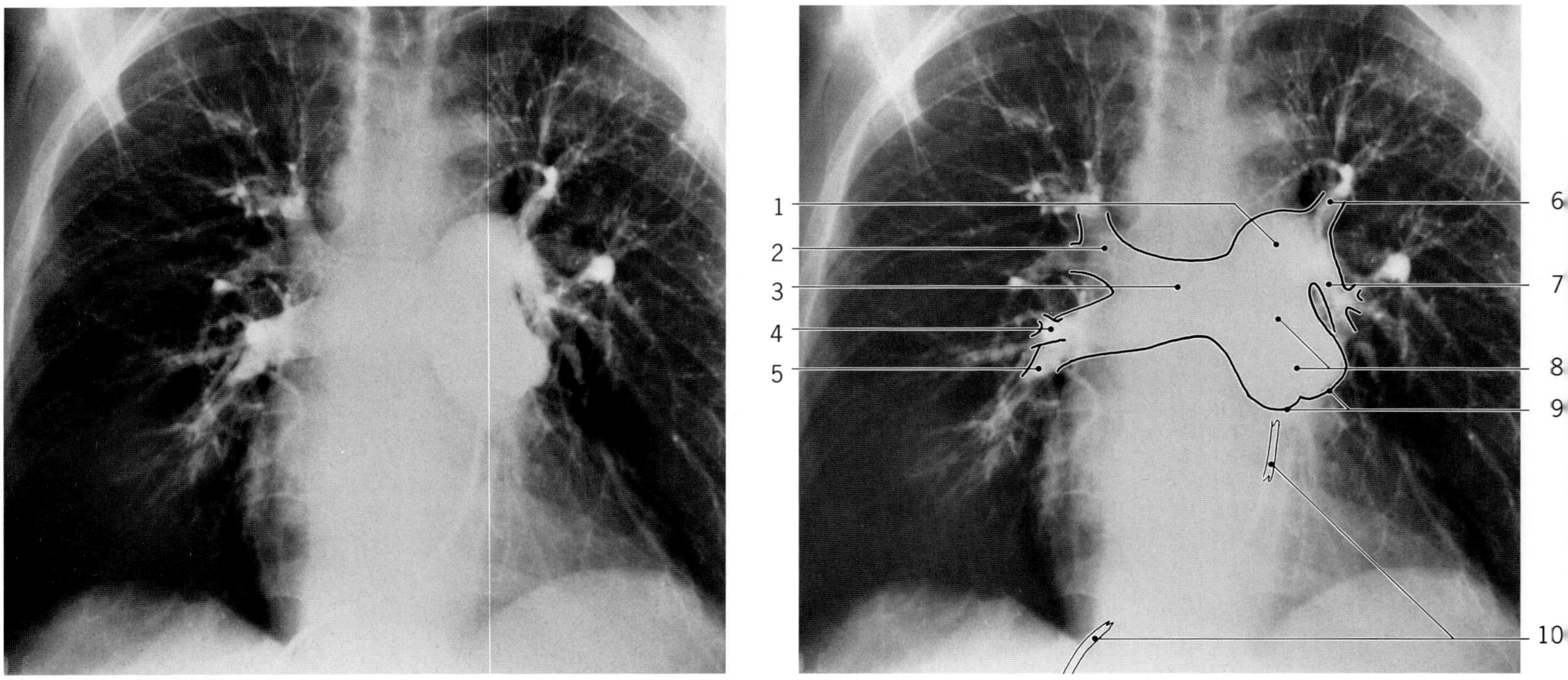

Pulmonary arteries, a-p X-ray, arteriography

1: Left pulmonary artery
2: Right upper lobe artery
3: Right pulmonary artery
4: Middle lobe artery
5: Right lower lobe artery
6: Left upper lobe artery
7: Left lower lobe artery
8: Pulmonary trunk
9: Pulmonary valve
10: Catheter

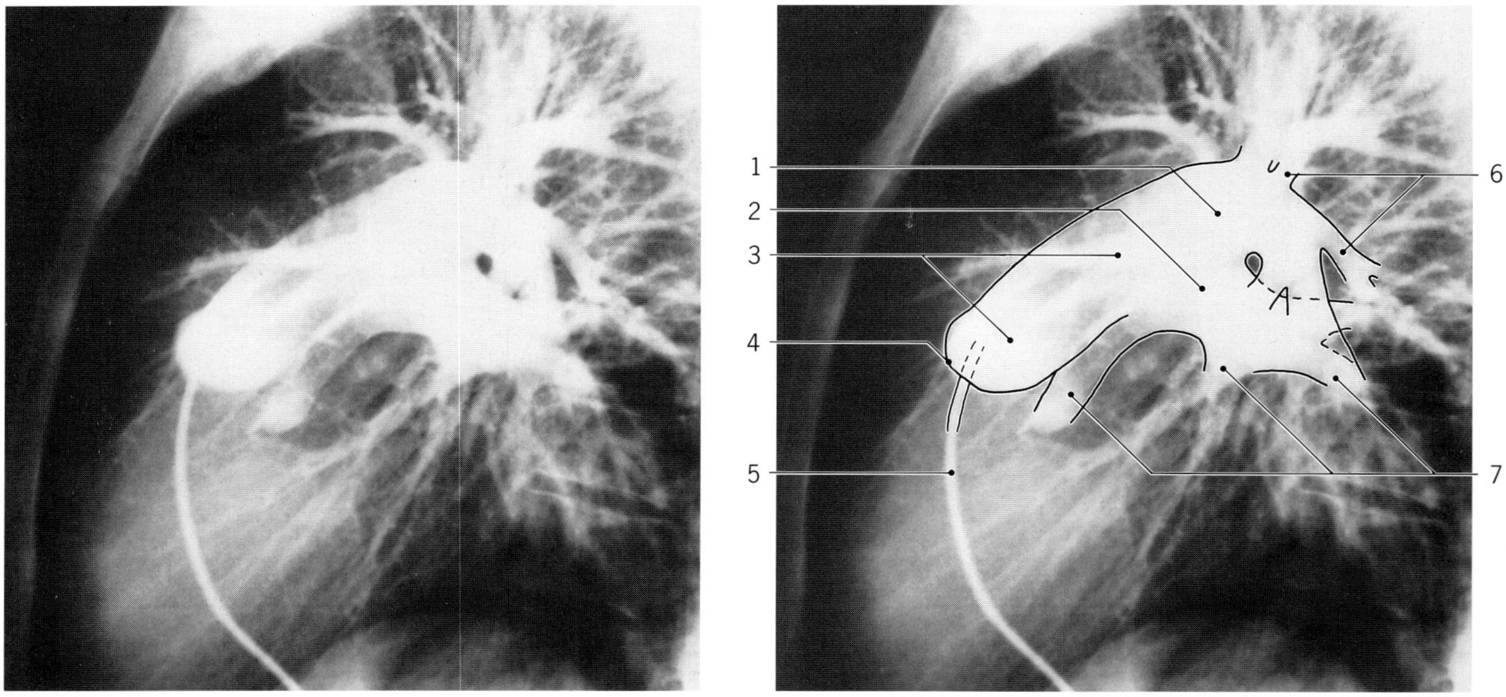

Pulmonary arteries, lateral X-ray, arteriography

1: Left pulmonary artery
2: Right pulmonary artery
3: Pulmonary trunk
4: Pulmonary valve
5: Catheter in right ventricle
6: Branches of left pulmonary artery
7: Branches of right pulmonary artery

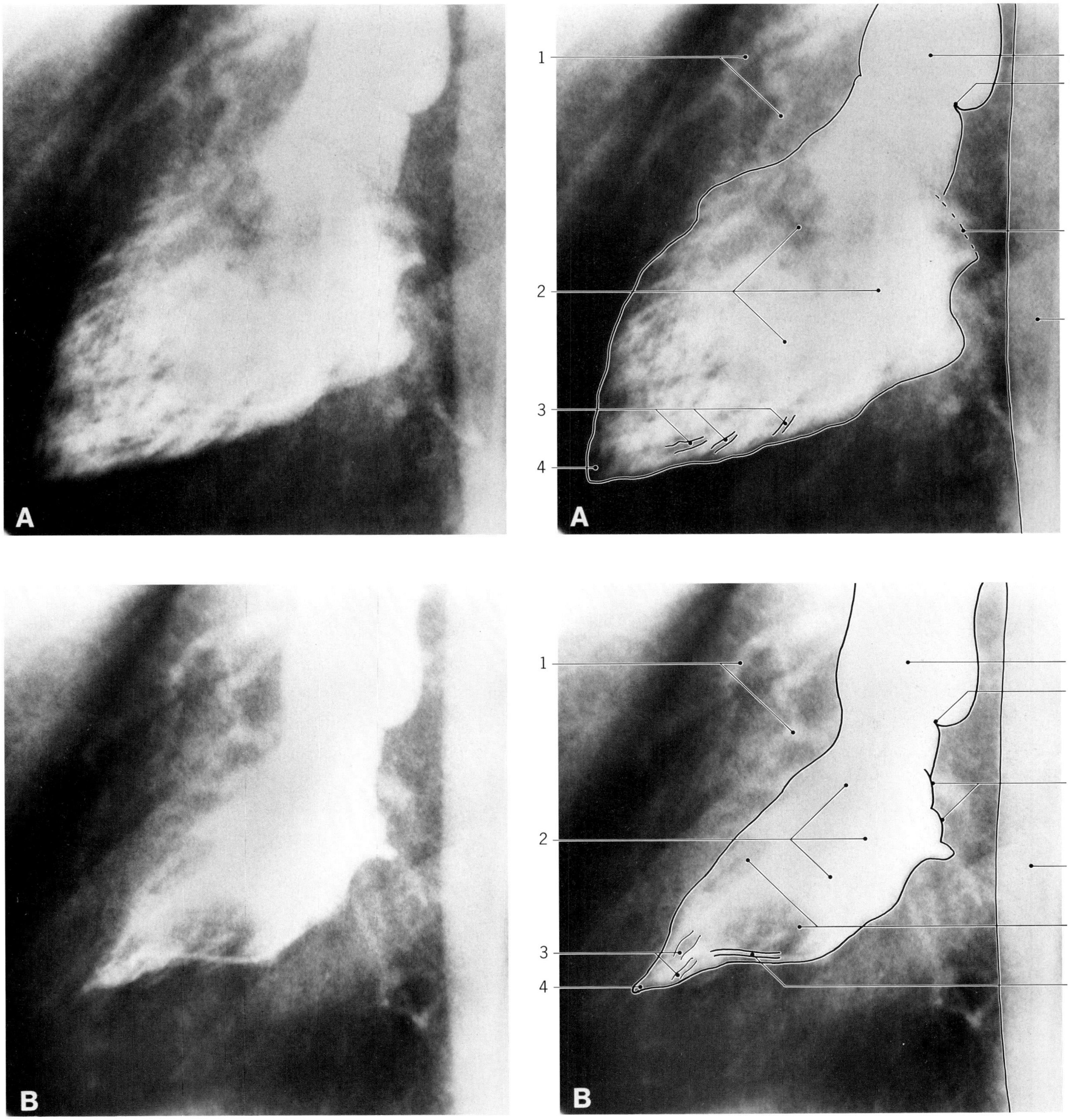

Left ventricle, lateral X-rays, cardiac angiography

A: Diastole, B: Systole

1: Coronary arteries
2: Left ventricle
3: Trabeculae carneae
4: Apex of left ventricle
5: Aortic bulb
6: Semilunar valve of aortic ostium
7: Mitral valve
8: Thoracic aorta
9: Anterior and posterior papillary muscle
10: Catheter

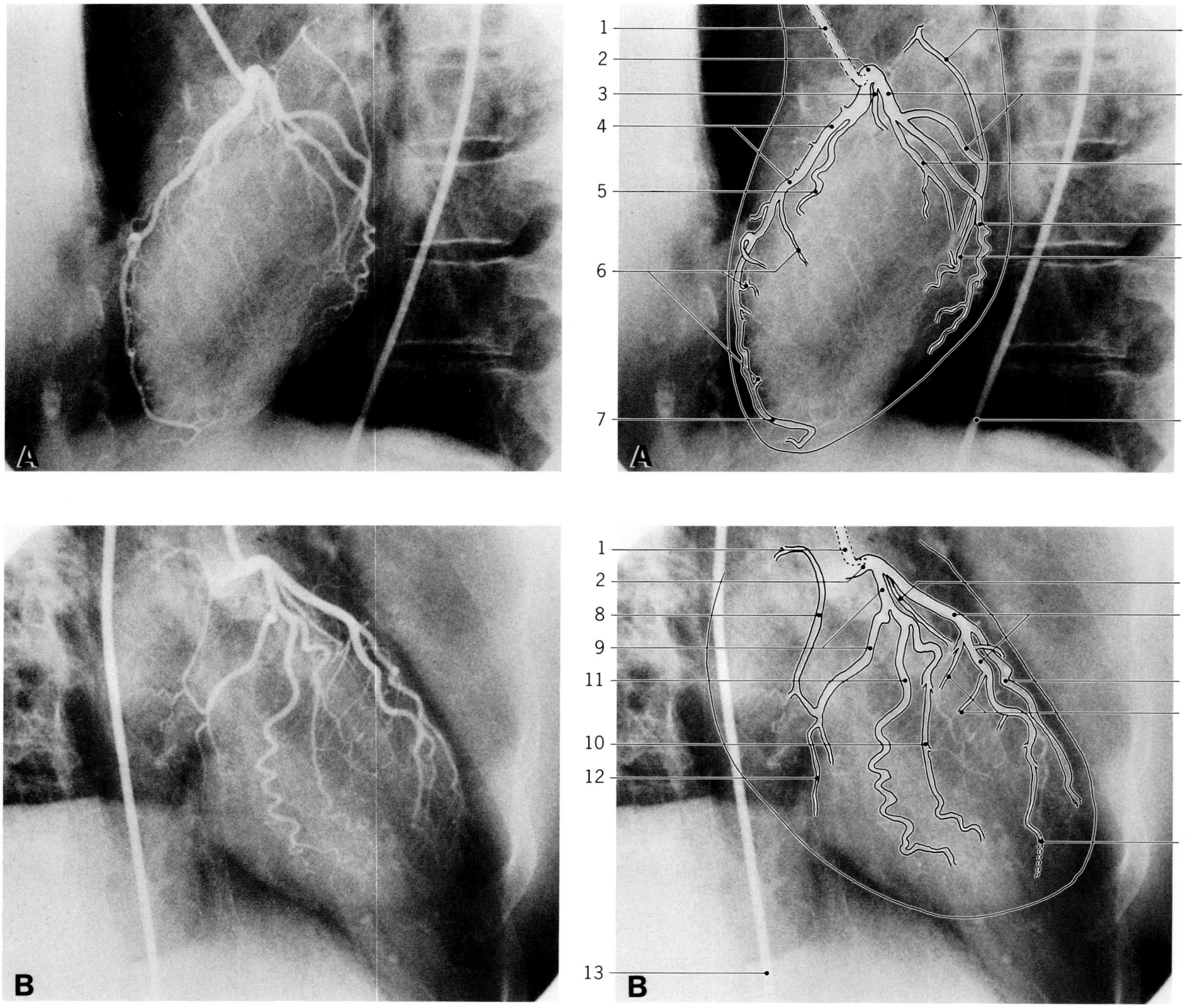

Left coronary artery, arteriography

A: left lateral X-ray. B: right anterior oblique (RAO) X-ray

1: Catheter with tip in orifice of left coronary artery
2: Left coronary artery, main stem
3: Intermediate ramus
4: Anterior interventricular artery (left anterior descendent, LAD)
5: Left diagonal artery
6: Anterior septal rami
7: LAD at apex of the heart
8: Atrial ramus
9: Circumflex artery
10: Anterior left ventricular branch (anterior marginal branch)
11: Obtuse marginal branch
12: Posterior left ventricular branch (posterior marginal branch)
13: Catheter in aorta

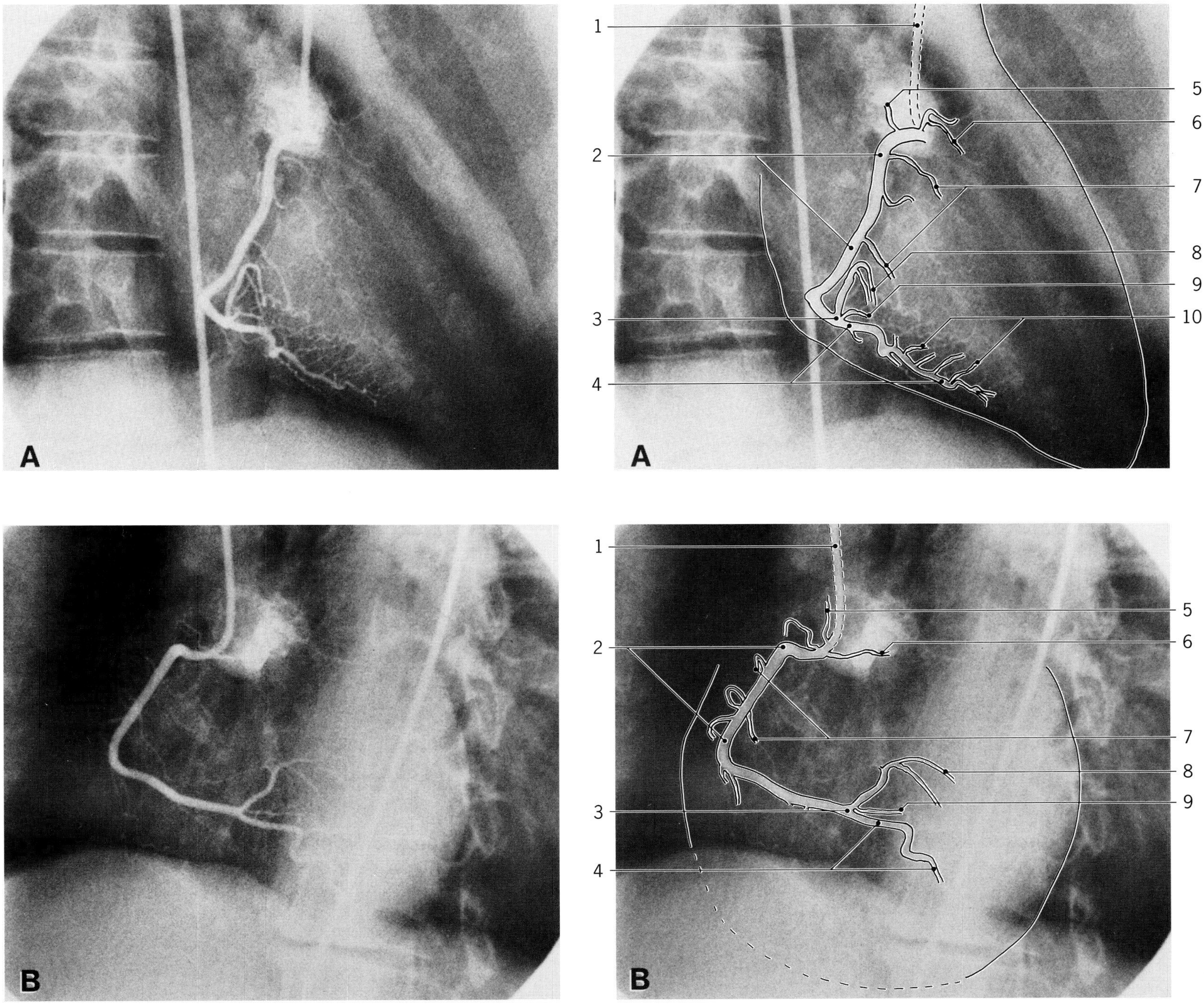

Right coronary artery, arteriography

A: right anterior oblique (RAO) X-ray. B: left anterior oblique (LAO) X-ray

1: Catheter with tip in orifice of right coronary artery
2: Right coronary artery
3: Crux of heart
4: Posterior interventricular artery
5: Sinus node artery
6: Conus artery
7: Anterior right ventricular rami (marginal branches)
8: Terminal left ventricular ramus
9: Atrio-ventricular node artery
10: Posterior septal rami

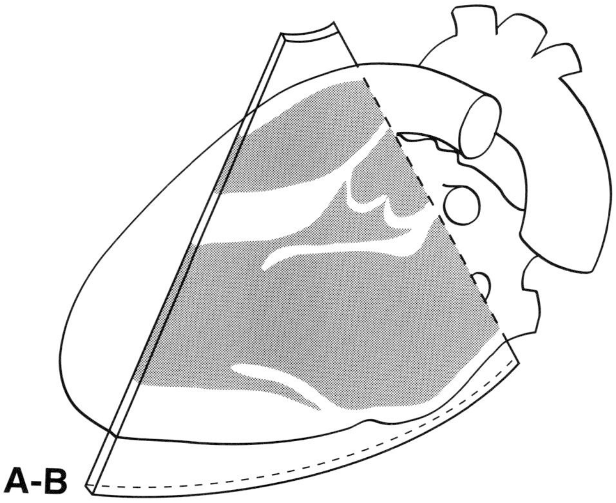

Orientation of parasternal, long axis sections A and B

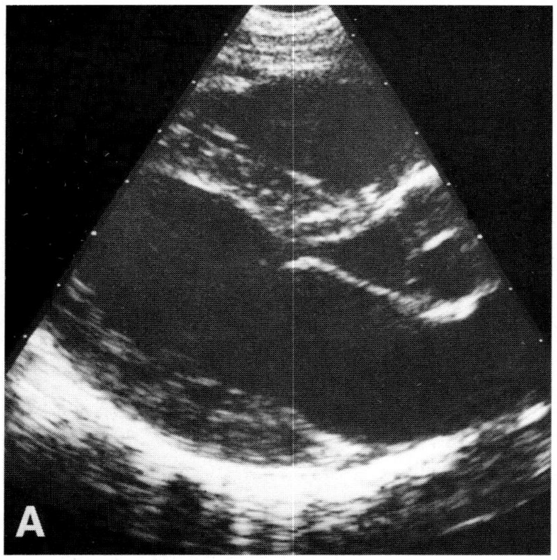

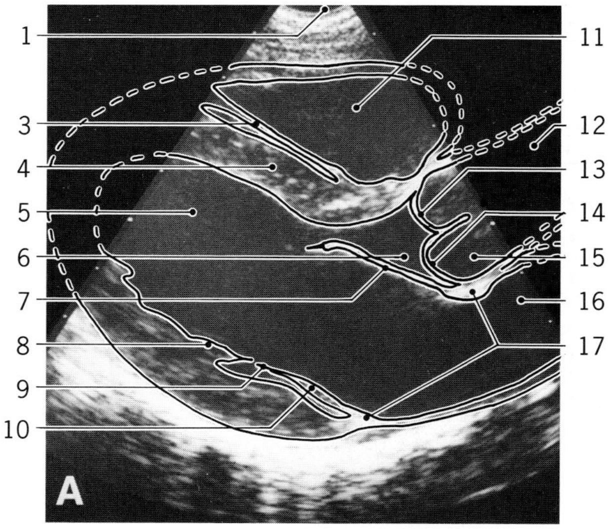

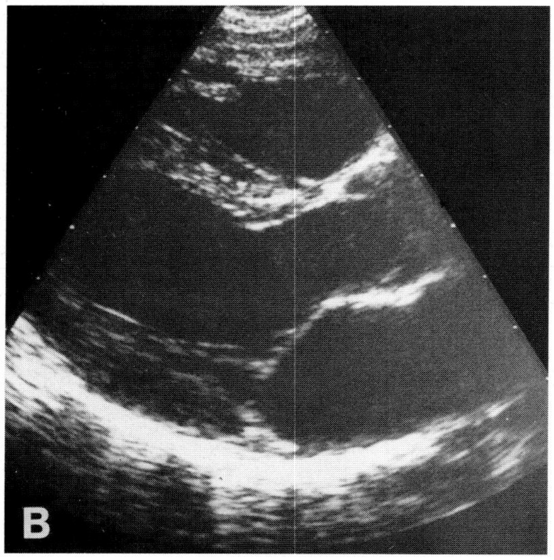

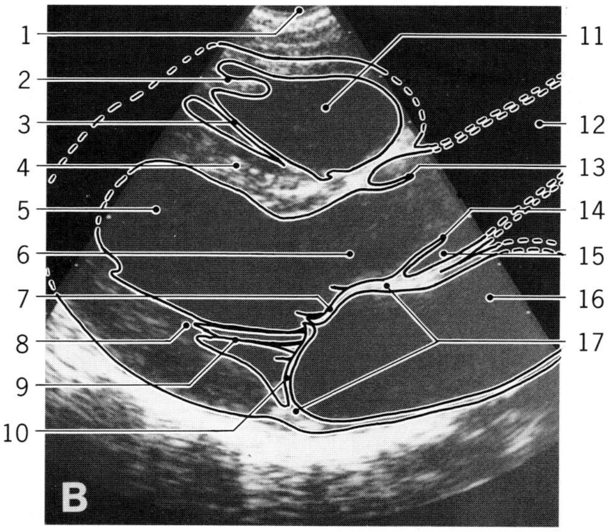

Mitral and aortic valve, parasternal, long axis section, US

A: diastole. B: systole

1: Probe over fourth left intercostal space
2: Anterior papillary muscle of right ventricle
3: Septomarginal trabecula (inconstant)
4: Interventricular septum
5: Left ventricle
6: Left ventricular outflow tract
7: Anterior cusp of mitral valve
8: Papillary muscle
9: Chorda tendinea
10: Posterior cusp of mitral valve
11: Right ventricle
12: Ascending aorta
13: Anterior semilunar cusp of aortic valve
14: Right semilunar cusp of aortic valve
15: Aortic sinus
16: Left atrium
17: Fibrous annulus of mitral ostium

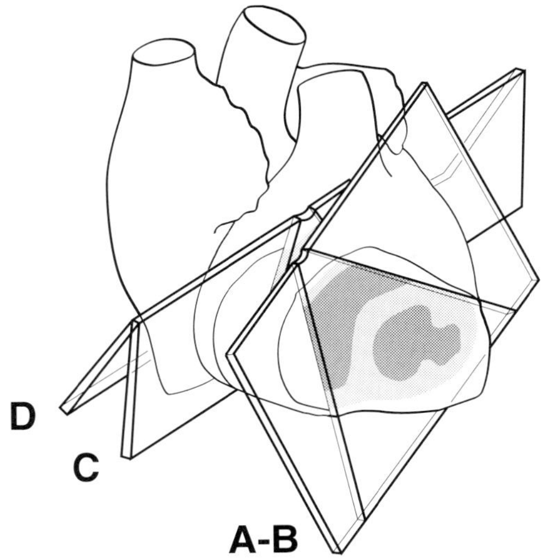

Orientation of parasternal, short axis sections A-D

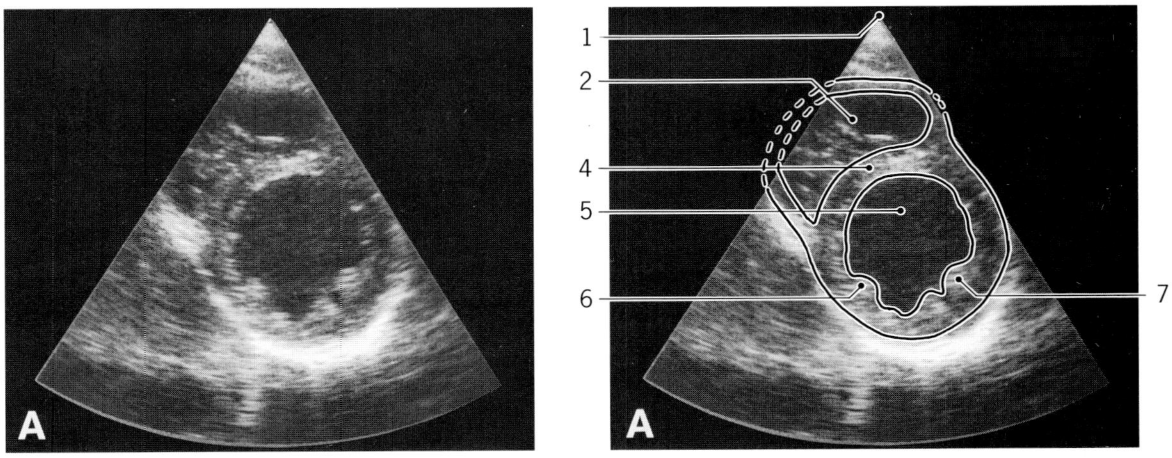

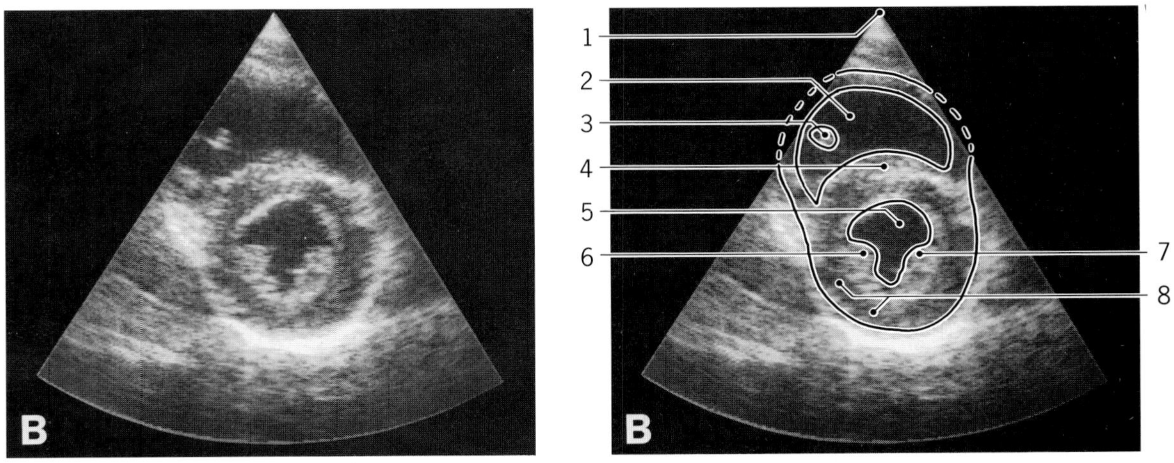

Right and left ventricle, parasternal, short axis sections, US

A: diastole. B: systole

1: Probe over third left intercostal space
2: Right ventricle
3: Anterior papillary muscle of right ventricle
4: Interventricular septum
5: Left ventricle
6: Posterior papillary muscle of left ventricle
7: Anterior papillary muscle of left ventricle
8: Posterior wall of left ventricle

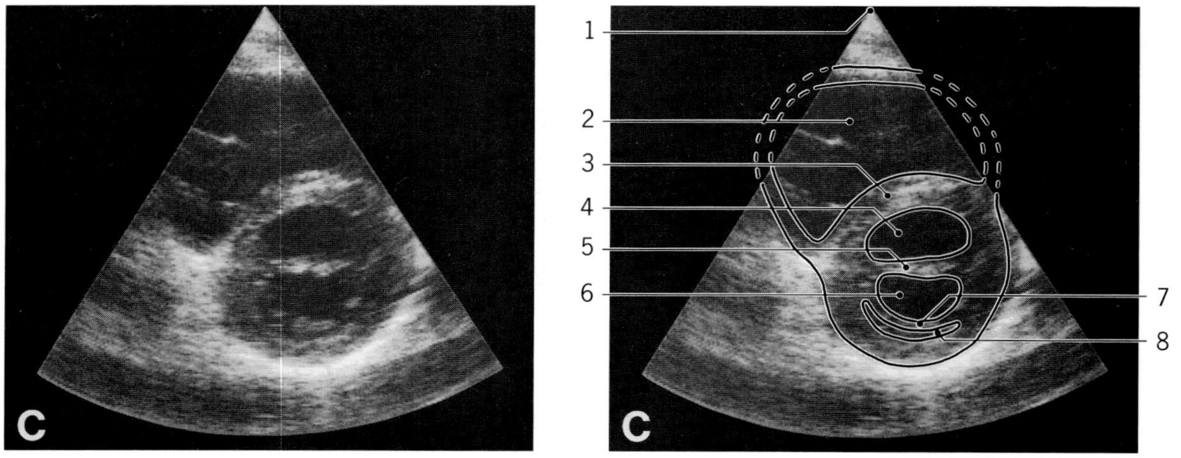

Mitral valve, parasternal, short axis section, US

Position of section C explained on previous page.

1: Probe over third intercostal space
2: Right ventricle
3: Interventricular septum
4: Left ventricular outflow tract
5: Anterior cusp of mitral valve
6: Mitral ostium
7: Posterior cusp of mitral valve
8: Blood between ventricular wall, and posterior cusp

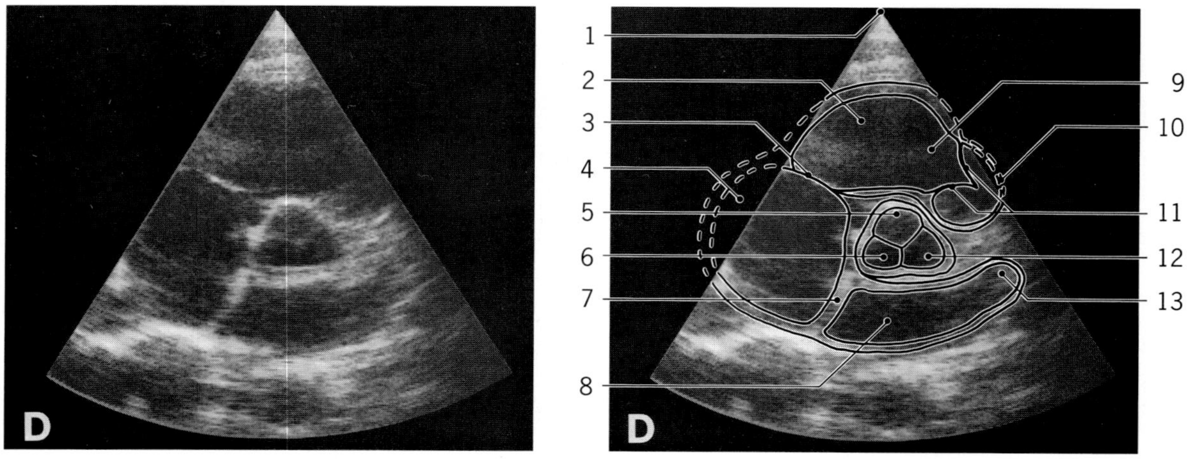

Aortic valve, parasternal, short axis section, US

Position of section D explained on previous page.

1: Probe over third intercostal space
2: Right ventricle
3: Tricuspid valve
4: Right atrium
5: Anterior semilunar cusp of aortic valve
6: Right semilunar cusp of aortic valve
7: Interatrial septum
8: Left atrium
9: Conus arteriosus
10: Pulmonary trunk
11: Pulmonary valve
12: Left semilunar cusp of aortic valve
13: Left auricle

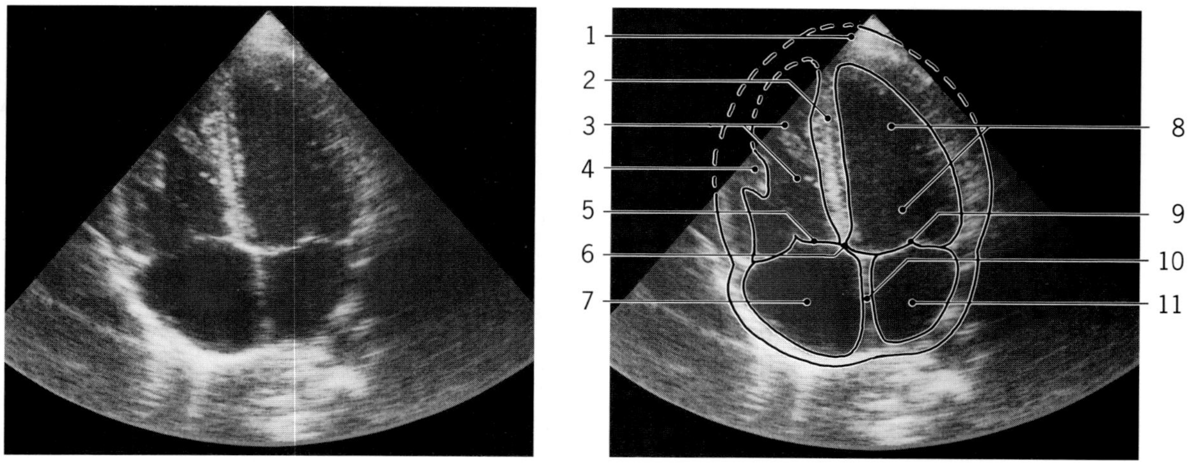

Cardiac chambers, subcostal, long axis section, US

1: Apex of heart
2: Interventricular septum
3: Right ventricle
4: Anterior papillary muscle
5: Tricuspid valve
6: Membraneous part of interventricular septum
7: Right atrium
8: Left ventricle
9: Mitral valve
10: Interatrial septum
11: Left atrium

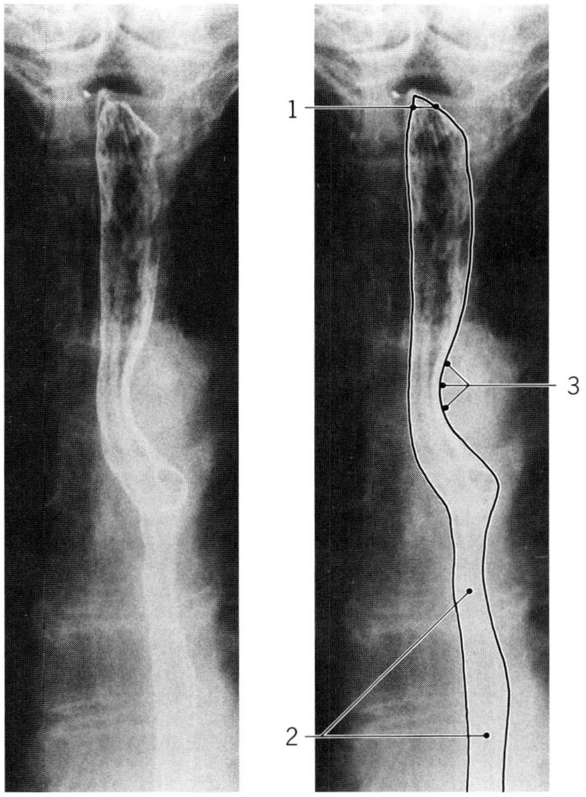

Oesophagus, a-p X-ray, barium swallow

1: Cricoesophageal sphinchter
2: Oesophagus, thoracic part
3: Impression from aortic arch

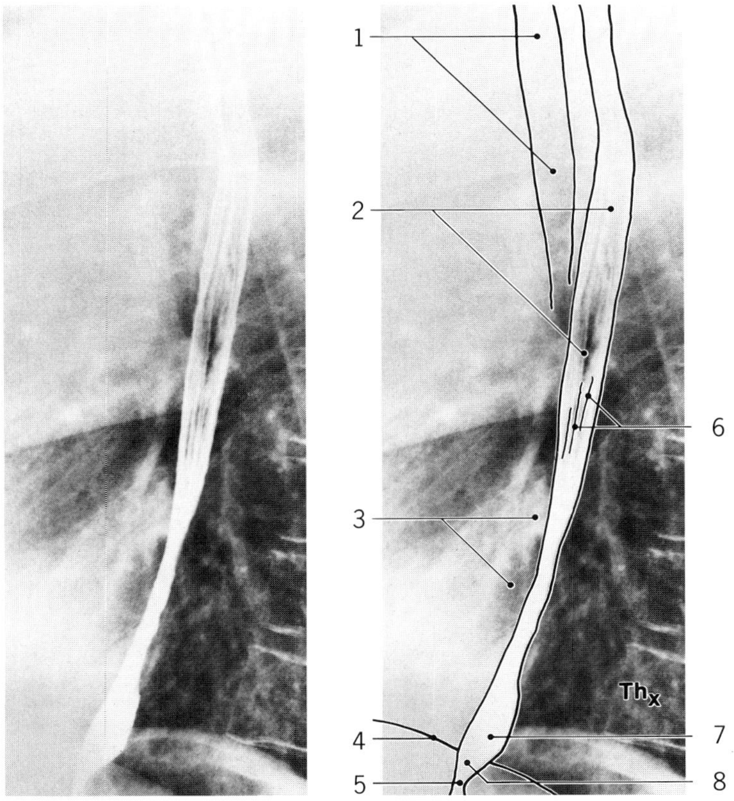

Oesophagus, lateral X-ray, barium swallow

1: Trachea
2: Oesophagus
3: Left atrium
4: Diaphragm
5: Cardia
6: Mucosal folds
7: "Ampulla phrenica" (radiology term)
8: Abdominal part of oesophagus

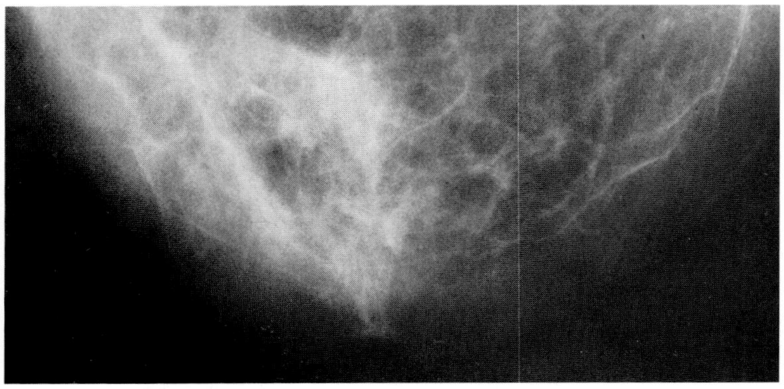

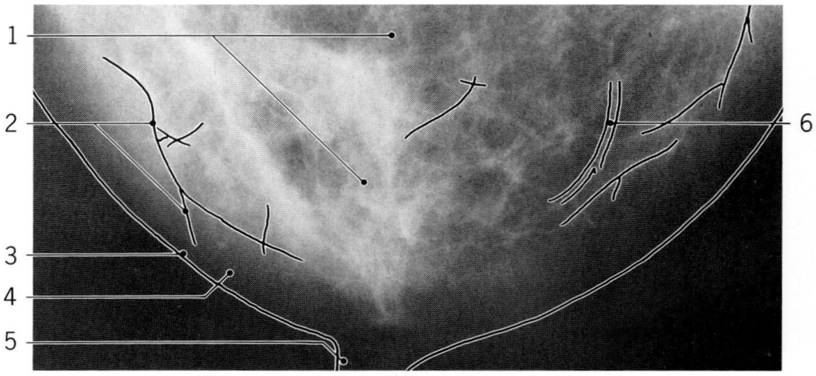

Breast, cranio-caudal (axial) X-ray, mammography

1: Body of mamma with glandular tissue
2: Connective tissue strands (suspensory ligament)
3: Skin
4: Subcutis
5: Nipple
6: Vein

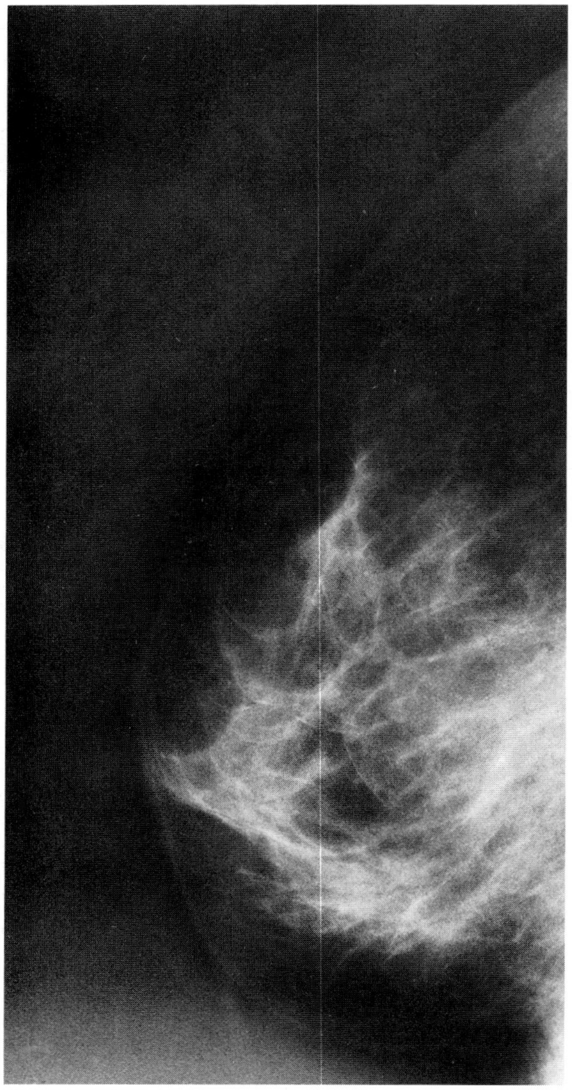

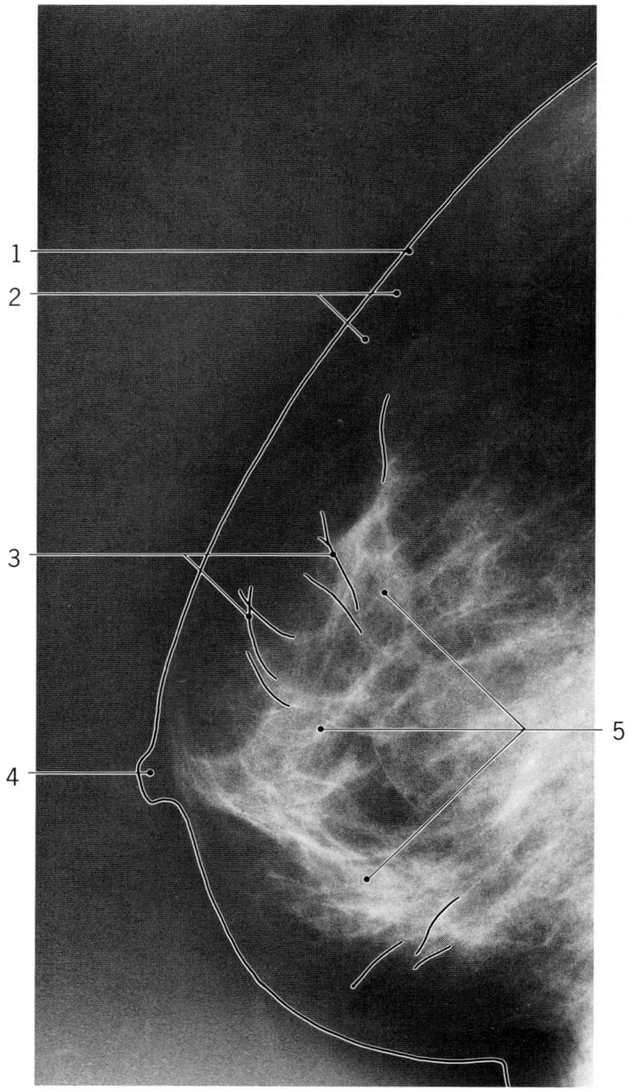

Breast, lateral X-ray, mammography

1: Skin
2: Subcutis
3: Connective tissue strands, (suspensory ligament)
4: Nipple
5: Body of mamma with glandular tissue

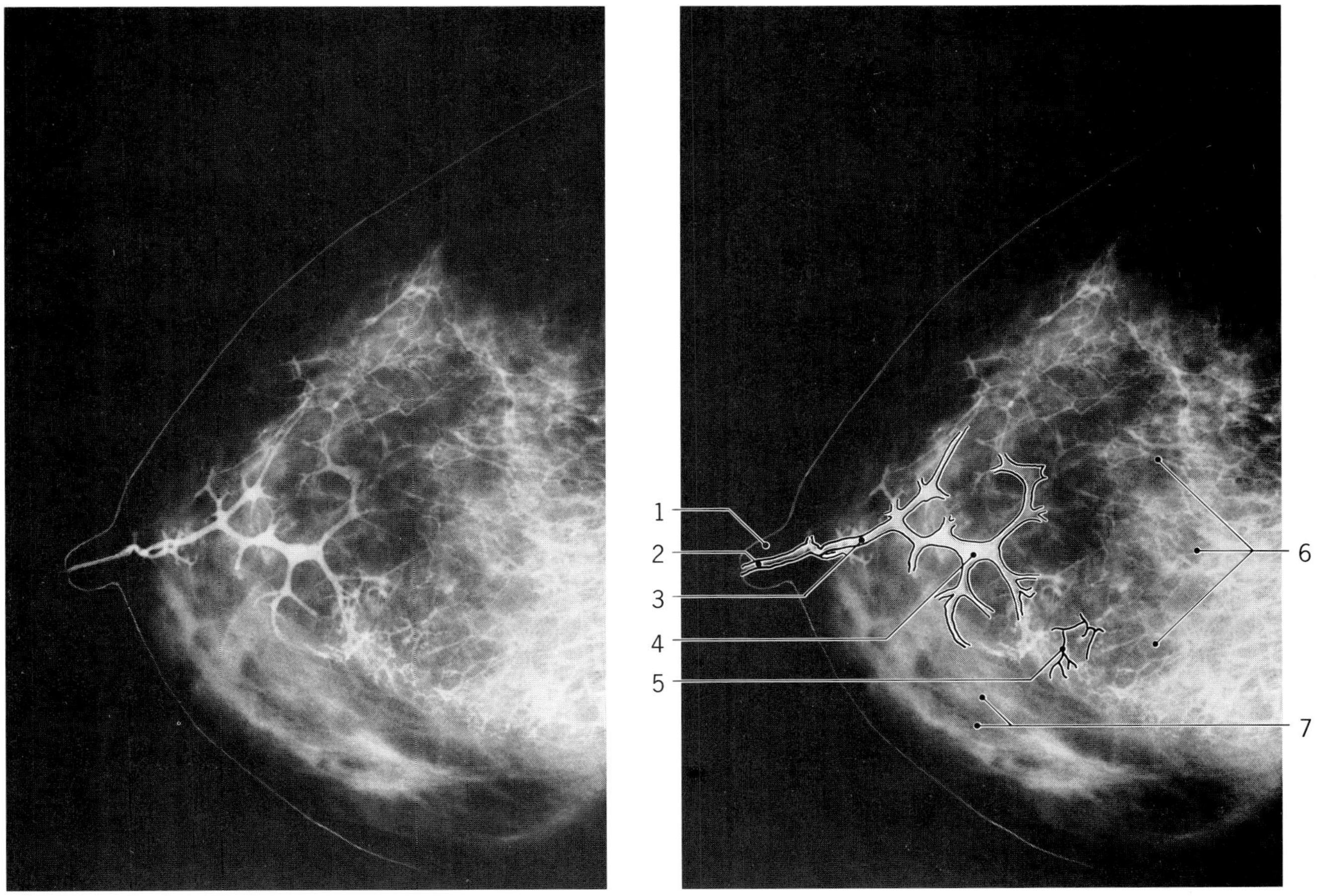

Breast, lateral X-ray, ductography

1: Nipple
2: Lactiferous duct
3: Lactiferous sinus
4: Major excretory duct
5: Minor excretory duct
6: Glandular tissue with contrast filling
7: Glandular tissue without contrast filling

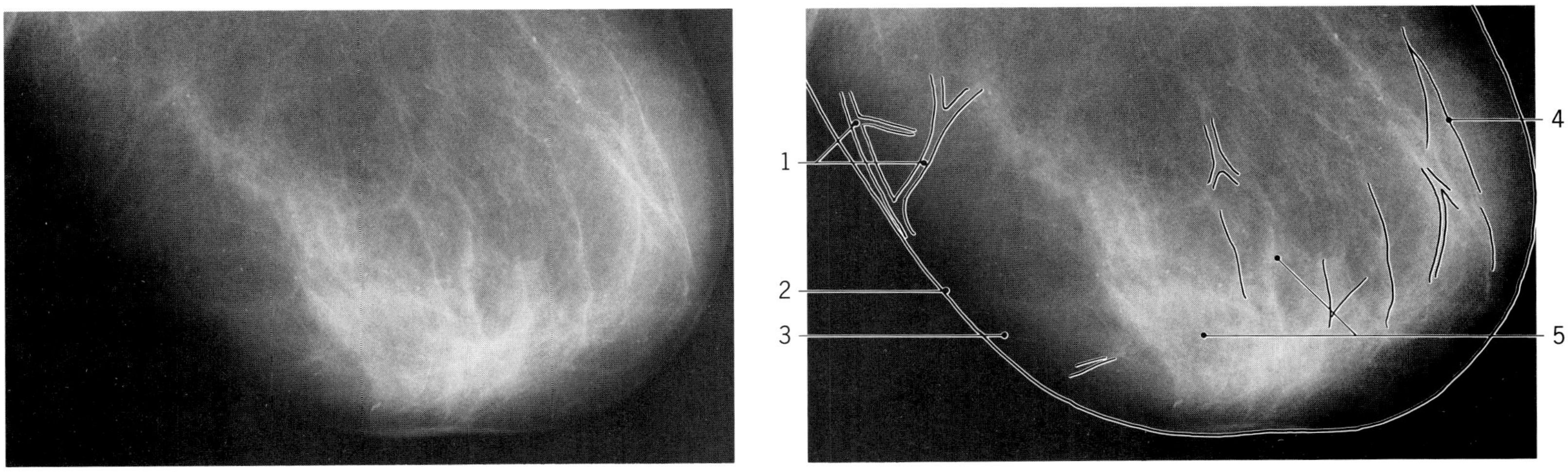

Breast, postmenopauseal, carnio-caudal (axial) X-ray, mammography

1: Veins
2: Skin
3: Subcutis
4: Connective tissue strand, (suspensory ligament)
5: Body of mamme with involuted glandular tissue

ABDOMEN

Axial CT-series

Stomach

Small intestine

Colon and rectum

Liver and pancreas

Spleen

Arteries

Veins

Lymphatics

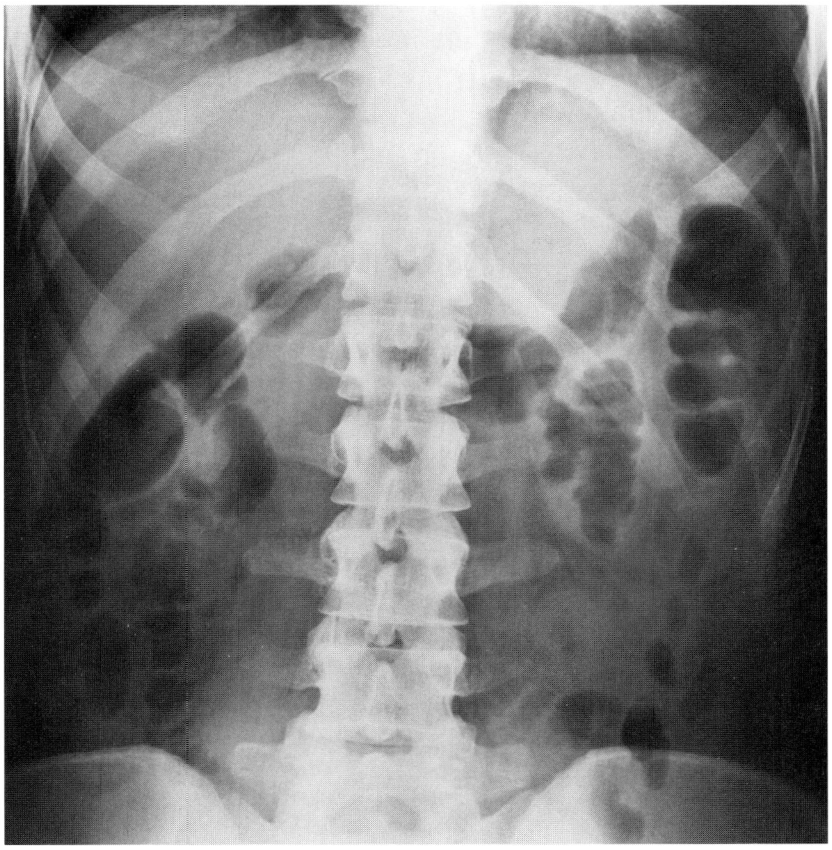

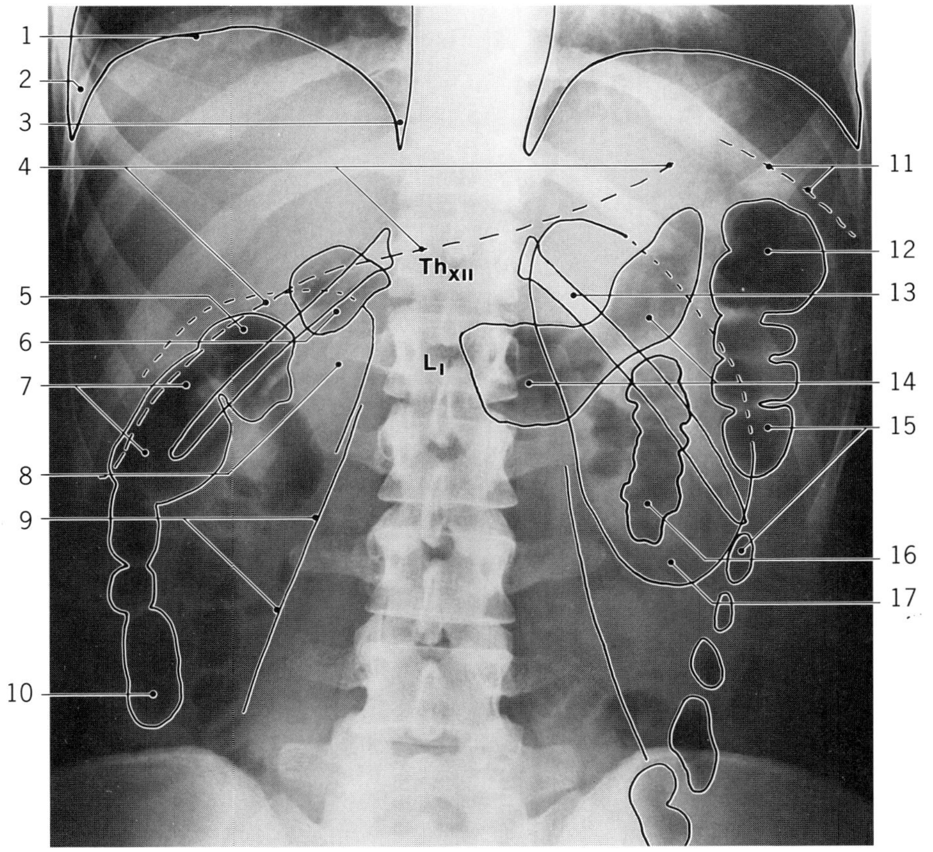

Abdomen, a-p X-ray, erect

The gastro-intestinal tract is outlined by its natural gas content

1: Diaphragm
2: Costodiaphragmatic sulcus
3: Mediastinodiaphragmatic sulcus
4: Lower border of liver
5: Hepatic flexure of colon
6: Duodenal cap (radiology term)
7: Ascending colon
8: Upper pole of right kidney
9: Psoas major (lateral contour)
10: Caecum
11: Lower border of spleen
12: Splenic flexure of colon
13: 12th rib
14: Stomach
15: Descending colon
16: Jejunum
17: Lower pole of left kidney

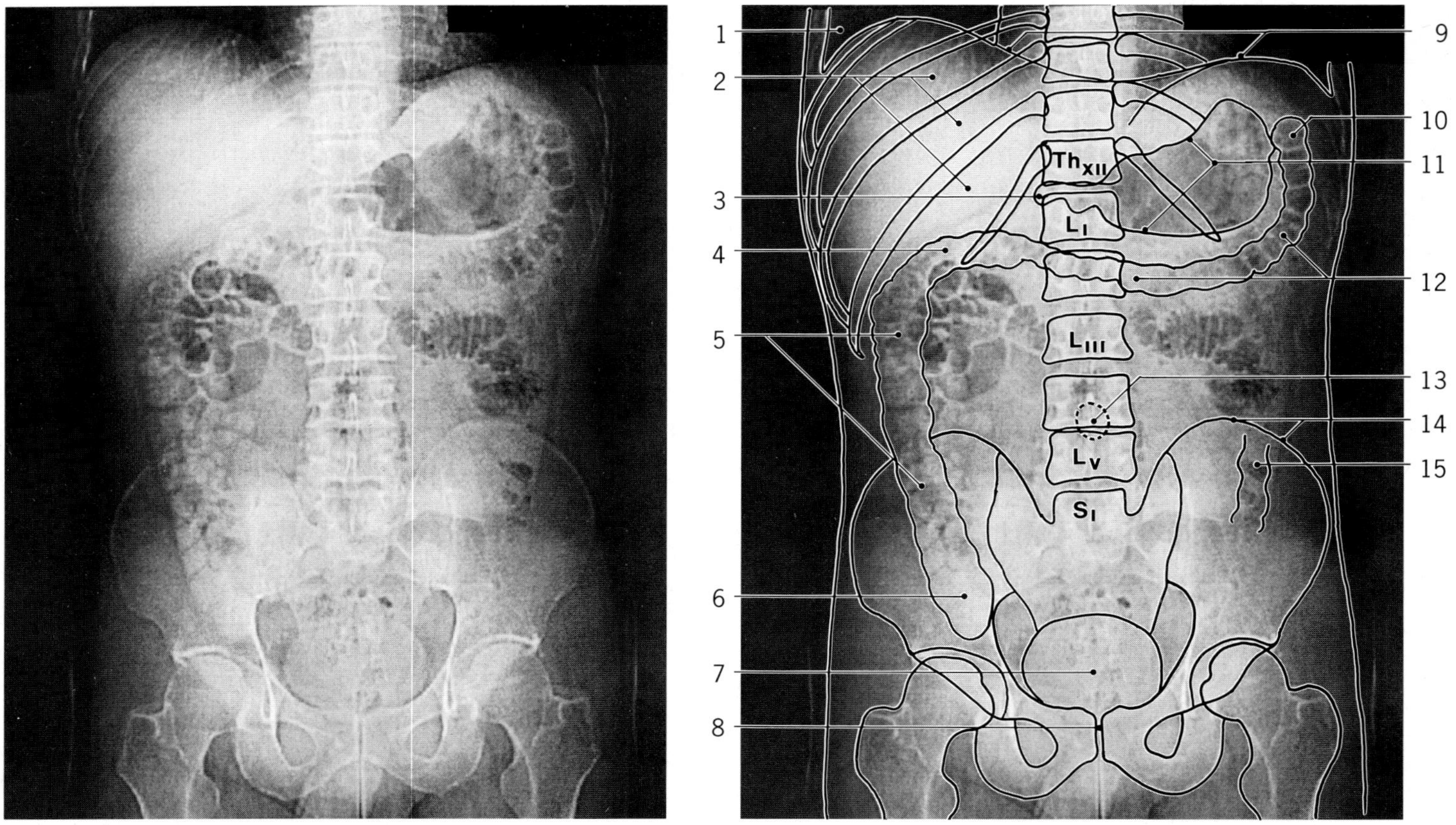

Scout view

1: Costodiaphragmatic sulcus
2: Liver
3: Duodenal cap
4: Hepatic flexure of colon
5: Ascending colon
6: Caecum
7: Urinary bladder
8: Symphysis pubis
9: Diaphragm
10: Splenic flexure of colon
11: Curvatures of stomach
12: Transverse colon
13: Position of umbilicus
14: Iliac crest
15: Descending colon

Scout view

Lines #1-45 indicate position of sections in the following CT series.

Consecutive sections, 10 mm thick.

The gastrointestinal tract is outlined by peroral contrast medium.

Intravenous watersoluble contrast has been given to outline the urinary tract.

Residues of contrast from an earlier lymphography are present in some iliac and lumbar lymph nodes

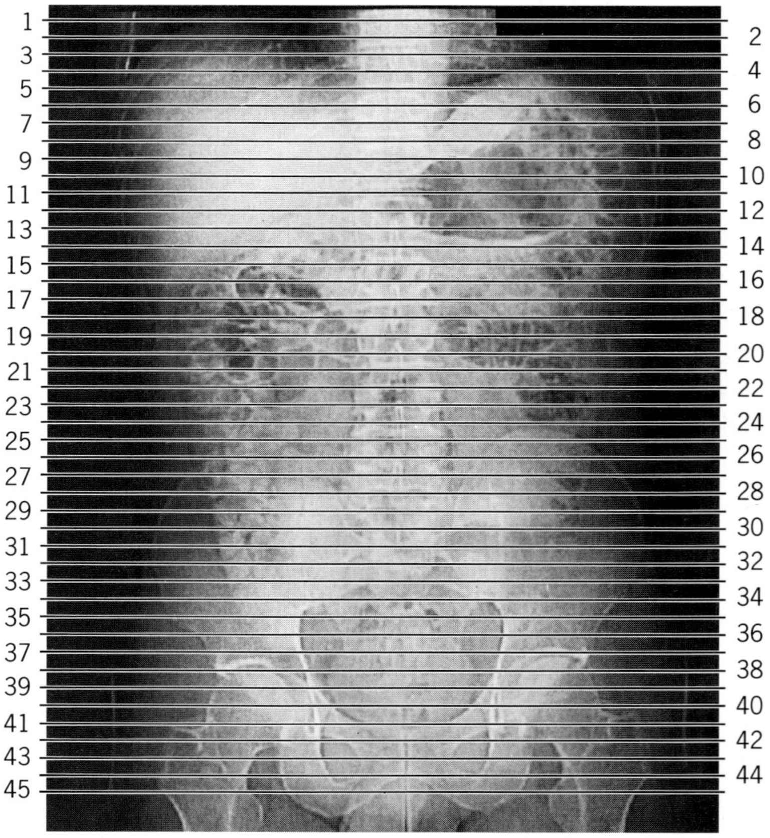

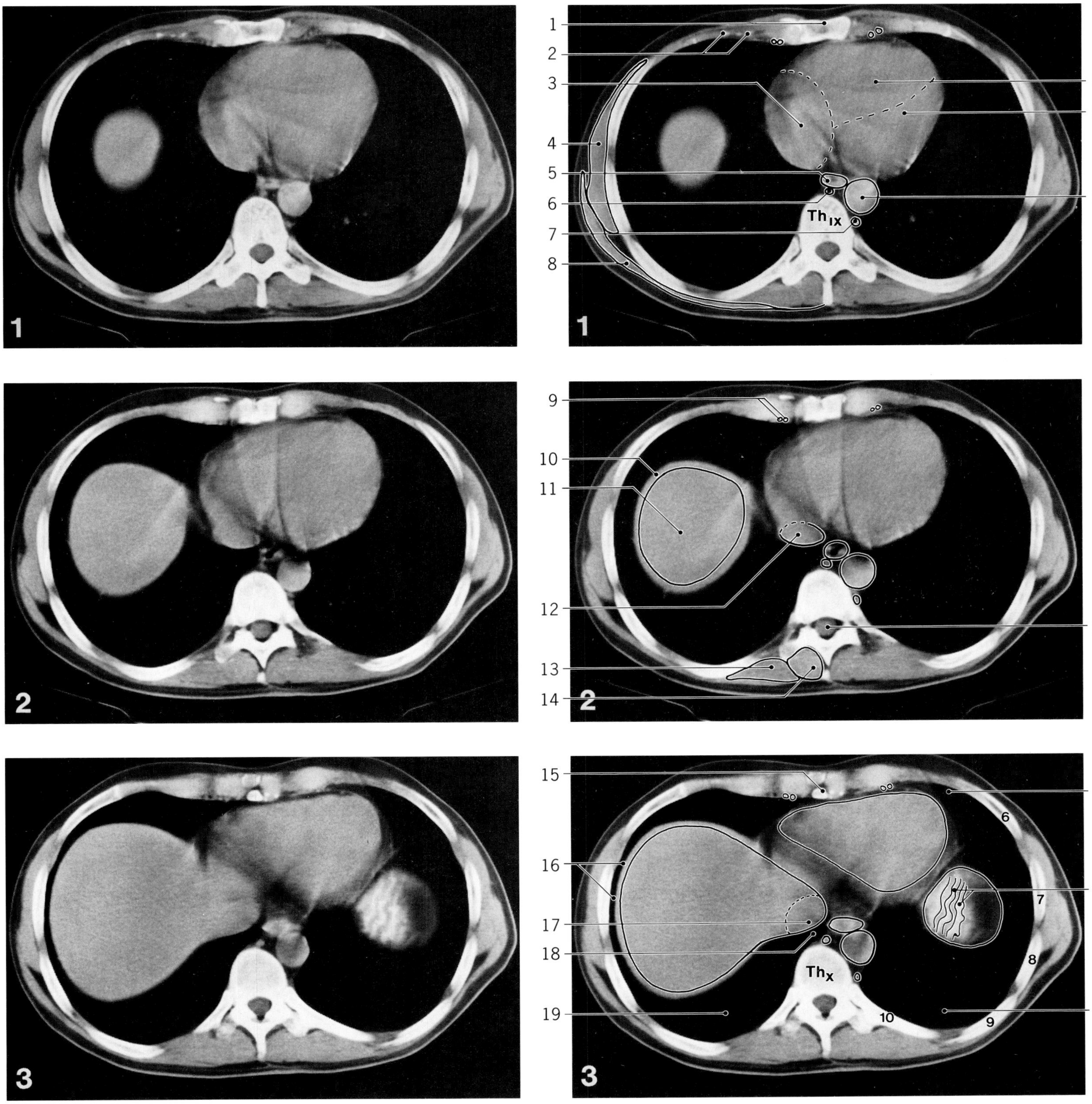

Abdomen, axial CT

Scout view on opposite page

1: Body of sternum
2: Calcified costal cartilage
3: Right atrium
4: Serratus anterior
5: Oesophagus
6: Azygos vein
7: Hemiazygos vein
8: Latissimus dorsi
9: Internal thoracic artery and vein
10: Diaphragm
11: Right lobe of liver
12: Inferior caval vein
13: Iliocostalis thoracis, and longissimus thoracis
14: Transversospinal muscles
15: Xiphoid process
16: Costodiaphragmatic groove
17: Inferior caval vein
18: Phrenico-mediastinal groove
19: Lower lobe of right lung
20: Right ventricle
21: Left ventricle
22: Thoracic aorta
23: Spinal cord
24: Lingula of left lung
25: Rugae in fundus of stomach
26: Lower lobe of left lung
Ribs are numbered.

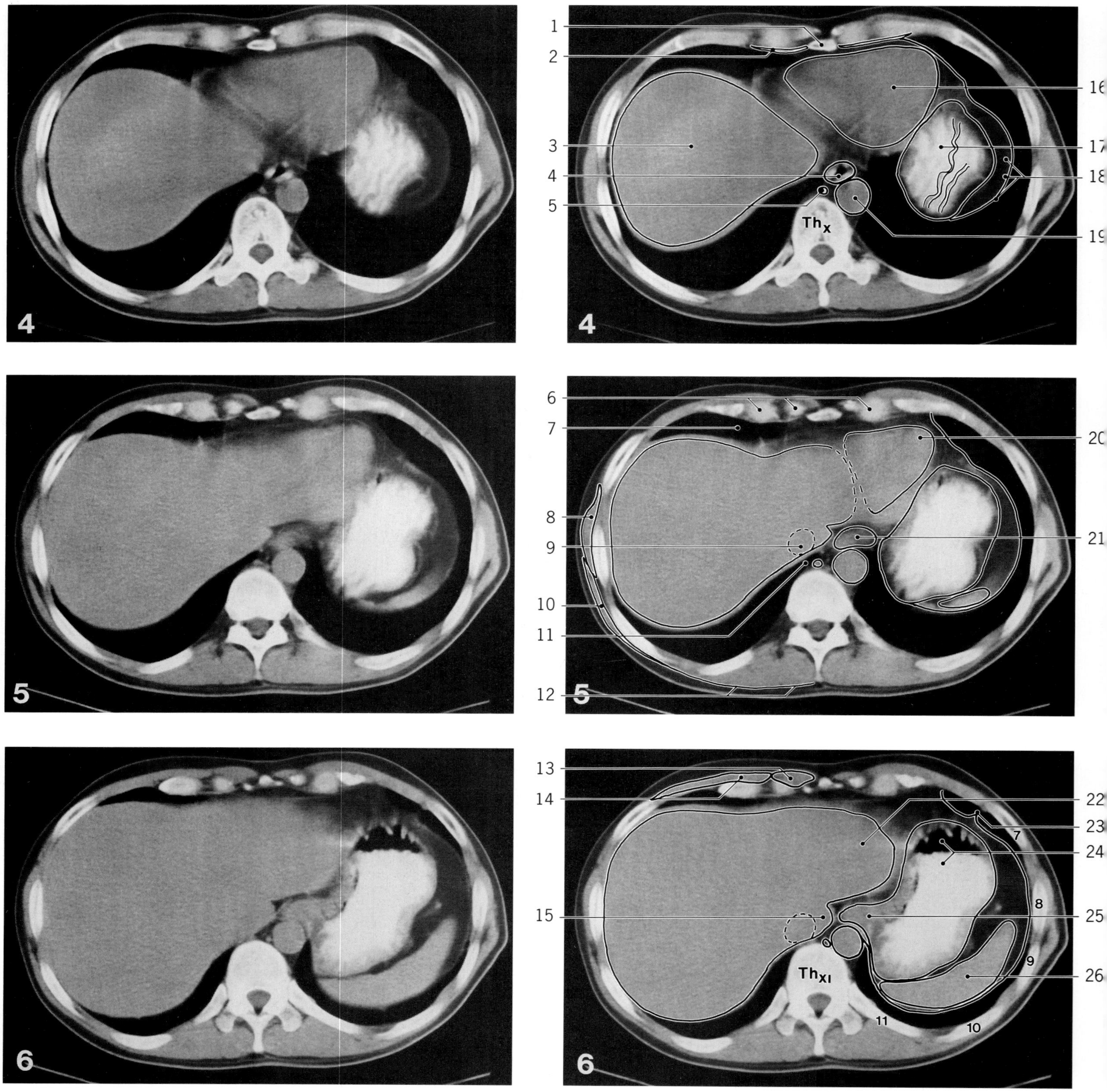

Abdomen, axial CT

Scout view on page 244

1: Xiphoid process
2: Transversus thoracis
3: Right lobe of liver
4: Oesophagus
5: Azygos vein
6: Costal cartilage
7: Costo-diaphragmatic groove with inferior margin of right lung
8: Serratus anterior
9: Inferior caval vein
10: Latissimus dorsi
11: Phrenico-mediastinal groove
12: Thoracolumbar fascia
13: Rectus abdominis
14: Obliquus externus abdominis
15: Caudate lobe of liver
16: Heart
17: Fundus of stomach with rugae
18: Parietal pleura, diaphragm, and parietal peritoneum
19: Thoracic aorta
20: Apex of heart
21: Oesophagus, abdominal part
22: Left lobe of liver
23: Oblique fissure of left lung
24: Fundus of stomach with air and barium
25: Cardia
26: Spleen
Ribs are numbered.

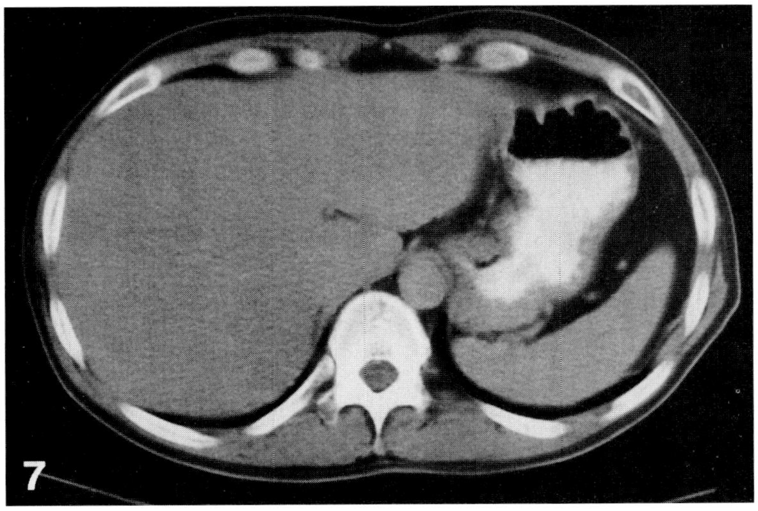

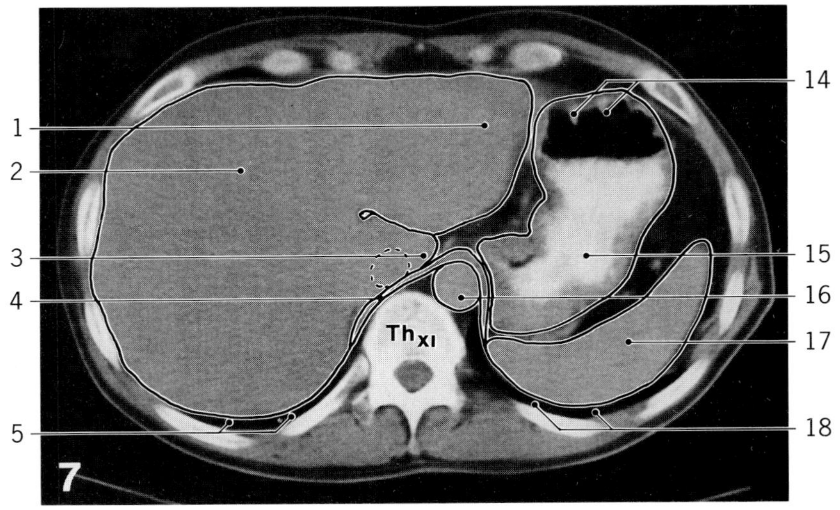

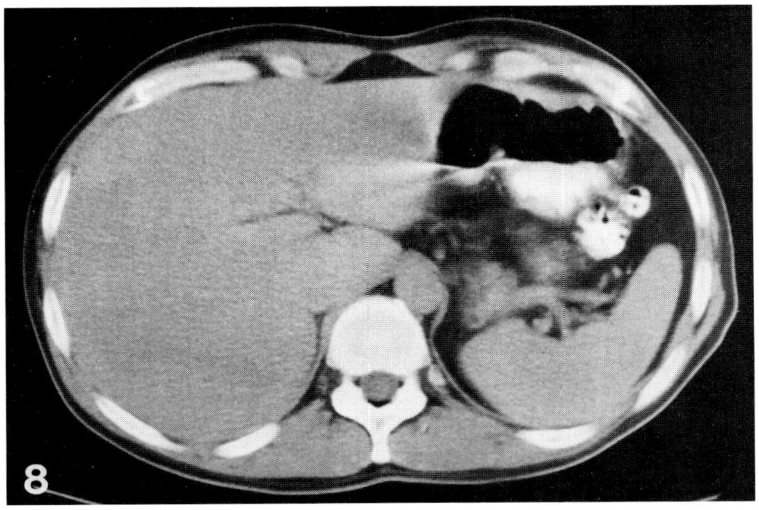

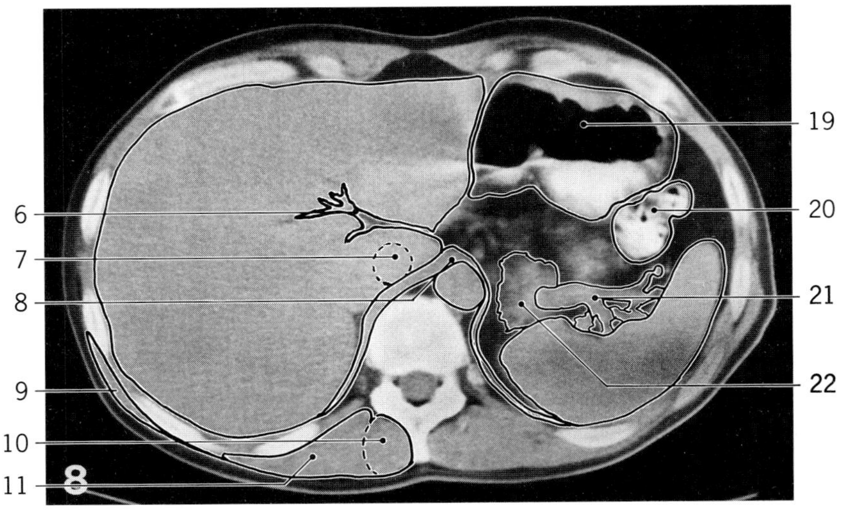

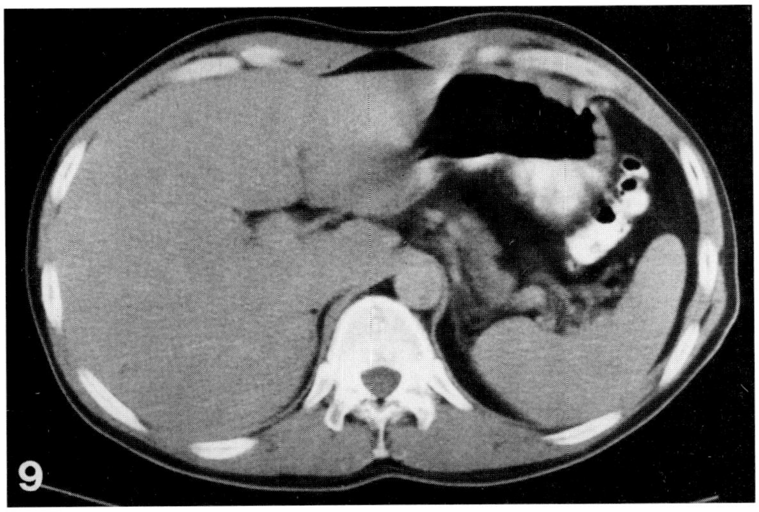

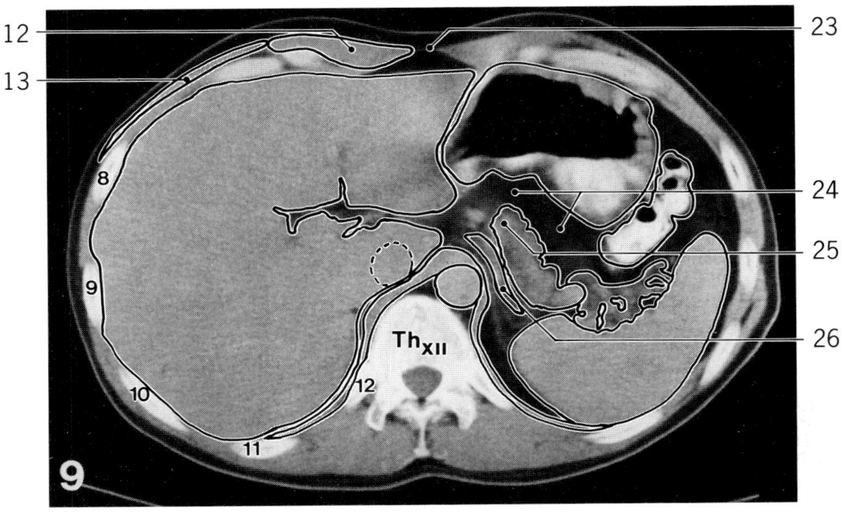

Abdomen, axial CT

Scout view on page 244

1: Left lobe of liver
2: Right lobe of liver
3: Caudate lobe of liver
4: Lumbar part of diaphragm
5: Inferior margin of left lung
6: Porta hepatis
7: Inferior caval vein
8: Right crus of diaphragm
9: Latissimus dorsi
10: Transversospinal muscles
11: Iliocostalis and longissimus
12: Rectus abdominis
13: Obliquus externus abdominis
14: Rugae in fundus of stomach
15: Body of stomach
16: Thoracic aorta
17: Spleen
18: Inferior margin of left lung
19: Air in body of stomach
20: Splenic flexure of colon
21: Splenic vessels
22: Tail of pancreas
23: Linea alba
24: Omental bursa with surrounding peritoneal fat
25: Body of pancreas
26: Splenic artery
Ribs are numbered.

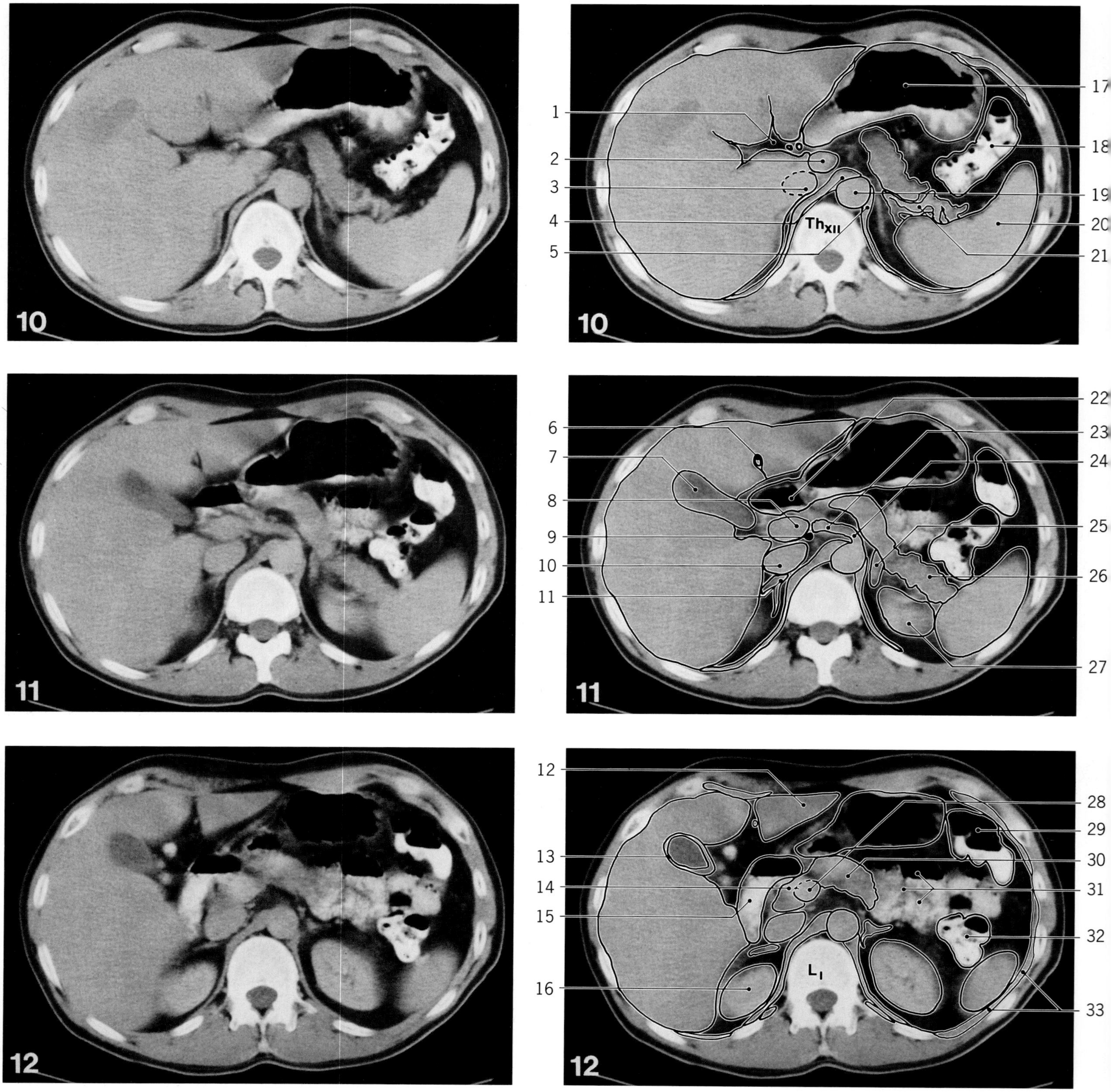

Abdomen, axial CT

Scout view on page 244

1: Porta hepatis
2: Portal vein
3: Inferior caval vein
4: Right crus of diaphragm
5: Left crus of diaphragm
6: Lig. teres hepatis
7: Gall bladder
8: Portal vein
9: Bile duct (choledochus)
10: Inferior caval vein
11: Right suprarenal gland
12: Left lobe of liver
13: Wall of gall bladder
14: Head of pancreas
15: Superior part of duodenum
16: Upper pole of right kidney
17: Body of stomach
18: Splenic flexure of colon
19: Abdominal aorta
20: Spleen
21: Splenic vessels
22: Duodenal "cap" (bulbus)
23: Common hepatic artery
24: Coeliac trunk
25: Left suprarenal gland
26: Tail of pancreas
27: Upper pole of left kidney
28: Portal vein behind pancreas
29: Transverse colon
30: Body of pancreas
31: Jejunum with air and barium
32: Descending colon
33: Diaphragm

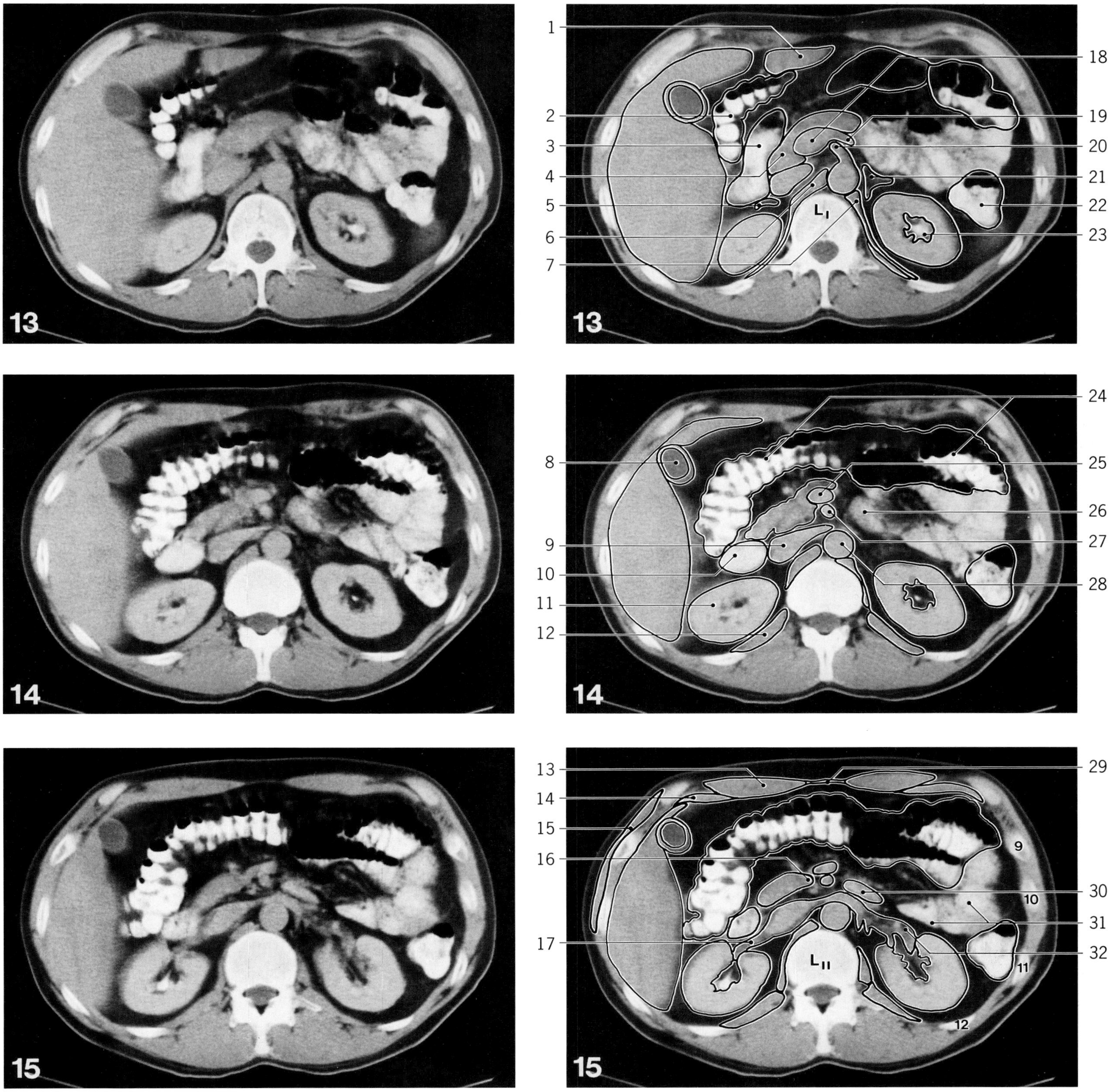

Abdomen, axial CT

Scout view on page 244

1: Left lobe of liver
2: Hepatic flexure of colon
3: Superior part of duodenum
4: Head of pancreas
5: Right suprarenal gland
6: Right crus of diaphragm
7: Left crus of diaphragm
8: Fundus of gall bladder
9: Inferior caval vein
10: Descending part of duodenum
11: Right kidney
12: Quadratus lumborum
13: Rectus abdominis
14: Transversus abdominis
15: Obliquus externus abdominis
16: Uncinate process of pancreas
17: Right renal vein
18: Portal vein
19: Splenic vein
20: Superior mesenteric artery
21: Left suprarenal gland
22: Descending colon
23: Sinus renalis
24: Transverse colon
25: Superior mesenteric vein
26: Duodenojejunal flexure
27: Superior mesenteric artery
28: Abdominal aorta
29: Linea alba
30: Ascending part of duodenum
31: Jejunum
32: Left renal vein

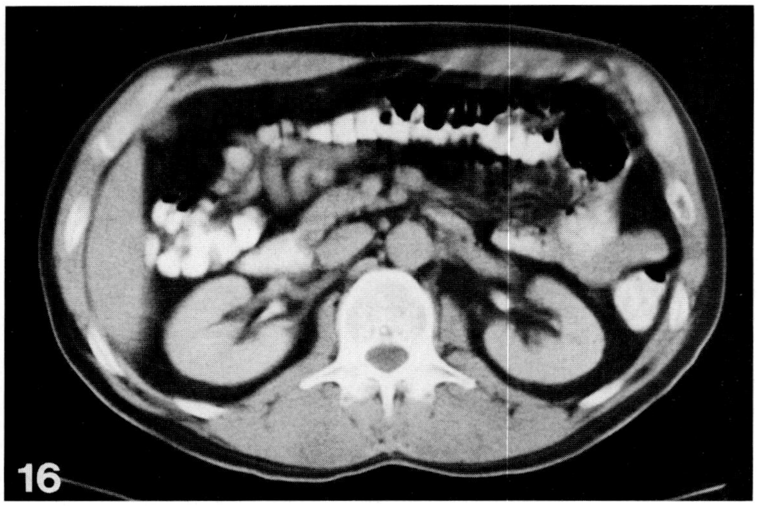

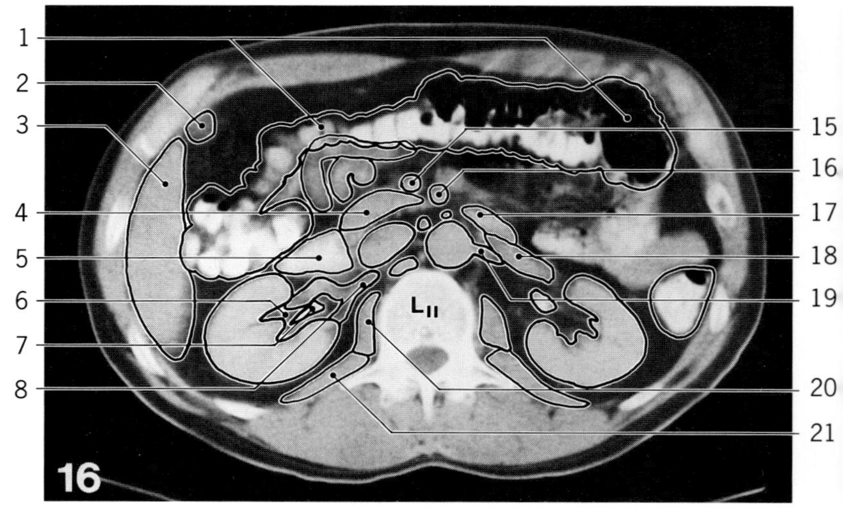

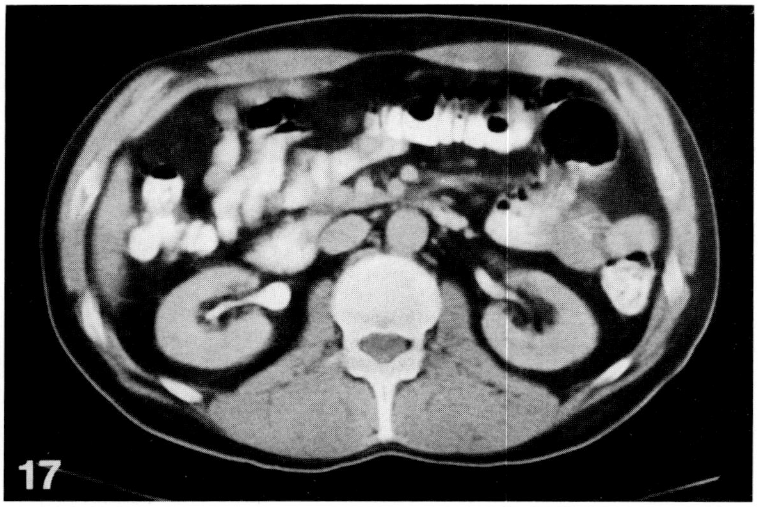

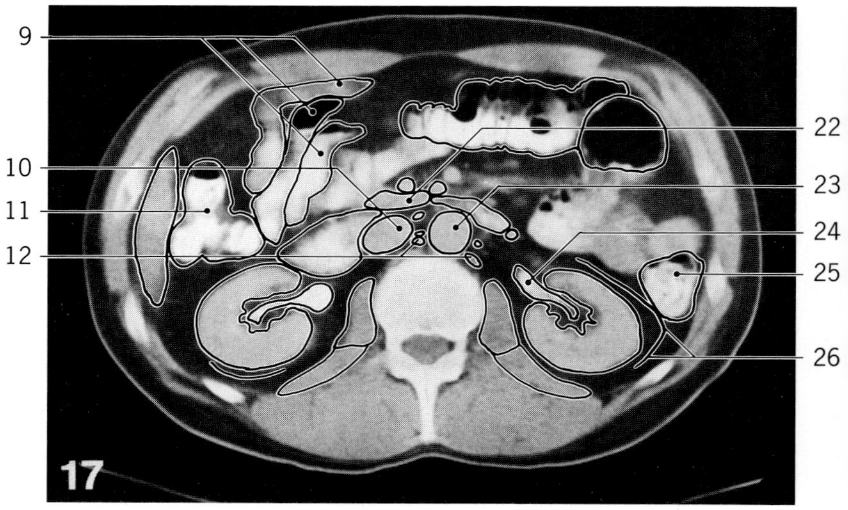

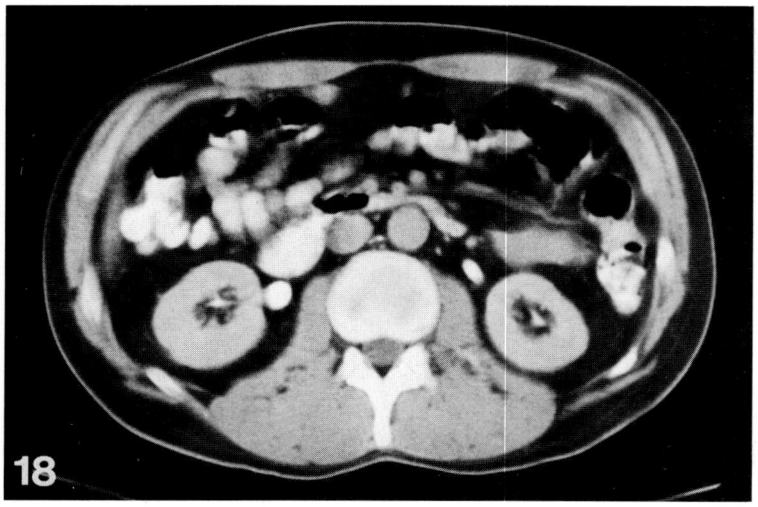

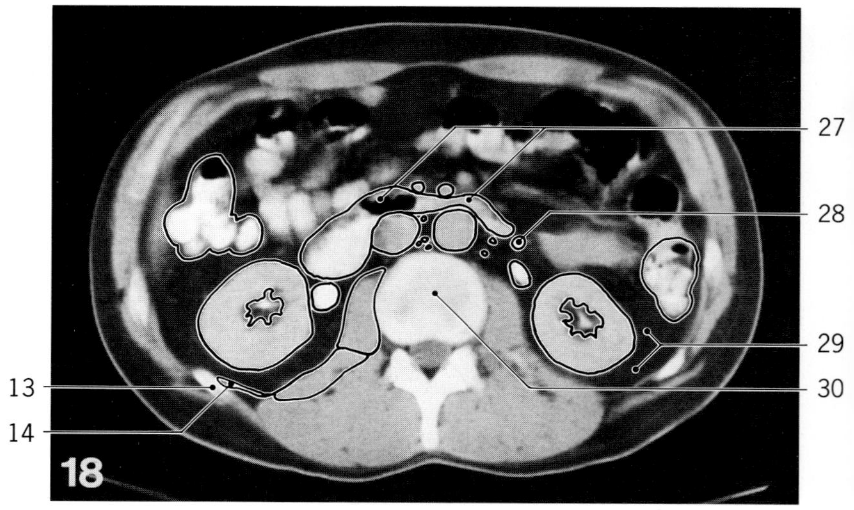

Abdomen, axial CT

Scout view on page 244

1: Transverse colon with air and contrast
2: Fundus of gall bladder
3: Right lobe of liver
4: Head of pancreas
5: Descending part of duodenum
6: Sinus renalis dxt.
7: Pelvis of right kidney
8: Right renal artery
9: Jejunum
10: Inferior caval vein
11: Ascending colon
12: Paraaortic lymph nodes
13: 12th rib
14: Lateral arcuate ligament
15: Superior mesenteric vein
16: Superior mesenteric artery
17: Ascending part of duodenum
18: Left renal vein
19: Left renal artery
20: Psoas major
21: Quadratus lumborum
22: Uncinate process of pancreas
23: Abdominal aorta
24: Pelvis of left kidney
25: Descending colon
26: Renal fascia
27: Horizontal part of duodenum
28: Inferior mesenteric vein
29: Retroperitoneal fat
30: Intervertebral disc L II - L III

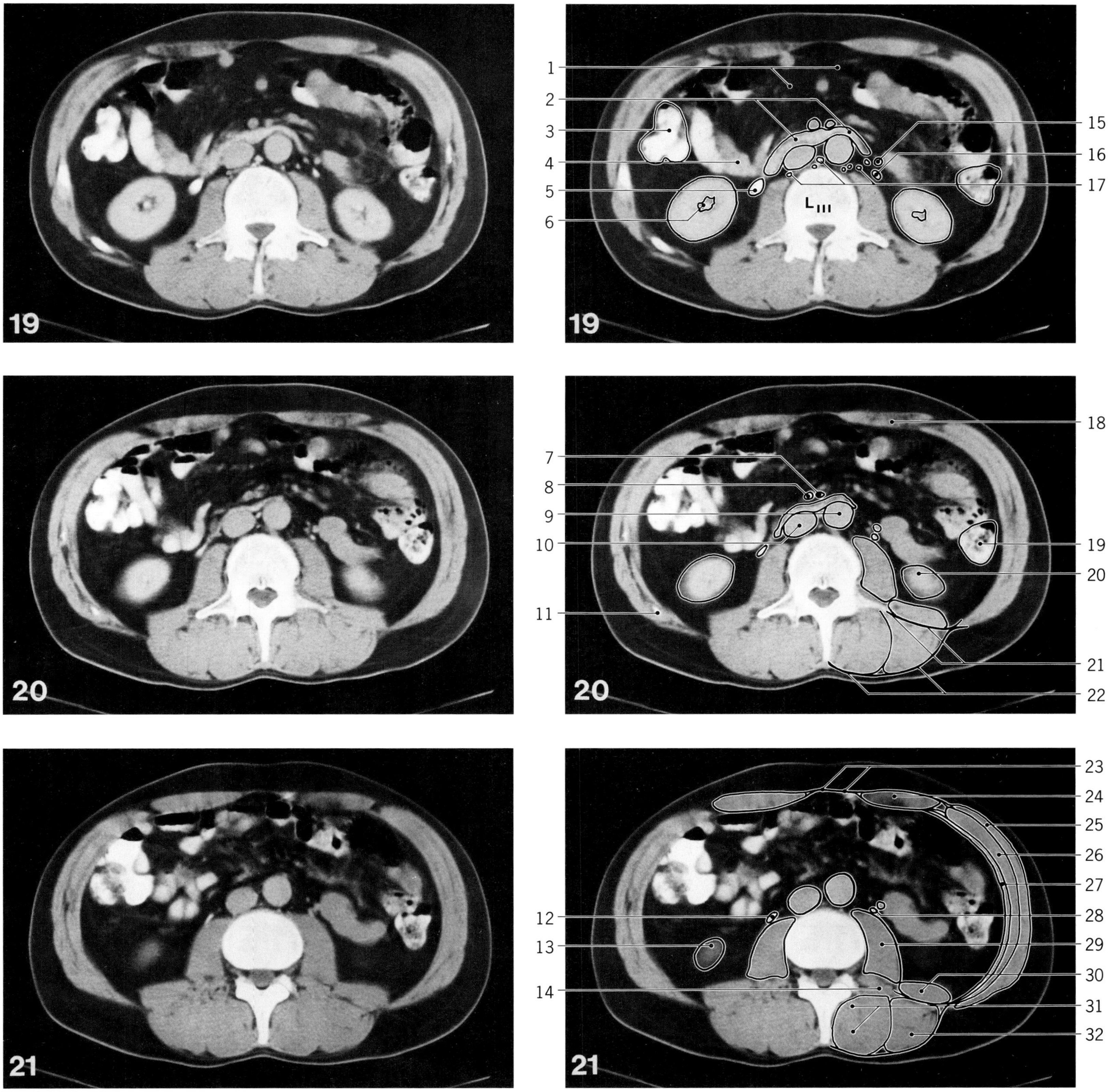

Abdomen, axial CT

Scout view on page 244

1: Mesenterial fat
2: Horizontal part of duodenum
3: Ascending colon
4: Jejunum
5: Pelvis of right kidney
6: Sinus renalis dxt.
7: Superior mesenteric artery
8: Superior mesenteric vein
9: Abdominal aorta
10: Inferior caval vein
11: 12th rib (tip)
12: Right ureter
13: Lower pole of right kidney
14: Intertransversarius muscle
15: Inferior mesenteric vein
16: Pelvis of left kidney
17: Lumbar lymph nodes
18: Tendinous intersection in rectus abdominis
19: Descending colon
20: Lower pole of left kidney
21: Lumbar aponeurosis
22: Thoracolumbar fascia
23: Linea alba
24: Rectus abdominis
25: Obliquus externus abdominis
26: Obliquus internus abdominis
27: Transversus abdominis
28: Left ureter
29: Psoas major
30: Quadratus lumborum
31: Transversospinal muscles
32: Iliocostalis lumborum, and longissimus thoracis

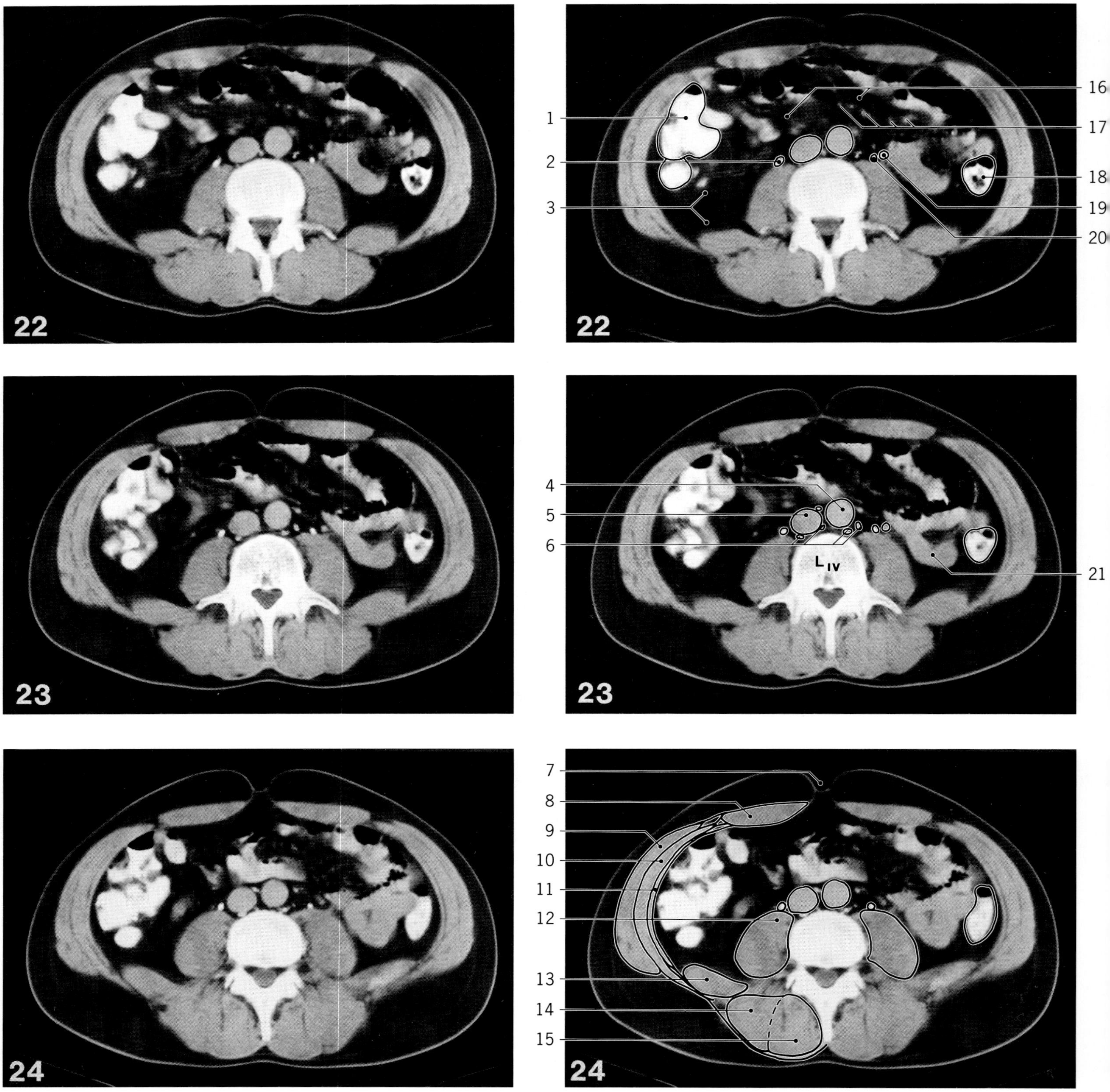

Abdomen, axial CT

Scout view on page 244

1: Ascending colon
2: Right ureter
3: Retroperitoneal fat
4: Abdominal aorta
5: Inferior caval vein
6: Paraaortic lymph nodes
7: Umbilicus
8: Rectus abdominis
9: Obliquus externus abdominis
10: Obliquus internus abdominis
11: Transversus abdominis
12: Psoas major
13: Quadratus lumborum
14: Erector spinae
15: Transversospinal muscles (mostly multifidi)
16: Mesenterial fat
17: Mesenterial vessels
18: Descending colon
19: Inferior mesenteric vein
20: Left ureter
21: Small intestinal loop

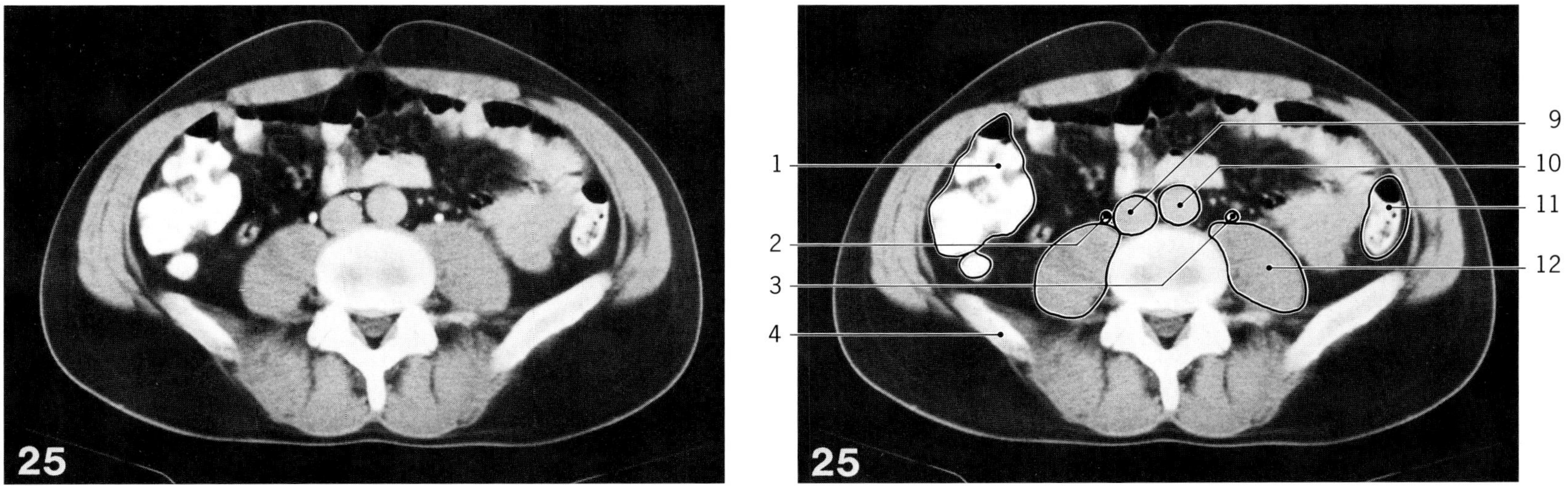

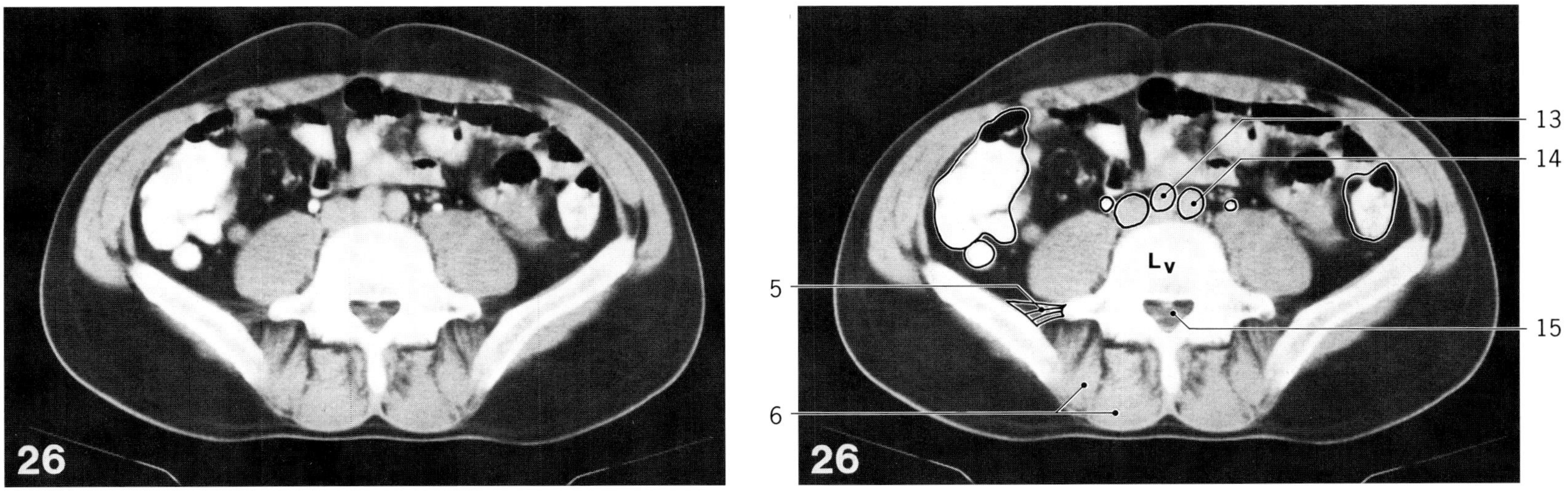

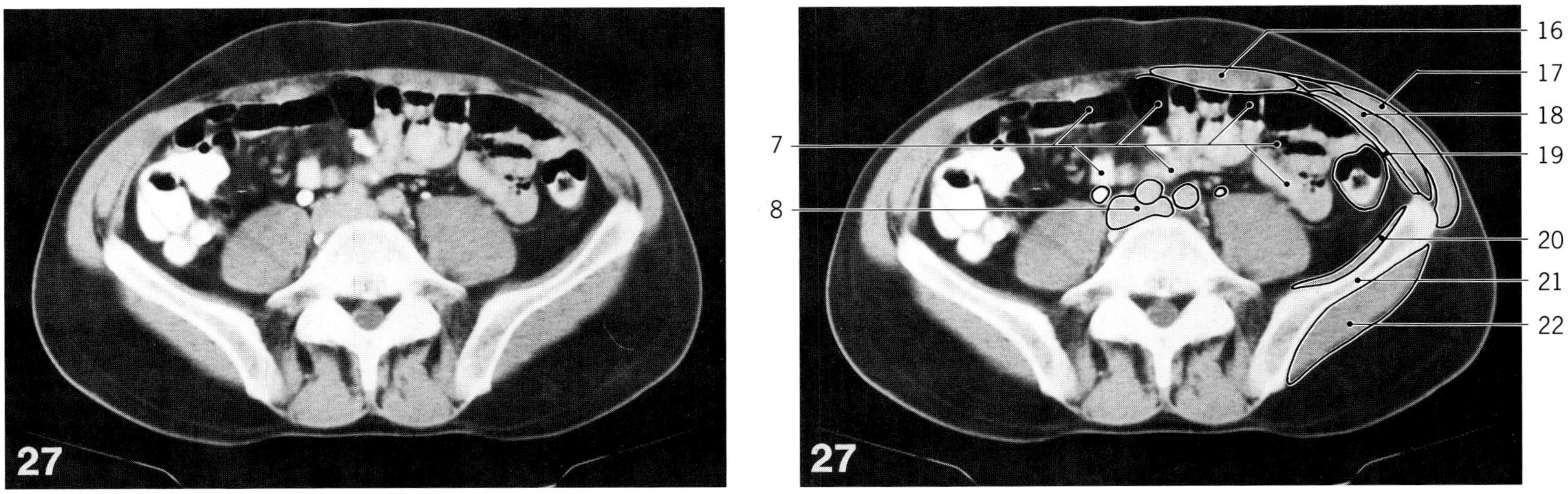

Abdomen, axial CT

Scout view on page 244

1: Ascending colon
2: Right ureter
3: Left ureter
4: Iliac crest
5: Iliolumbar ligament
6: Erector spinae
7: Small intestine with barium and air
8: Inferior caval vein (bifurcation)
9: Inferior caval vein
10: Abdominal aorta
11: Descending colon
12: Psoas major
13: Right common iliac artery
14: Left common iliac artery
15: Cauda equina
16: Rectus abdominis
17: Obliquus externus abdominis
18: Obliquus internus abdominis
19: Transversus abdominis
20: Iliacus
21: Wing of ilium
22: Gluteus medius

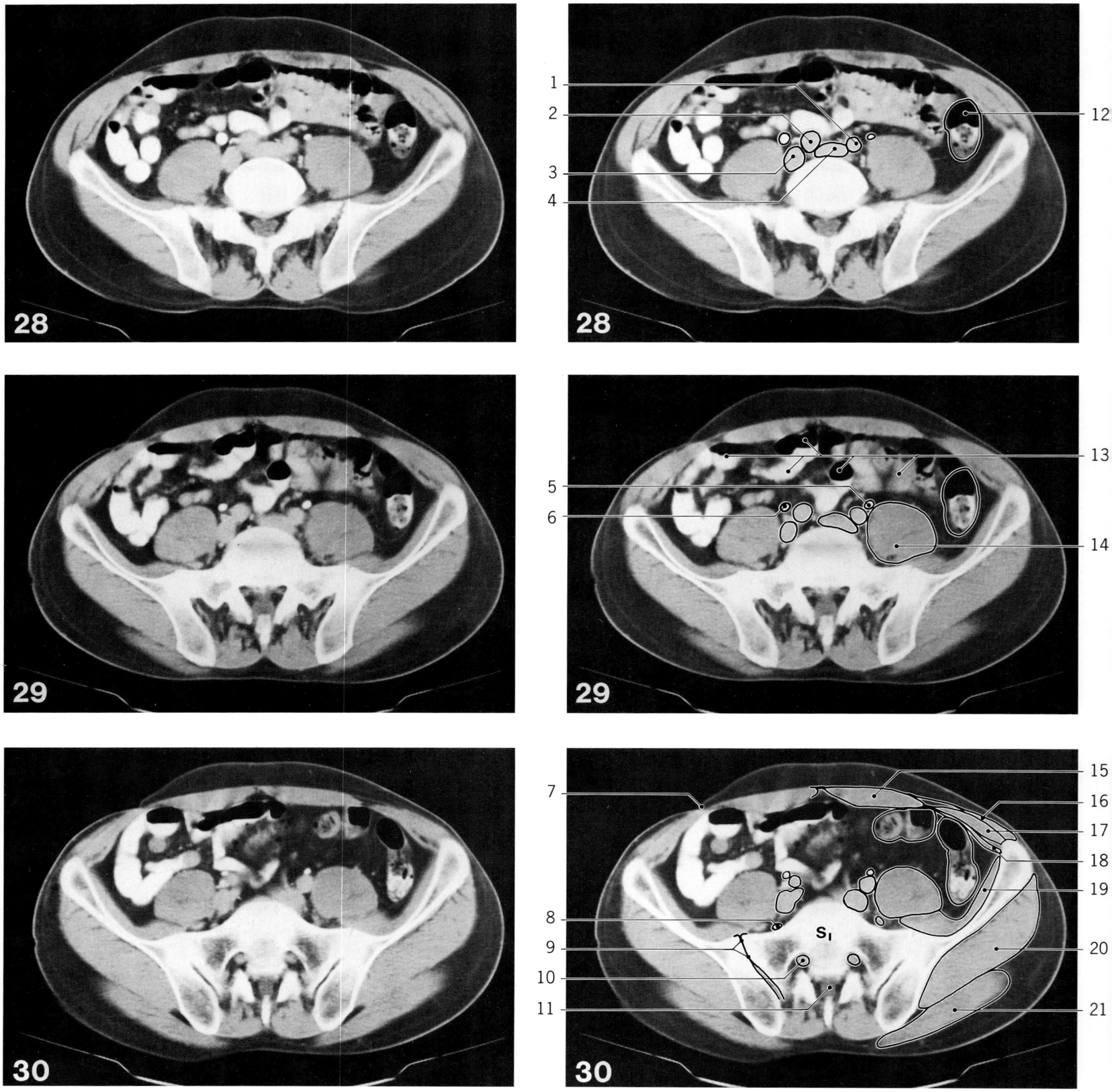

Abdomen, axial CT

Scout view on page 244

1: Left common iliac artery
2: Right common iliac artery
3: Right common iliac vein
4: Left common iliac vein
5: Left ureter
6: Right ureter
7: Appendectomy scar
8: Lumbosacral trunk
9: Sacro-iliac joint
10: Spinal nerve root S I
11: Cauda equina in sacral canal
12: Descending colon
13: Small intestine
14: Psoas major
15: Rectus abdominis
16: Obliquus externus abdominis
17: Obliquus internus abdominis
18: Transversus abdominis
19: Iliacus
20: Gluteus medius
21: Gluteus maximus

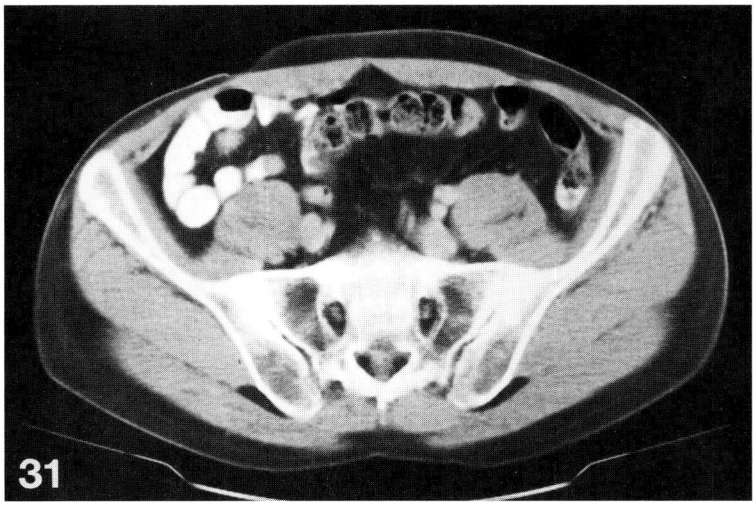

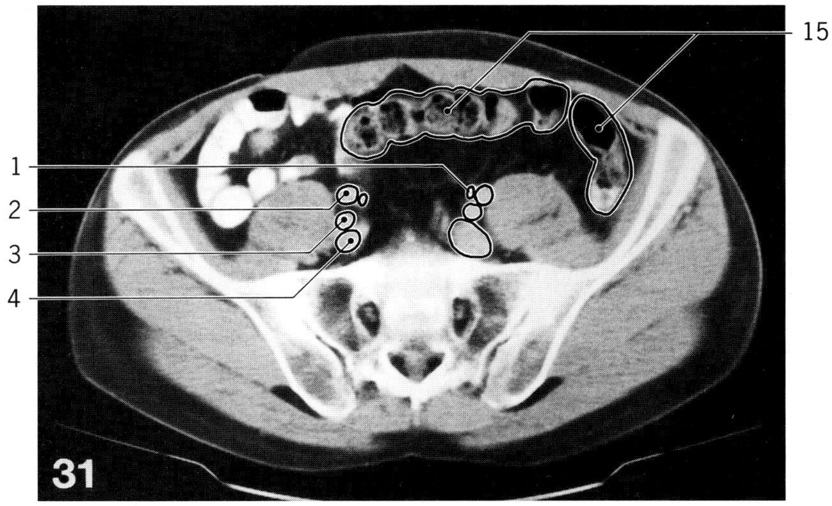

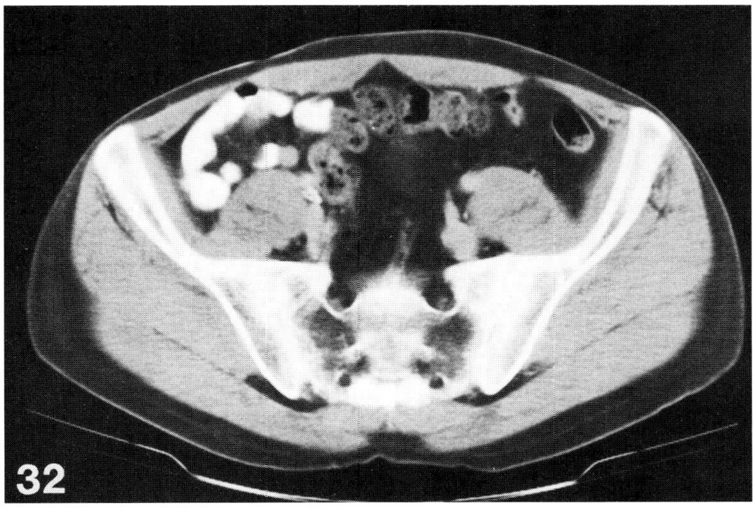

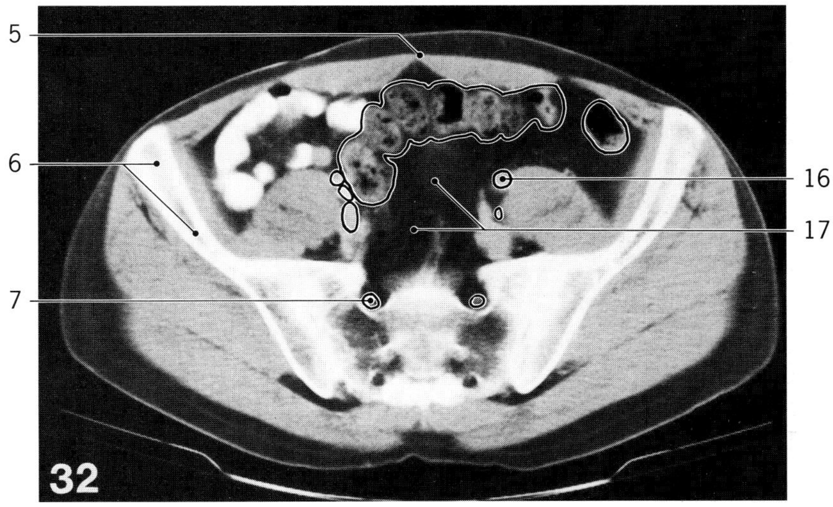

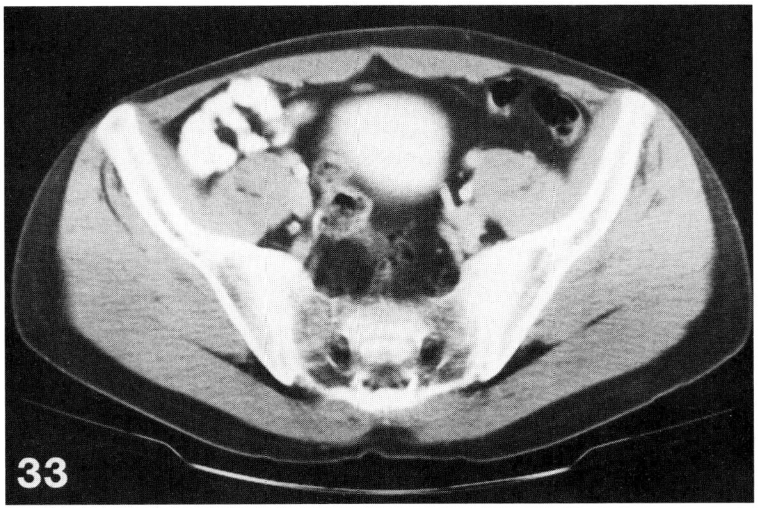

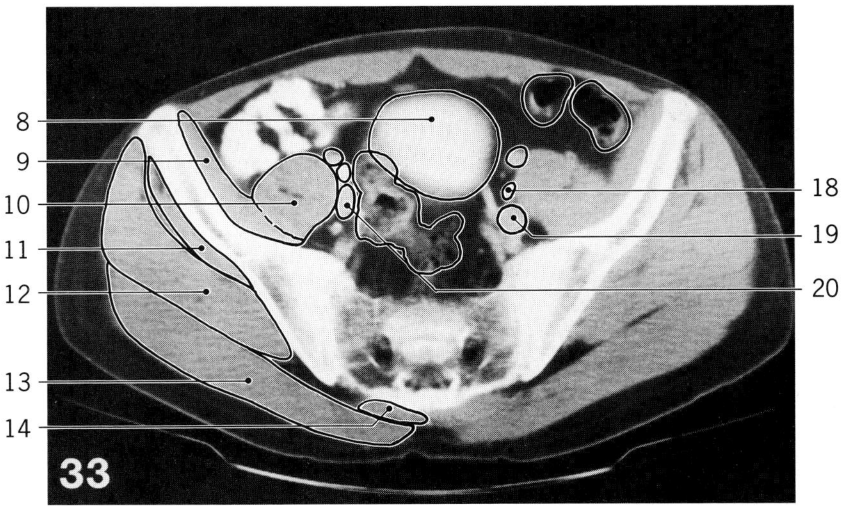

Abdomen, axial CT

Scout view on page 244

1: Left ureter
2: Right external iliac artery
3: Right internal iliac artery
4: Right common iliac vein
5: Linea alba
6: Ilium (wing)
7: Spinal nerve S I in pelvic sacral foramen
8: Urinary bladder
9: Iliacus
10: Psoas major
11: Gluteus minimus
12: Gluteus medius
13: Gluteus maximus
14: Erector spinae (origin)
15: Sigmoid colon
16: Left external iliac artery
17: Mesenterial fat
18: Left ureter
19: Left external iliac vein
20: Right external iliac vein

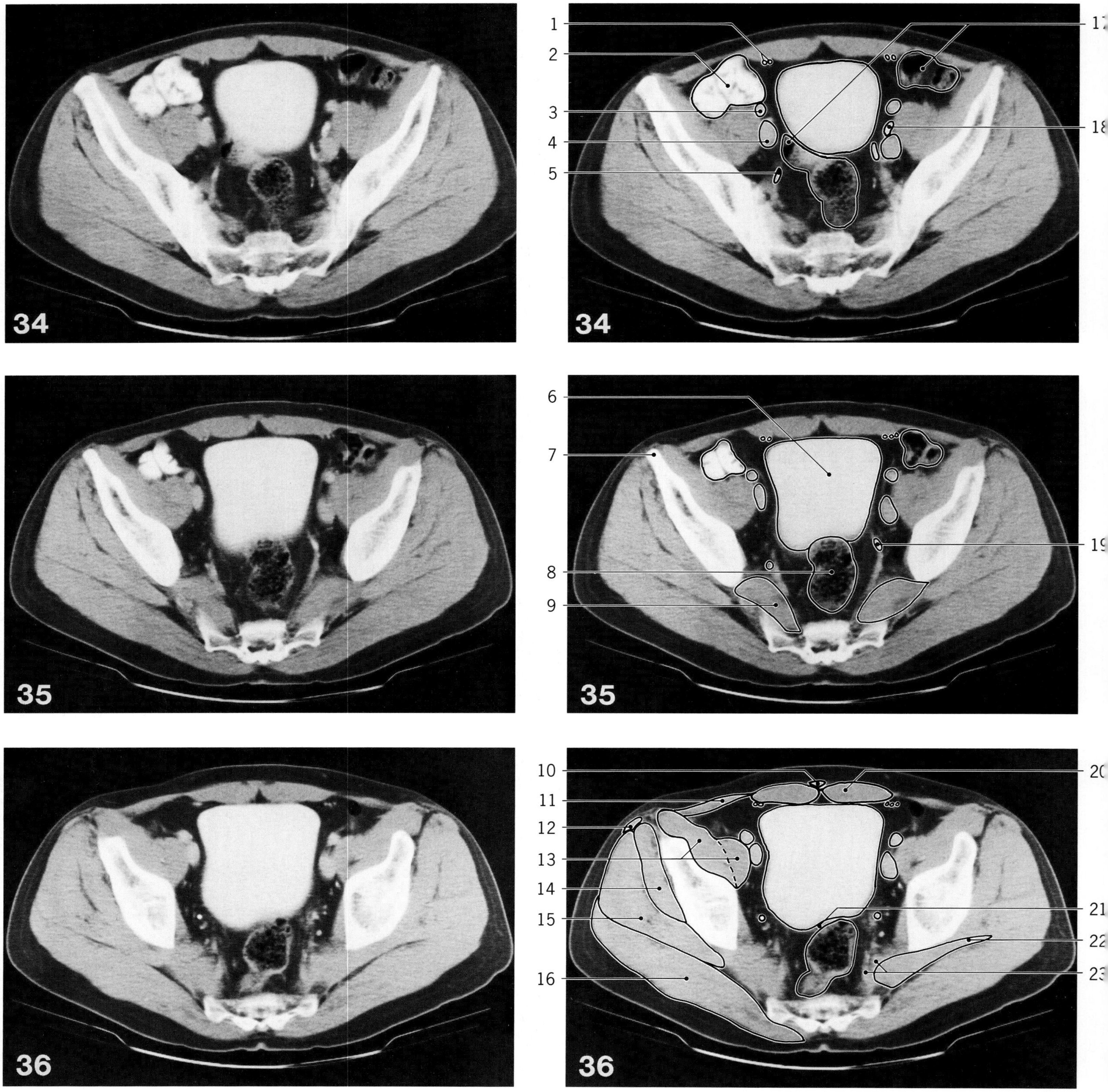

Male pelvis, axial CT

Scout view on page 244

1: Inferior epigastric artery and vein
2: Caecum
3: Right external iliac artery
4: Right external iliac vein
5: Right ureter
6: Urinary bladder
7: Anterior superior iliac spine
8: Rectum
9: Piriformis
10: Pyramidalis muscle
11: Obliquus externus, - internus, and - transversus abdominis
12: Tensor fasciae latae (origin)
13: Iliopsoas
14: Gluteus minimus
15: Gluteus medius
16: Gluteus maximus
17: Sigmoid colon
18: External iliac lymph node with contrast medium
19: Left ureter
20: Rectus abdominis
21: Rectovesical fold
22: Piriformis (tendon)
23: Sacral plexus

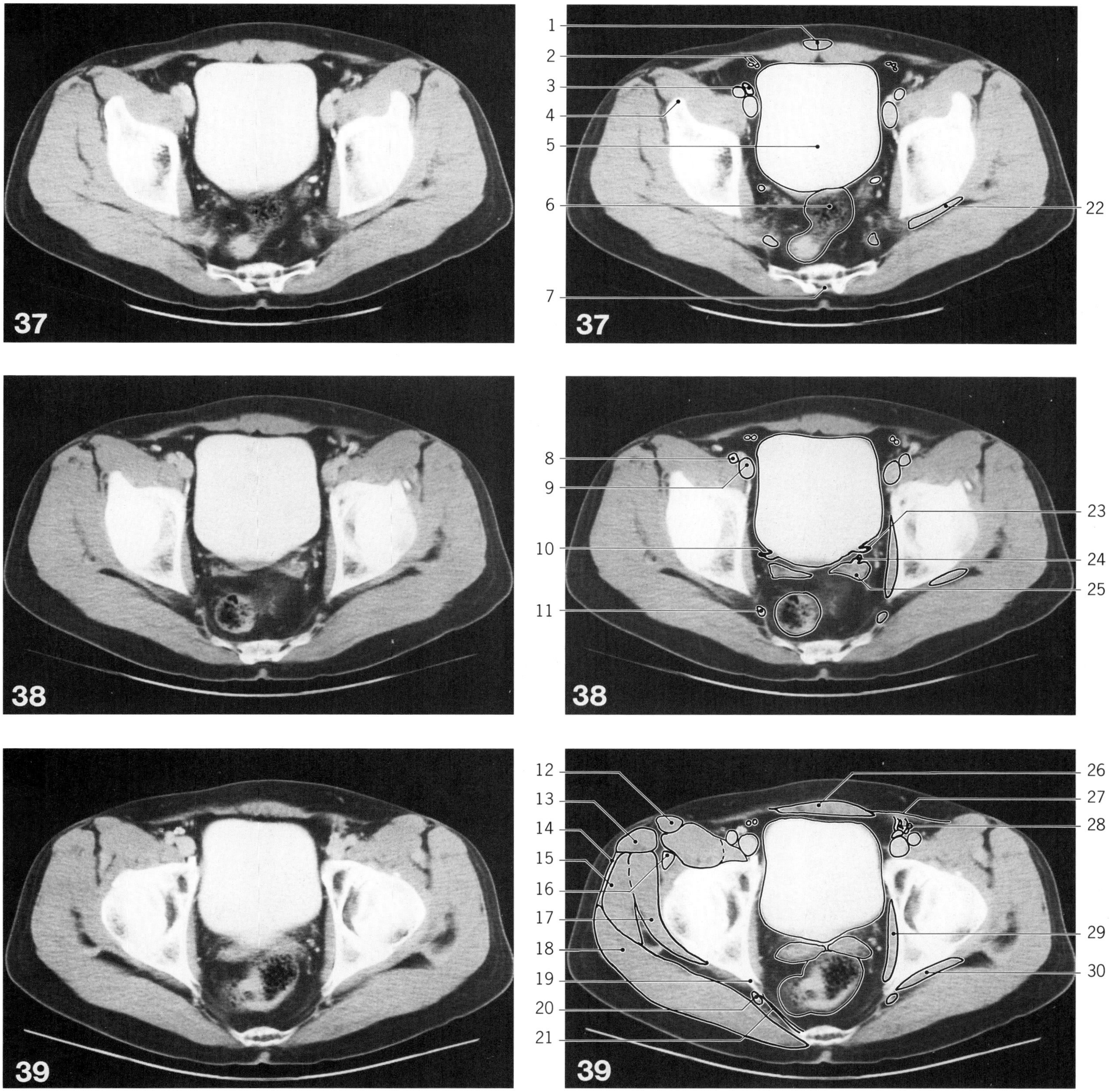

Male pelvis, axial CT

Scout view on page 244

1: Pyramidalis muscle
2: Inferior epigastric artery and vein
3: Lymph node with contrast medium
4: Anterior inferior iliac spine
5: Urinary bladder
6: Rectum
7: Hiatus sacralis
8: Right external iliac artery
9: Right external iliac vein
10: Right ureter
11: Sciatic nerve in infrapiriform foramen
12: Sartorius
13: Tensor fasciae latae
14: Iliotibial tract
15: Gluteus medius
16: Rectus femoris
17: Gluteus minimus
18: Gluteus maximus
19: Ischial spine
20: Sciatic nerve
21: Sacrospinous ligament
22: Piriformis (tendon)
23: Left ureter
24: Ductus deferens
25: Seminal vesicle
26: Rectus abdominis
27: Obliquus externus abdominis (aponeurosis)
28: Inferior epigastric vessels, testicular vessels and deferent duct
29: Obturatorius internus
30: Gemellus superior

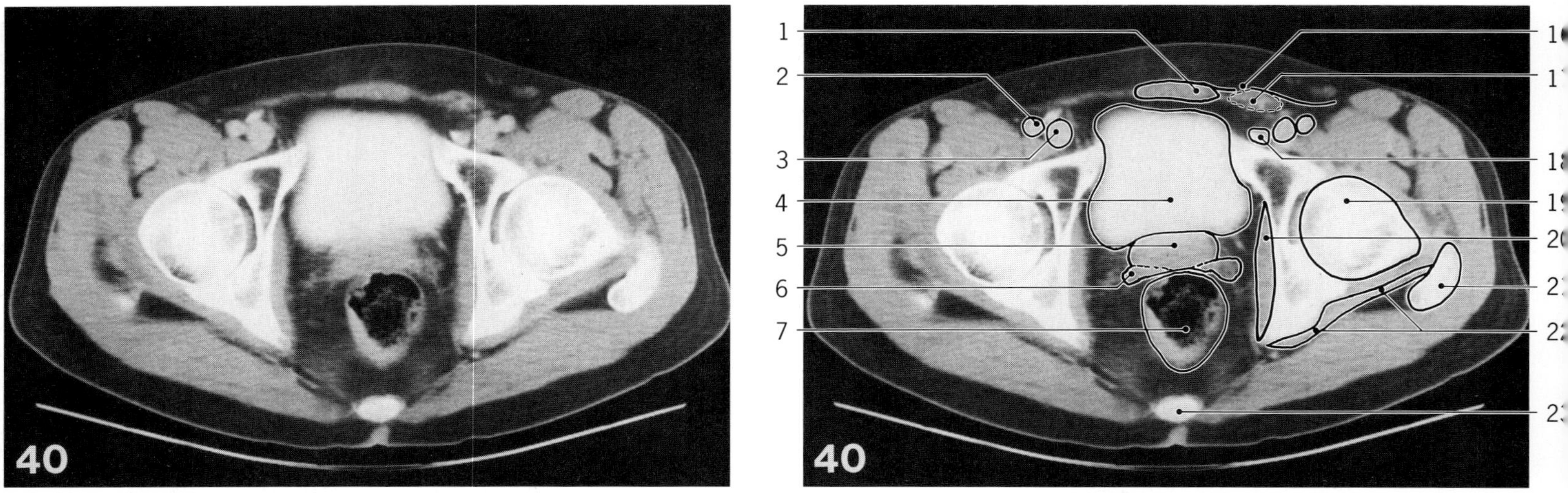

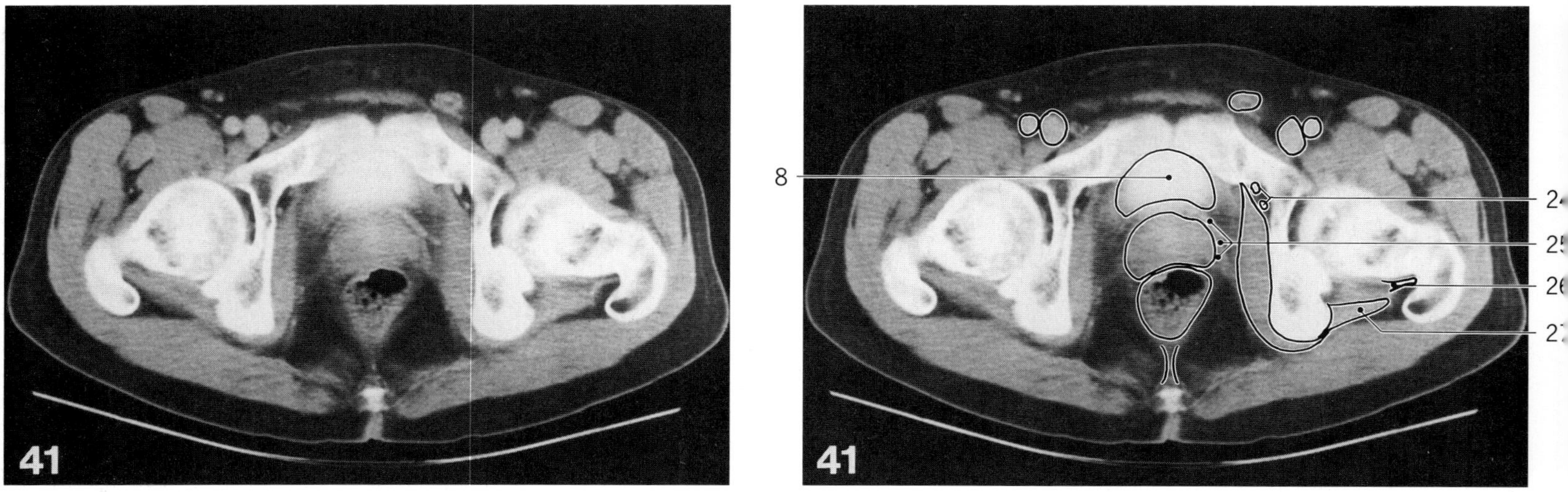

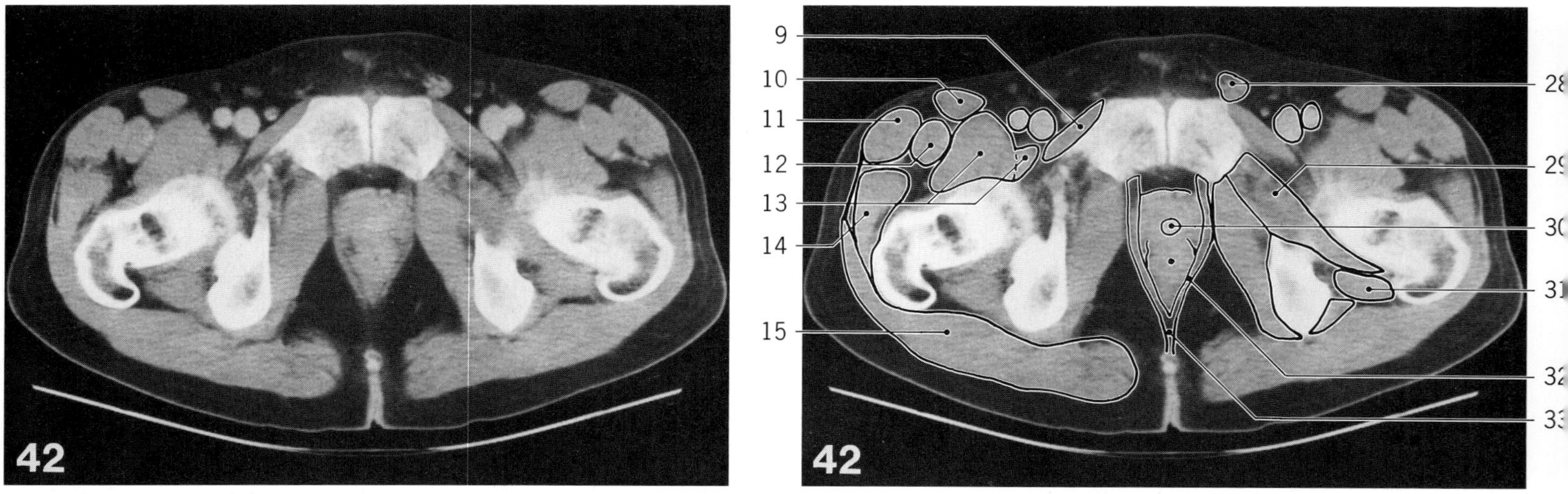

Male pelvis, axial CT

Scout view on page 244

1: Rectus abdominis (tendon)
2: Right external iliac artery
3: Right external iliac vein
4: Urinary bladder
5: Prostate
6: Seminal vesicle
7: Rectum
8: Fundus of urinary bladder
9: Pectineus
10: Sartorius
11: Tensor fasciae latae
12: Rectus femoris
13: Iliopsoas
14: Gluteus medius and minimus
15: Gluteus maximus
16: Superficial inguinal annulus
17: Spermatic cord
18: Deep inguinal lymph node
19: Head of femur
20: Obturatorius internus
21: Greater trochanter
22: Gemellus superior, and obturatorius internus (tendon)
23: Coccyx
24: Obturator artery and nerve
25: Prostatic venous plexus
26: Obturatorius externus (tendon)
27: Gemellus inferior
28: Spermatic cord (removed on right side)
29: Obturatorius externus
30: Prostatic part of urethra
31: Quadratus femoris
32: Levator ani
33: Anococcygeal ligament

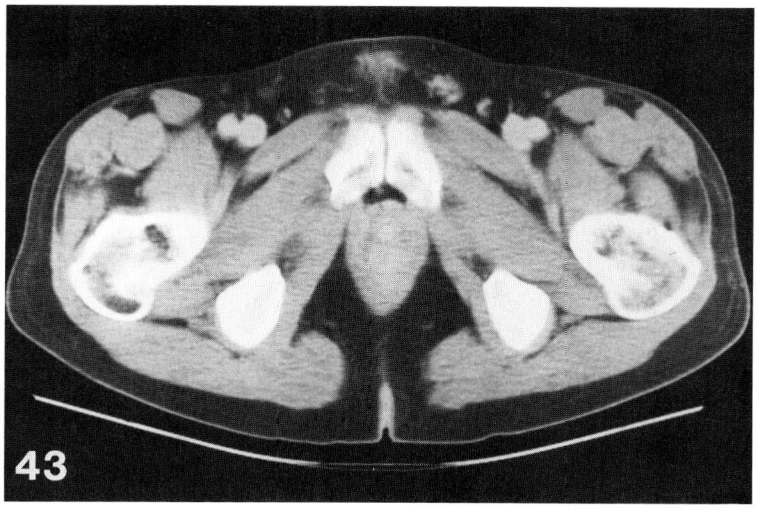

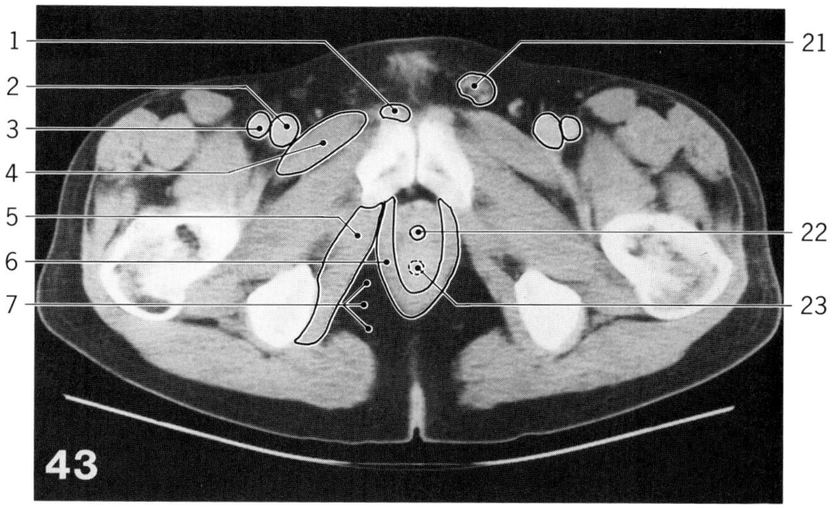

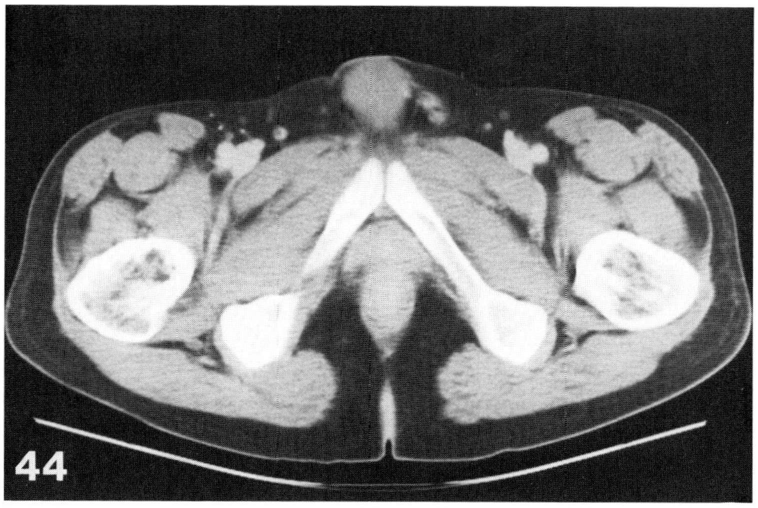

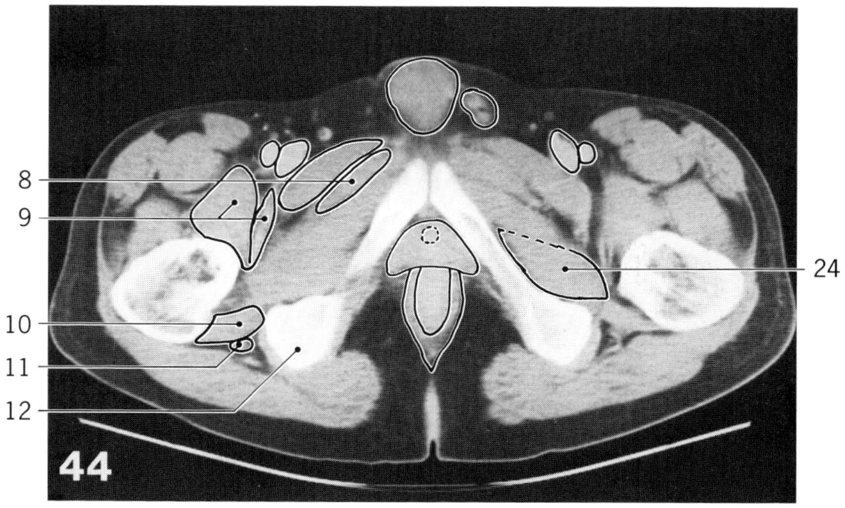

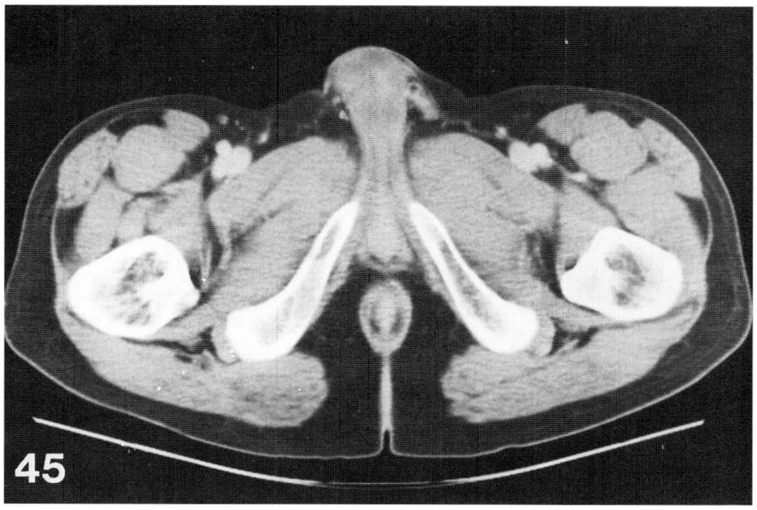

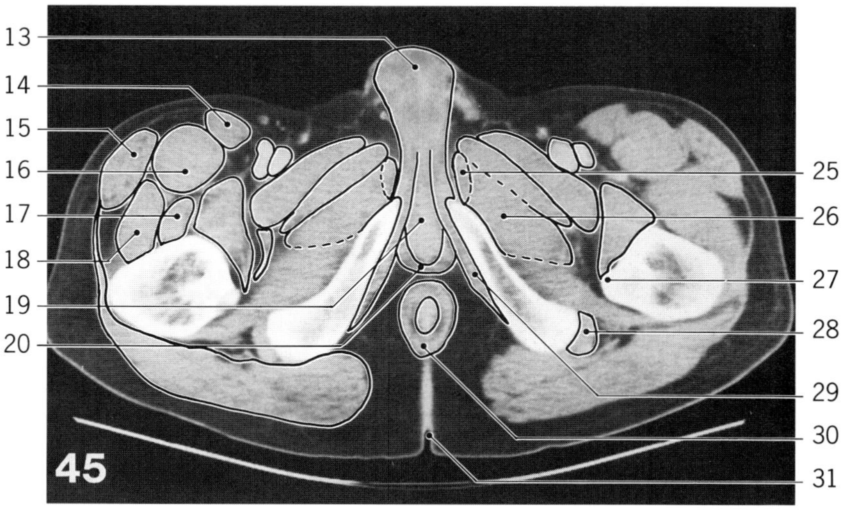

Male pelvis, axial CT

Scout view on page 244

1: Adductor longus (origin)
2: Femoral vein
3: Femoral artery
4: Pectineus
5: Obturatorius internus
6: Puborectalis
7: Ischiorectal fossa
8: Adductor longus
9: Iliopsoas
10: Quadratus femoris
11: Sciatic nerve
12: Ischial tuberosity
13: Penis
14: Sartorius
15: Tensor fasciae latae
16: Rectus femoris
17: Vastus intermedius
18: Vastus lateralis
19: Bulb of penis
20: Bulbocavernosus
21: Spermatic cord (removed on right side)
22: Prostatic part of urethra
23: Anal canal
24: Obturatorius externus
25: Gracilis
26: Adductor brevis
27: Lesser trochanter
28: Biceps femoris (origin)
29: Crus penis and ischiocavernosus
30: Anal sphincter muscles
31: Crena ani

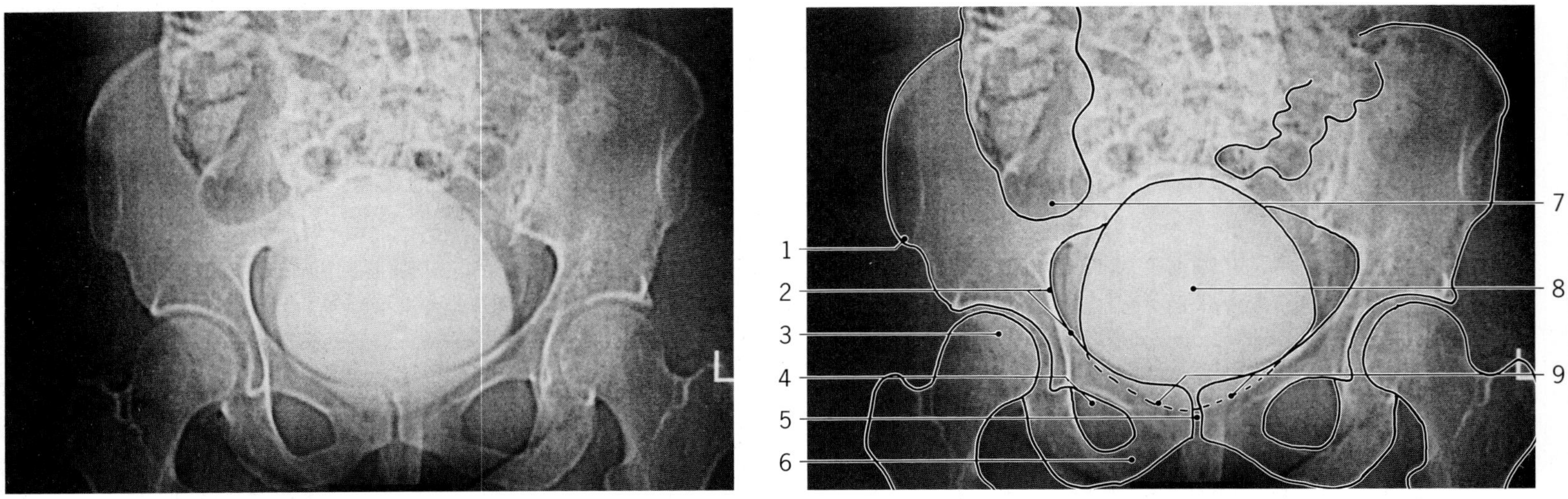

Scout view

1: Anterior superior iliac spine
2: Linea terminalis
3: Head of femur
4: Obturator foramen
5: Symphysis pubis
6: Inferior ramus of pubis
7: Caecum
8: Urinary bladder
9: Fundus of bladder

Scout view

Lines #1-9 indicate positions of sections in the following CT series

Consecutive sections, 10 mm thick.

Intravenous watersoluble contrast has been given to outline the urinary tract

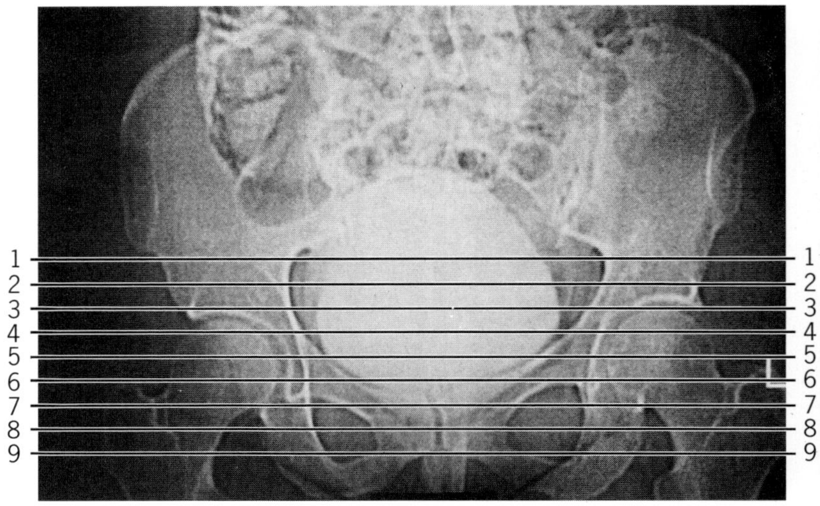

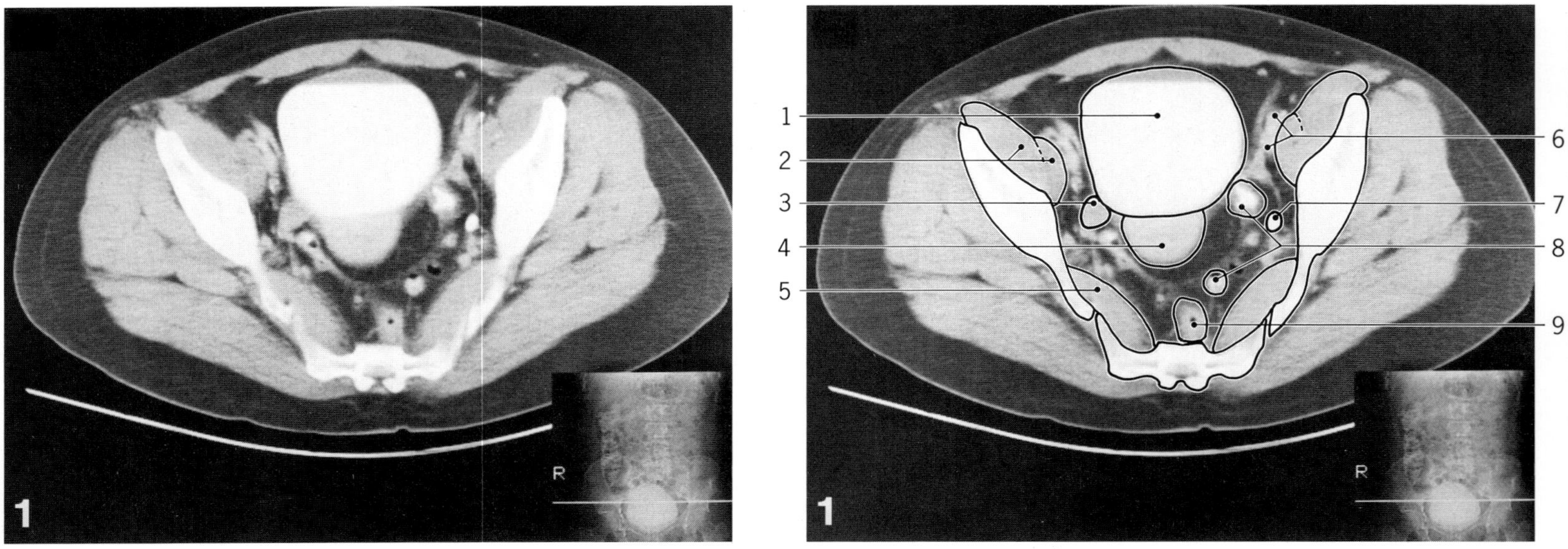

Female pelvis, axial CT

Scout view above

1: Urinary bladder
2: Iliopsoas
3: Right ovary
4: Corpus uteri
5: Piriformis
6: External iliac artery and vein
7: Left ureter
8: Sigmoid colon
9: Rectum

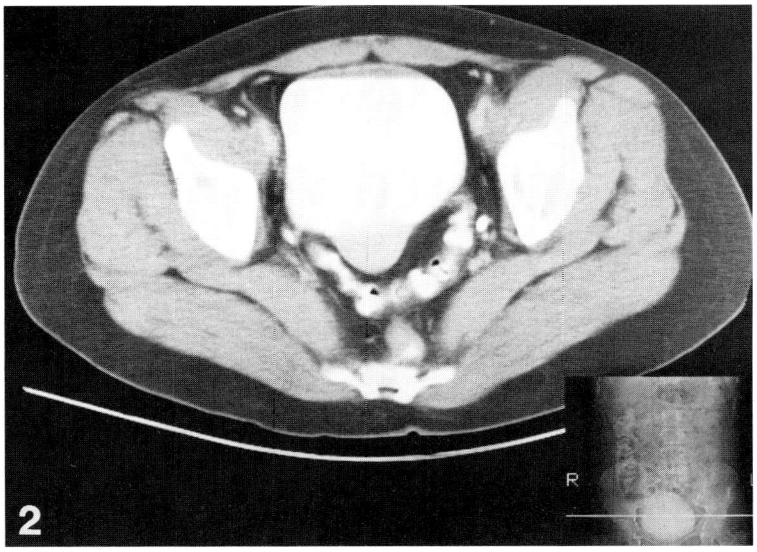

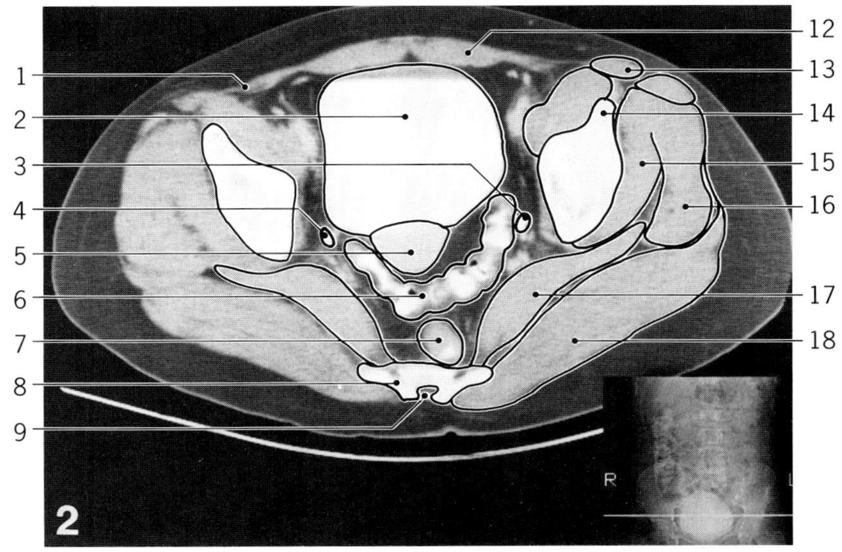

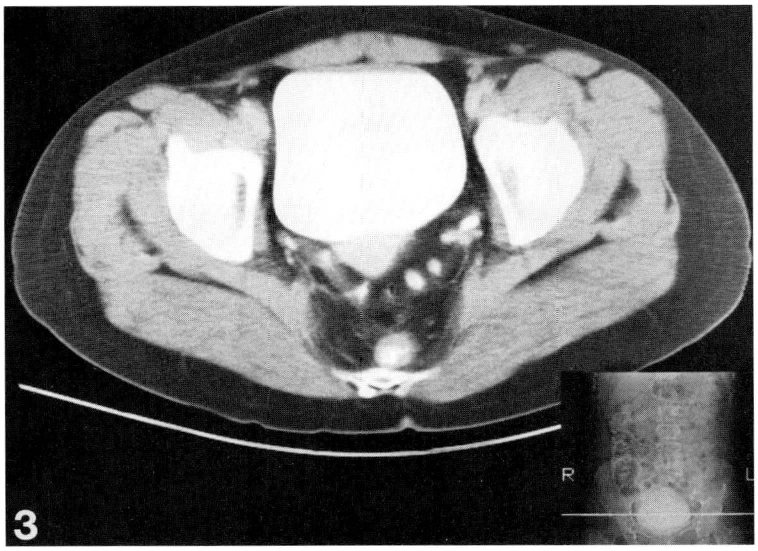

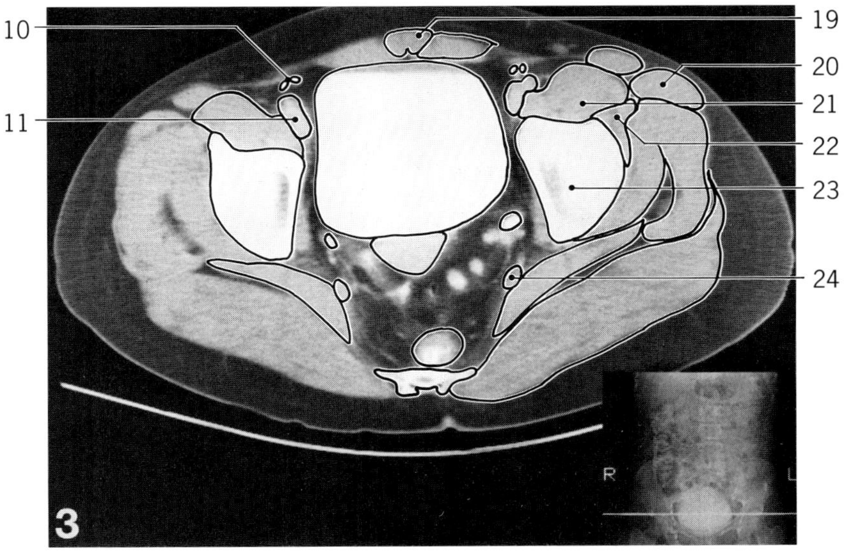

Female pelvis, axial CT

Scout view on opposite page.

1: Inguinal ligament
2: Urinary bladder
3: Left ureter
4: Right ureter
5: Corpus uteri
6: Sigmoid colon
7: Rectum
8: Sacrum
9: Hiatus sacralis
10: Inferior epigastric artery and vein
11: External iliac artery and vein
12: Rectus abdominis
13: Sartorius
14: Anterior inferior iliac spine
15: Gluteus minimus
16: Gluteus medius
17: Piriformis
18: Gluteus maximus
19: Pyramidalis muscle
20: Tensor fasciae latae
21: Iliopsoas
22: Rectus femoris
23: Body of ilium
24: Sciatic nerve

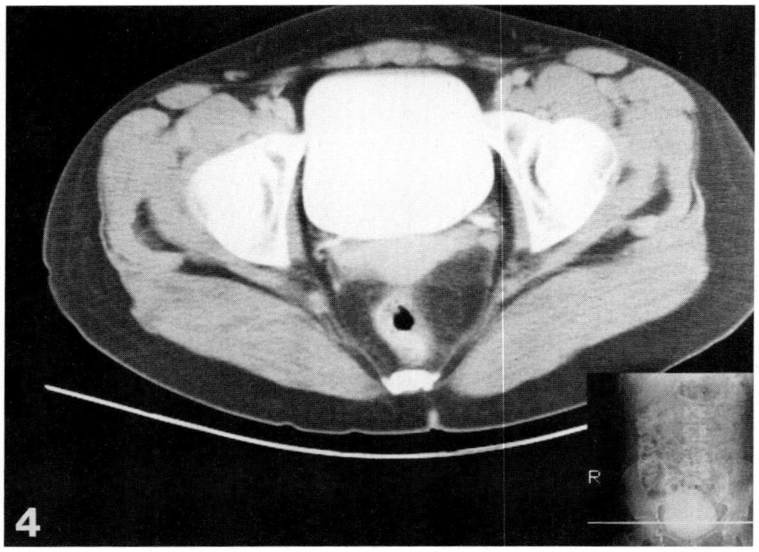

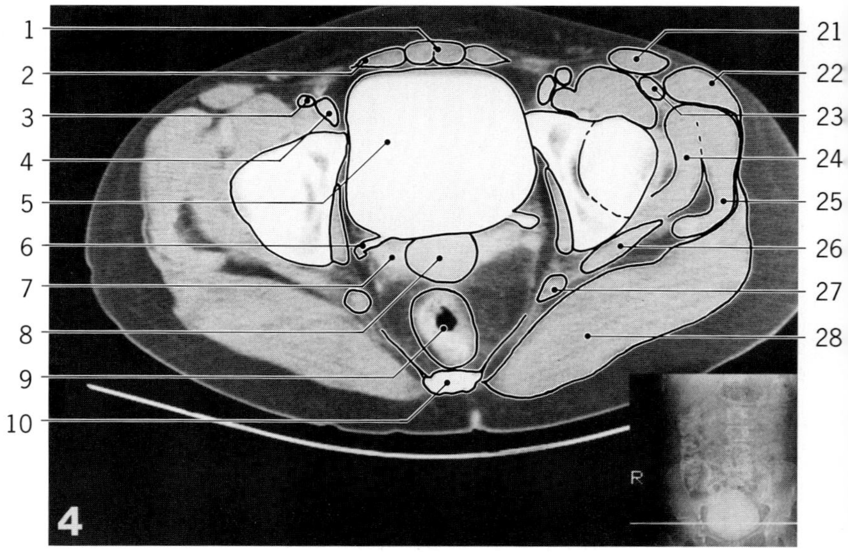

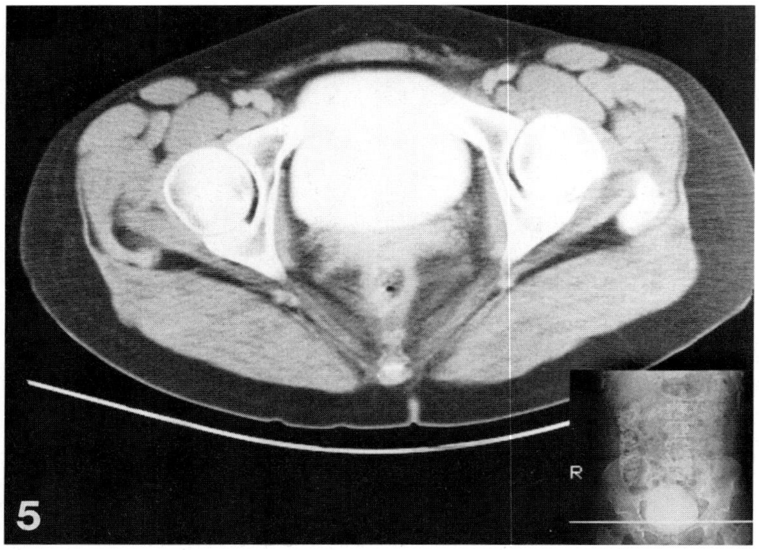

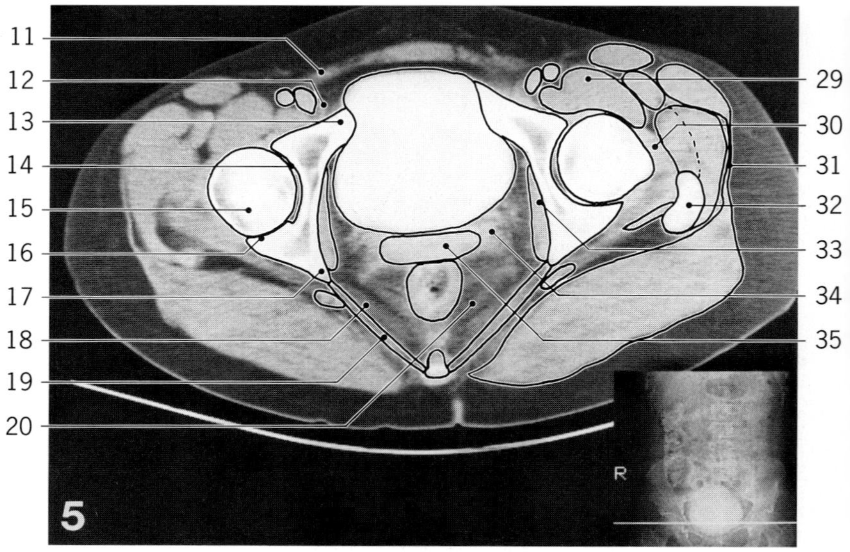

Female pelvis, axial CT

Scout view on page 260

1: Pyramidalis
2: Rectus abdominis
3: External iliac artery
4: External iliac vein
5: Urinary bladder
6: Right ureter
7: Parametrium
8: Cervix uteri
9: Rectum
10: Coccyx
11: Inguinal ligament
12: Deep inguinal lymph node
13: Superior ramus of pubis
14: Acetabular fossa
15: Head of femur
16: Lunate surface
17: Ischial spine
18: Coccygeus muscle
19: Sacrospinous ligament
20: Levator ani
21: Sartorius
22: Tensor fasciae latae
23: Rectus femoris
24: Gluteus minimus
25: Gluteus medius
26: Piriformis
27: Sciatic nerve
28: Gluteus maximus
29: Iliopsoas
30: Iliofemoral ligament
31: Iliotibial tract
32: Greater trochanter
33: Obturatorius internus
34: Vaginal venous plexus
35: Vagina

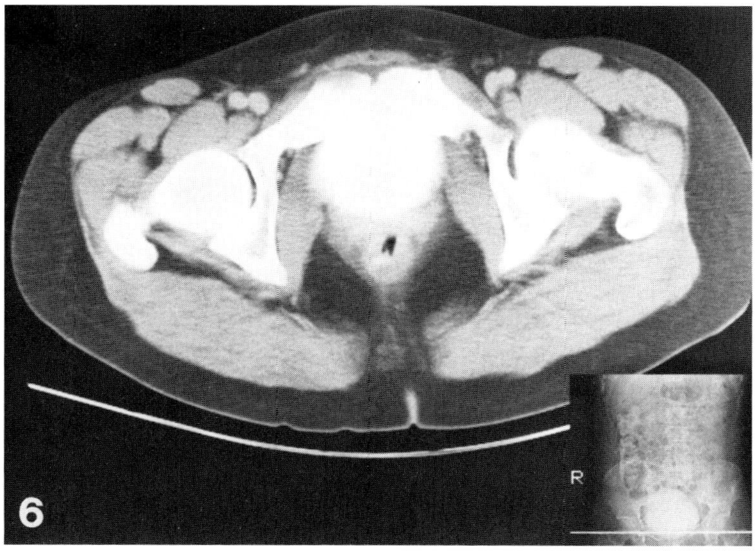

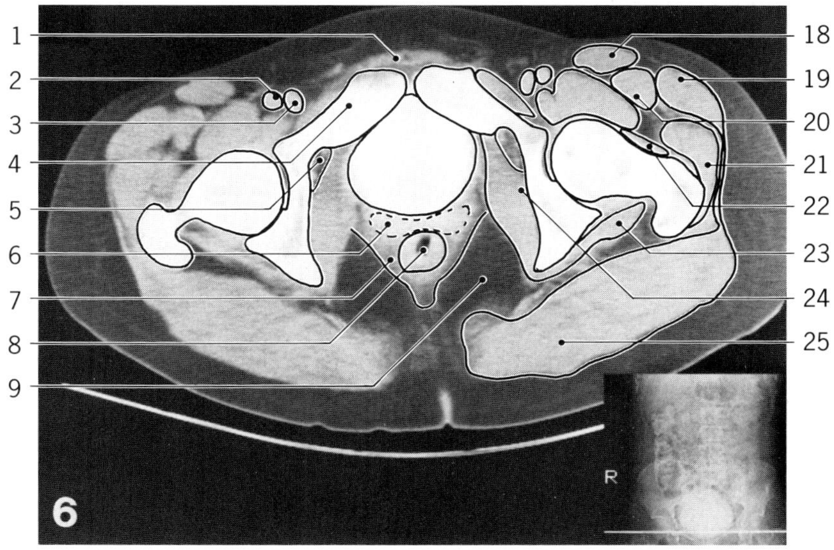

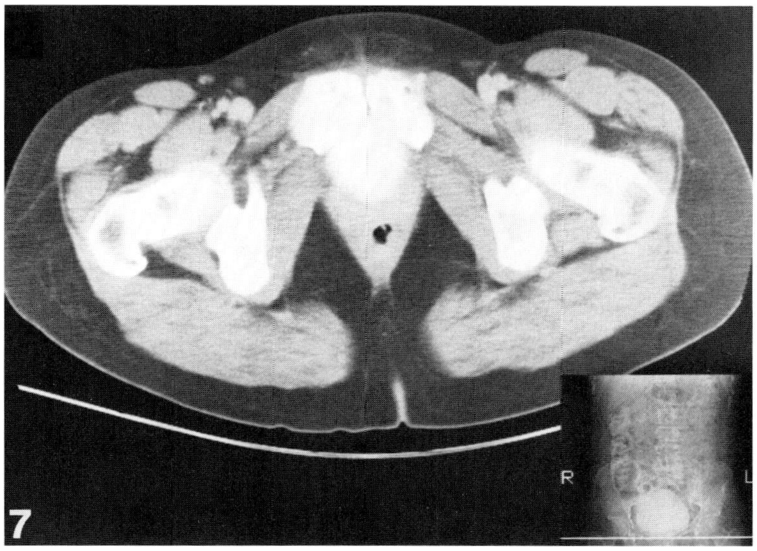

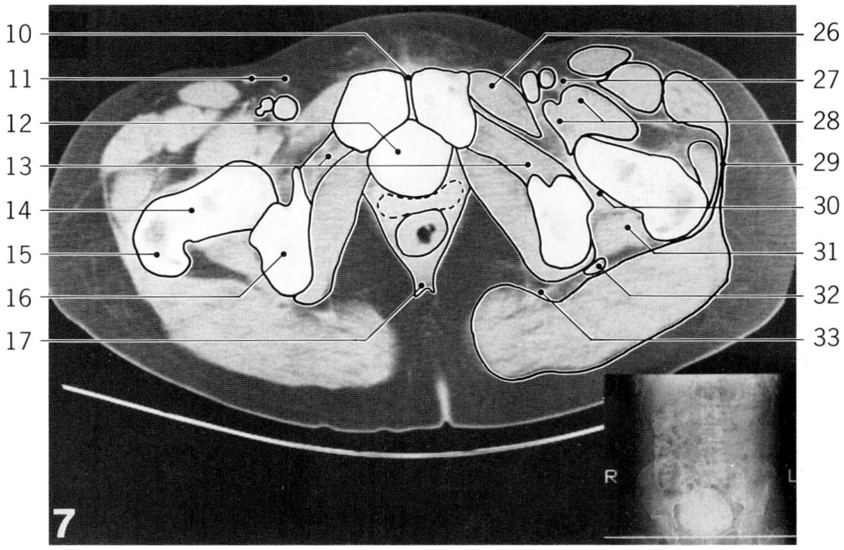

Female pelvis, axial CT

Scout view on page 260

1: Rectus abdominis, and pyramidalis
2: Femoral artery
3: Femoral vein
4: Superior ramus of pubis
5: Pudendal canal
6: Vagina
7: Levator ani
8: Rectum
9: Ischiorectal fossa
10: Symphysis pubica
11: Superficial inguinal lymph nodes
12: Fundus of urinary bladder
13: Obturatorius externus
14: Neck of femur
15: Greater trochanter
16: Body of ischium
17: Anococcygeal ligament
18: Sartorius
19: Tensor fasciae latae
20: Rectus femoris
21: Gluteus medius and minimus
22: Iliofemoral ligament
23: Gemelli and tendon of obturatorius internus
24: Obturatorius internus
25: Gluteus maximus
26: Pectineus
27: Femoral nerve
28: Iliopsoas
29: Iliotibial tract
30: Ischiofemoral ligament
31: Quadratus femoris
32: Sciatic nerve
33: Sacrotuberal ligament

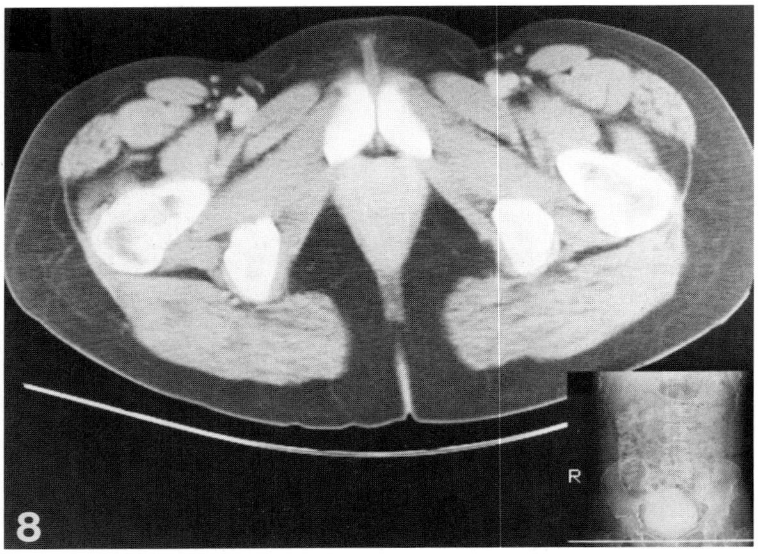

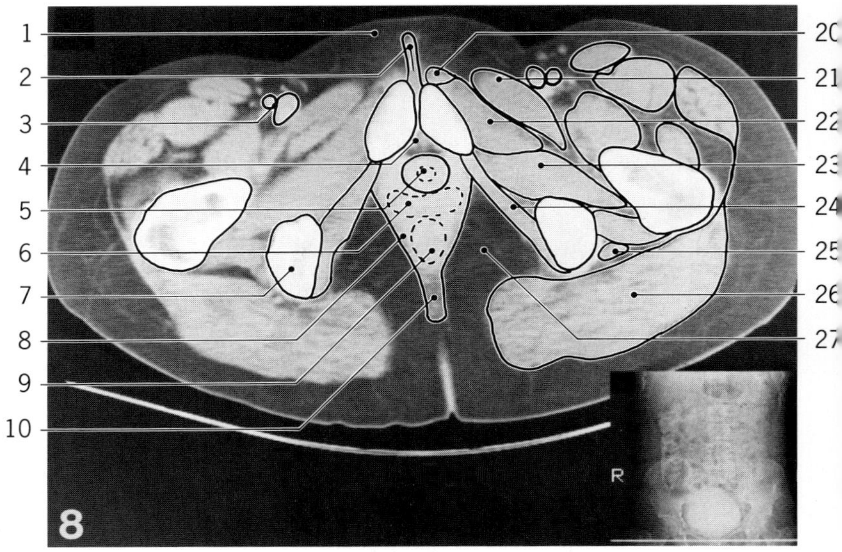

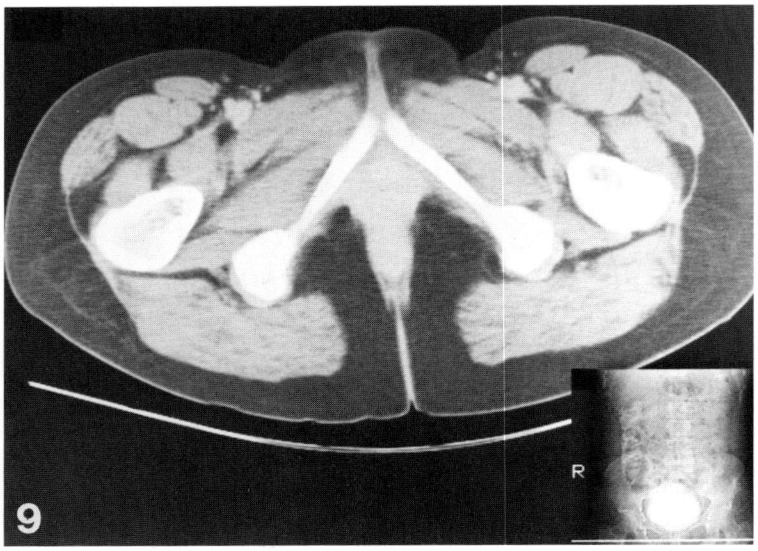

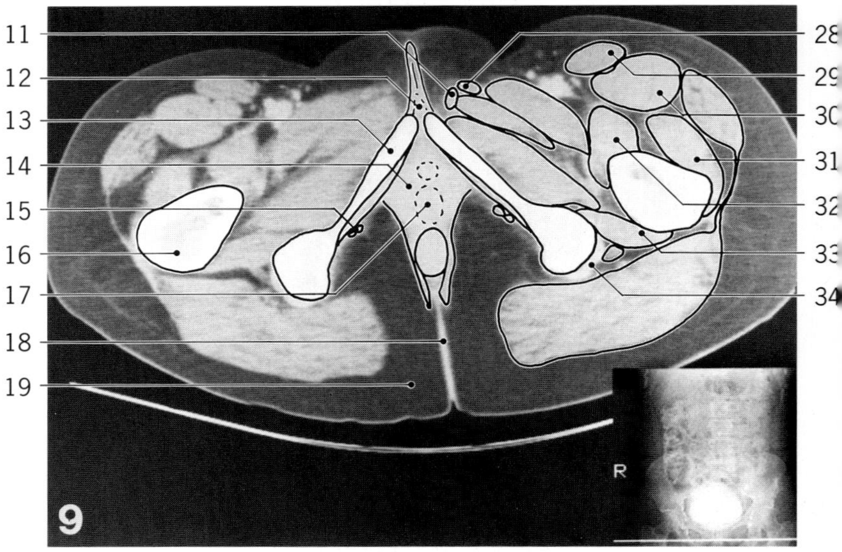

Female pelvis, axial CT

Scout view on page 260

1: Mons pubis (Veneris)
2: Rima pudendi
3: Femoral artery and vein
4: Subarcuate lacuna
5: Urethra feminina, and sphinchter urethrae externa
6: Vagina
7: Ischial tuberosity
8: Levator ani
9: Anal canal
10: Anococcygeal ligament
11: Gracilis
12: Clitoris
13: Inferior ramus of pubis
14: Bulb of vestibule
15: Internal pudendal artery and vein, and pudendal nerve
16: Femur
17: Vestibule of vagina
18: Crena ani
19: Subcutaneous fat
20: Adductor longus (origin)
21: Pectineus
22: Adductor brevis
23: Obturatorius externus
24: Obturatorius internus
25: Sciatic nerve
26: Gluteus maximus
27: Ischiorectal fossa
28: Adductor longus (tendon)
29: Sartorius
30: Rectus femoris
31: Vastus lateralis
32: Iliopsoas
33: Quadratus femoris
34: Common origin of semimembranosus, semitendinosus, and biceps femoris

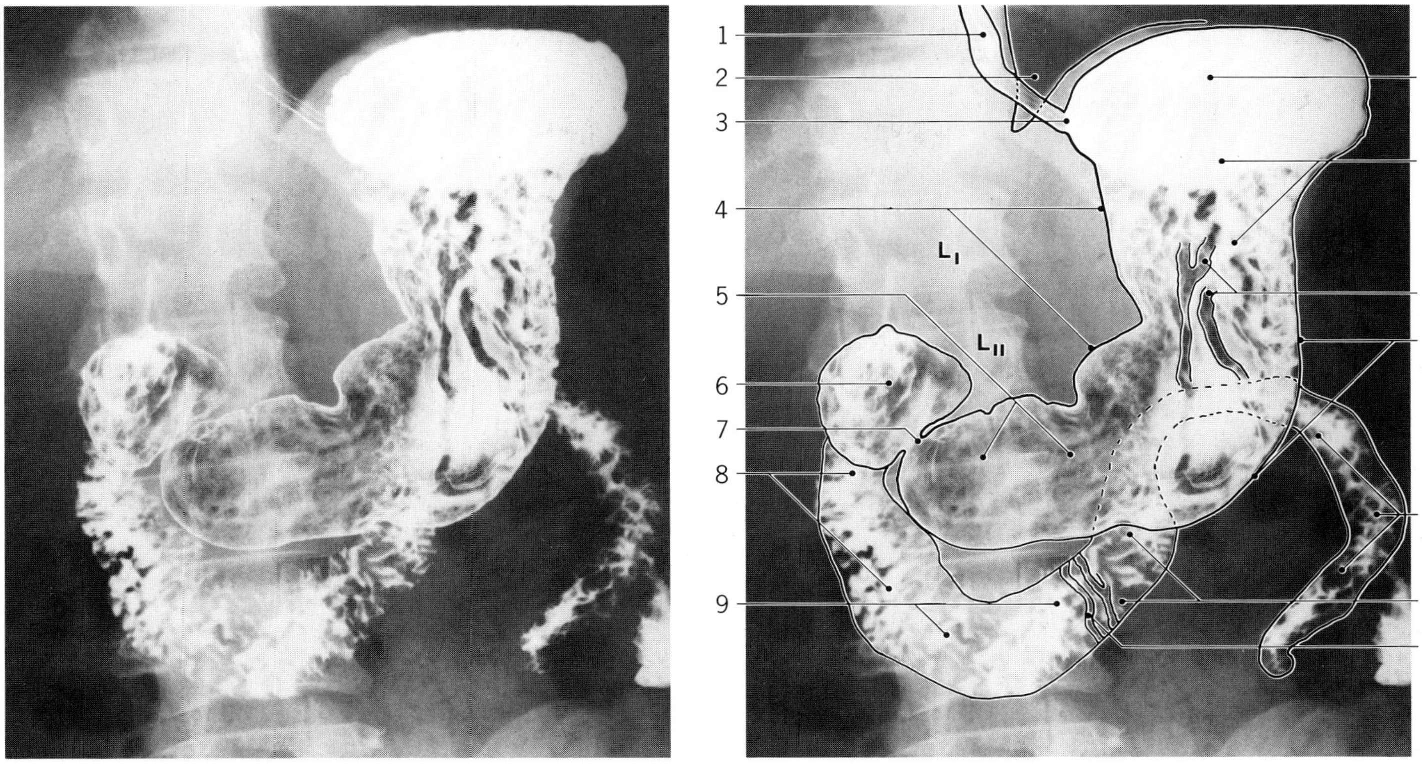

Stomach and duodenum, oblique X-ray, barium meal, double contrast

1: Oesophagus
2: Left lung
3: Cardia
4: Lesser curvature of stomach
5: Pyloric antrum
6: Duodenal "cap" (bulbus)
7: Pyloric orifice
8: Descending part of duodenum
9: Horizontal part of duodenum
10: Fundus of stomach
11: Body of stomach
12: Rugae gastricae
13: Greater curvature of stomach
14: Jejunum
15: Ascending part of duodenum
16: Plica circularis (Kerkring)

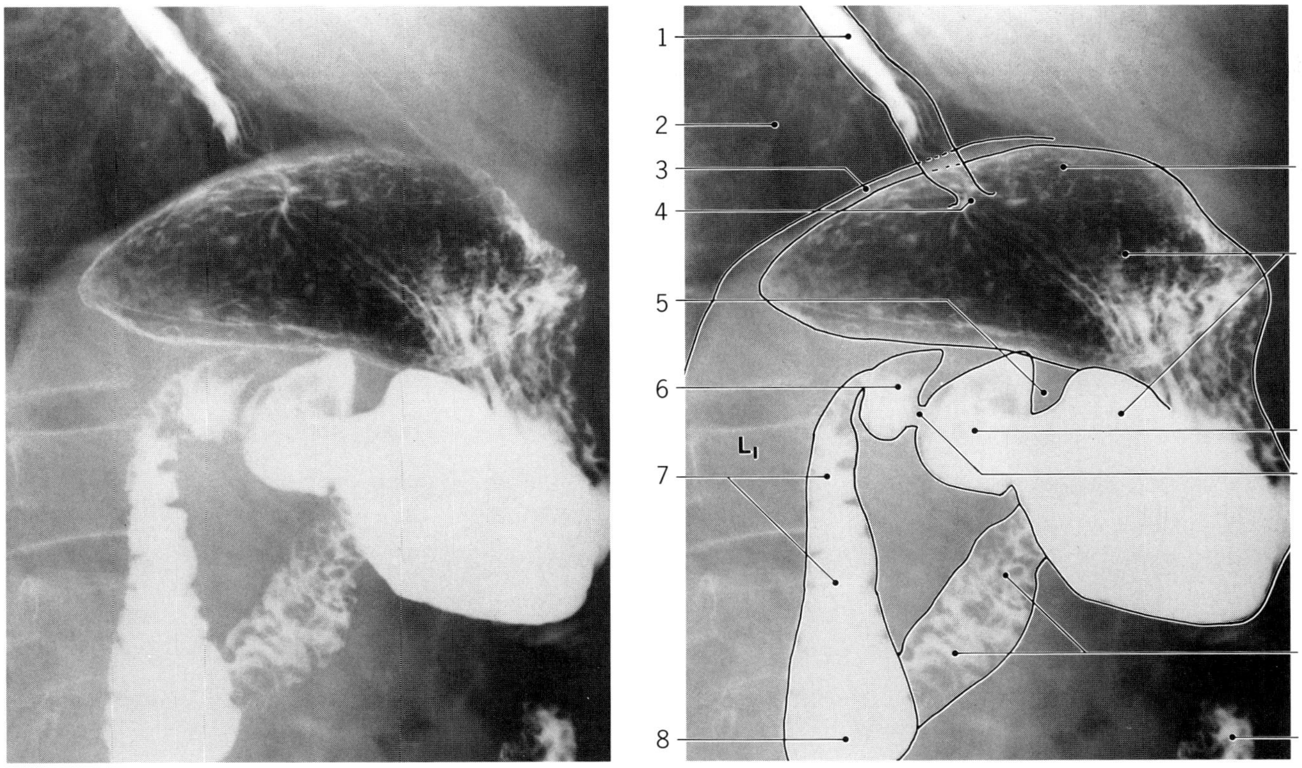

Stomach and duodenum, lateral X-ray, barium meal, double contrast

1: Oesophagus
2: Lung
3: Diaphragm and gastric wall
4: Cardia
5: Contraction furrow
6: Duodenal "cap" (bulbus)
7: Descending part of duodenum
8: Horizontal part of duodenum
9: Fundus of stomach
10: Body of stomach
11: Pyloric antrum
12: Pyloric orifice
13: Ascending part of duodenum
14: Jejunum

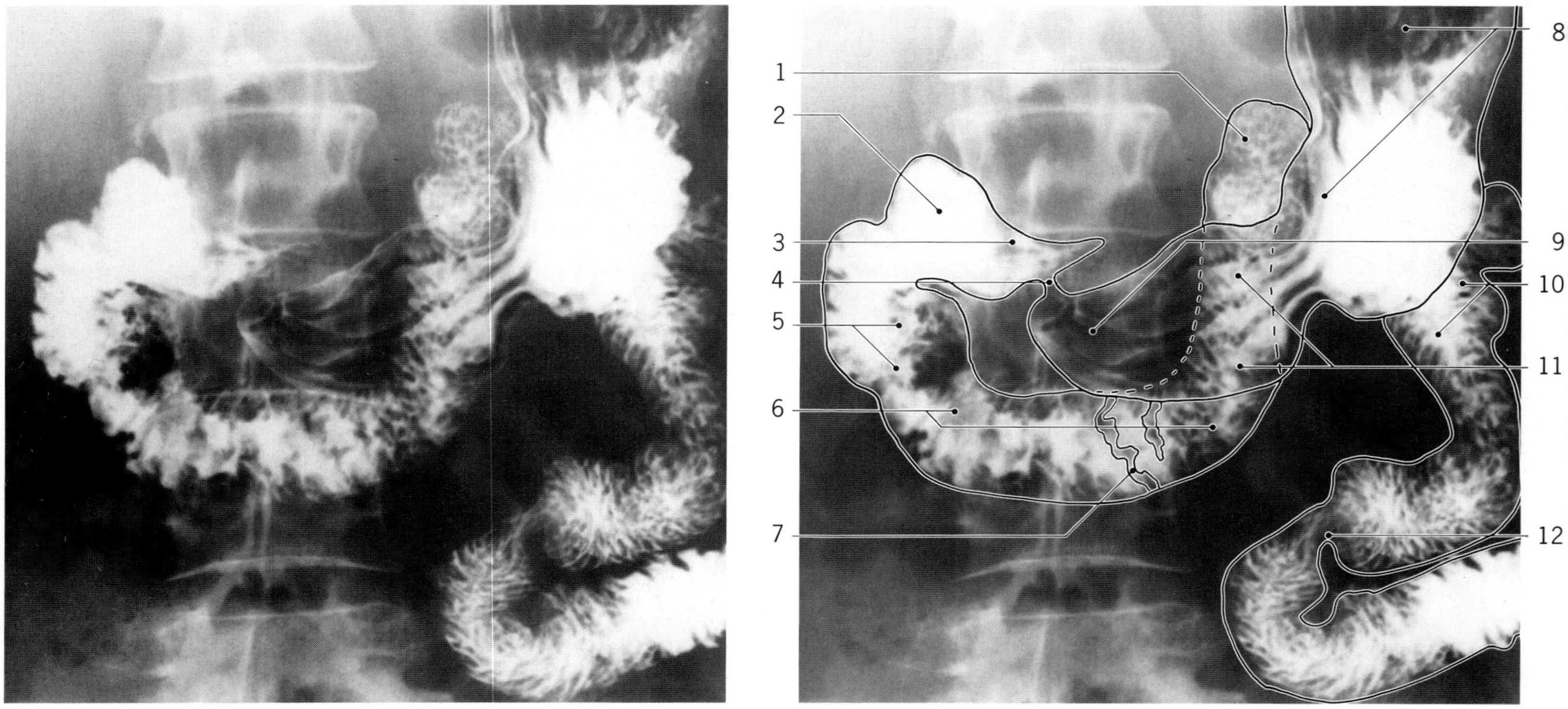

Duodenum, a-p X-ray, barium meal, double contrast

1: Duodenojejunal flexure
2: Superior part of duodenum
3: Duodenal cap (bulbus)
4: Pyloric canal
5: Descending part of duodenum
6: Horizontal part of duodenum
7: Plica circularis (Kerkring)
8: Body of stomach
9: Pyloric antrum
10: Jejunum
11: Ascending part of duodenum
12: Peristaltic contraction in jejunum

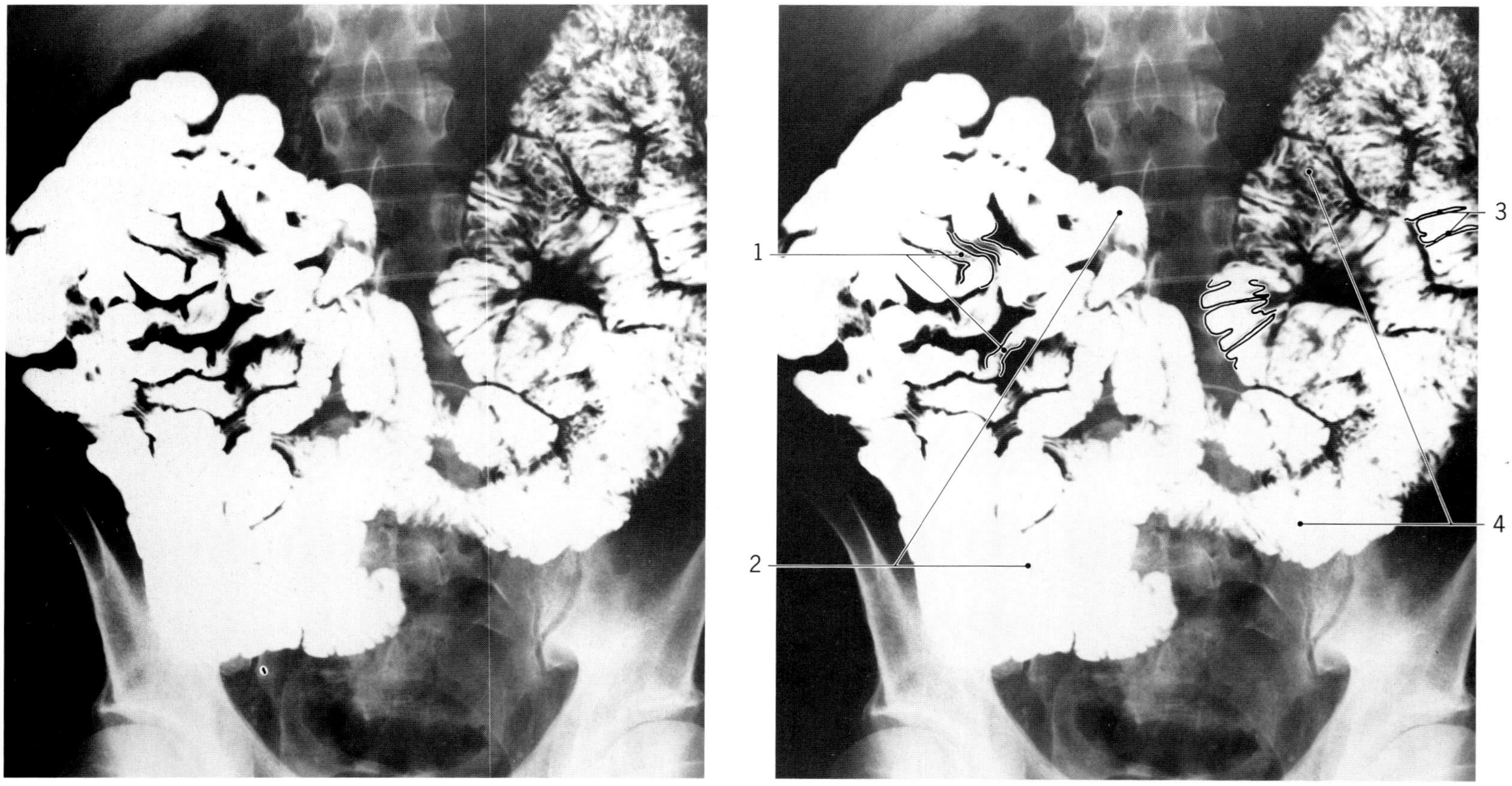

Jejunum and ileum, a-p X-ray, barium meal

1: Peristaltic contractions in ileum
2: Ileum
3: Plicae circulares in jejunum
4: Jejunum

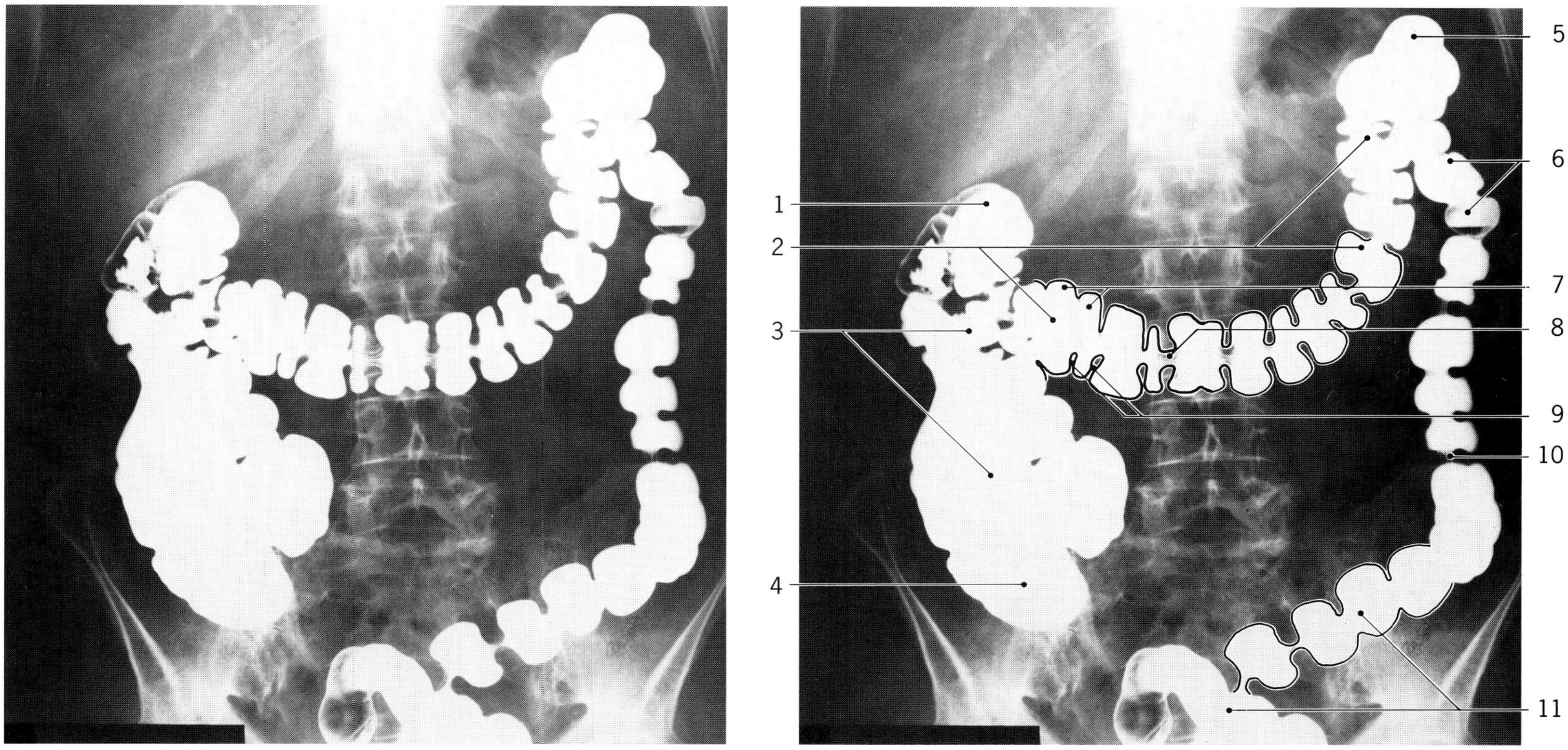

Colon, a-p X-ray, barium enema, single contrast

1: Hepatic flexure of colon
2: Transverse colon
3: Ascending colon
4: Caecum
5: Splenic flexure of colon
6: Descending colon
7: Haustra
8: Peristaltic contraction
9: Semilunar folds
10: Peristaltic contraction
11: Sigmoid colon

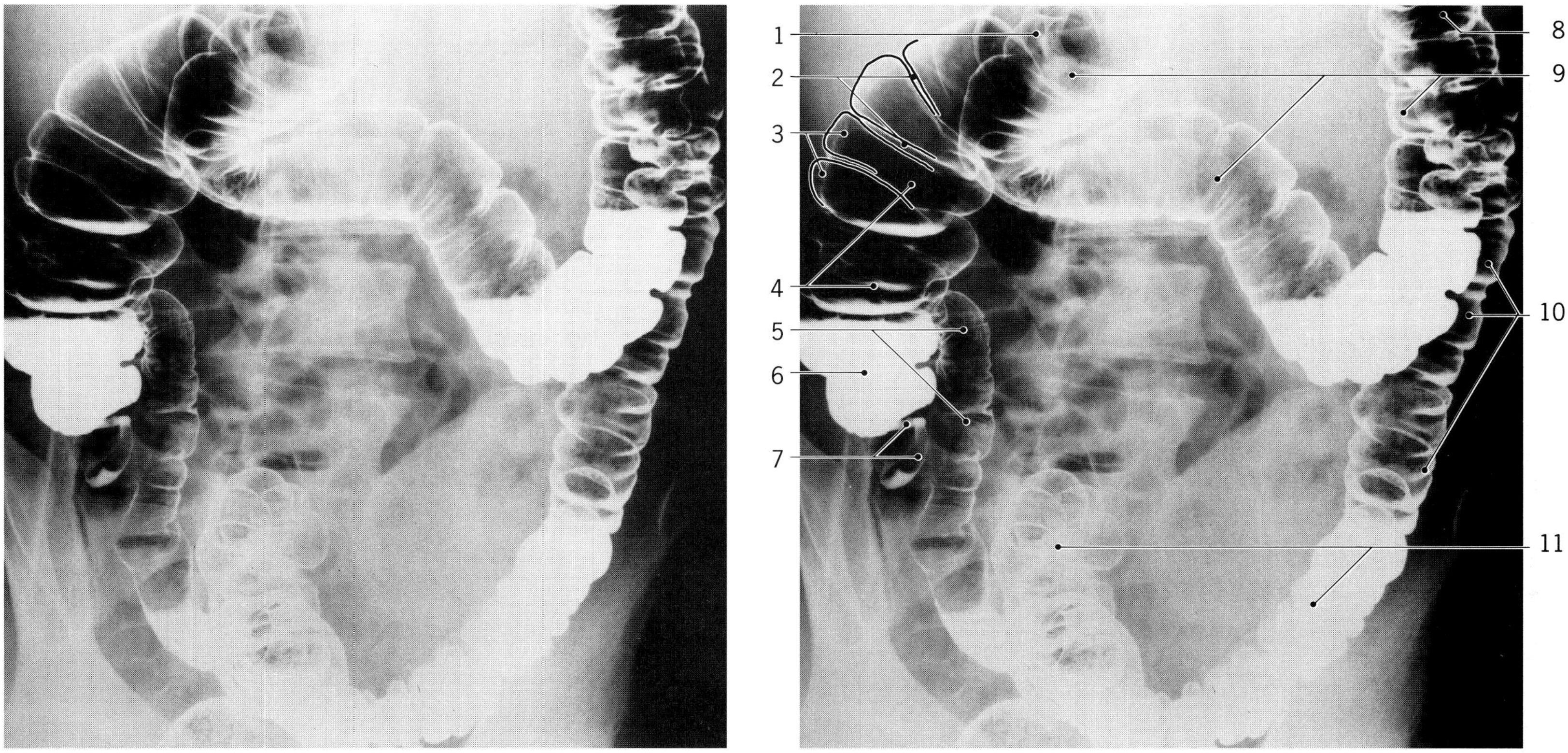

Colon, a-p X-ray, double contrast

1: Hepatic flexure of colon
2: Semilunar folds
3: Haustra
4: Ascending colon
5: Terminal ileum
6: Caecum
7: Vermiform appendix
8: Splenic flexure of colon
9: Transverse colon
10: Descending colon
11: Sigmoid colon

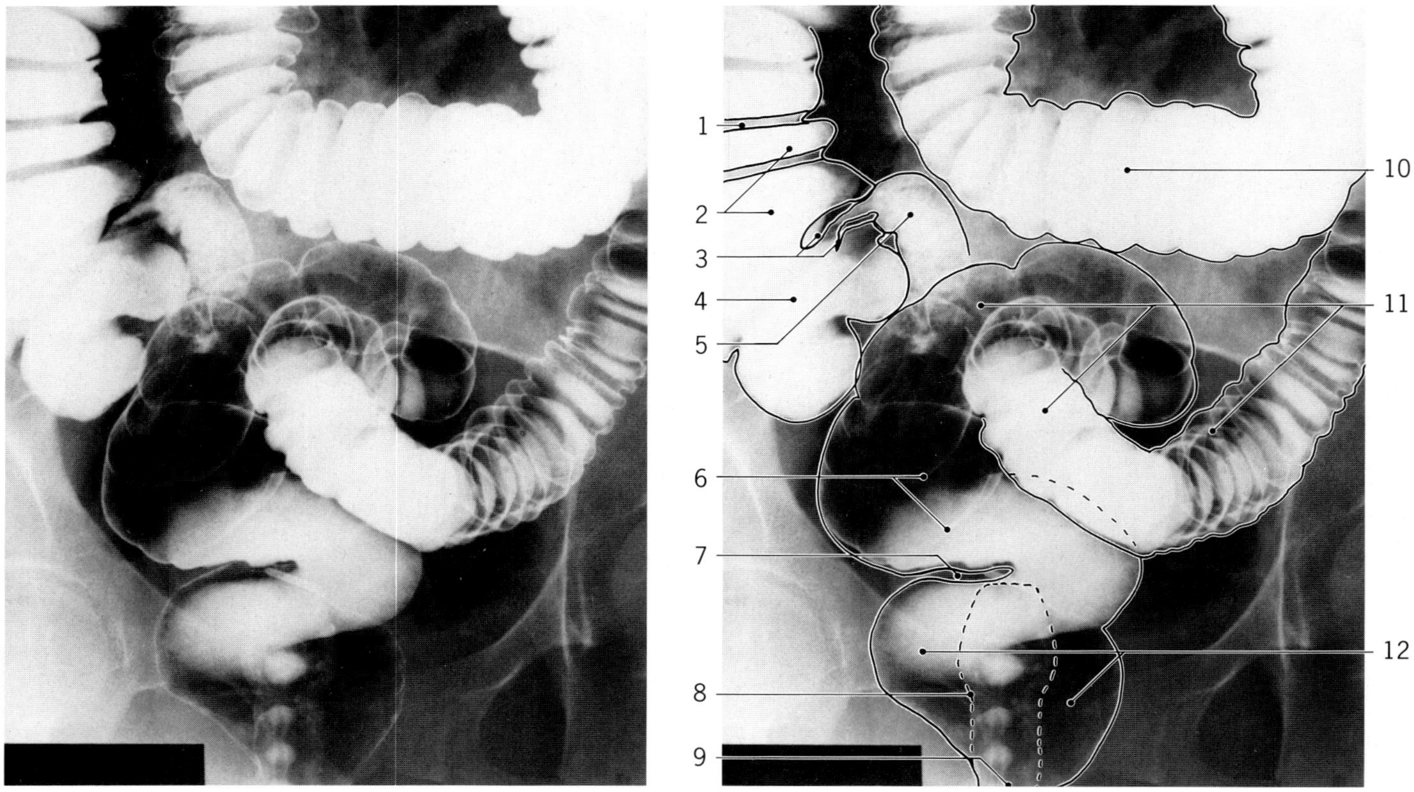

Rectum, a-p X-ray, double contrast

1: Semilunar fold
2: Ascending colon
3: Ileocaecal valve
4: Caecum
5: Terminal ileum
6: Rectum
7: Transverse fold of rectum
8: Tube
9: Anal canal
10: Transverse colon
11: Sigmoid colon
12: Rectal ampulla

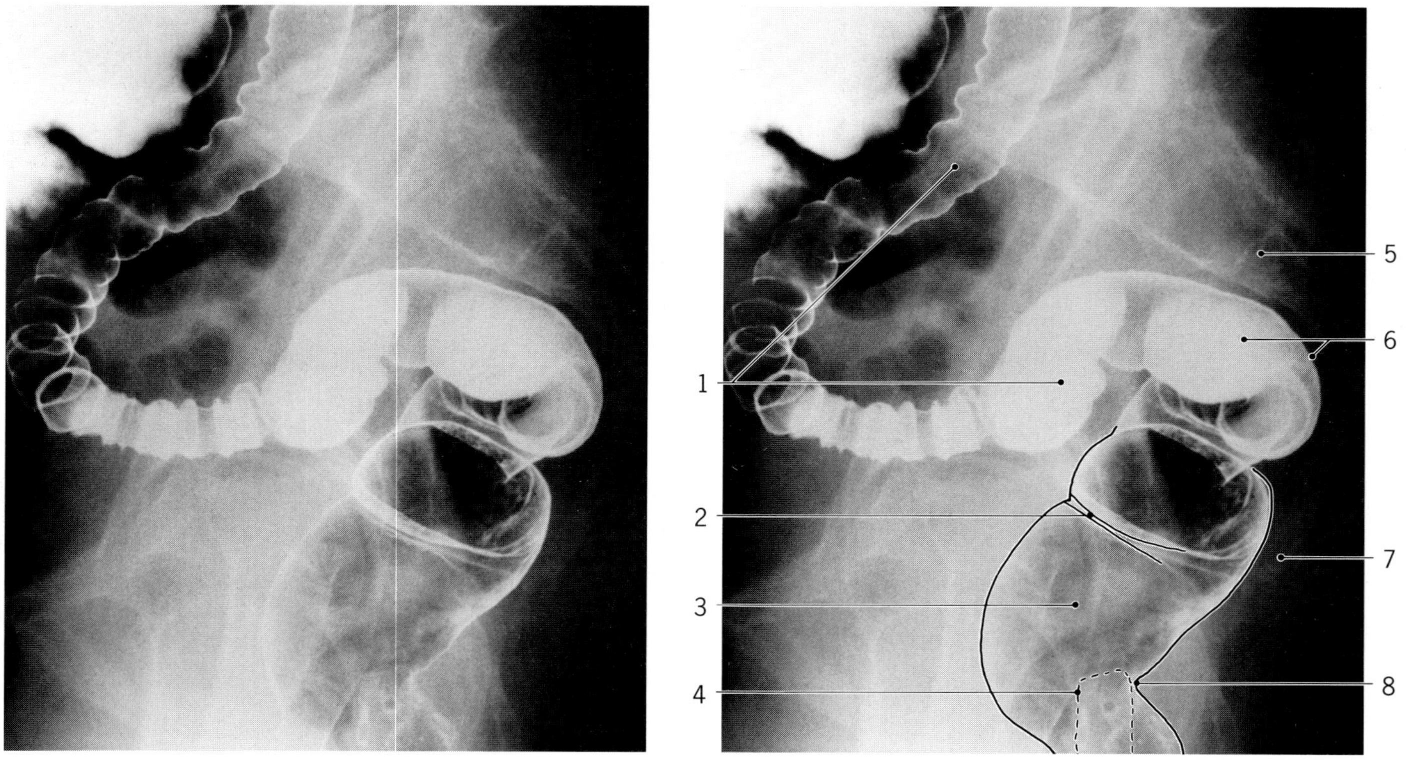

Rectum, lateral X-ray, double contrast

1: Sigmoid colon
2: Transverse fold of rectum
3: Rectal ampulla
4: Tube
5: Sacrum
6: Sacral flexure of rectum
7: Coccyx
8: Perineal flexure of rectum

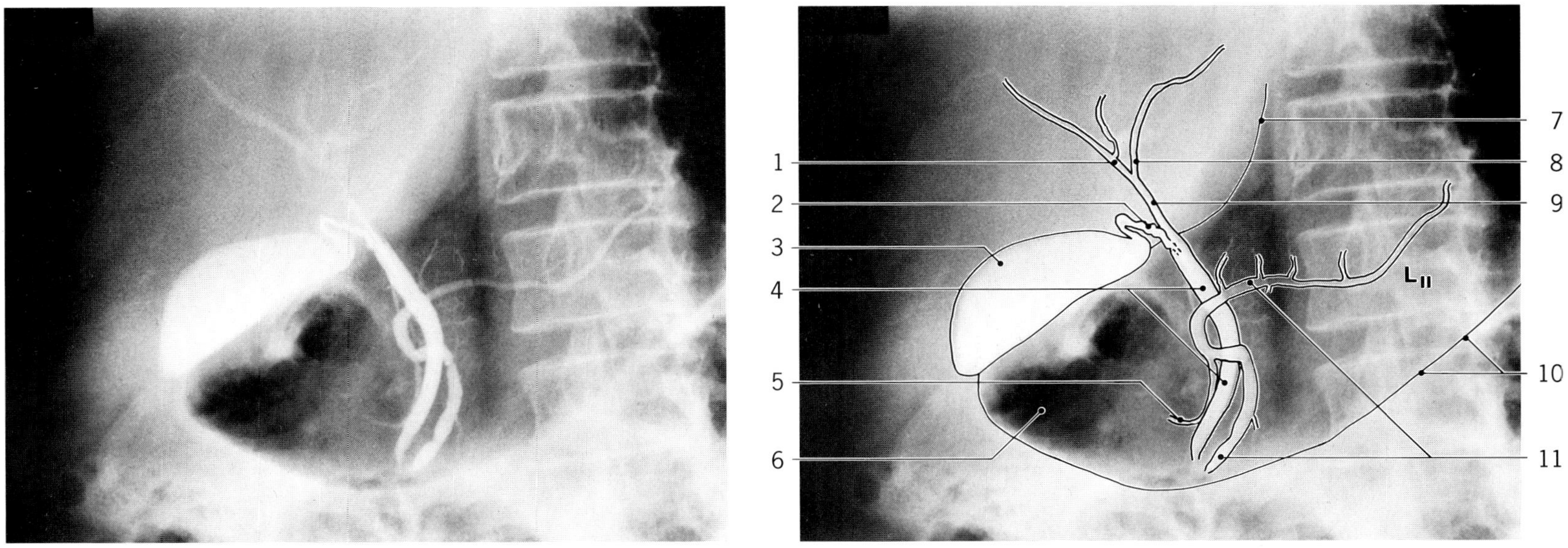

Biliary tract, a-p X-ray, endoscopic retrograde cholangio-pancreatography (ERCP)

1: Right hepatic duct
2: Cystic duct
3: Gall bladder
4: Bile duct (choledochus)
5: Accessory pancreatic duct
6: Pyloric antrum (air-filled)
7: Lesser curvature of stomach
8: Left hepatic duct
9: Common hepatic duct
10: Greater curvature of stomach
11: Pancreatic duct

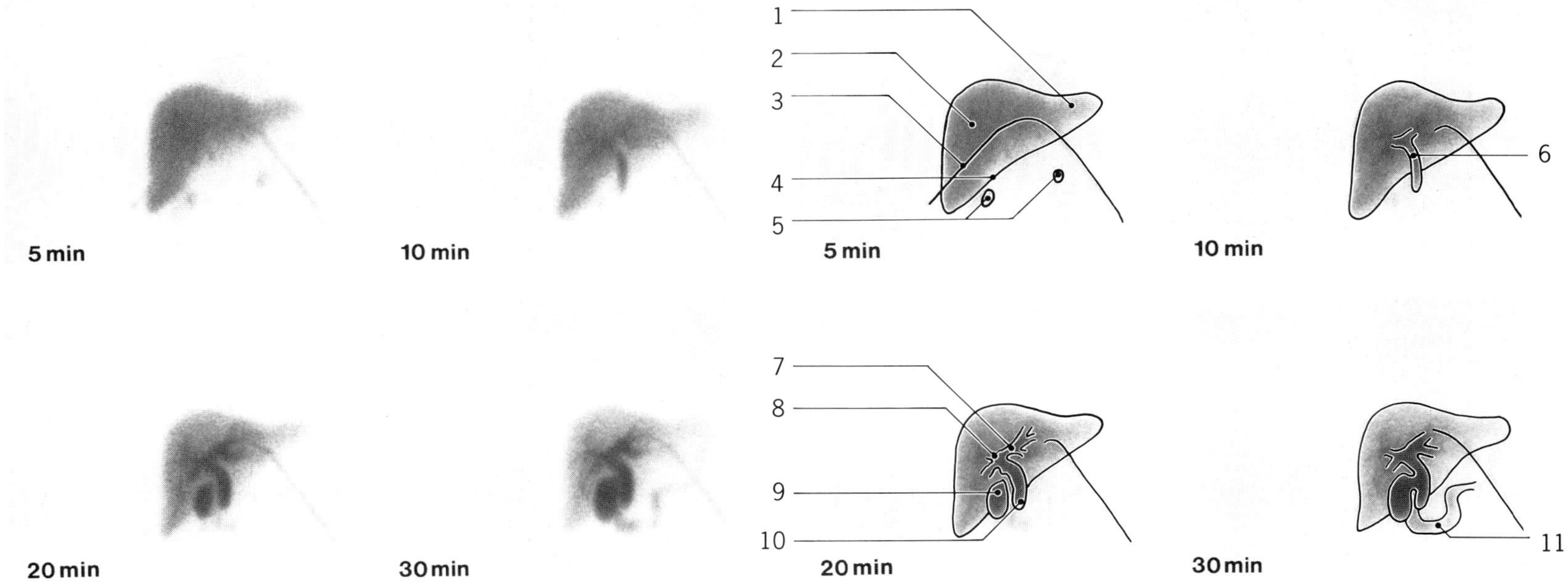

Biliary tract, ^{99m}Tc-HIDA, scintigraphy, anterior view

Biliary excretion of HIDA, 5, 10, 20 and 30 minutes after i.v. injection

1: Left lobe of liver
2: Right lobe of liver
3: Mark on rib curvature
4: Inferior margin of liver
5: Right and left renal pelvis
6: Common hepatic duct
7: Left hepatic duct
8: Right hepatic duct
9: Gall bladder
10: Bile duct (choledochus)
11: Duodenum

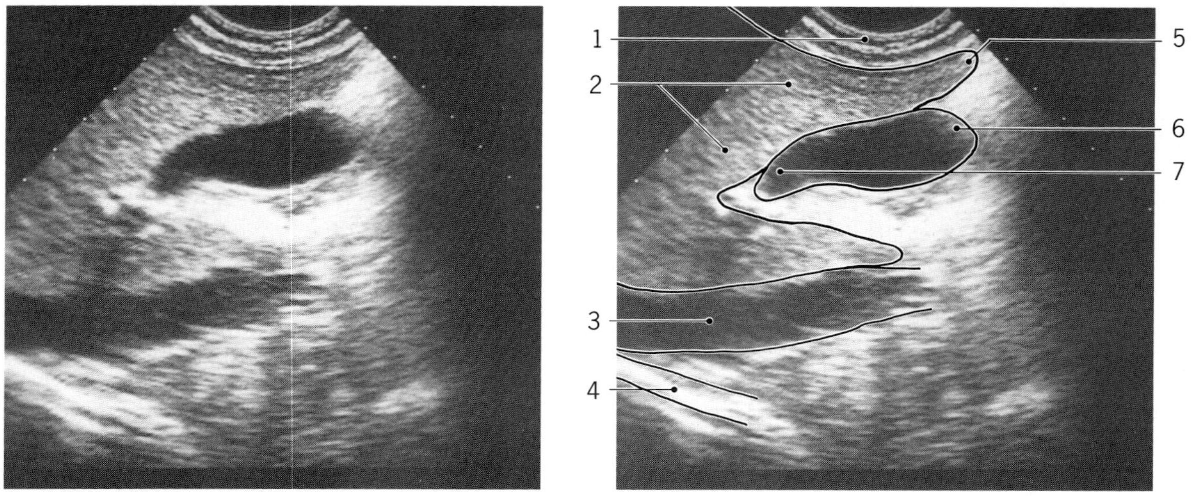

Gall bladder, subcostal sagittal section, US, deep inspiration

1: Anterior abdominal wall
2: Liver
3: Inferior caval vein
4: Diaphragm
5: Inferior margin of liver
6: Fundus of gall bladder
7: Neck of gall bladder

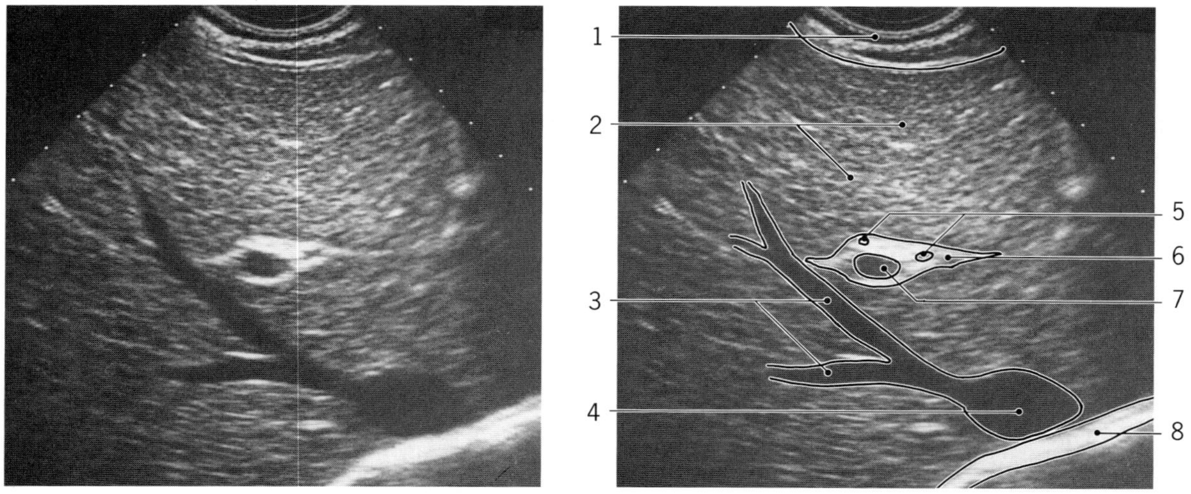

Liver, subcostal, tilted transverse section, US

1: Anterior abdominal wall
2: Liver
3: Hepatic veins
4: Inferior caval vein
5: Hepatic artery and bile duct in portal tract
6: Connective tissue of portal tract
7: Portal vein
8: Diaphragm

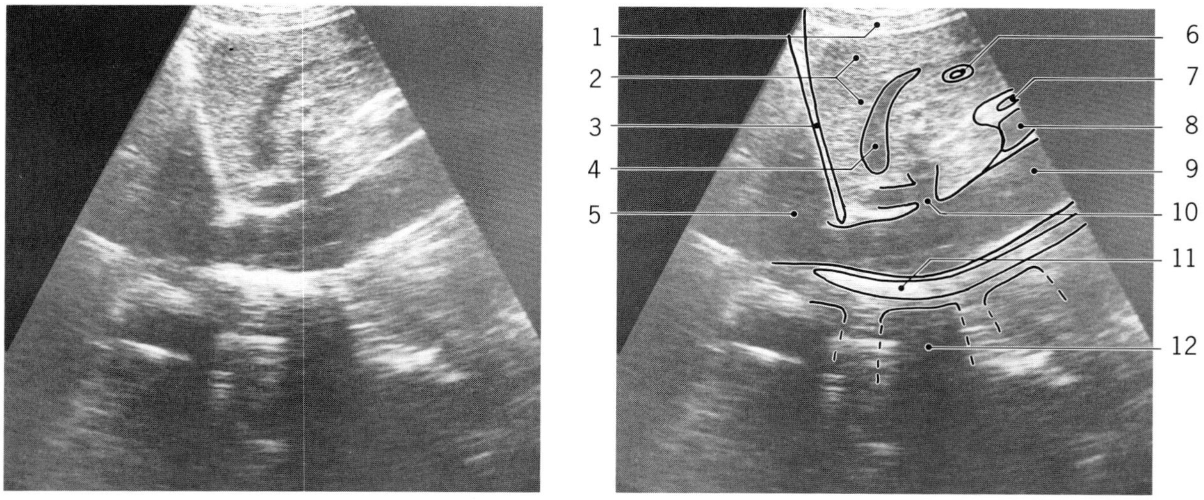

Liver, subcostal sagittal section, US

1: Anterior abdominal wall
2: Liver
3: Diaphragm
4: Hepatic vein
5: Right atrium
6: Portal tract
7: Hepatic artery proper
8: Portal vein
9: Inferior caval vein
10: Orifice of hepatic veins
11: Right crus of diaphragm
12: Vertebral body with acoustic shadow

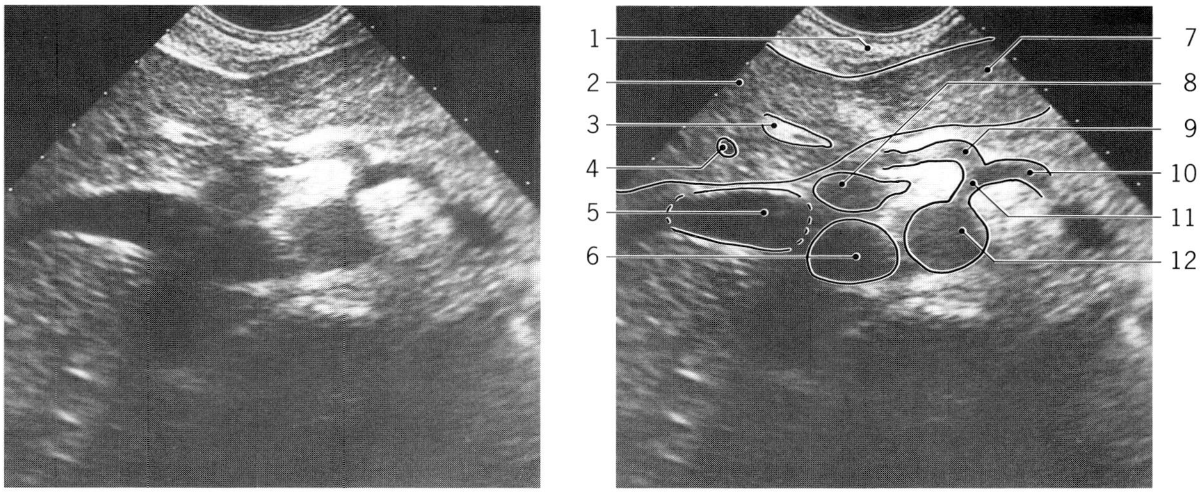

Upper abdomen, transverse section, US

1: Anterior abdominal wall
2: Right lobe of liver
3: Portal tract
4: Hepatic vein
5: Gall bladder
6: Inferior caval vein
7: Left lobe of liver
8: Portal vein
9: Common hepatic artery
10: Splenic artery
11: Coeliac trunk
12: Abdominal aorta

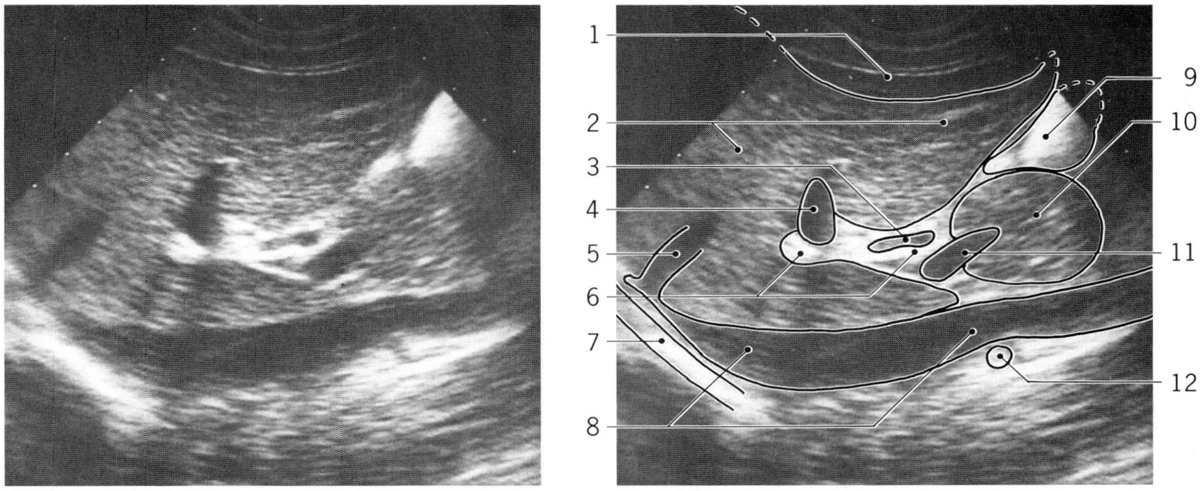

Upper abdomen, vertical section, US, deep inspiration

1: Anterior abdominal wall
2: Liver
3: Hepatic artery proper and bile duct
4: Right branch of portal vein
5: Hepatic vein
6: Porta hepatis
7: Diaphragm
8: Inferior caval vein
9: Stomach (pyloric antrum)
10: Head of pancreas
11: Portal vein
12: Right renal artery

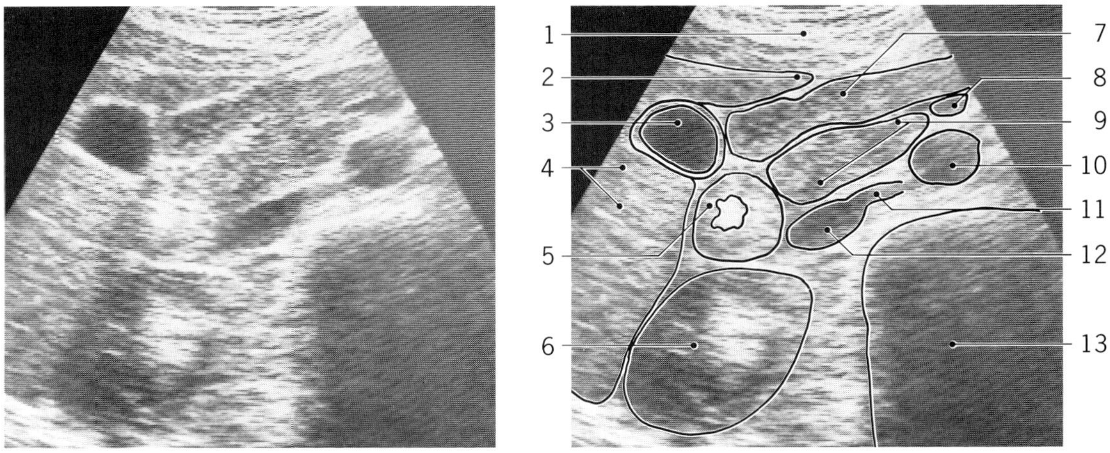

Upper abdomen, transverse section, US

1: Anterior abdominal wall
2: Inferior margin of liver
3: Gall bladder
4: Right lobe of liver
5: Descending part of duodenum
6: Right kidney
7: Stomach
8: Superior mesenteric artery
9: Pancreas
10: Abdominal aorta
11: Left renal vein
12: Inferior caval vein
13: Vertebral body

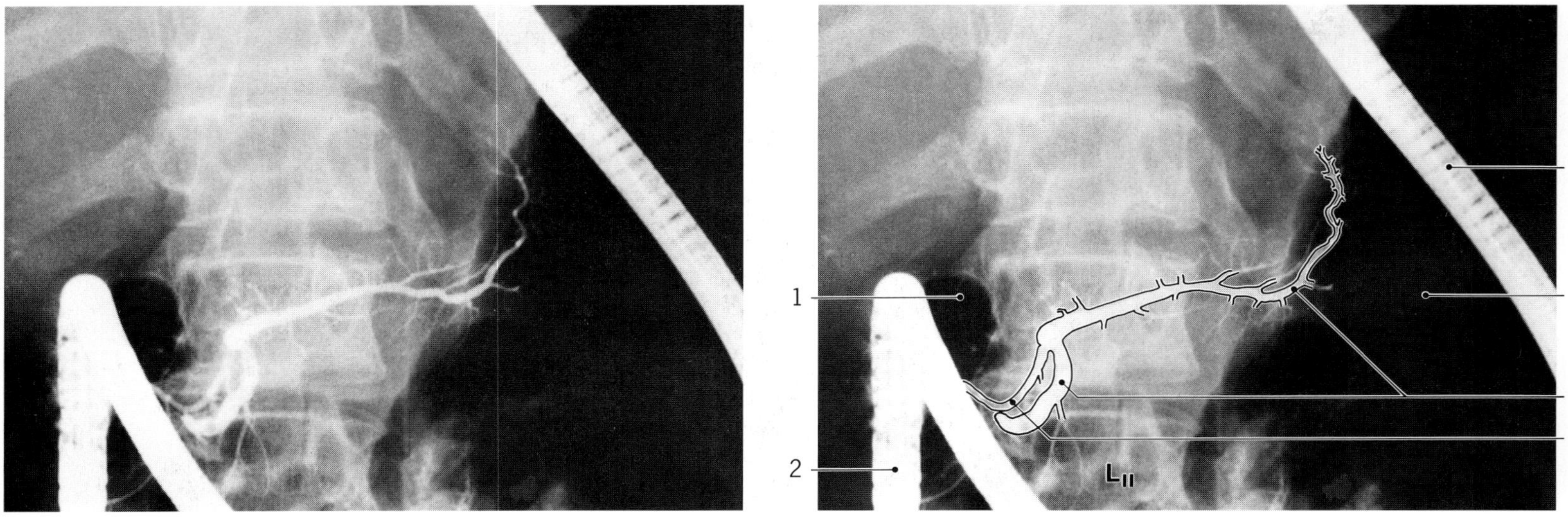

Pancreatic ducts, a-p X-ray, endoscopic retrograde pancreatography

1: Duodenal "cap" (with air)
2: Endoscope in descending part of duodenum
3: Endoscope in stomach
4: Body of stomach (inflated)
5: Pancreatic duct
6: Accessory pancreatic duct

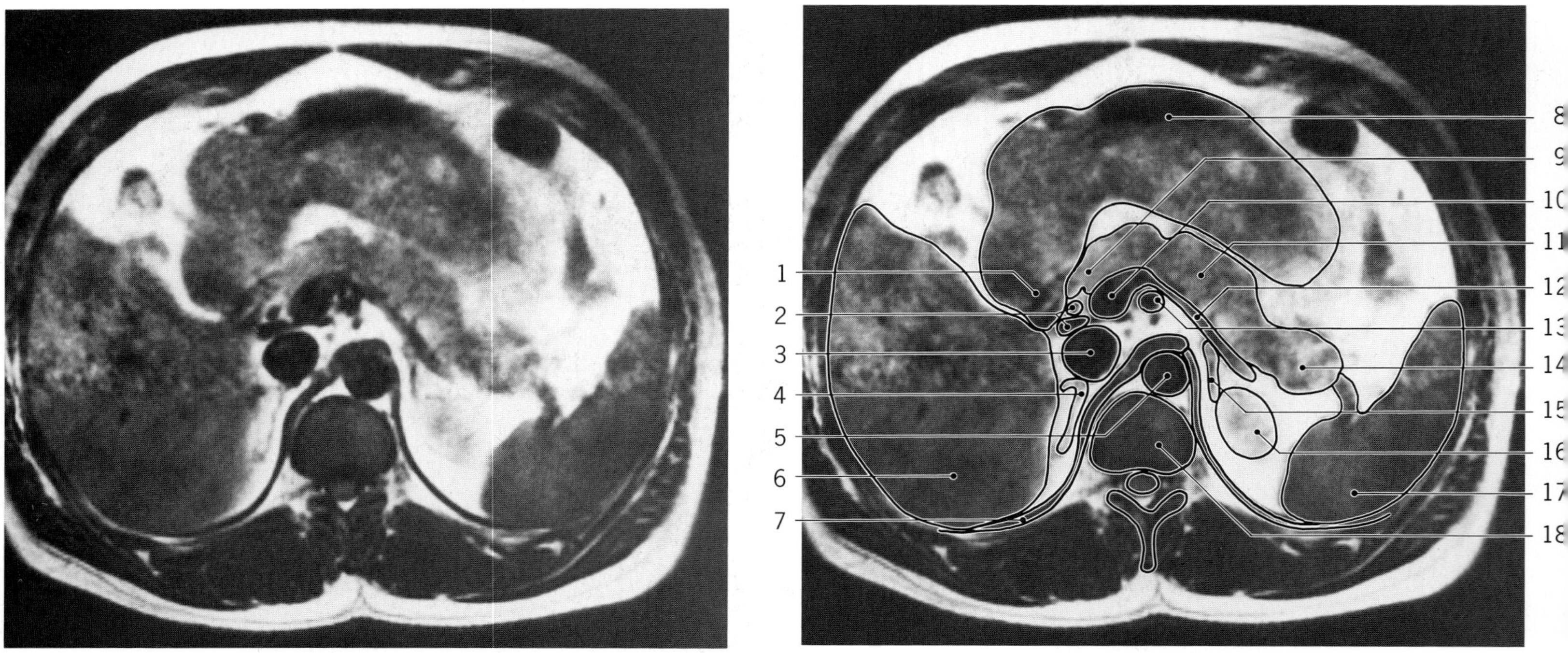

Upper abdomen with pancreas, axial MR

1: Duodenum
2: Bile duct and hepatic artery proper
3: Inferior caval vein
4: Right suprarenal gland
5: Aorta in aortic aperture of diaphragm
6: Liver
7: Lumbar part of diaphragm
8: Stomach
9: Head of pancreas
10: Portal vein
11: Body of pancreas
12: Splenic vein
13: Superior mesenteric artery
14: Tail of pancreas
15: Left suprarenal gland
16: Upper pole of left kidney
17: Spleen
18: Intervertebral disc Th XII - L I

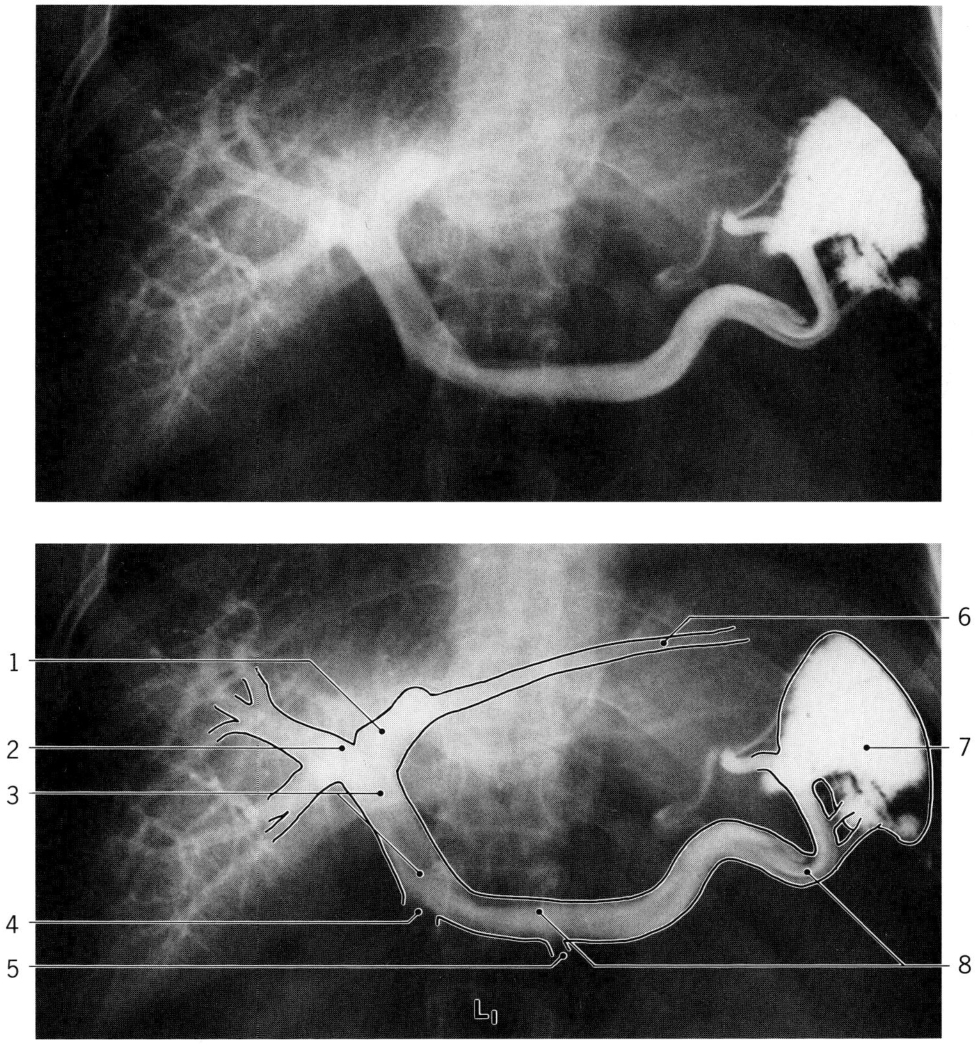

Spleen and liver, a-p X-ray, spleno-portography

1: Left branch of portal vein
2: Right branch of portal vein
3: Portal vein
4: Superior mesenteric vein (entrance)
5: Inferior mesenteric vein (entrance)
6: Portal branch in left lobe of liver
7: Spleen
8: Splenic vein

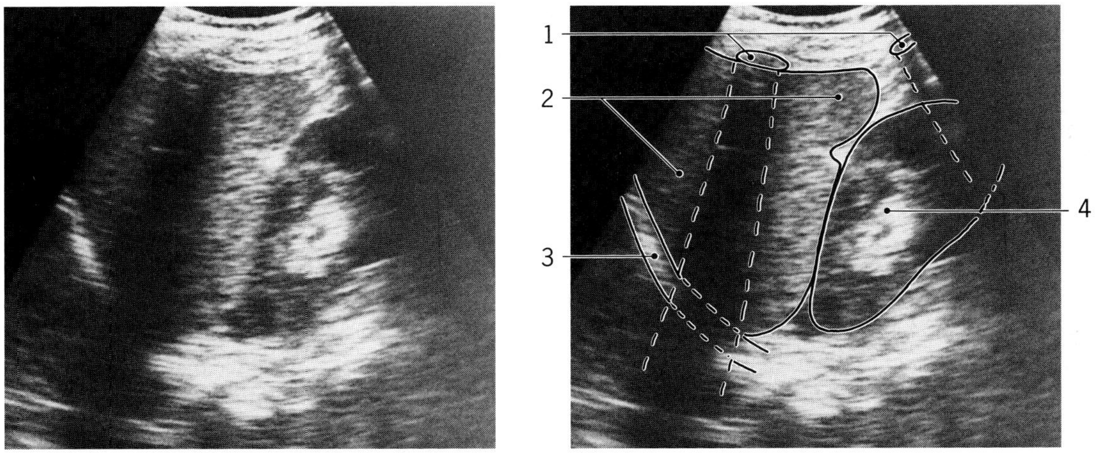

Spleen, intercostal sagittal section, US

1: 11th and 12th ribs with acoustic shadows
2: Spleen
3: Diaphragm
4: Left kidney

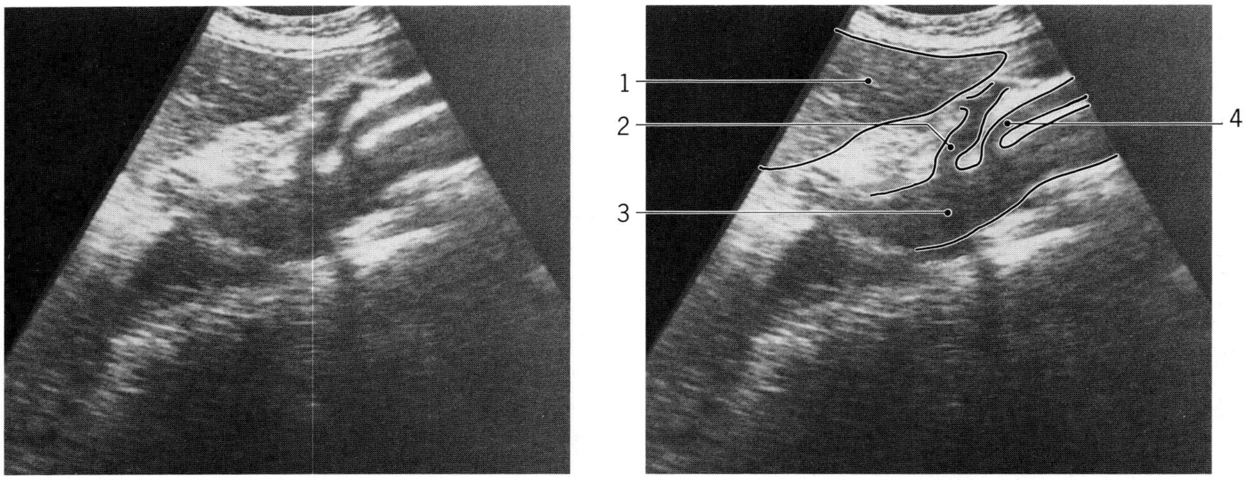

Abdominal aorta, sagittal section, US

1: Liver
2: Coeliac trunk
3: Abdominal aorta
4: Superior mesenteric artery

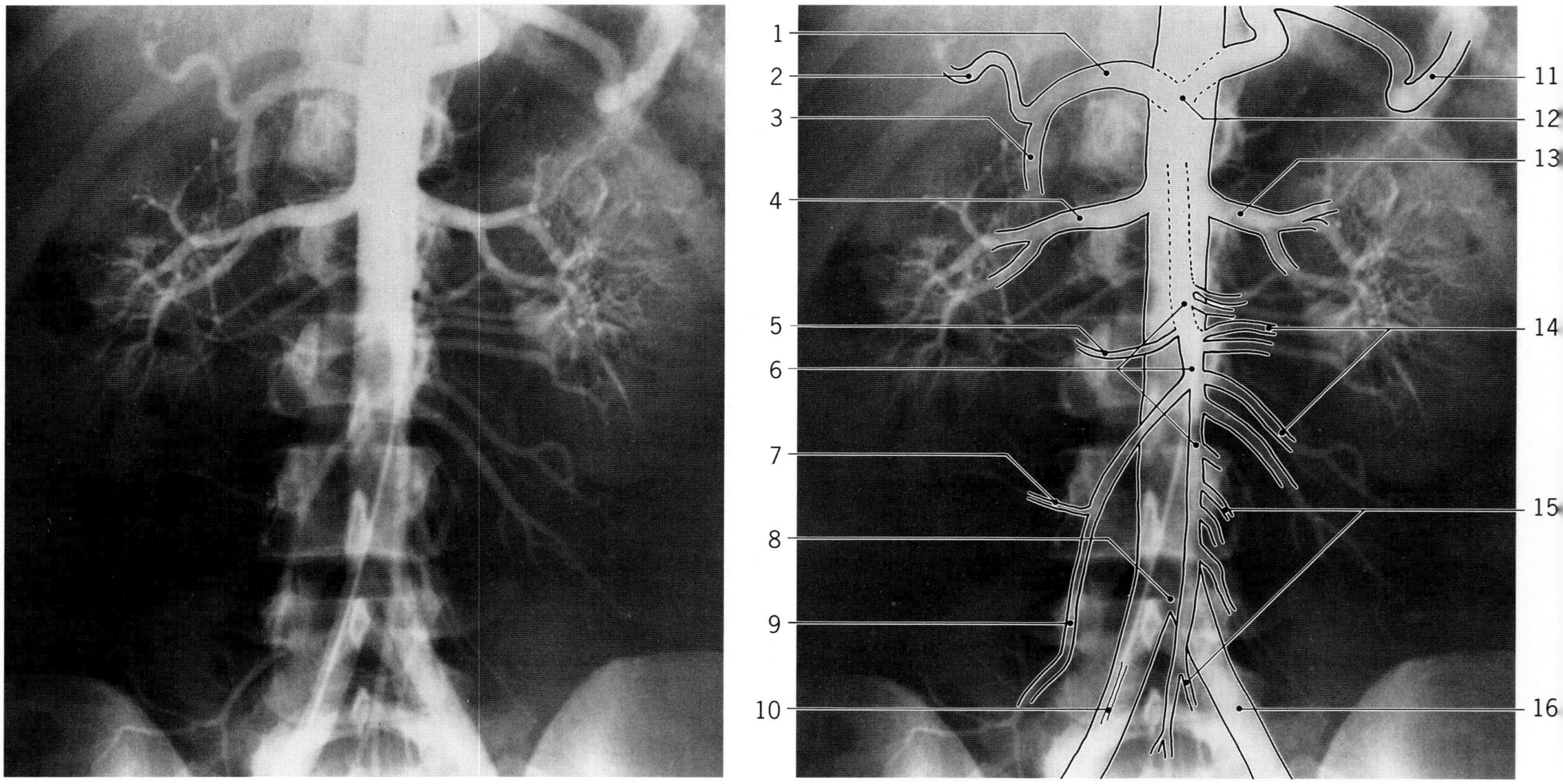

Abdominal aorta, a-p X-ray, aortography

1: Common hepatic artery
2: Hepatic artery proper
3: Gastroduodenal artery
4: Right renal artery
5: Middle colic artery
6: Superior mesenteric artery
7: Right colic artery
8: Aortic bifurcation
9: Iliocolic artery
10: Catheter
11: Splenic artery
12: Coeliac trunk
13: Left renal artery
14: Jejunal arteries
15: Ileal arteries
16: Left common iliac artery

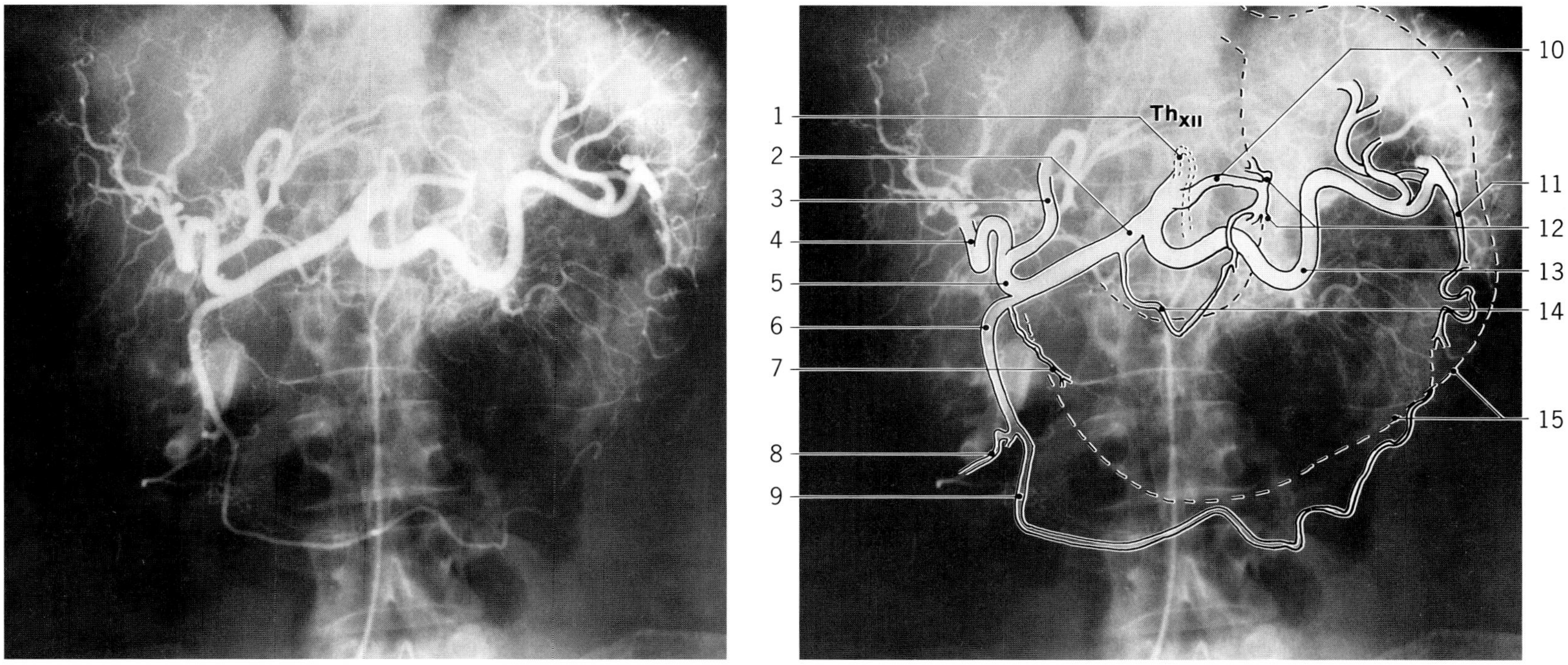

Coeliac trunk, a-p X-ray, arteriography (arterial phase)

1: Catheter tip in coeliac trunk
2: Common hepatic artery
3: Left branch of hepatic artery
4: Right branch of hepatic artery
5: Hepatic artery proper
6: Gastroduodenal artery
7: Supraduodenal artery
8: Superior pancreatico-duodenal artery
9: Right gastroepiploic artery
10: Left gastric artery
11: Left gastro-epiploic artery
12: Branches of left gastric artery
13: Splenic artery
14: Right gastric artery
15: Contour of ventricle (stippled)

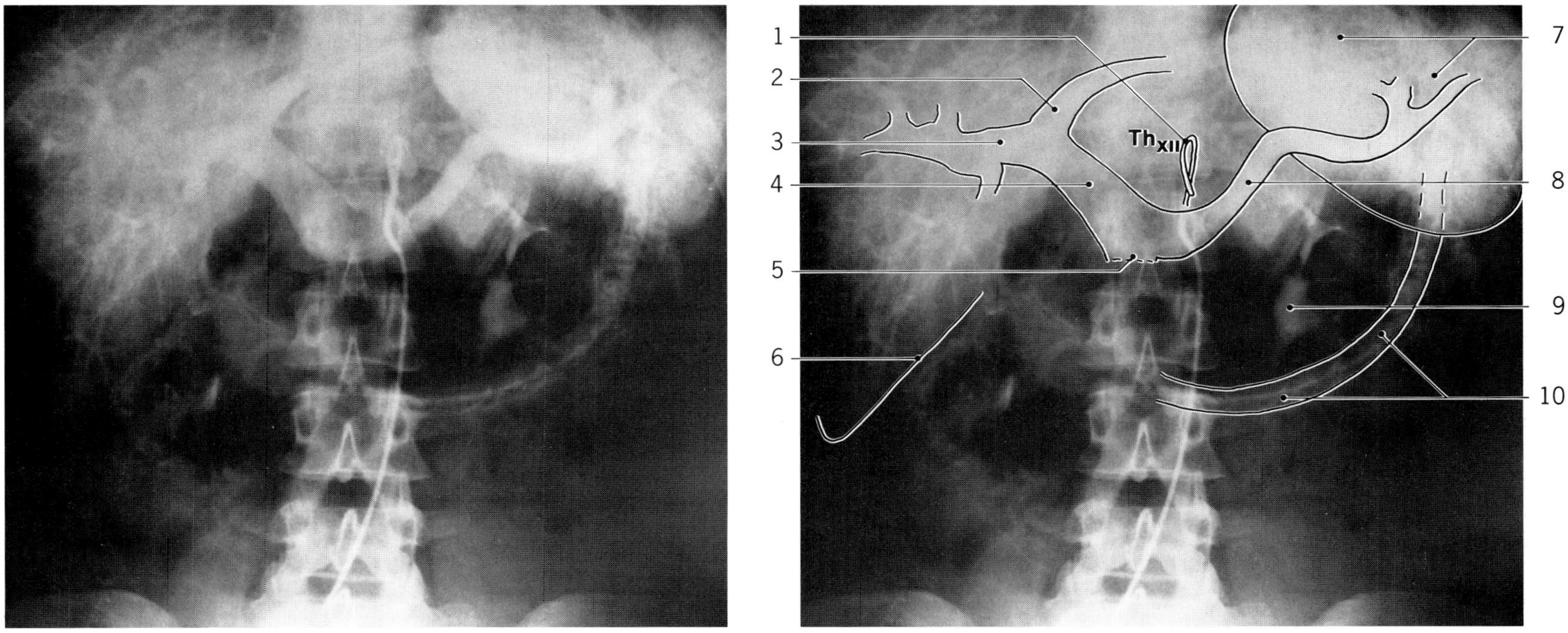

Portal vein, a-p X-ray, venous phase of coeliac arteriography (see above)

1: Catheter in coeliac trunk
2: Left branch of portal vein
3: Right branch of portal vein
4: Portal vein
5: Superior mesenteric vein (entrance)
6: Lower margin of liver
7: Spleen
8: Splenic vein
9: Pelvis of left kidney
10: Gastric wall (greater curvature)

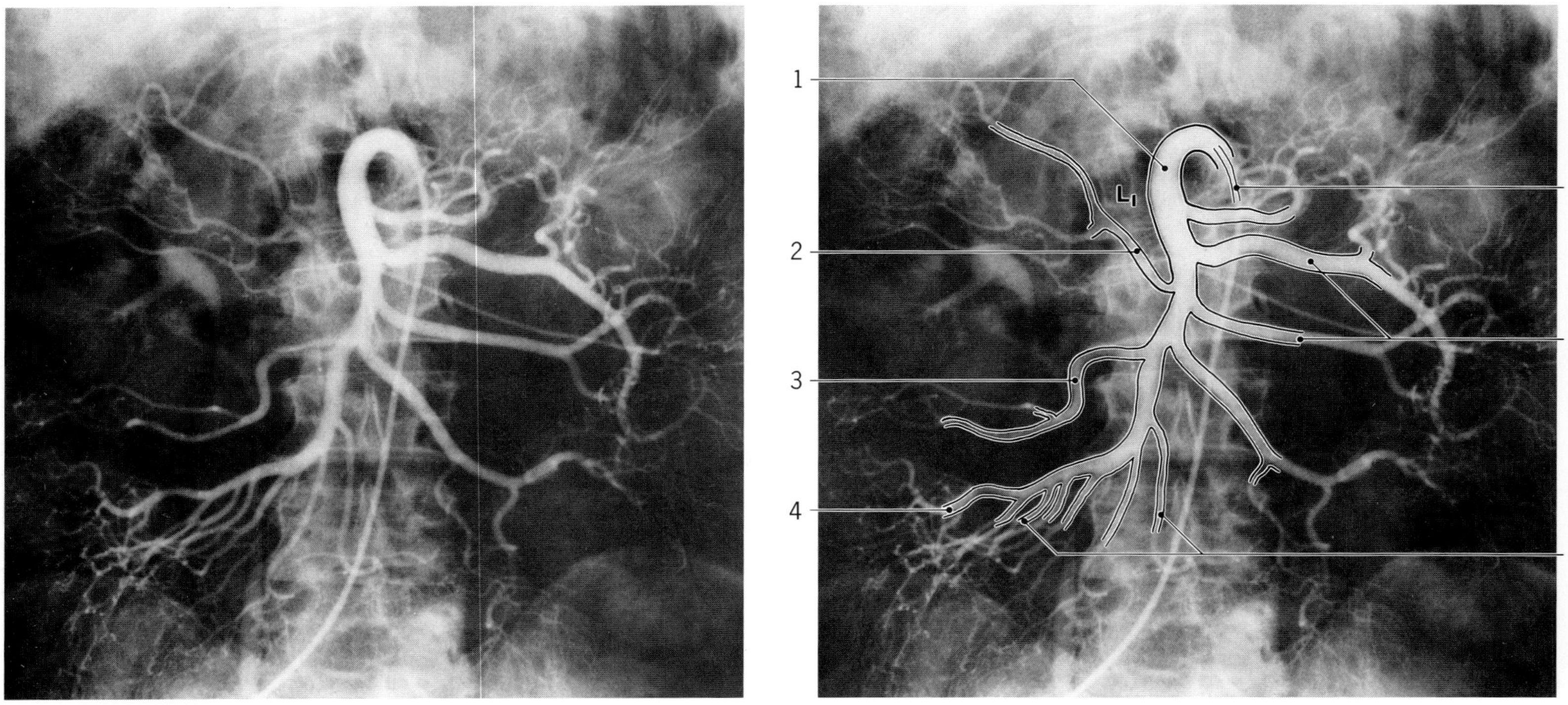

Superior mesenteric artery, a-p X-ray, arteriography

1: Superior mesenteric artery
2: Middle colic artery
3: Right colic artery
4: Ileocolic artery
5: Catheter
6: Jejunal arteries
7: Ileal arteries

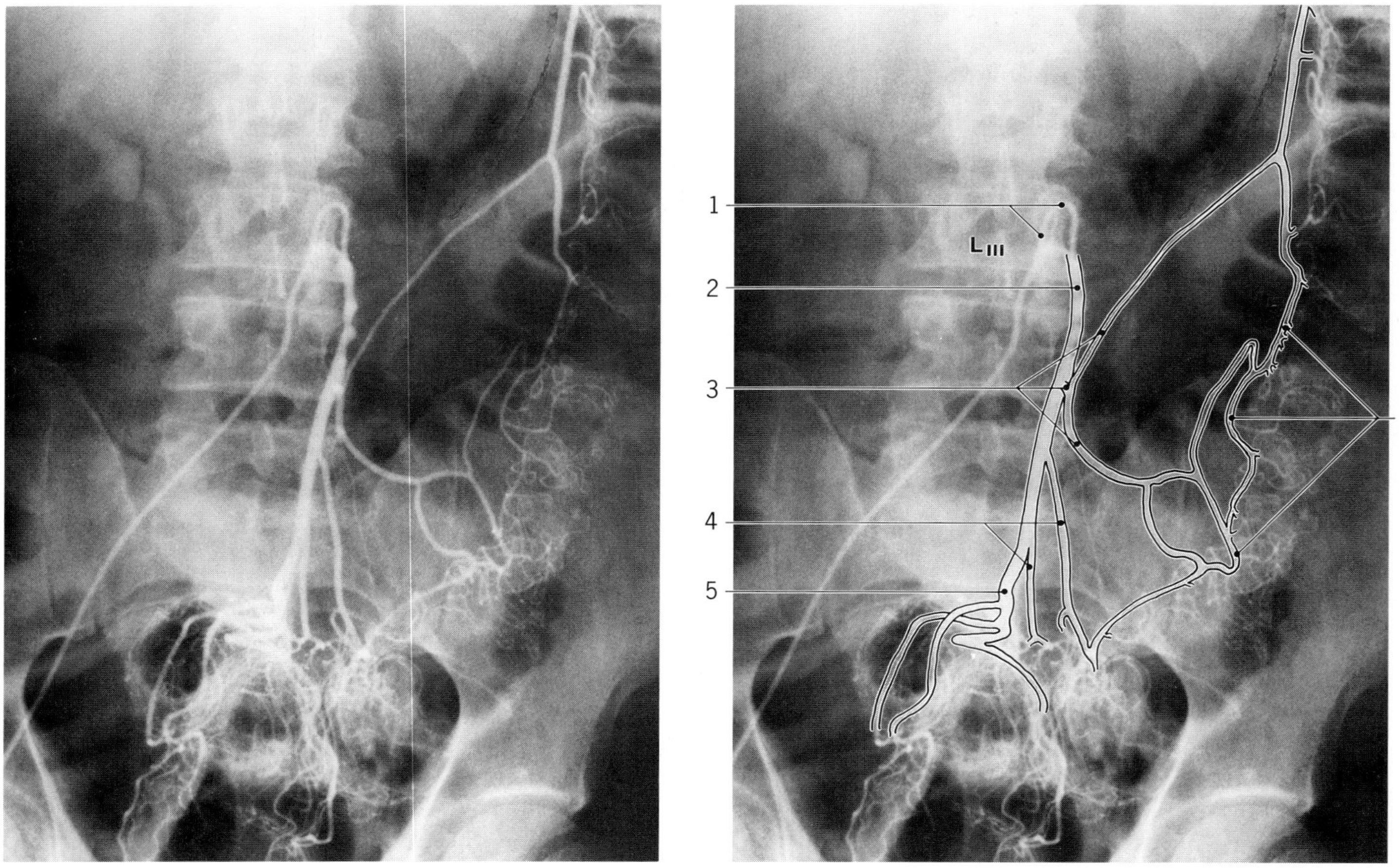

Inferior mesenteric artery, a-p X-ray, arteriography

1: Catheter
2: Inferior mesenteric artery
3: Left colic artery
4: Sigmoid arteries
5: Superior rectal artery
6: Marginal artery of colon

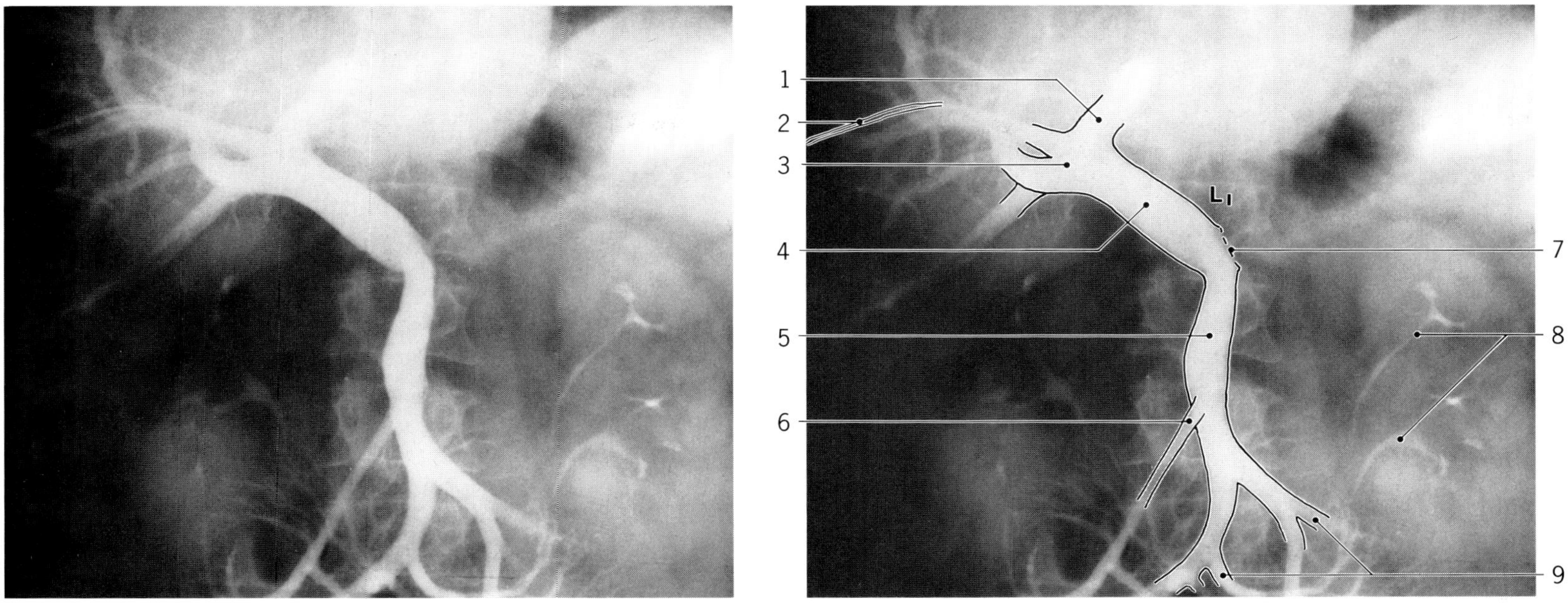

Superior mesenteric vein, a-p X-ray, transhepatic phlebography

1: Left branch of portal vein
2: Transhepatic catheter
3: Right branch of portal vein
4: Portal vein
5: Superior mesenteric vein
6: Middle colic vein
7: Splenic vein (entrance)
8: Pelvis of left kidney (duplex)
9: Jejunal veins

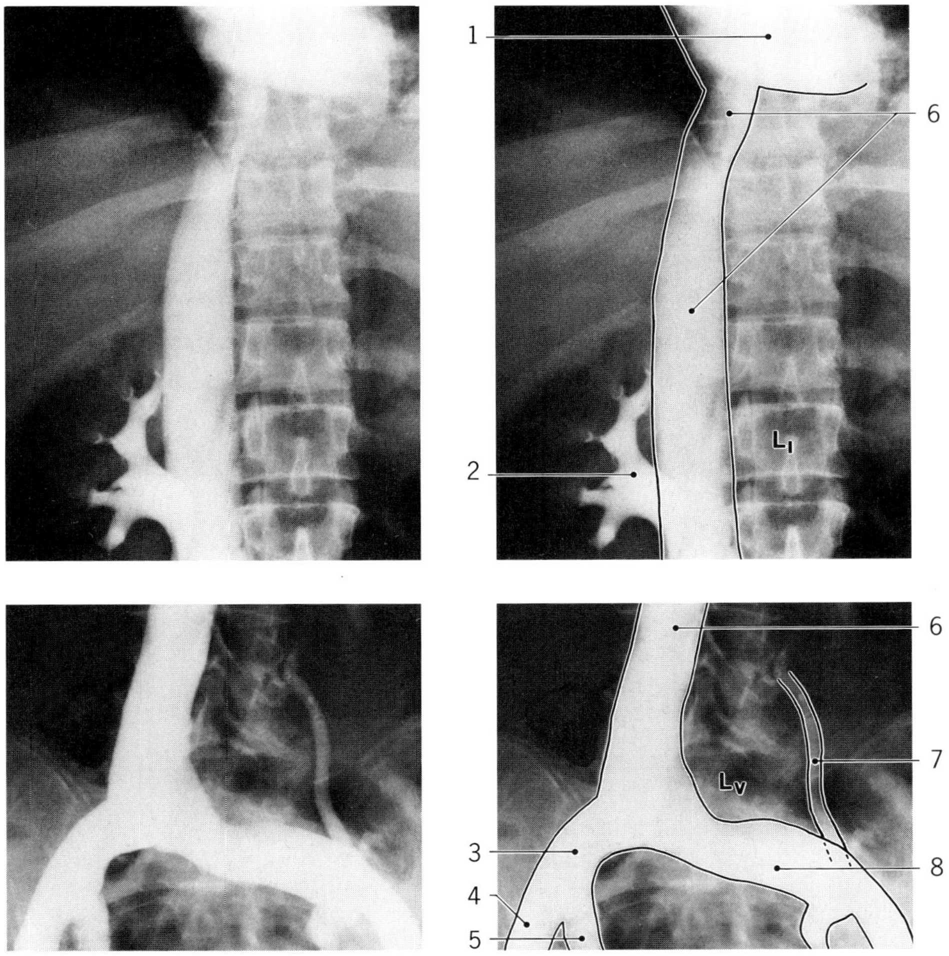

Inferior caval vein, a-p X-ray, phlebography

1: Right atrium
2: Pelvis of right kidney
3: Right common iliac vein
4: Right external iliac vein
5: Right internal iliac vein
6: Inferior caval vein
7: Left ureter
8: Left common iliac vein

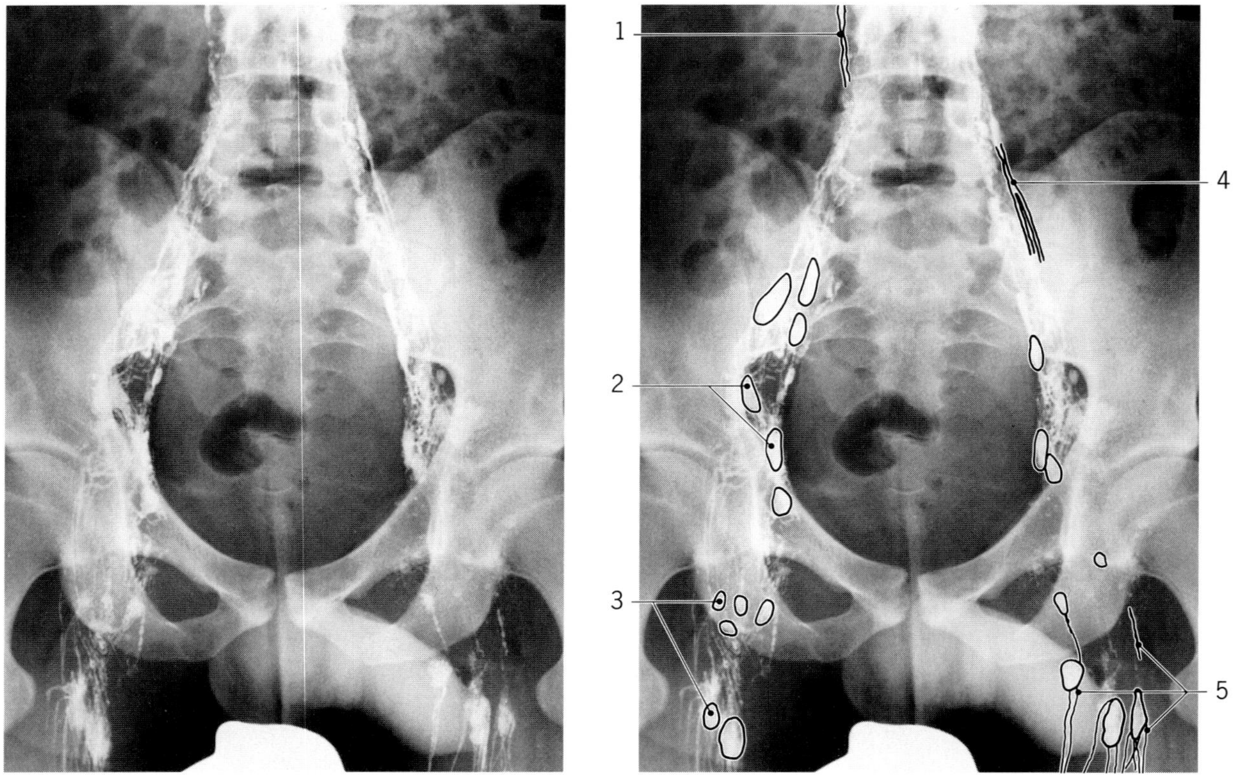

Lumbar lymph system, a-p X-ray, lymphography, first day

Bilateral infusion of contrast medium via lymphatic vessels on feet

1: Right lumbar trunk
2: External iliac lymph nodes
3: Superficial inguinal lymph nodes
4: Major iliolumbar lymphatic vessels
5: Afferent and efferent lymphatic vessels of superficial inguinal lymph nodes

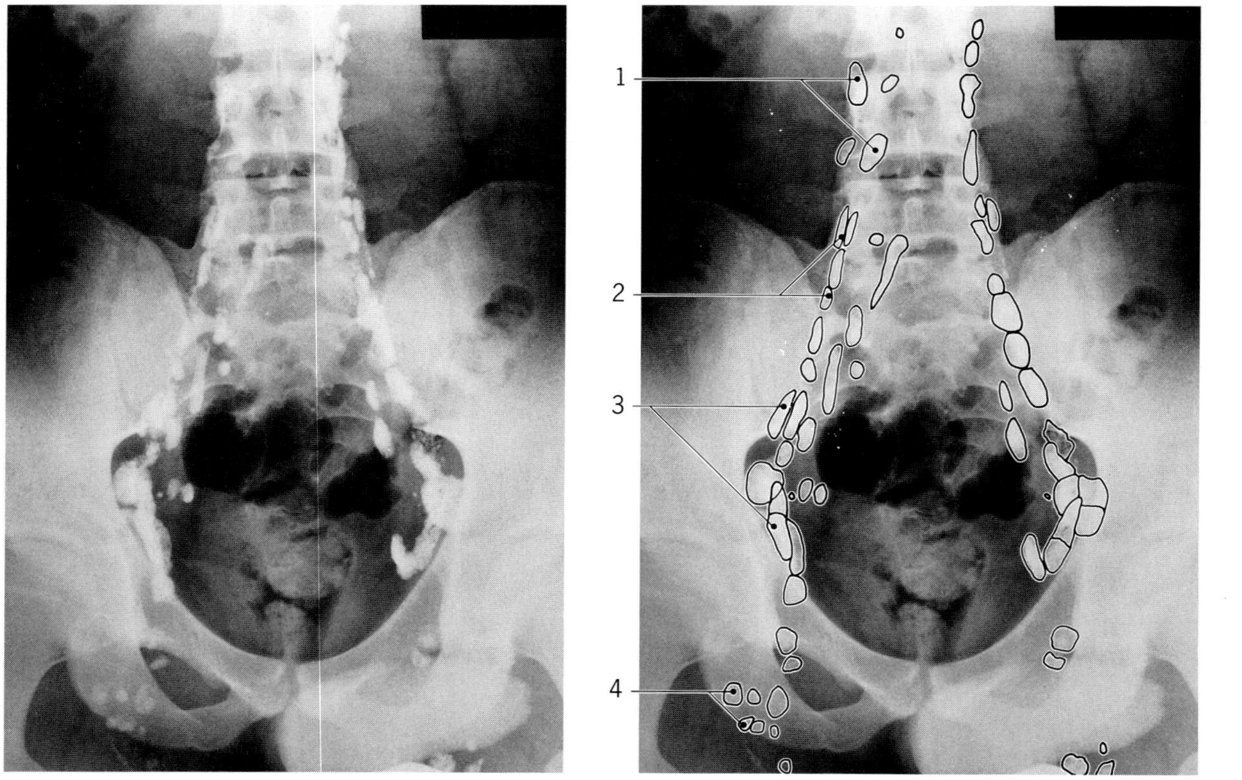

Lumbar lymph nodes, a-p, lymphography, second day

1: Lumbar (paraaortic) lymph nodes
2: Common iliac lymph nodes
3: External iliac lymph nodes
4: Superficial inguinal lymph nodes

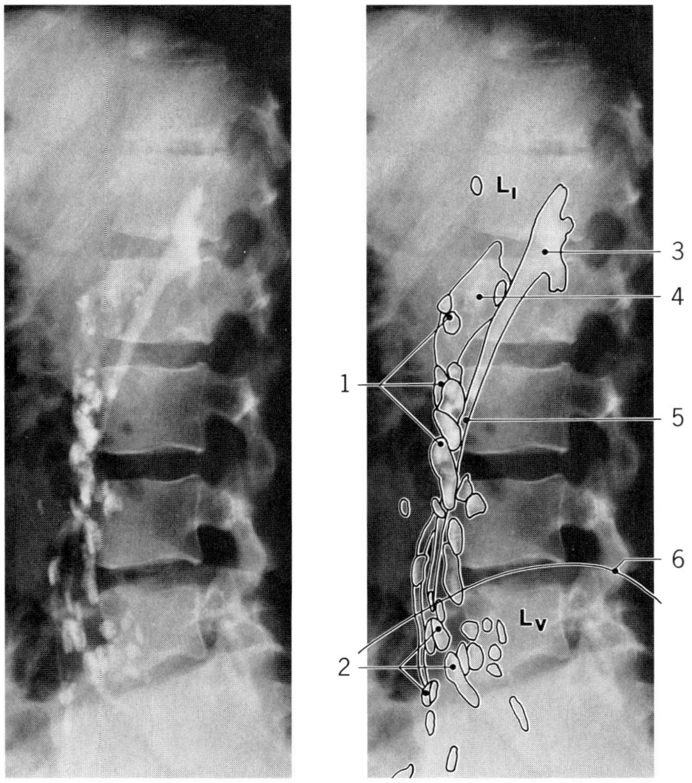

Lumbar lymph nodes, lateral X-ray, lymphography (second day), and intravenous urography

1: Lumbar (paraaortic) lymph nodes
2: Common iliac lymph nodes
3: Pelvis of left kidney
4: Pelvis of right kidney
5: Left ureter
6: Iliac crest

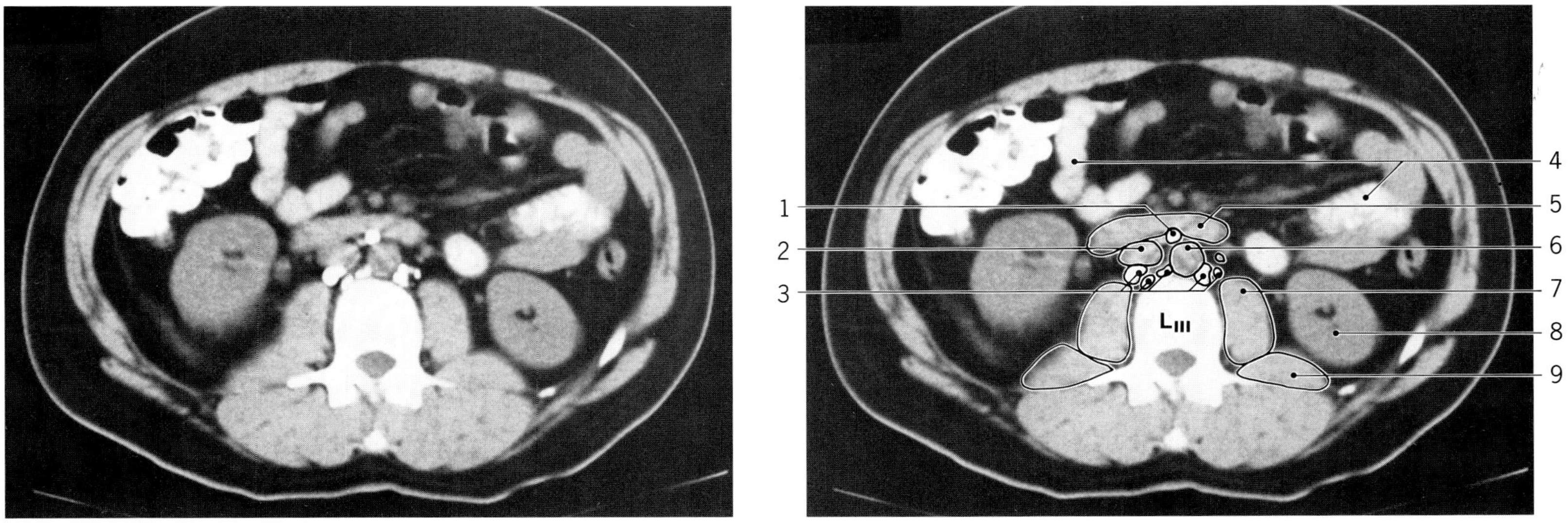

Lumbar lymph nodes, axial CT, after lymphography and peroral contrast

1: Lumbar (preaortic) lymph node
2: Inferior caval vein
3: Lumbar (paraaortic) lymph nodes
4: Small intestine
5: Horizontal part of duodenum
6: Abdominal aorta
7: Psoas major
8: Left kidney
9: Quadratus lumborum

Urogenital system

Kidney

Urinary bladder and urethra

Male genital organs

Female genital organs

Pregnancy

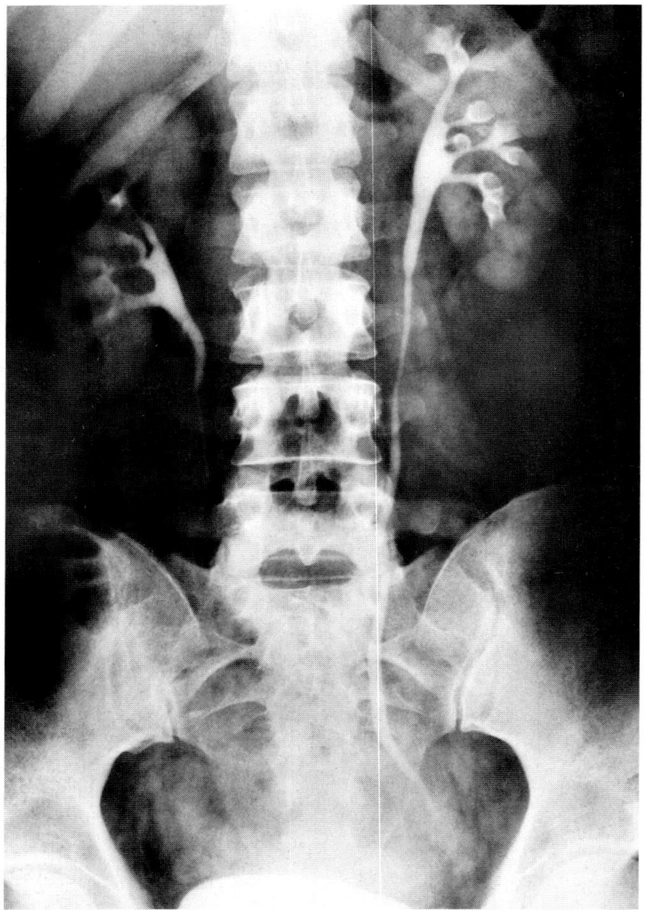

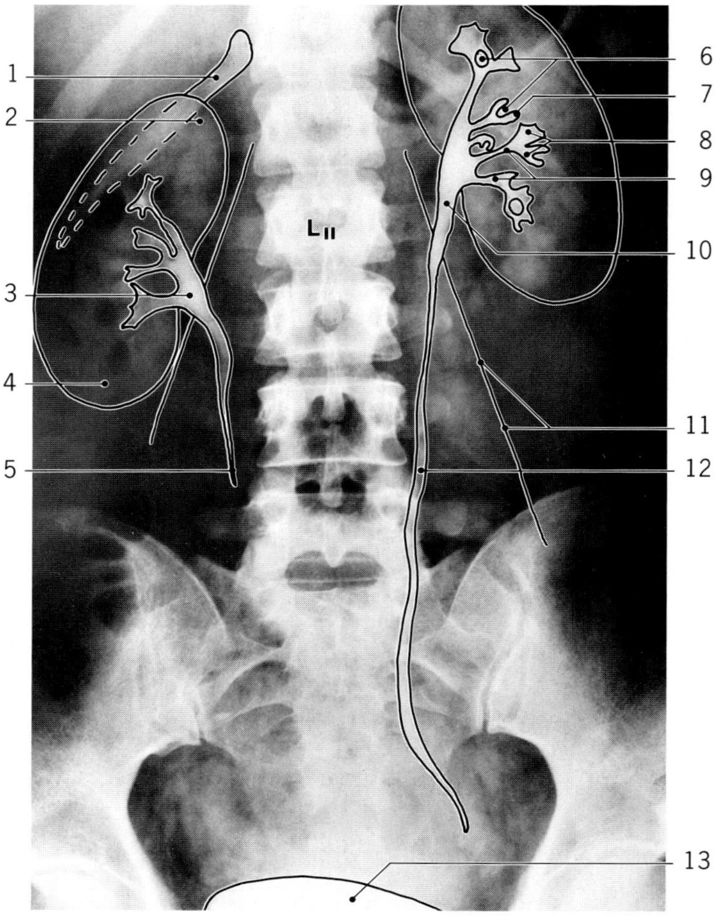

Urinary tract, a-p X-ray, i.v. urography

15 min after intravenous contrast

1: 12th rib
2: Upper pole of right kidney
3: Pelvis of right kidney
4: Lower pole of right kidney
5: Right ureter
6: Renal papillae
7: Fornix of minor calyx
8: Minor calices
9: Major calices
10: Pelvis of left kidney
11: Psoas major (lateral contour)
12: Left ureter
13: Urinary bladder

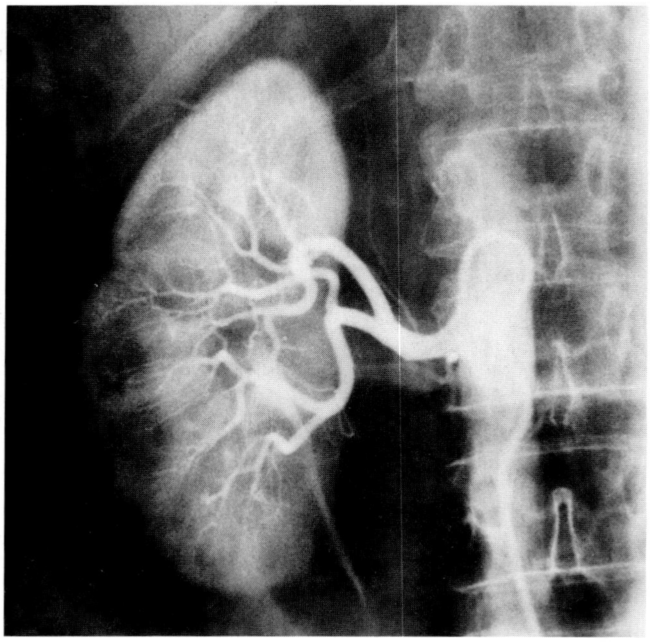

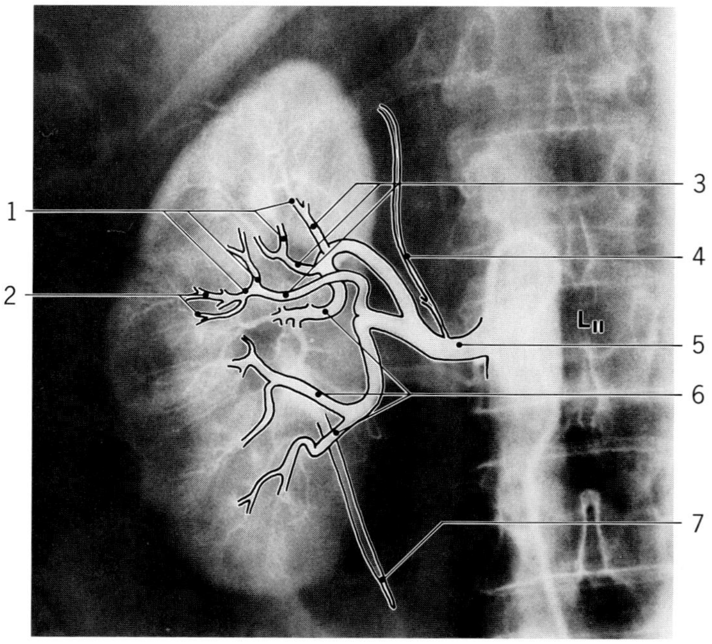

Renal artery, a-p X-ray, arteriography

1: Arcuate arteries
2: Interlobular arteries
3: Interlobar arteries
4: Inferior suprarenal artery
5: Right renal artery
6: Segmental arteries
7: Right ureter

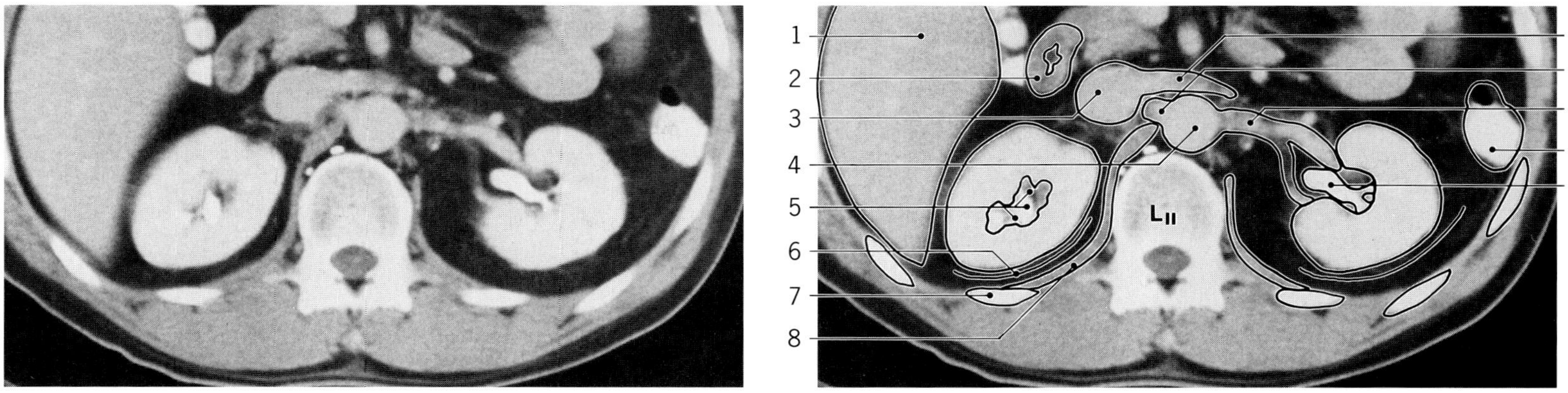

Kidneys, axial CT, with intravenous and peroral contrast

1: Liver
2: Descending part of duodenum
3: Inferior caval vein
4: Abdominal aorta
5: Renal sinus
6: Renal fascia
7: 12th rib
8: Lumbar part of diaphragm
9: Left renal vein
10: Right renal artery
11: Left renal artery
12: Descending colon
13: Pelvis of left kidney

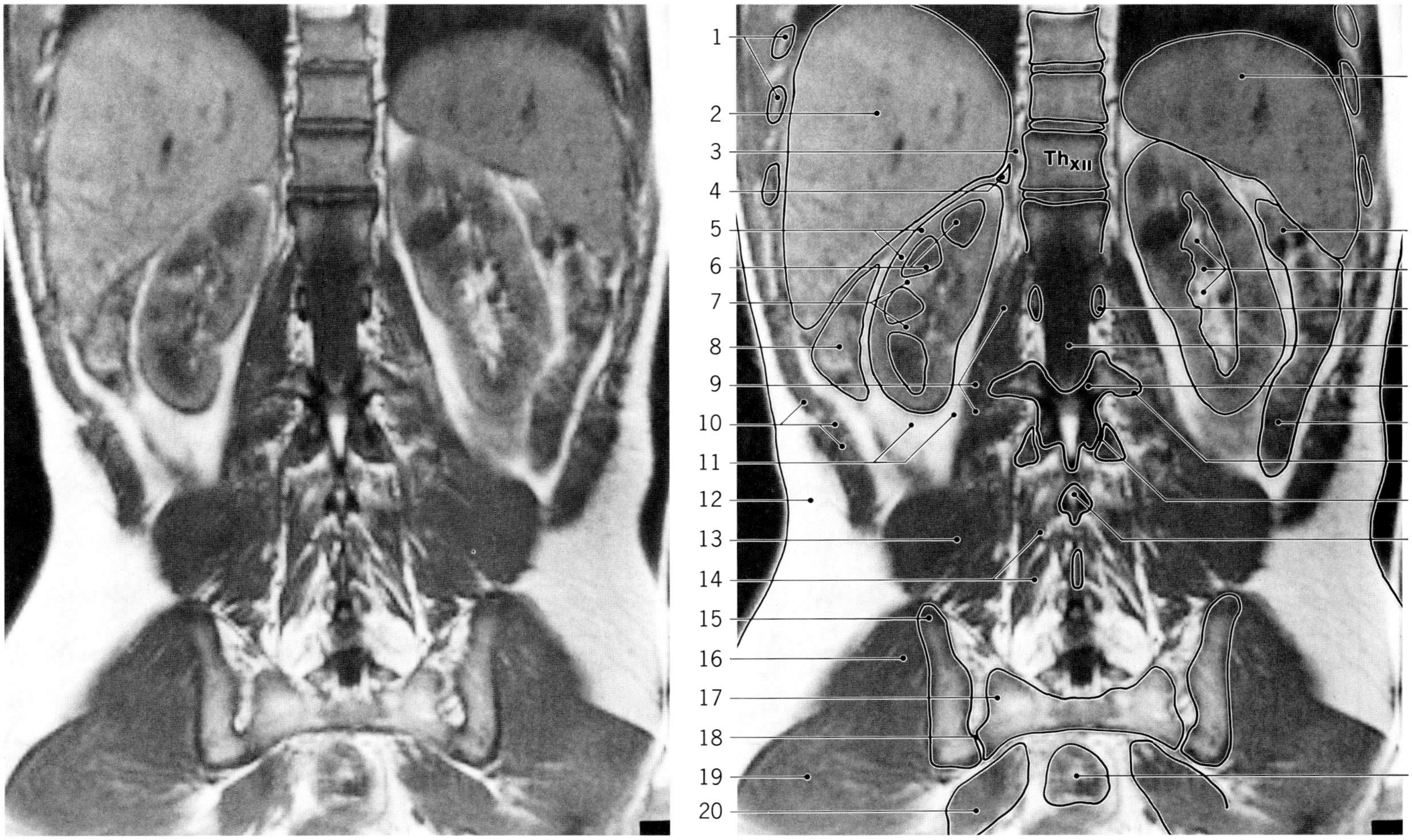

Kidneys, coronal MR, T1 weighted recording

1: Ribs
2: Liver
3: Lumbar part of diaphragm
4: Right suprarenal gland
5: Renal cortex
6: Renal pyramids
7: Renal columns
8: Ascending colon
9: Psoas major
10: Abdominal wall muscles
11: Perirenal fat
12: Subcutaneous fat
13: Quadratus lumborum
14: Transversospinal muscles
15: Iliac crest
16: Gluteus medius
17: Ala of sacrum
18: Sacro-iliac joint
19: Gluteus maximus
20: Piriformis
21: Spleen
22: Splenic flexure of colon
23: Renal sinus
24: Pedicle of vertebral arch L II
25: Vertebral canal
26: Lamina of vertebral arch L III
27: Descending colon
28: Transverse process of L III
29: Zygapophyseal (facet) joint L III - L IV
30: Spinous process of L IV
31: Rectum

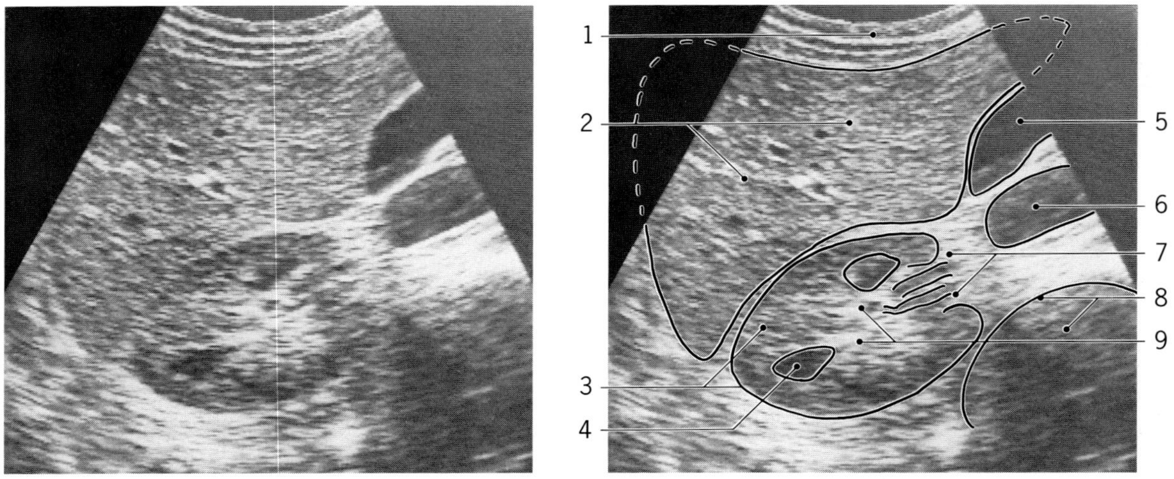

Kidney, oblique section, US

1: Anterior abdominal wall
2: Right lobe of liver
3: Right kidney
4: Renal pyramid
5: Portal vein
6: Inferior caval vein
7: Hilum of right kidney
8: Vertebral column (lumbar)
9: Renal sinus

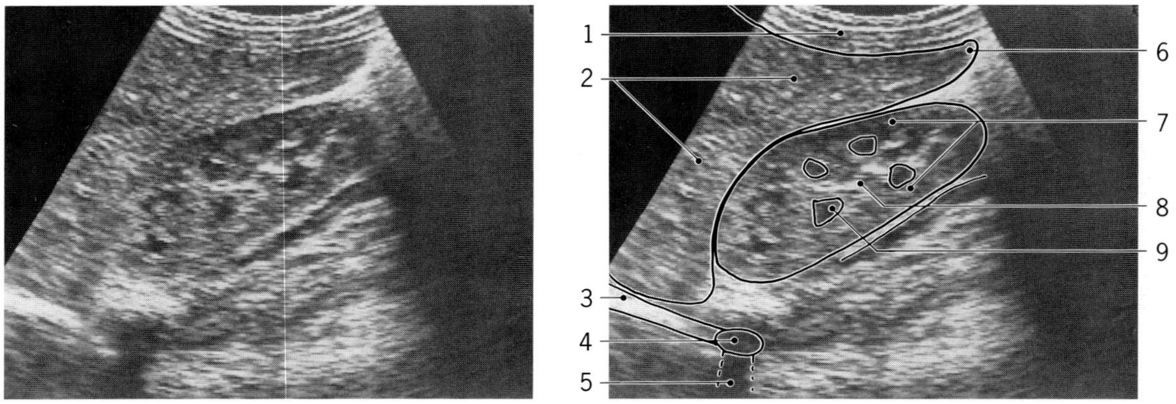

Kidney, longitudinal section, US

1: Abdominal wall
2: Right lobe of liver
3: Diaphragm
4: 12th rib
5: Acoustic shadow of rib
6: Inferior margin of liver
7: Right kidney
8: Renal sinus
9: Renal pyramid

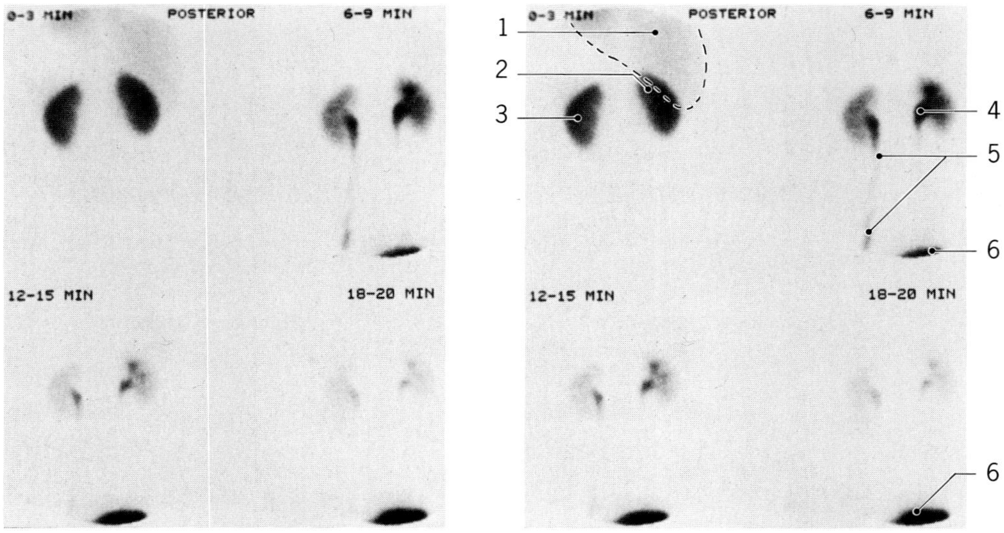

Kidneys, ^{131}J-hippuran, scintigraphy (renography), posterior view

Four samplings at intervals indicated after i.v. injection of ^{131}J-hippurate

1: Liver
2: Right kidney
3: Left kidney (usually more cranial than the right)
4: Renal pelvis
5: Ureter
6: Urinary bladder

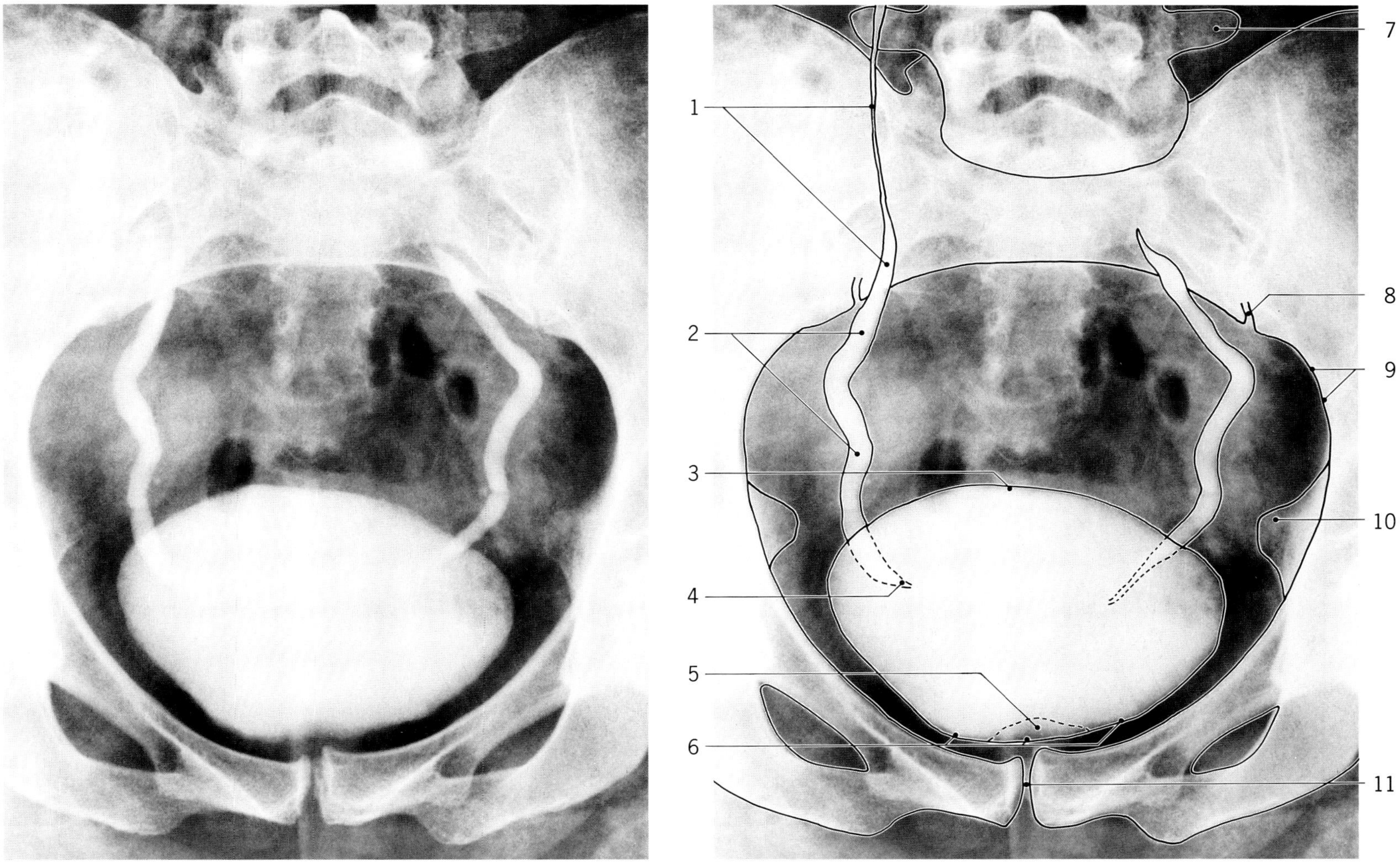

Urinary bladder, male, a-p, tilted X-ray, i.v. urography

20 min after intravenous contrast

1: Abdominal part of ureter
2: Pelvic part of ureter
3: Apex of urinary bladder
4: Intramural part of ureter
5: Impression of prostate
6: Fundus of urinary bladder
7: Transverse process of L V
8: Sacro-iliac joint
9: Linea arcuata
10: Ischial spine
11: Pubic symphysis

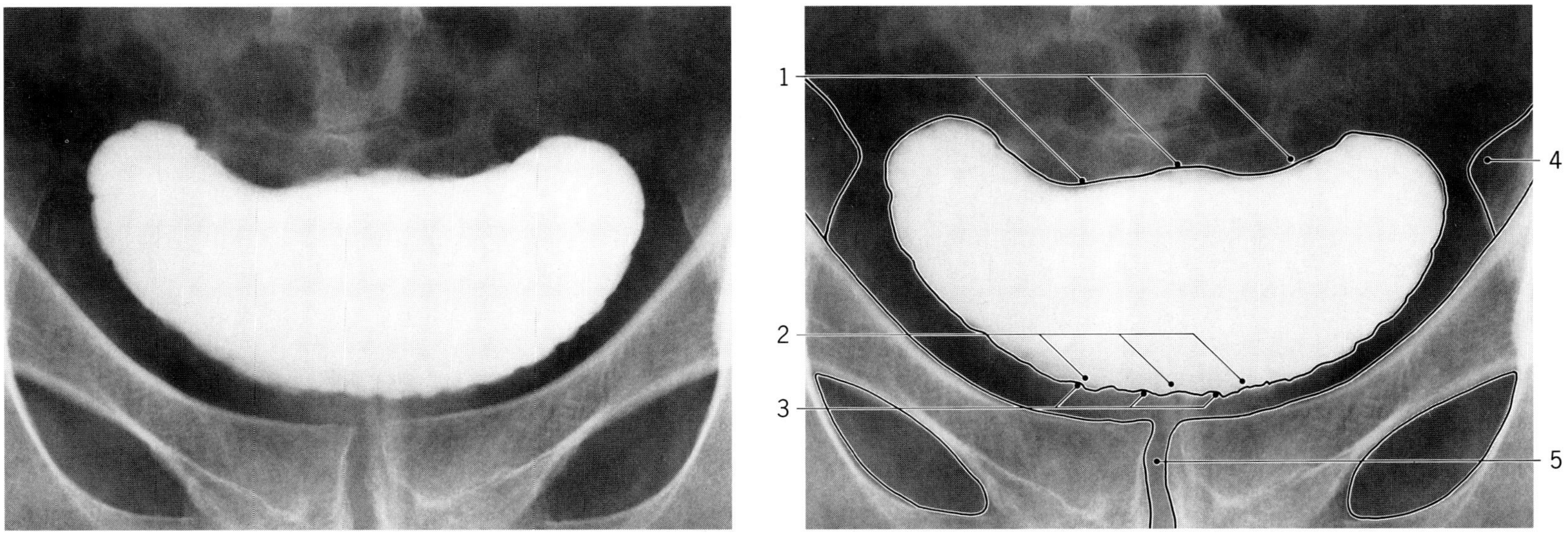

Urinary bladder, female, a-p, tilted X-ray, i.v. urography

1: Impression of uterus
2: Fundus of urinary bladder
3: Contours of trabecular muscle in bladder wall
4: Ischial spine
5: Pubic symphysis

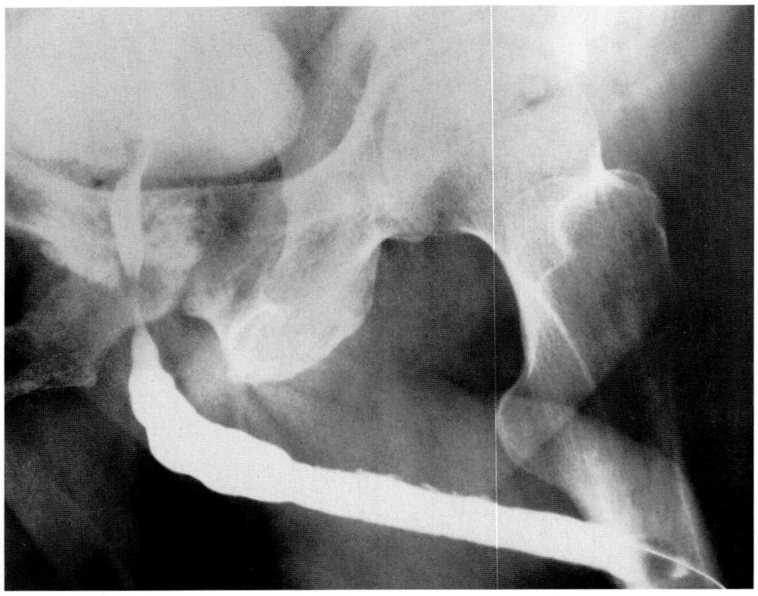

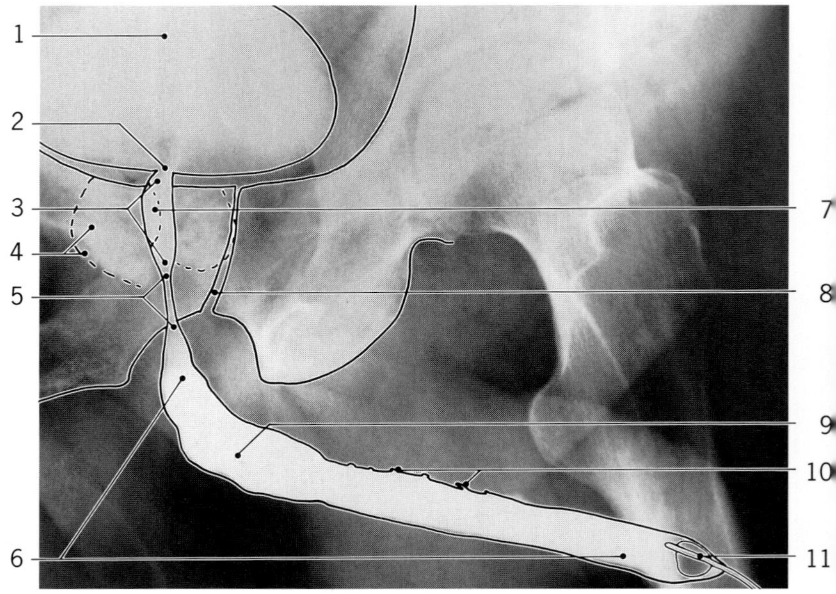

Urethra, male, oblique X-ray, urethrography

1: Urinary bladder
2: Internal urethral orifice
3: Prostatic part of urethra
4: Overflow of contrast medium into prostatic glands
5: Membranous part of urethra
6: Spongious part of urethra
7: Site of colliculus seminalis (verumontanum)
8: Pubic symphysis
9: Urethral bulb
10: Urethral lacunae
11: Balloon catheter in navicular fossa

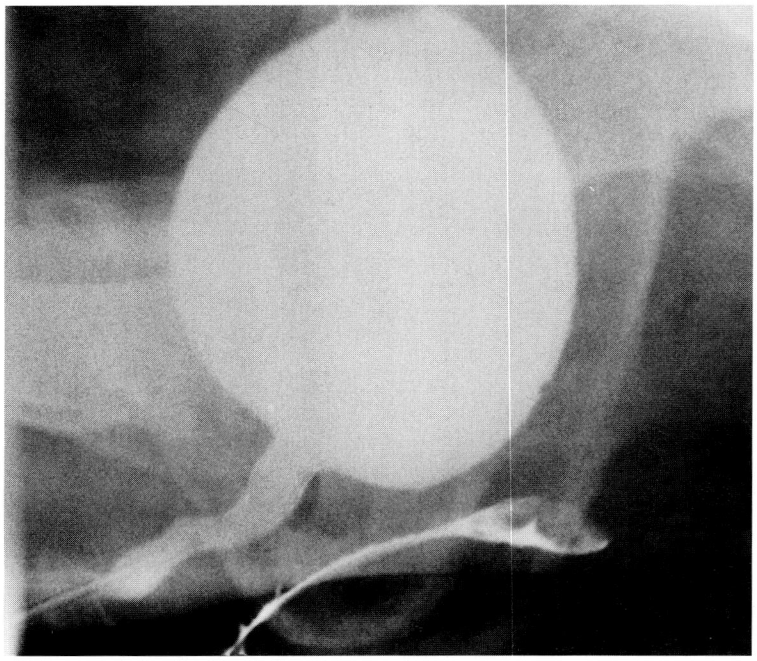

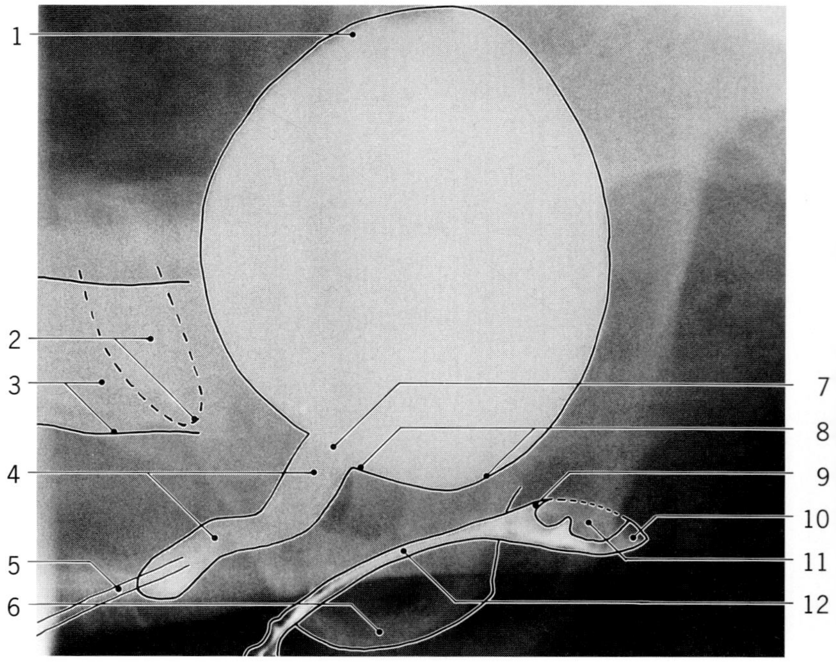

Urethra, female, lateral X-ray, kolpo-cysto-urethrography, micturating

1: Apex of urinary bladder
2: Pubic symphysis
3: Femoral bone
4: Urethra
5: Catheter
6: Ischial tuberosity
7: Internal urethral orifice
8: Trigone of bladder
9: Anterior fornix of vagina
10: Posterior fornix of vagina
11: Vaginal part of cervix uteri
12: Vagina

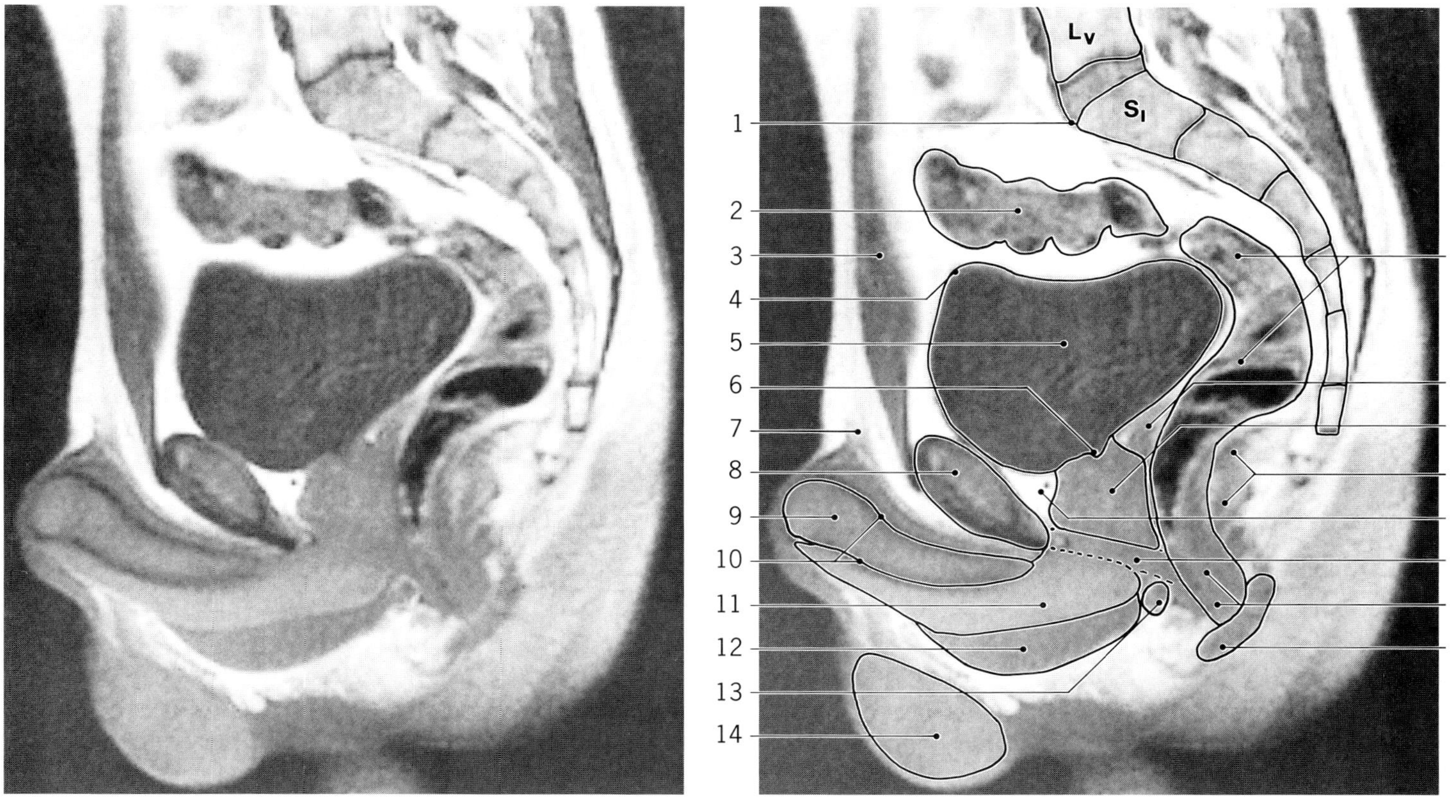

Male pelvis, median MR

T1 weighted recording

1: Promontory
2: Sigmoid colon
3: Rectus abdominis
4: Apex of urinary bladder
5: Urinary bladder
6: Internal orifice of urethra
7: Fundiform ligament of penis
8: Pubic symphysis
9: Corpus cavernosum
10: Tunica albuginea
11: Bulb of penis
12: Bulbospongiosus muscle
13: Bulbo-urethral gland (Cowper)
14: Testis
15: Rectum
16: Ampulla of deferent duct
17: Prostate
18: Levator ani
19: Retropubic space (cavum Retzii)
20: Urogenital diaphragm
21: Anal canal
22: Sphinchter ani externus, subcutaneous part

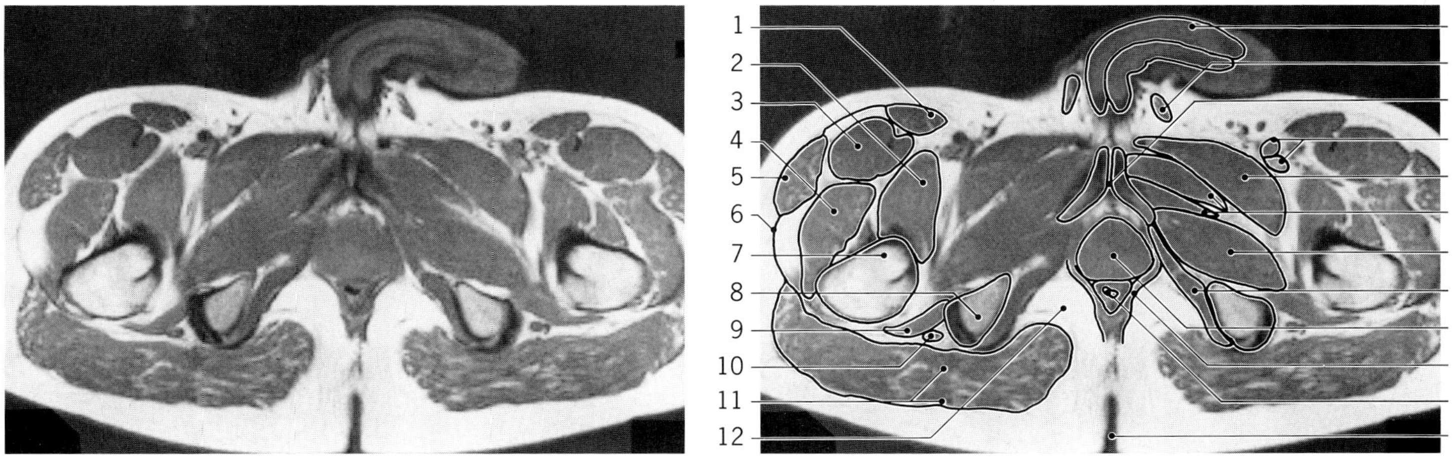

Male pelvis, axial MR

T1 weighted recording

1: Sartorius
2: Iliopsoas
3: Rectus femoris
4: Vastus lateralis
5: Tensor fasciae latae
6: Iliotibial tract
7: Femoral bone
8: Ischial tuberosity
9: Quadratus femoris
10: Sciatic nerve
11: Gluteus maximus
12: Ischiorectal fossa
13: Corpus cavernosum
14: Spermatic cord
15: Pubic symphysis
16: Femoral artery and vein
17: Pectineus
18: Adductor longus and brevis
19: Obturatorius externus
20: Obturatorius internus
21: Prostate
22: Levator ani
23: Rectum
24: Crena ani

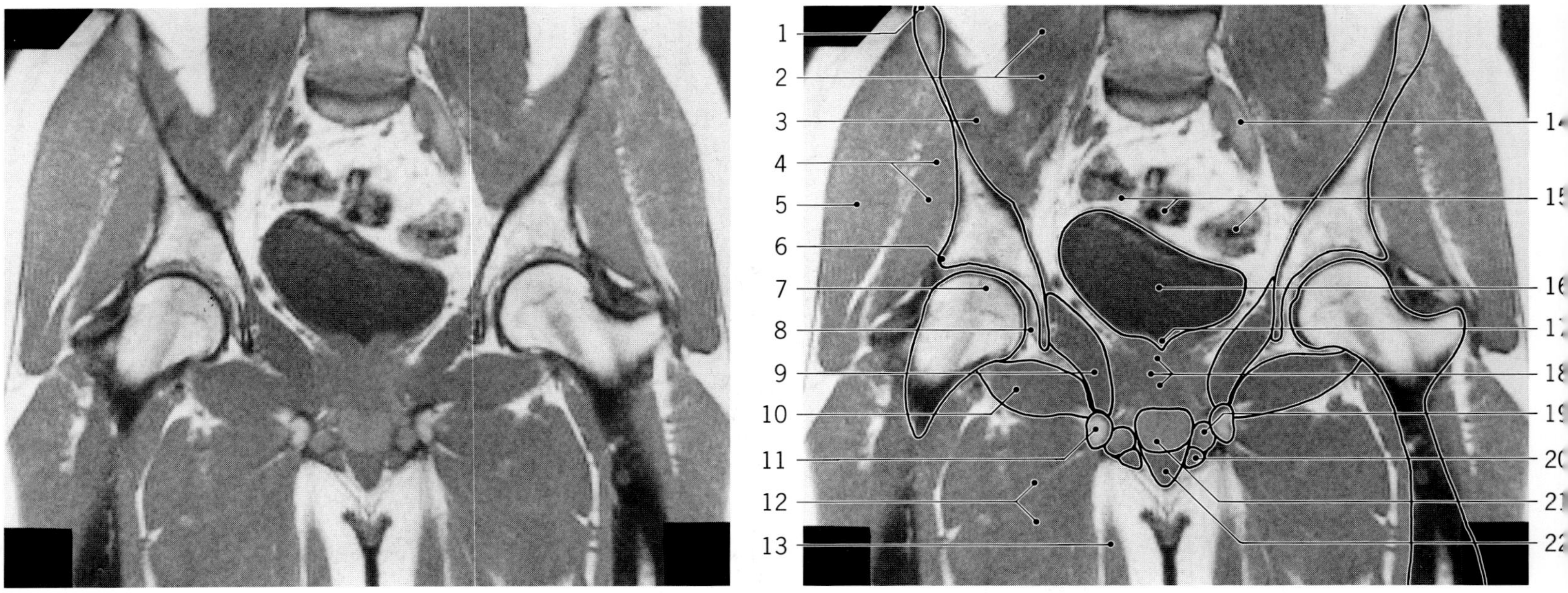

Male pelvis, coronal MR

T1 weighted recording

1: Iliac crest
2: Psoas major
3: Iliacus
4: Gluteus minimus
5: Gluteus medius
6: Acetabular rim
7: Femoral head
8: Acetabular fossa
9: Obturatorius internus
10: Obturatorius externus
11: Inferior ramus of pubis
12: Adductor muscles
13: Gracilis
14: Left common iliac vein
15: Sigmoid colon
16: Urinary bladder
17: Internal orifice of urethra
18: Prostate
19: Crus penis
20: Ischiocavernosus muscle
21: Bulb of penis
22: Bulbospongiosus muscle

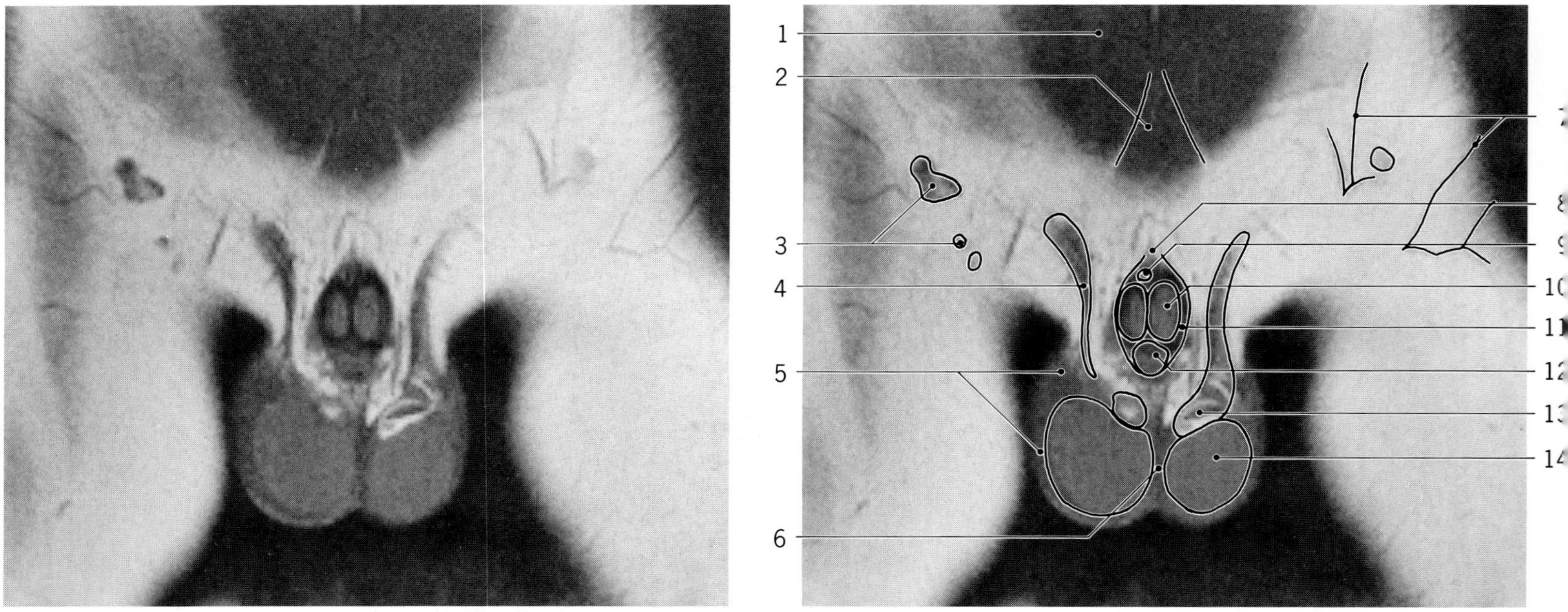

Penis and scrotum, coronal MR

T1 weighted recording

1: Rectus abdominis
2: Pyramidalis muscle
3: Superficial inguinal lymph nodes
4: Spermatic cord
5: Scrotum
6: Septum of scrotum
7: Superficial vessels
8: Suspensory ligament of penis
9: Deep dorsal vein of penis
10: Corpus cavernosum
11: Deep fascia of penis
12: Corpus spongiosum
13: Epididymis
14: Testis

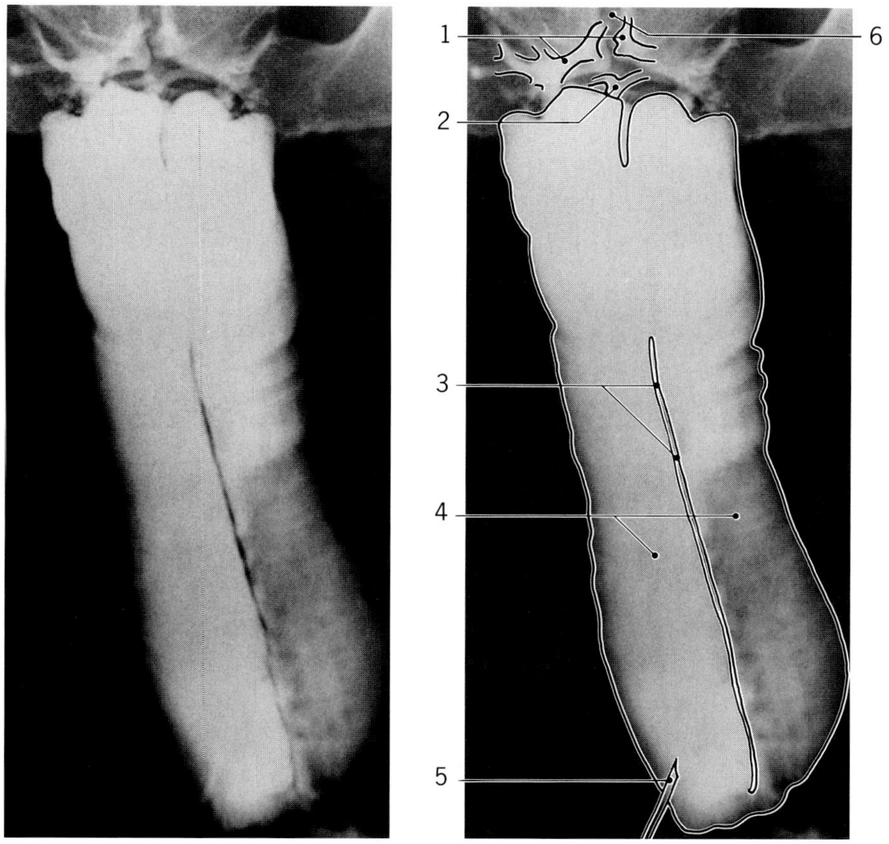

Penis, a-p X-ray, cavernosography

1: Prostatic venous plexus
2: Deep dorsal vein of penis
3: Septum of penis
4: Corpora cavernosa
5: Injection site
6: Pubic symphysis

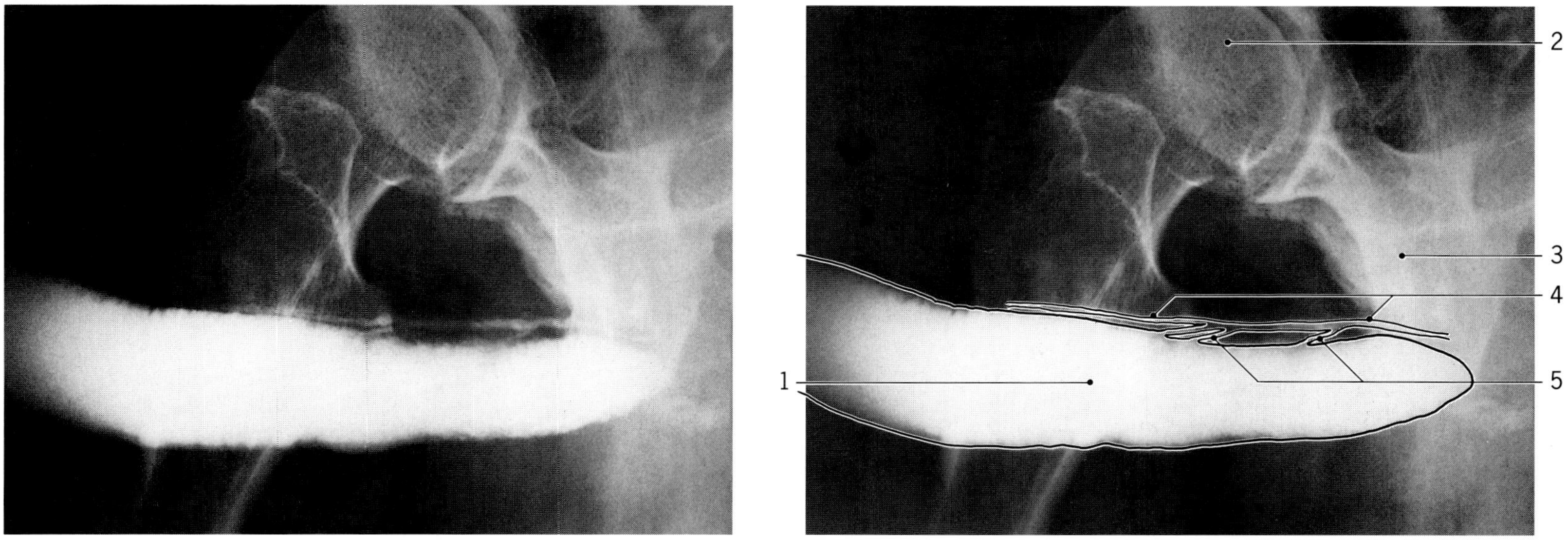

Penis, lateral X-ray, cavernosography

1: Corpus cavernosum
2: Femoral head
3: Pubic symphysis
4: Deep dorsal vein of penis
5: Emissary veins of penis

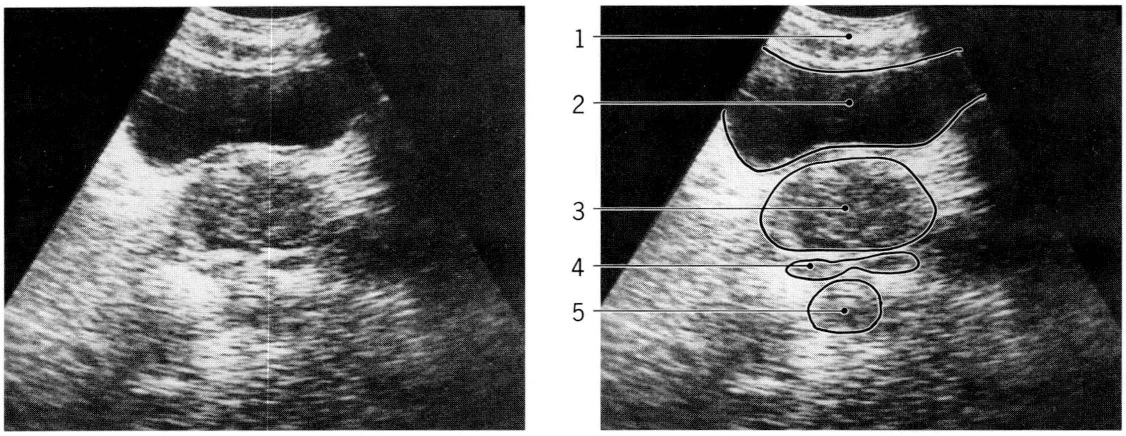

Prostate, tilted transverse section, US

1: Anterior abdominal wall
2: Urinary bladder
3: Prostate
4: Seminal vesicle
5: Rectum

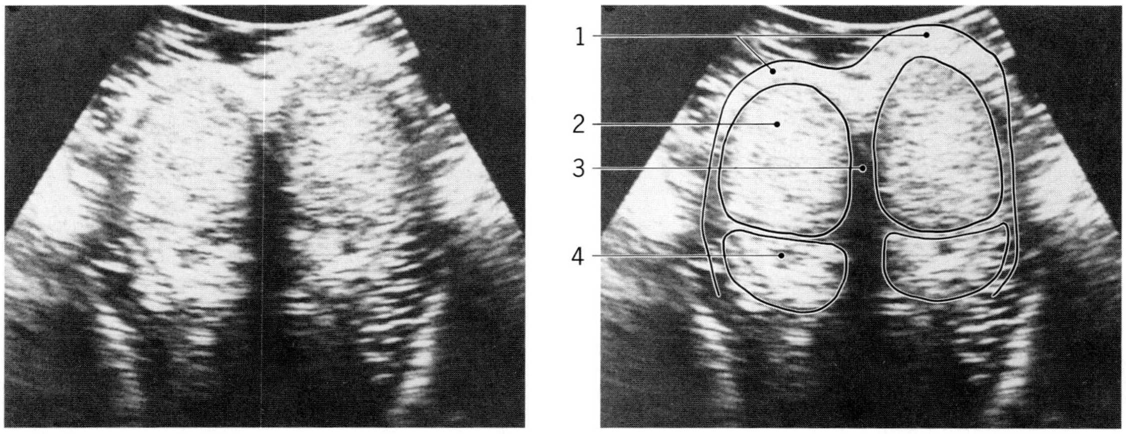

Testes, cross section, US

1: Scrotum (ventral)
2: Testis
3: Septum of scrotum
4: Epididymis

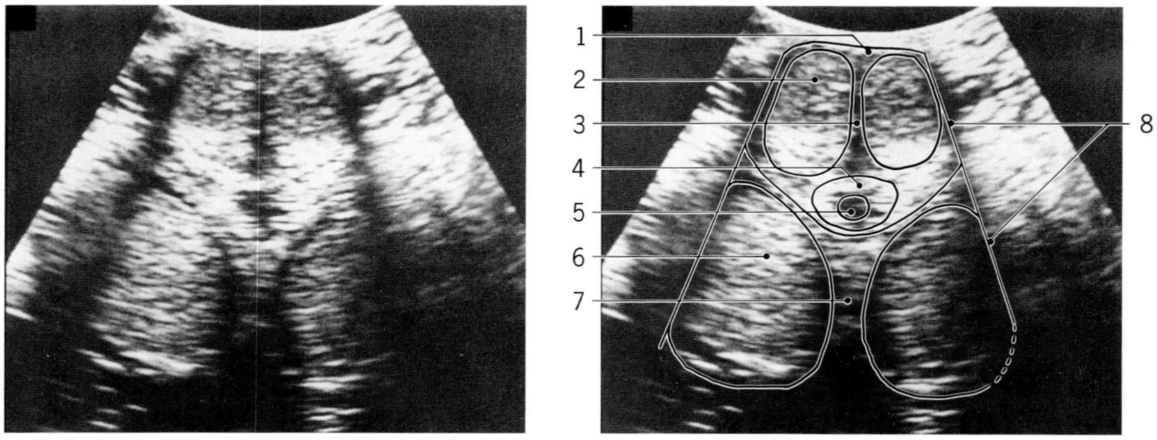

Penis, cross section, US

1: Dorsum penis
2: Corpus cavernosum
3: Septum of penis
4: Corpus spongiosum
5: Urethra
6: Testis
7: Septum of scrotum
8: Artefactual shadow

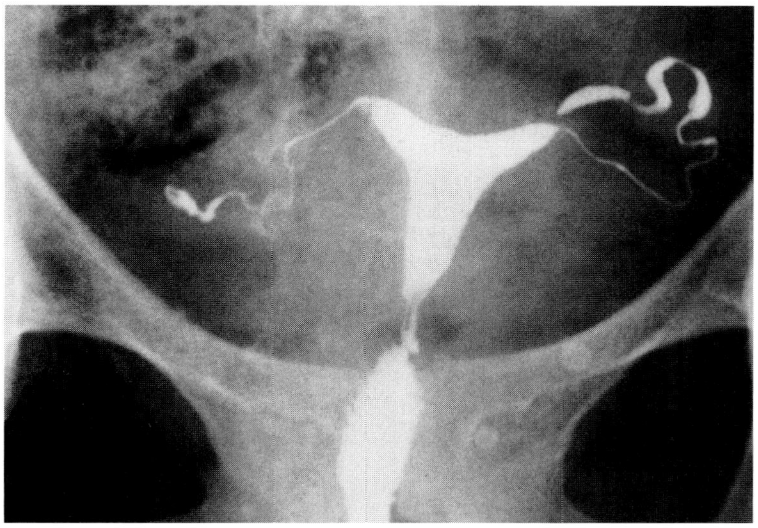

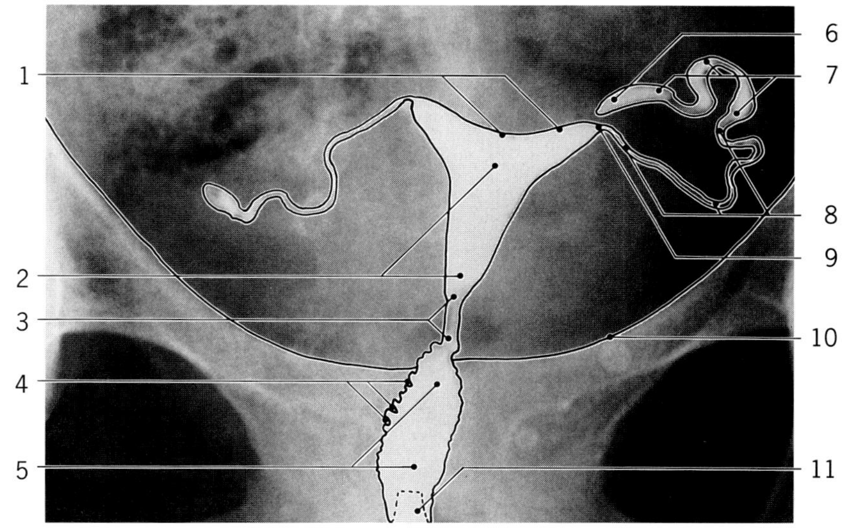

Uterus, a-p X-ray, hysterosalpingography (HSG)

1: Fundus of uterine cavity
2: Uterine cavity
3: Isthmus ("lower uterine segment")
4: Palmate folds of cervix
5: Canal of cervix (dilated and stretched)
6: Infundibulum of uterine tube
7: Ampulla of uterine tube
8: Isthmus of uterine tube
9: Uterine ostium of uterine tube
10: Pecten of pubis
11: Tube

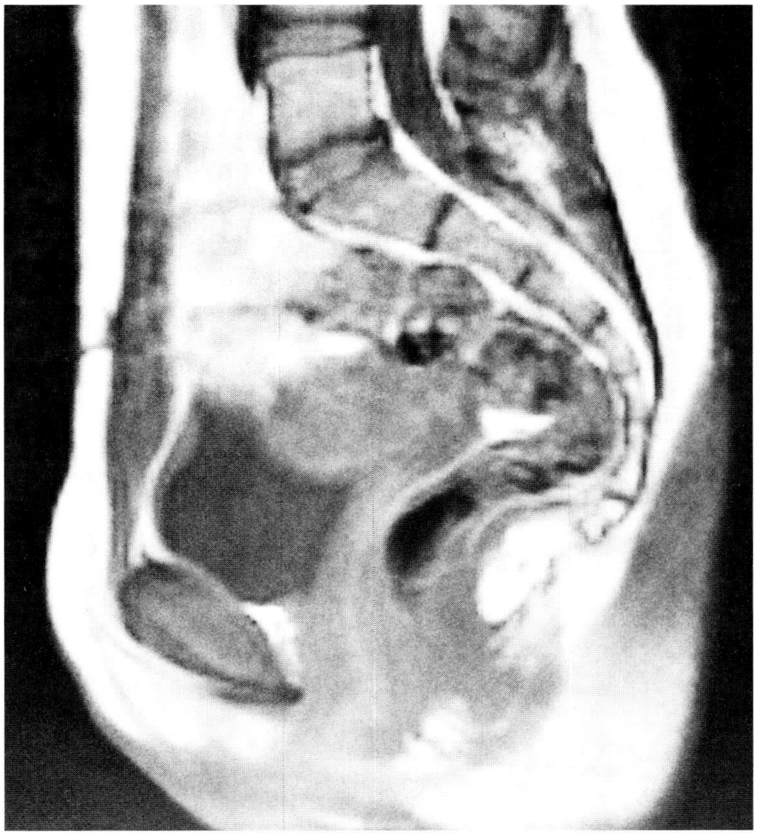

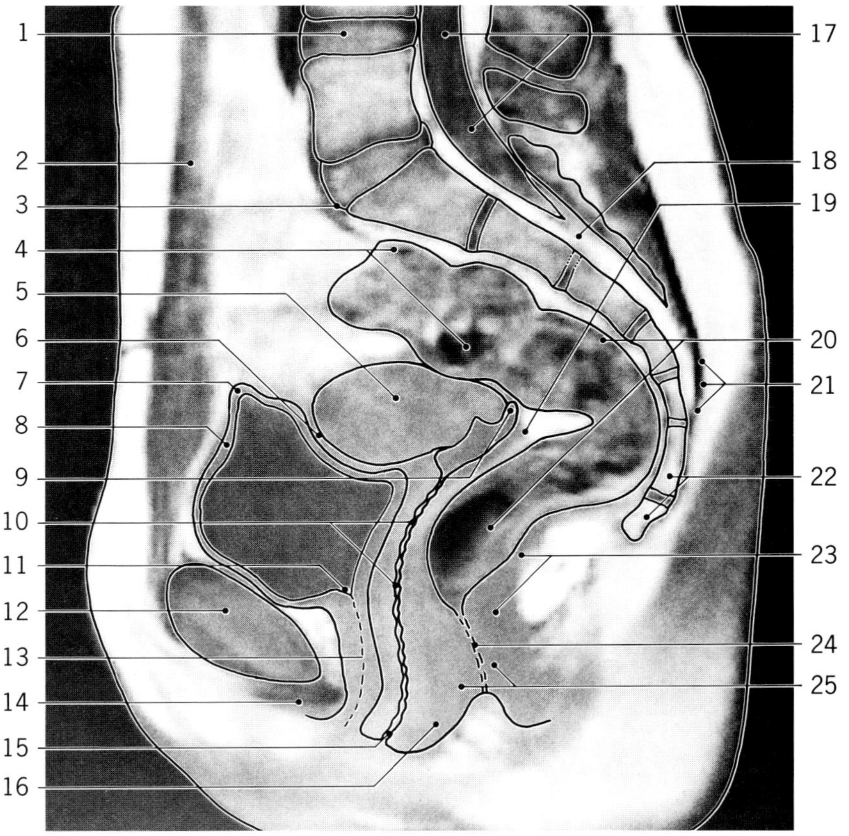

Female pelvis, median MR

T_1 weighted recording

1: Intervertebral disc
2: Rectus abdominis
3: Promontory
4: Sigmoid colon
5: Uterus
6: Vesico-uterine pouch
7: Apex of urinary bladder
8: Wall of urinary bladder
9: Posterior fornix of vagina
10: Vagina
11: Internal orifice of urethra
12: Pubic symphysis
13: Urethra
14: Clitoris
15: Vaginal orifice
16: Perineum
17: Dural sac with cauda equina
18: Sacral canal
19: Recto-uterine pouch (fossa Douglasi)
20: Rectum
21: Lumbar aponeurosis
covering sacral hiatus
22: Coccyx
23: Levator ani
24: Anal canal
25: Sphinchter ani externus

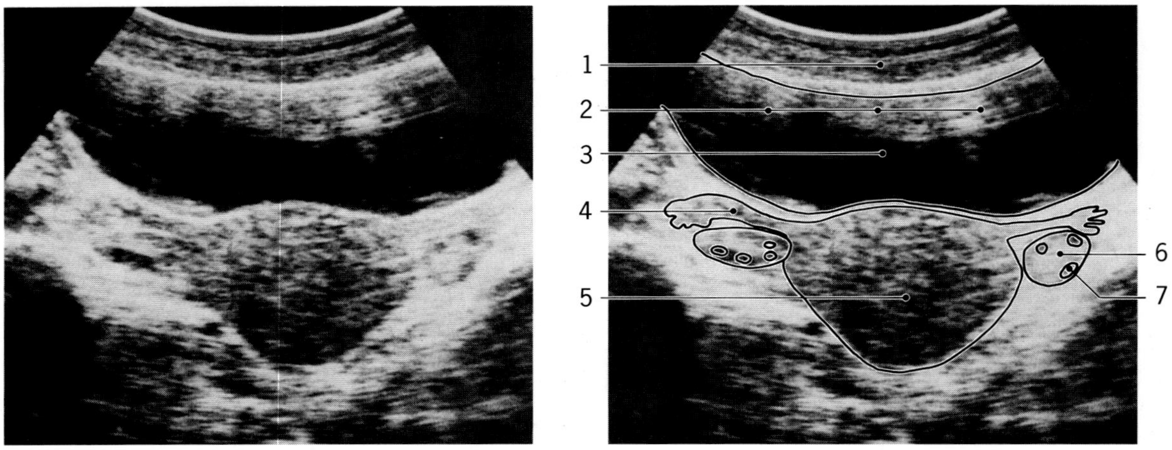

Uterus and ovaries, transverse section, US

1: Anterior abdominal wall
2: Artefacts in lumen of bladder
3: Urinary bladder
4: Uterine tube
5: Corpus uteri
6: Ovary
7: Ovarian follicles

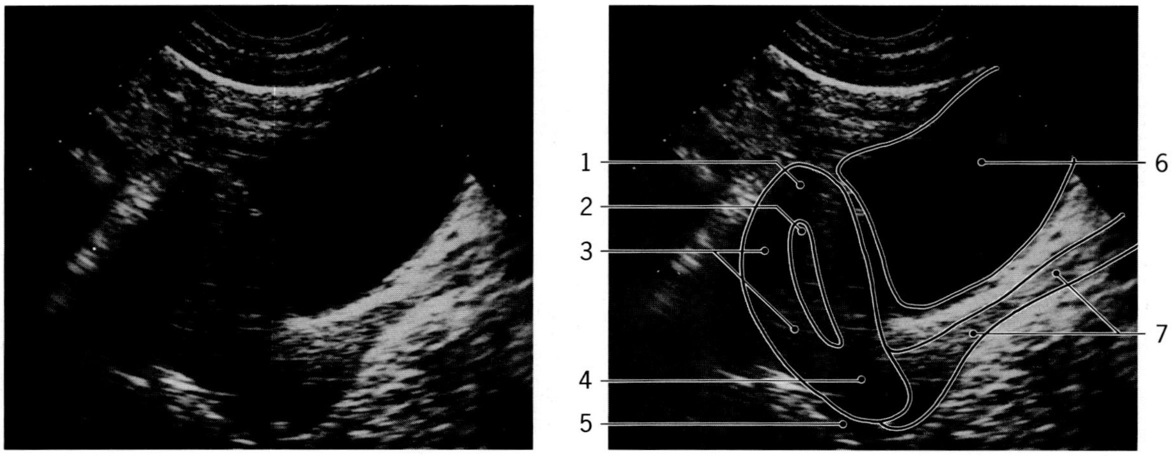

Uterus, longitudinal section, US

1: Fundus of uterus
2: Endometrium lining uterine cavity
3: Corpus uteri
4: Cervix uteri
5: Recto-uterine pouch (fossa Douglasi)
6: Urinary bladder
7: Vagina

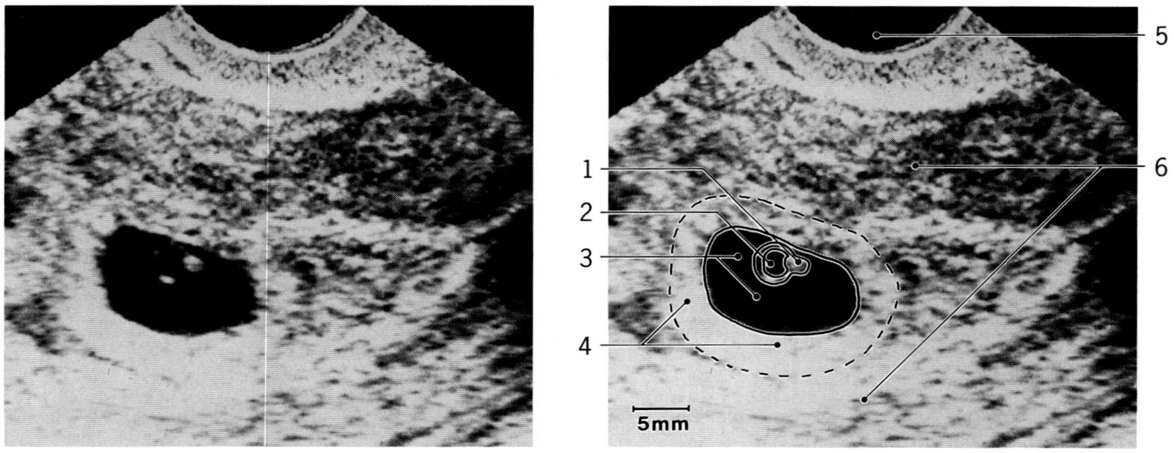

Embryon, 5 weeks gestational age, transvaginal US

1: Embryon
2: Yolk sac
3: Extraembryonic coelom ("gestation sac")
4: Decidua
5: Probe in vagina
6: Uterus

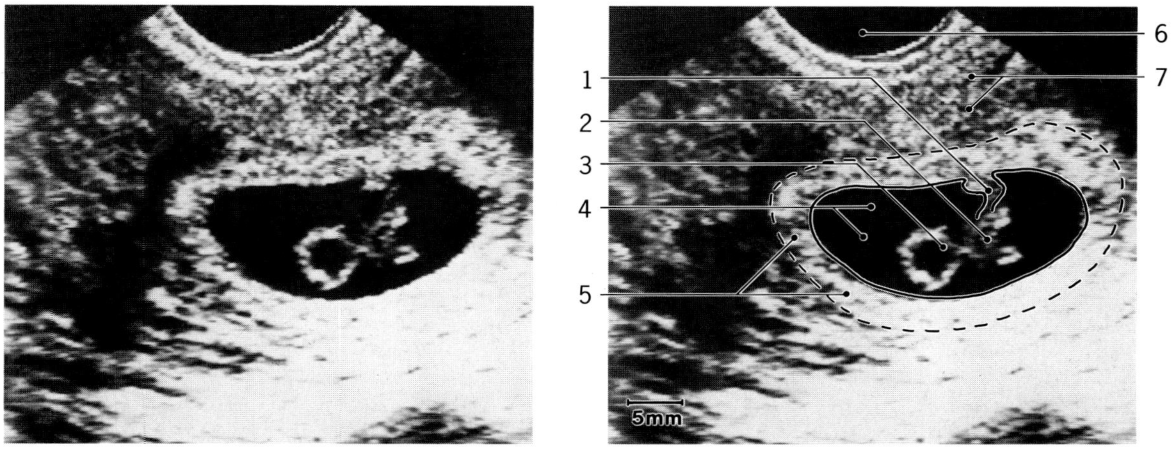

Embryon, 7 weeks gestational age, transvaginal US

1: Body stalk
2: Embryon
3: Yolk sac
4: Extraembryonic coelom ("gestation sac")
5: Decidua
6: Probe in vagina
7: Uterus

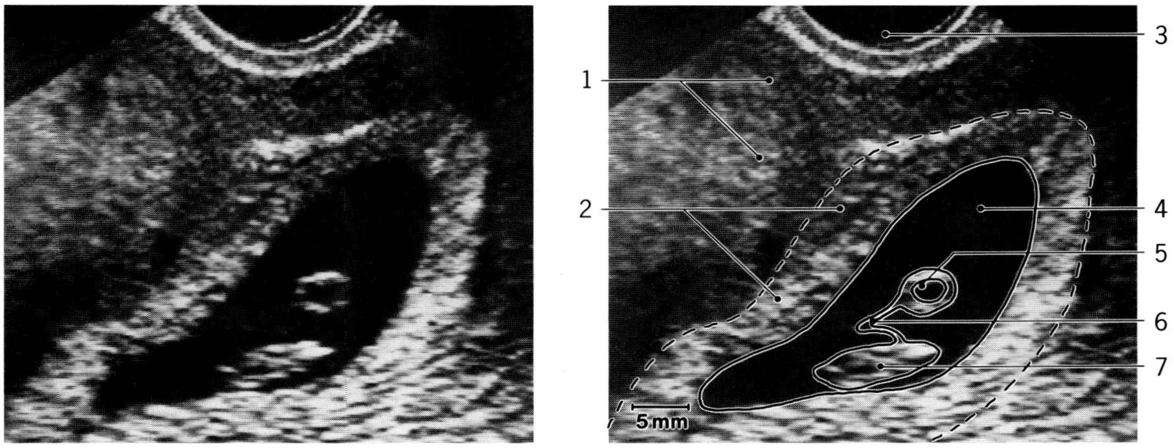

Embryon, 7 weeks gestational age, transvaginal US

1: Myometrium
2: Decidua
3: Probe in vagina
4: Extraembryonic coelom
5: Yolk sac
6: Vitello-intestinal duct
7: Embryon

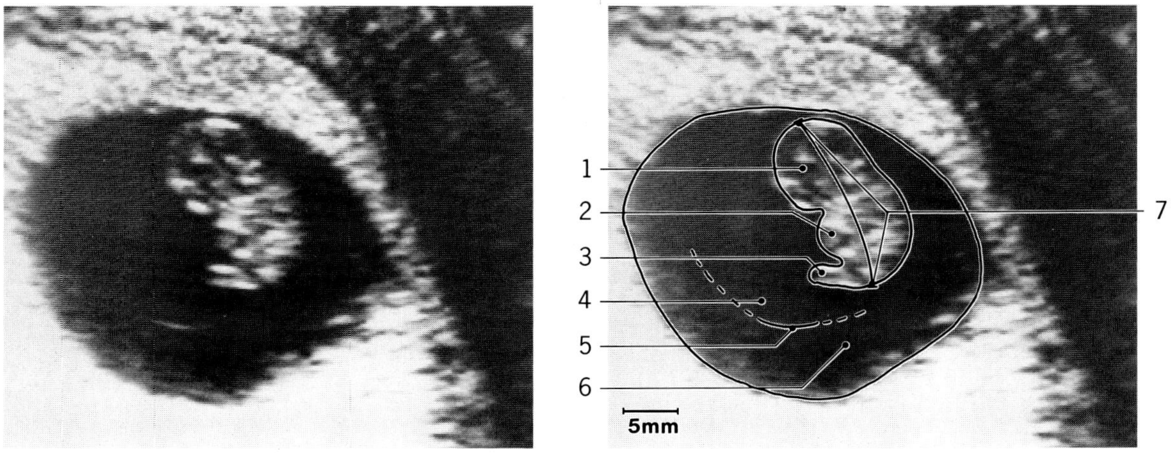

Embryon, 8 weeks gestational age, transvaginal US

1: Head of embryon
2: Pericardial swelling
3: Tail
4: Amniotic cavity
5: Amniotic membrane
6: Extraembryonic coelom
7: Crown-rump length (CRL = 17 mm)

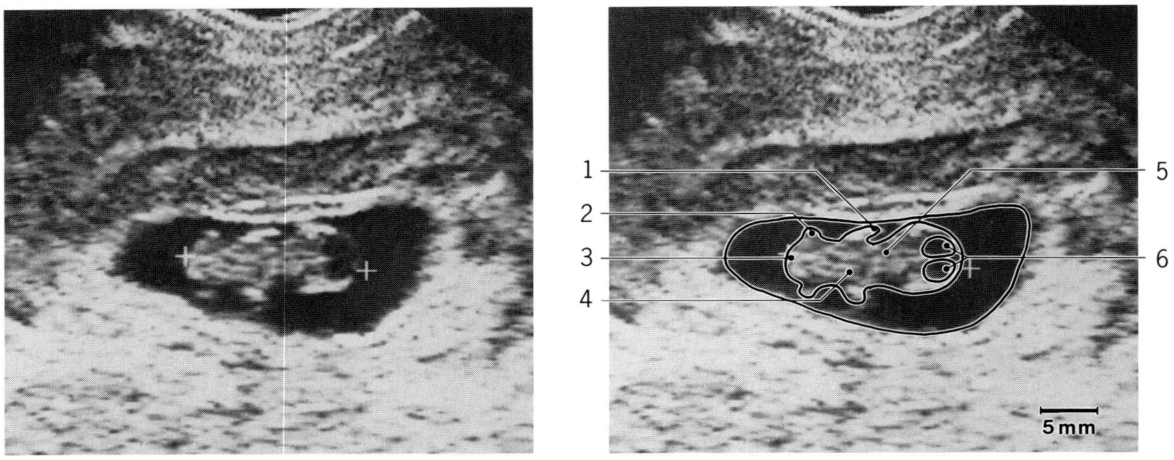

Embryon, 8 weeks gestational age, transvaginal US

1: Upper limb of embryon
2: Lower limb of embryon
3: Rump
4: Trunk
5: Neck
6: Ventricles of brain

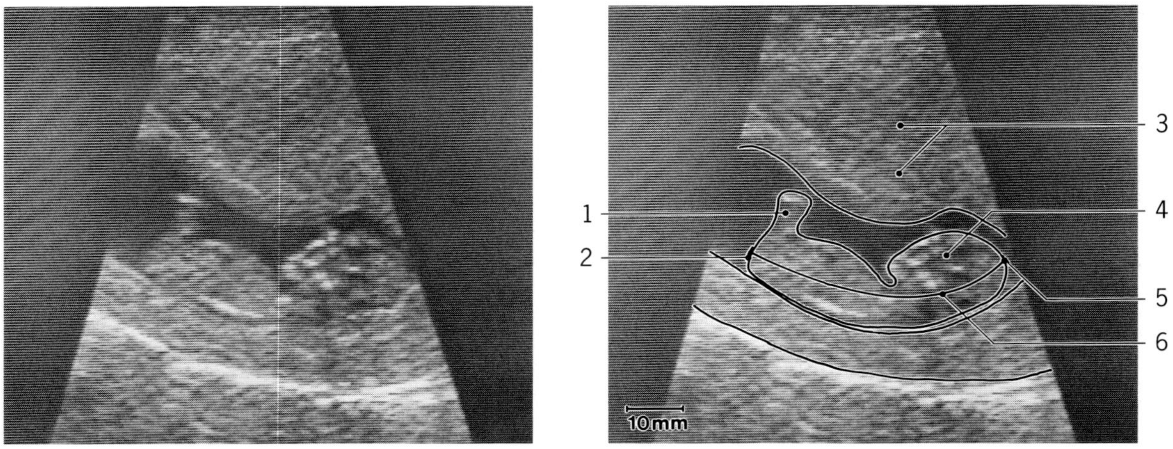

Fetus, 12 weeks gestational age, transabdominal US

1: Lower limb of fetus
2: Rump
3: Placenta
4: Face of fetus
5: "Crown"
6: Crown-rump length (CRL = 50 mm)

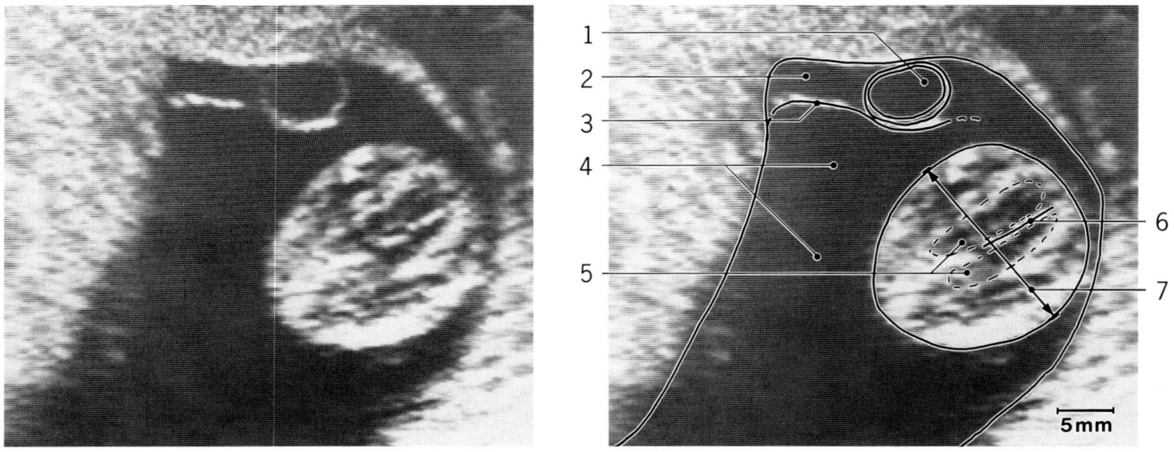

Fetus, 12 weeks gestational age, transvaginal US

1: Yolk sac
2: Extraembryonic coelom
3: Amniotic membrane
4: Amniotic cavity
5: Ventricles of brain
6: Falx cerebri
7: Biparietal diameter (BPD = 17 mm)

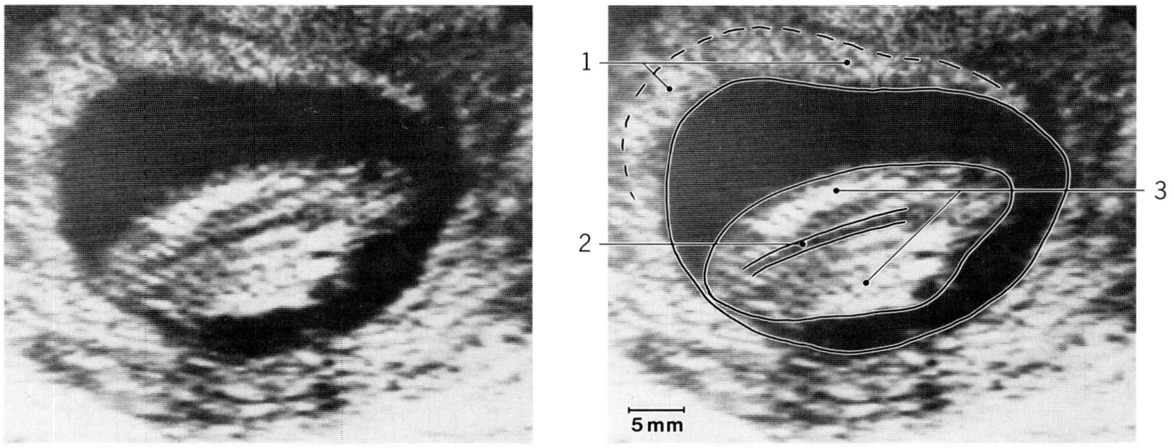

Fetus, 12 weeks gestational age, transvaginal US

1: Placenta
2: Vertebral canal
3: Trunk of fetus

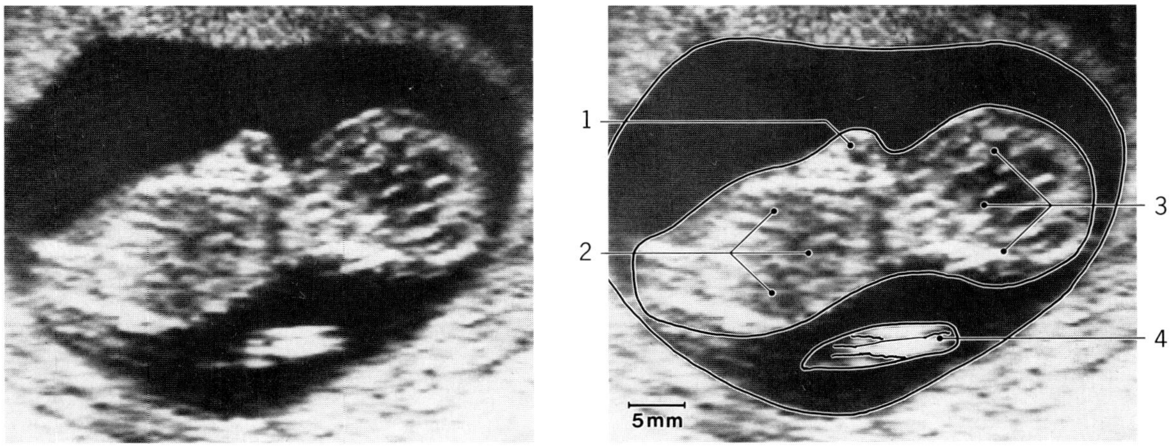

Fetus, 12 weeks gestational age, transvaginal US

1: Shoulder
2: Trunk
3: Head
4: Umbilical cord

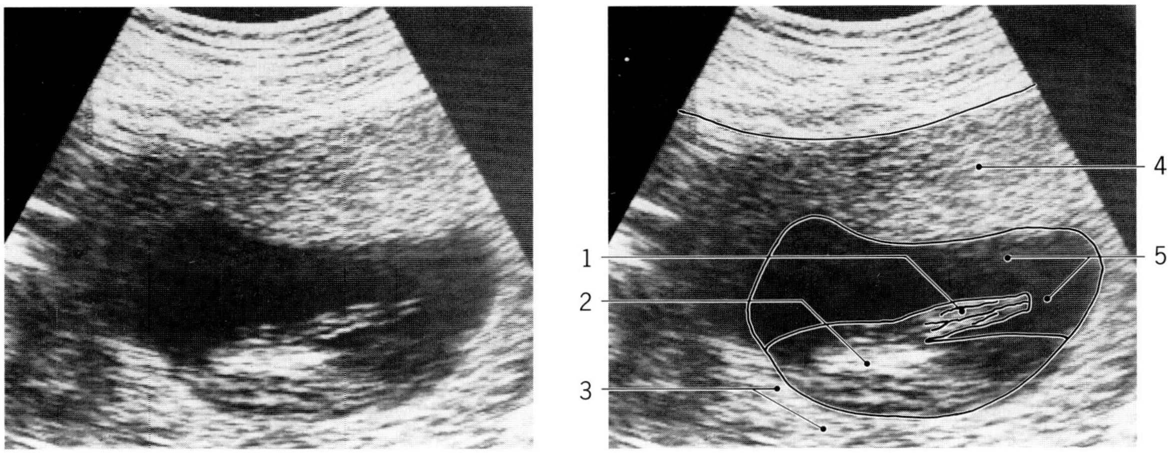

Placenta, 12 weeks gestational age, transabdominal US

1: Umbilical cord
2: Placenta
3: Decidua basalis
4: Myometrium
5: Amniotic cavity

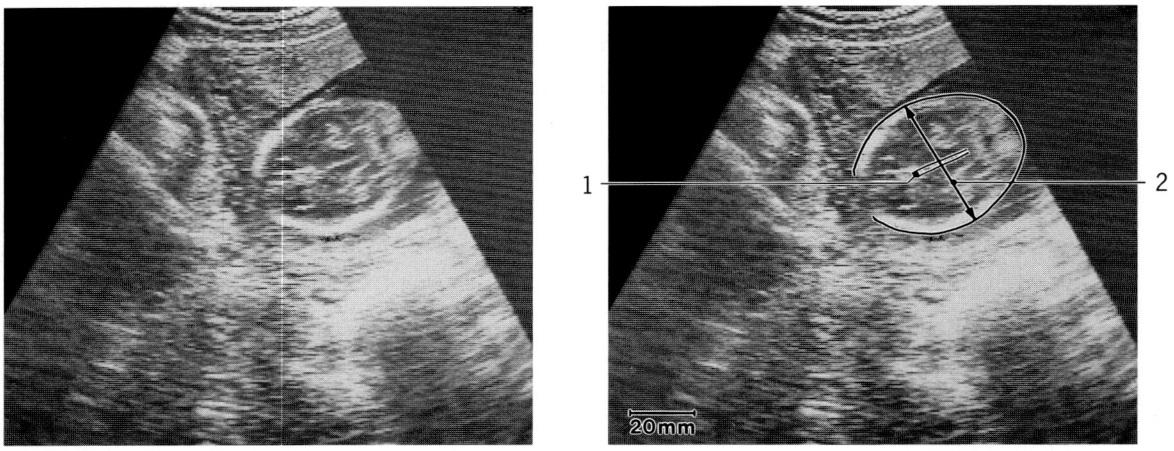

Fetus, 18 weeks gestational age, transabdominal US

1: Falx cerebri
2: Biparietal diameter (BPD = 42 mm)

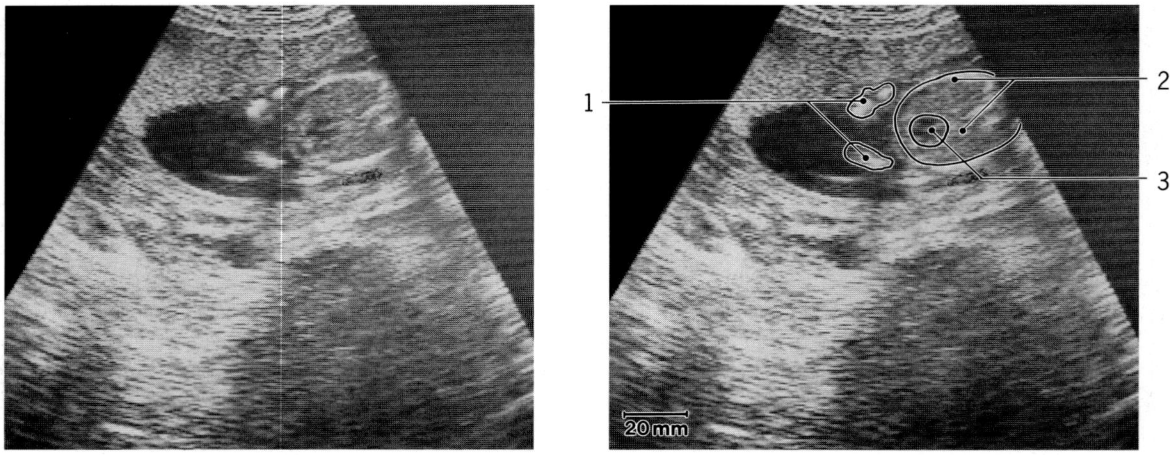

Fetus, 18 weeks gestational age, transabdominal US

1: Limbs
2: Thorax (cross section)
3: Heart

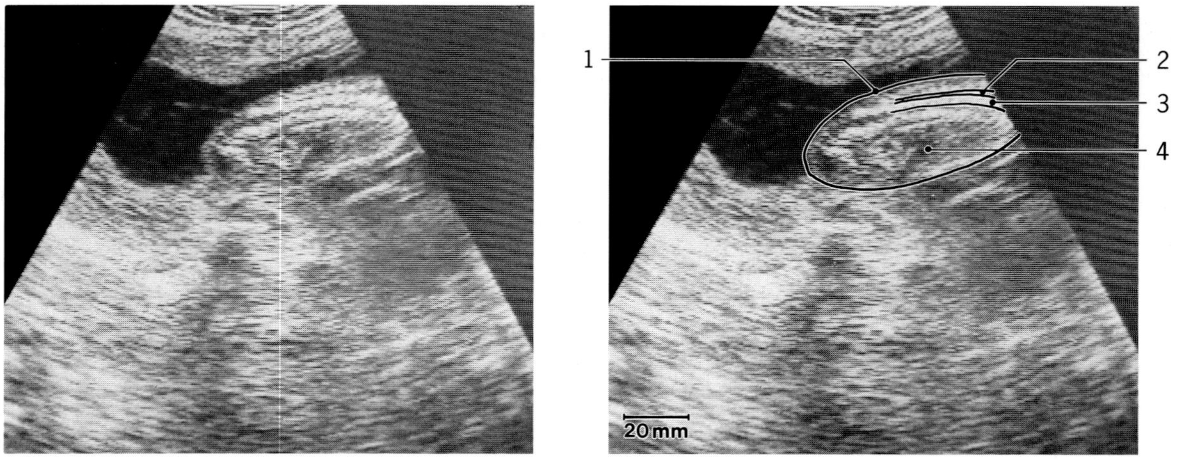

Fetus, 18 weeks gestational age, transabdominal US

1: Back of fetus
2: Vertebral canal
3: Vertebral column
4: Abdomen of fetus

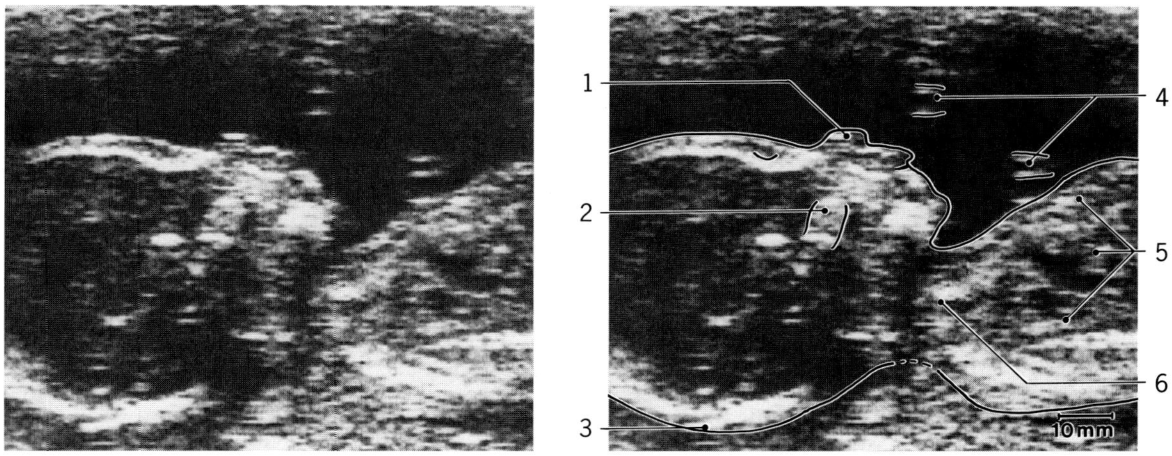

Fetus, 20 weeks gestational age, transabdominal US

1: Nose
2: Maxilla
3: Occiput
4: Umbilical cord
5: Thorax
6: Neck

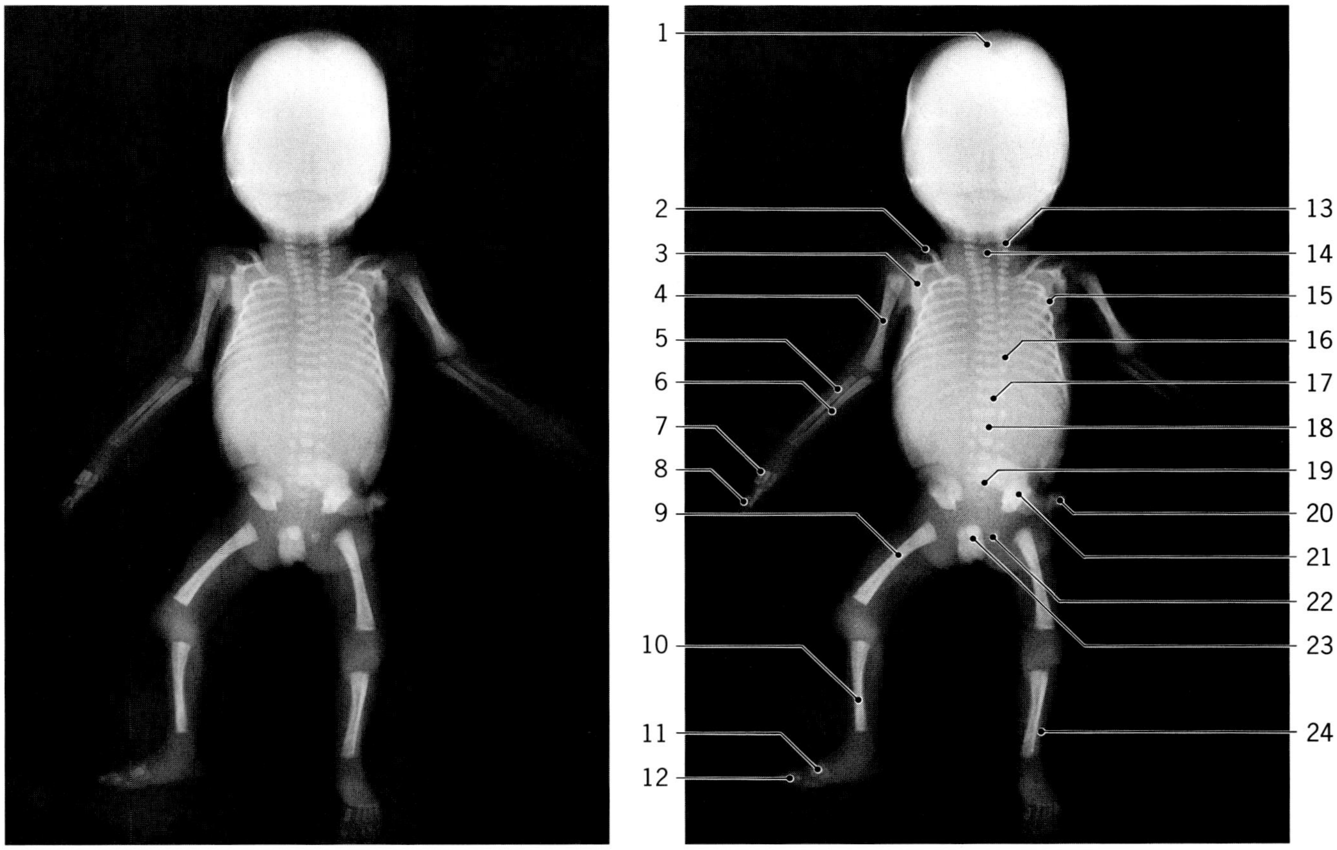

Fetus, 18 weeks, CRL = 140 mm, stillborn, a-p X-ray

1: Anterior fontanelle
2: Clavicle
3: Scapula
4: Humerus (diaphysis)
5: Radius (diaphysis)
6: Ulna (diaphysis)
7: Metacarpal bone (diaphysis)
8: Phalanx (diaphysis)
9: Femur (diaphysis)
10: Tibia and fibula (diaphyses)
11: Metatarsal bone (diaphysis)
12: Phalanx (diaphysis)
13: Arch of cervical vertebra (ossification center)
14: Body of cervical vertebra (ossification center)
15: Third rib
16: Arch of ninth thoracic vertebra (ossification center)
17: Body of 12th thoracic vertebra (ossification center)
18: Body of second lumbar vertebra (ossification center)
19: Body of first sacral vertebra (ossification center)
20: Umbilical cord
21: Ilium
22: Pubis
23: Penis
24: Fibula (diaphysis)

Dictionary

Short dictionary of examination procedures in diagnostic imaging

angiocardiography X-ray examination of the heart and the adjacent great vessels. Contrast medium is usually injected into the right ventricle through a catheter introduced via the femoral vein by the Seldinger technique. The passage of contrast is recorded on a rapid sequence of images, e.g. by cineradiography.

angiography Imaging of arteries (arteriography, q.v.), veins (phlebography, q.v.) or lymphatics (lymphography, q.v.).

antegrade pyelography X-ray examination of the urinary tract after puncture and injection of contrast medium into the renal pelvis, often guided by ultrasound.

aortography X-ray examination of the aorta and its branches. Water soluble contrast medium is injected through a catheter, usually introduced by the Seldinger technique via the femoral artery (transfemoral aortography). The abdominal aorta can also be punctured directly (lumbar aortography).

arteriography Imaging of arteries. Water soluble contrast medium is injected through a cannula inserted by direct puncture of an artery or by the Seldinger technique. A rapid sequence of single radiographs or a cineradiographic recording is taken in order to image the passage of contrast medium through the arterial branches. The latest exposures taken, when the contrast medium collects on the venous side, are denoted the venous phase.

arthrography Examination of a joint after injection of water- soluble contrast medium or air, often both (double contrast), into the synovial cavity.

axial In or along the axis (midline) of the body. The term is used in conventional X-ray examinations for a positioning where the X-rays pass along, and the film is positioned perpendicular to the long axis of the body. Used in computed tomography and magnetic resonance imaging to denote a cross section (i.e. transverse section) of the body, an "axial section".

B-mode imaging "Brightness" mode of ultrasound imaging. See p. 49.

barium A suspension of barium sulphate in a watery medium. Used as a contrast medium to visualize the digestive tract. See p. 29.

barium enema X-ray examination of the colon and the rectum after introduction of barium through the anus. The colon is cleaned before the examination by laxatives and/or a cleaning enema.

barium meal X-ray examination of the stomach and the duodenum after ingestion of barium.

barium swallow X-ray examination of the oesophagus while swallowing barium.

biliary tree scintigraphy Imaging the biliary tree and the gall bladder by isotopes. Often performed with ^{99m}Tc labelled imino-diacetic acid derivates, e.g. ^{99m}Tc-HIDA.

biligraphy Cholangiography, q.v.

biparietal diameter (BPD) The maximum distance between the parietal bones of the skull, measured perpendicular to the falx cerebri. Used in ultrasound sonography to determine the age of a fetus.

bite-wing radiography Intra-oral dental X-ray film. The patient bites over a wing which projects from the film packing.

BPD Biparietal diameter, q.v.

bronchography X-ray imaging of the bronchial tree after introduction of contrast medium, often through a catheter placed in a main bronchus.

cardioangiography Angiocardiography, q.v.

cavernosography X-ray examination of the cavernous bodies of the penis after direct injection of contrast medium. The venous drainage is also visualized.

cavography Angiographic X-ray examination of the caval vein. Contrast is usually injected simultaneously in both femoral veins.

cholangiogram X-ray imaging of the gall bladder and bile ducts.

cholangiography Imaging of the biliary tree by contrast injected intravenously (intravenous cholangiography) or directly into a bile duct. This can be performed percutaneously (percutanous transhepatic cholangiography q.v.), through an endoscope (endoscopic retrograde cholangiography) or through a tube inserted in a duct during surgery (per-operative or post-operative cholangiography).

cholecystography, intravenous X-ray examination of the biliary ducts and the gallbladder after intravenous injection of a special water-soluble contrast medium that is excreted with bile.

cholecystography, oral X-ray examination of the gallbladder after oral intake of a contrast medium which is excreted with the bile. The examination depends on the function of the small bowel, the liver and the gallbladder. Emptying of the gallbladder can be studied after a fatty meal.

cholecysto-scintigraphy Biliary tree scintigraphy, q.v.

cineangiography Examination of arteries using cineradiography during intravascular injection of contrast medium.

cineradiography Recording of the live image from the X-ray fluorescent screen on film or videotape.

cisternography X-ray or computed tomography imaging of the intracranial cisterns after introduction of a small amount of air or contrast medium into the subarachnoid cavity via a lumbar puncture.

colloid scintigraphy Scintigraphic imaging after intravenous injection of colloid particles labelled with a radioisotope, often ^{99m}Tc. The colloid will be taken up by macrophages. Especially the liver and the spleen can be visualized.

color-flow Doppler imaging An ultrasonic imaging technique in which a color-coded image of Doppler shifts is superimposed on an ordinary greytone ultrasound sonogram. Used especially for cardiovascular examinations.

computed tomography (CT) CT-scanning. Tomographic X-ray imaging technique. See p. 25.

contrast media Media, used to improve imaging of organs or cavities. See pp. 29 and 36.

coronal section Used in radiology to denote a tomographic image of a frontal section.

coronary arteriography Imaging of the coronary arteries by selective injection of contrast medium. Usually performed by the Seldinger technique through the femoral artery or through the brachial artery.

CT Computed tomography, q.v.

cystography Examination of the urinary bladder using water- soluble contrast medium.

cystourethrography X-ray examination of the bladder and the urethra. Water-soluble contrast medium is instilled into the bladder, and the bladder and the urethra are studied during voiding.

dacryocystography or dacryography X-ray examination of the lachcrymal cannaliculi, -sac, and -

canal after cannulation and injection of contrast medium into the two lachcrymal points.

digital subtraction angiography (DSA) Angiography using digital subtraction. Computer image processing technique for improved imaging of vessels after injection of contrast medium. The image contrast is improved by subtraction of images taken just before and during contrast injection, whereby image details common to both images cancel out. See p. 24.

discography Imaging of an intervertebral disc after direct puncture and injection of contrast medium into the nucleus pulposus.

Doppler effect See p. 50.

Doppler-scanning Ultrasound examination using Doppler effect.

double contrast examination Use of positive and negative contrast media in combination, often barium and air. Particularly used for examination of the colon where a barium enema is followed by insufflation of air.

DSA Digital subtraction angiography, q.v.

ductography X-ray examination of a duct, e.g. in the breast. Contrast is injected through the opening of the duct.

duplex scanning Ultrasound imaging combined with simultaneous measurement of flow velocity by Doppler shift at a selected site in the image. See p. 51.

"echo" Synonymous with ultrasound examination.

echocardiography Ultrasonic cardiography. Ultrasound examination of the heart. The real time live image is often supplemented with one-dimensional scanning (M-mode), to give quantitative information on the motion of the cardiac walls and valves. Duplex scanning and color-flow Doppler imaging yield additional information on velocities and directions of blood flow.

encephalography Imaging the brain. Can be performed with air (pneumoencephalography q.v.), or with contrast medium introduced into the subarachnoid space and the brain ventricles (ventriculography). The imaging technique can be conventional radiography, conventional tomography or computed tomography.

endoluminal ultrasound scanning Examination in which the ultrasound generator and receiver (the probe) is placed in the lumen of an organ, e.g. transesophageal echocardiography or transvaginal scanning of the uterus, or transrectal scanning of the prostate.

endoscopic retrograde cholangio-pancreatography (ERCP) X-ray examination during retrograde injection of contrast medium into the biliary tract (cholangio-) and the pancreatic duct (pancreato-). A catheter is passed into the ampulla Vateri via an endoscope placed in the duodenum.

endoscopy Direct visual examination of an organ by viewing through a tube-shaped optical instrument. The tube is often constructed with fiber optics. Commonly used for examination of the respiratory tract, esophagus, stomach, duodenum, colon, peritoneal and pleural cavity, and joint cavities.

ERCP Endoscopic retrograde cholangio-pancreatography, q.v.

fluoroscopy X-ray imaging on a screen coated with a thin layer of a material that fluoresces proportional to the intensity of incident X-rays. The screen is positioned instead of the photographic film and is viewed directly or via a video camera. See p. 24.

gadolinium-DTPA. Gadolinium chelated with diethylene-triamine-penta-acetate. Contrast medium used in magnetic resonance imaging. See p. 36.

galactography Mammary ductography. X-ray examination of mammary ducts after injection of contrast into the duct system.

gestational age The age of a pregnancy defined from the first day of the last menstruation.

HIDA scintigraphy Biliary tree scintigraphy, q.v.

hippuran scintigraphy Radiosotope examination of the urinary tract using ^{123}J- or ^{131}J - hippuran which is rapidly excreted by the kidneys.

Hounsfield unit Unit of X-ray attenuation, expressed relative to water. See p. 27.

hypotonic duodenography X-ray examination of the duodenum after relaxation of the intestinal wall, often obtained by intravenous injection of glucagon. Especially used for examination of the head of the pancreas.

hysterosalpingography (HSG) X-ray examination where iodine contrast medium is injected through the external uterine orifice and passed through the uterus and the salpinges into the peritoneal cavity.

infusion excretory urography X-ray imaging of the kidneys during continuous intravenous infusion of water soluble contrast medium.

intravenous biligraphy Cholangiography, intravenous, q.v.

intravenous urography Urography, q.v.

isotope scintigraphy Examination using γ-emitting radioisotopes targeted to specific organs or tissues. The time dependent accumulation and/or wash-out in a particular organ is recorded with a gamma-detector or visualized with a gamma-camera. See p. 52.

IVP Intravenous pyelography, i.e. urography, q.v.

kolpo-cysto-urethrography (KCU) X-ray examination of the female bladder, urethra and vagina during rest, coughing and voiding. Contrast medium is introduced into the bladder and vagina.

left anterior oblique(LAO) Oblique X-ray projection with the anterior part of the left side of the patient nearest to the film.

left lateral Lateral projection with the left side of the patient nearest to the film.

lung perfusion scintigraphy Radioisotope examination of the blood perfusion of the lungs after intravenous injection of a tracer (often ^{99m}Tc-labelled albumin).

lung ventilation scintigraphy Radioisotope examination of the ventilation of the lungs after inhalation of a radioactive gas (often ^{133} Xe or ^{81m} Kr).

lymphangiography Lymphography, q.v.

lymphography X-ray examination of lymphatic vessels and lymph nodes after injection of an oil-based contrast medium containing iodine. Inguinal, external iliac and lumbar nodes are visualized after injection of contrast in a lymph vessel on both feet. Axillary nodes are similarly visualized after injection on the hand. X-rays taken a few hours after the injection (the early phase) show lymphatic vessels. X-rays taken the next day or later show only the lymph nodes.

M-mode "Motion" mode of ultrasound scanning. See p. 50.

magnetic resonance imaging MR. MRI. NMR. See p. 31.

mammography X-ray examination of the breast at low kV (20-30kV) to obtain good differentiation in soft tissue imaging. To reduce the X-ray dose highly efficient intensifier screens are used.

MDP-scanning Methylene diphosphonate scintigraphy, q.v.

median Midsagittal, q.v.

methylene diphosphonate scintigraphy MDP scintigraphy. Radioisotope examination of bone using ^{99m}Tc-labelled methylene diphosphonate, which concentrates in bone tissue in proportion to the mineral metabolism in the bone. Thus, it concentrates especially around growthplates of the long bones.

micturating cystography X-ray examination of the bladder during voiding.

midsagittal Median. Sagittal section in the midline of the body.

MR Magnetic resonance imaging. See p. 31.

myelography Imaging of the spinal cord. Water soluble contrast medium is injected in the subarachnoid space either by lumbar or by suboccipital injection. The subarachnoid space is subsequently imaged by X-ray or computed tomography (computed myelography).

nephrotomography Imaging the kidneys by tomography, especially used for demonstration of calcifications.

orthopantomography Panorama, q.v.

panorama X-ray examination of the teeth and the adjacent bones by a special tomographic technique.

percutaneus transhepatic cholangiography (PTC) X-ray contrast examination of the biliary tract after percutaneous cannulation of a biliary duct in the liver.

percutaneous transhepatic portography X-ray contrast examination of the portal vein and/or its branches after cannulation of a portal branch by percutaneous liver puncture. The vein is cannulated by the Seldinger method.

perfusion lung scanning Lung perfusion scintigraphy, q.v.

PET Positron emission tomography, q.v.

phlebography Imaging of veins. Contrast medium is usually injected by direct puncture of a peripheral vein distal to the region imaged on X-ray. Selective phlebography can also be performed by Seldinger technique.

plain film X-ray examination without use of contrast media. Plain films of the abdomen are usually taken in both supine and upright position to observe changes in the distribution of gases in the abdominal viscera.

pneumoencephalography X-ray examination of the brain, especially the ventricles, after injection of air in the subarachnoidal space usually via a lumbar puncture. By a series of positional manipulations of the patient, the air is manoeuvered into the brain ventricles.

portal phlebography X-ray examination of the portal vein. Can be performed after injection of contrast medium in the spleen (splenic phlebography, splenoportography); during the venous phase of splenic arteriography (arterioportography), or after catheterization of the portal vein by percutaneous liver puncture.

portography Portal phlebography, q.v.

positron emission tomography (PET) Radioisotope imaging technique utilizing positron-emitting isotopes. See p. 53.

PTC Percutaneus transhepatic cholangiography, q.v.

radiculography X-ray examination of spinal nerve roots after injection of water soluble contrast medium in the subarachnoid space.

radiogram Radiograph. An image made by X-rays.

radioisotope imaging Scintigraphy, q.v.

radiolucent Material or structure that is easily penetrated by X-rays, such an object appears dark on the film.

radionuclide Radioactive isotope.

radiopaque Material or structure that absorbs and scatters X-rays. Such an object appears light on the film.

renal arteriography Selective arteriography of the renal artery and its branches.

renography Scintigraphic and quantitative examination of the renal excretion of a radiolabelled pharmaceutical, e.g. hippuran, -^{99m}Tc.

retrograde urethrography Urethrography, q.v.

retrograde pyelography X-ray examination of the renal pelvis, calyces and ureter after injection of water-soluble contrast medium, through a catheter positioned in the ureter via a cystoscope.

right anterior oblique(RAO) Oblique projection with the anterior part of the right side of the patient nearest to the film.

right lateral Lateral projection with the right side of the patient nearest to the film.

Roentgenogram An X-ray film.

Roentgenography Imaging by X-ray.

sagittal section Section parallel to the median plane of the body.

salpingogram Hystero-salpingography, q.v.

scintigraphy Imaging of the intensity and distribution of radioactivity in organs and tissues after administration of a radioactive tracer substance. See p. 51.

scout view Survey image used for orientation in CT scanning. See p. 26.

Seldinger technique Method of introducing a fine tube (catheter). After puncture of, for example, an artery by a cannula, a flexible guide wire is introduced through the cannula, which is then withdrawn. A radiopaque catheter is placed over the wire, which guides it into the artery. A catheter inserted in this way may subsequently be guided into smaller vessels aided by fluoroscopic observation of the catheter. This technique permits selective catheterization of small vessels and other narrow hollow structures.

selective arteriography X-ray examination of a selected artery, often performed by placing a tube (catheter) in a small artery by the Seldinger technique.

sialography Imaging of a salivary gland and its ducts, often performed by dilatation of the external orifice of the duct, followed by catheterization and injection of contrast medium.

single contrast X-ray examination using either a positive or a negative contrast medium.

small bowel enema X-ray imaging of the small bowel after infusion of contrast through a tube placed in the duodenum.

sonography Ultrasound, q.v.

SPECT Single photon emisssion computed tomography. See p. 53.

splenoportography X-ray examination of the spleen and the portal vein by percutaneous injection of contrast medium into the spleen.

subtraction imaging Photographic or digital method of improving the contrast in diagnostic X-ray imaging, e.g. removing bone shadows from arteriography images (see digital subtraction angiography).

tomography Imaging an imaginary section or slice at a predetermined level in the body. In conventional X-ray performed by simultaneous and opposite motion of the X-ray tube and film during the period of exposure. See p. 22. See also computed tomography and magnetic resonance imaging, pp. 25 and 31.

transhepatic catheterization Percutaneous transhepatic portography/cholangiography, q.v.

transesophageal Examination performed via the esophagus.

transrectal Examination performed via the rectum.

transvaginal Examination performed via the vagina.

ultrasound (sonography) Imaging based on reflection of high- frequency sound waves. See p. 45.

urethrography X-ray examination of the urethra. Water soluble contrast medium is injected through the external orifice, or the urethra is examined during voiding. See also cysto-urethro-graphy.

urography Intravenous urography. Intravenous pyelography. IVP. X-ray examination of the kidneys, the ureters and the bladder after intravenous injection of a water-soluble contrast medium that is excreted by the kidneys. The contrast medium is concentrated in the urine and visualizes the kidney parenchyma, calyces, pelvis, ureters and bladder, in that order. Besides providing images of the urinary tract, the examination provides information on the renal excretory function.

venography Phlebography, q.v.

venous arteriography Vizualizing arteries after intravenous injection of contrast medium, especially used for imaging with digital subtraction and computed tomography.

ventilation scintigraphy Lung ventilation scintigraphy, q.v.

ventriculography 1. X-ray of the brain after introduction of contrast medium in the cerebral ventricles usually via lumbar puncture. 2. X-ray examination of the cardiac ventricles with contrast medium injected through a catheter.

vesiculography X-ray examination of the male seminal vesicles and deferent ducts after injection of contrast medium in the ejaculatory ducts.

xeroradiography A special process for recording of X-ray images using metal plates coated with a semiconductor, such as selenium, analogous to xerographic photocopying. Especially used for soft tissue imaging.

INDEX

Abbreviations used in diagnostic imaging

X-ray Conventional X-ray and digital subtraction

CT Computed tomography

MR Magnetic resonance

US Ultrasound sonography

Sc Scintigraphy

Nomenclature in english according to Gray's Anatomy

(Williams PL, Warwick R, eds. Gray's Anatomy. 36th ed, Churchill Livingstone, 1980)

The index is supplemented with latin entries in *italics*

(Nomina Anatomica. 6th ed, Churchill Livingstone, 1989)

A

B

D

E

F

I

M

R